Pain After Surgery

IASP Mission Statement

The International Association for the Study of Pain brings together scientists, clinicians, health-care providers, and policymakers to stimulate and support the study of pain and translate that knowledge into improved pain relief worldwide.

Pain After Surgery

Editors:

Daniel B. Carr, MD, MA
Professor
Public Health and Community Medicine, Anesthesiology, and Medicine
Founding Director, Program on Pain Research, Education and Policy
Tufts University School of Medicine
Boston, Massachusetts

Lars Arendt-Nielsen, dr.med.sci., Ph.D.
Professor
Department of Health Science and Technology
Center for Sensory-Motor Interaction (SMI)
Translation Pain Biomarkers
Aalborg University
Aalborg, Denmark

Kris C. P. Vissers, MD, Ph.D., FIPP
Professor
Pain and Palliative Medicine
Chairman
Academic Center of Pain and Palliative Medicine
Radboud University Medical Center
Nijmegen, Netherlands

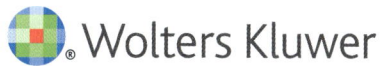

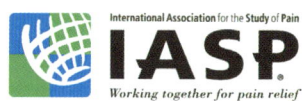

Philadelphia • Baltimore • New York • London
Buenos Aires • Hong Kong • Sydney • Tokyo

Acquisitions Editor: Keith Donnellan
Development Editor: Sean McGuire
Production Coordinator: Sadie Buckallew
Design Coordinator: Joan Wendt
Manufacturing Coordinator: Beth Welsh
Marketing Manager: Stacy Malyil
Prepress Vendor: TNQ Technologies

Copyright © 2019 IASP Press®
International Association for the Study of Pain®

All rights reserved. This book is protected by copyright. No part of this book may be reproduced or transmitted in any form or by any means, including as photocopies or scanned-in or other electronic copies, or utilized by any information storage and retrieval system without written permission from the copyright owner, except for brief quotations embodied in critical articles and reviews. Materials appearing in this book prepared by individuals as part of their official duties as US government employees are not covered by the abovementioned copyright. To request permission, please contact Wolters Kluwer Health at Two Commerce Square, 2001 Market Street, Philadelphia, PA 19103, via email at permissions@lww.com, or via our website at lww.com (products and services).

9 8 7 6 5 4 3 2 1

Printed in China

Library of Congress Cataloging-in-Publication Data

Names: Carr, Daniel B., editor. | Arendt-Nielsen, Lars, editor. | Vissers, Kris C. P., editor. | International Association for the Study of Pain, issuing body.
Title: Pain after surgery / editors, Daniel B. Carr, Lars Arendt-Nielsen, Kris C. P. Vissers.
Description: Philadelphia : Wolters Kluwer, [2019] | Includes bibliographical references.
Identifiers: LCCN 2018021917 | ISBN 9781975111410 (paperback)
Subjects: | MESH: Pain, Postoperative | Pain Management | Analgesics—therapeutic use | Pain Measurement
Classification: LCC RB127 | NLM WO 184 | DDC 616/.0472—dc23 LC record available at https://lccn.loc.gov/2018021917

This work is provided "as is," and the publisher disclaims any and all warranties, express or implied, including any warranties as to accuracy, comprehensiveness, or currency of the content of this work.

This work is no substitute for individual patient assessment based upon health care professionals' examination of each patient and consideration of, among other things, age, weight, gender, current or prior medical conditions, medication history, laboratory data, and other factors unique to the patient. The publisher does not provide medical advice or guidance, and this work is merely a reference tool. Health care professionals, and not the publisher, are solely responsible for the use of this work, including all medical judgments and for any resulting diagnosis and treatments.

Given continuous, rapid advances in medical science and health information, independent professional verification of medical diagnoses, indications, appropriate pharmaceutical selections and dosages, and treatment options should be made and health care professionals should consult a variety of sources. When prescribing medication, health care professionals are advised to consult the product information sheet (the manufacturer's package insert) accompanying each drug to verify, among other things, the conditions of use, warnings, and side effects and identify any changes in dosage schedule or contraindications, particularly if the medication to be administered is new, infrequently used, or has a narrow therapeutic range. To the maximum extent permitted under applicable law, no responsibility is assumed by the publisher for any injury and/or damage to persons or property, as a matter of products liability, negligence law, or otherwise, or from any reference to or use by any person of this work.

LWW.com

PREFACE

Pain after surgery continues to be a major humanitarian, medical, social, and financial challenge. Our knowledge regarding the mechanisms underlying acute postoperative pain as well as the development and maintenance of chronic pain after surgical intervention remains limited. As a result, clinical approaches to the treatment and management of the continuum of pain after surgery are still very much in their infancy. Furthermore, the ability to predict which patients will develop chronic postoperative pain is likewise in its infancy.

This volume is an updated and expanded version of the 11th International Association for the Study of Pain (IASP) Research Symposium titled "Brain and Pain: Researching Pain Persistence after Surgery." The editors of the first edition of the present book organized a research symposium in the setting of the Netherlands Olympic Training Centre in Papendal in November 2013. Top researchers in this field gathered to address what was known—and what was still missing—regarding chronic pain development and maintenance after surgery.

The present, second edition of this book (*Pain After Surgery*) was timed to coincide with the 2017 Global Year Against Pain After Surgery, a collaborative effort of IASP and the European Pain Federation (EFIC). Its title has been revised slightly to align it with the theme of this Global Year. During 2017, IASP developed and posted 14 related Fact Sheets in multiple languages, and *PAIN Reports* published related articles, including the proceedings of a Satellite Symposium held at the 2016 World Congress on Pain, organized by the Acute Pain Special Interest Group (SIG) on the topic, "Are Perioperative Opioids Obsolete?" Previous chapters have been elaborated and expanded with new advances surveyed by initial and new authors. The aim of this expanded text is to provide an in-depth, comprehensive view of basic and clinical research into the continuum of acute and persistent pain after surgery. Global interest in better understanding and improving short- and long-term management of pain after surgery is reflected in the numerous formal statements of support for the 2017 Global Year Against Pain After Surgery provided by over a dozen organizations worldwide.

This second edition has two major emphases. *First*, it presents an up-to-date view of the scientific research regarding changes in central nervous system (CNS) function accompanying and following surgery, as a model of chronic pain development. *Second*, it aims to translate the scientific understanding presented into a basis for effective clinical management of acute and persistent pain after surgery.

Major issues addressed by the book in the context of pain after surgery include the following:

1. Understanding the extensive range of available research tools and methods
2. Achieving integrated approaches to deal with the inherent complexity of pain after surgery
3. Implementing translational research methodologies while understanding their limitations
4. Implementing a comprehensive "menu" of pharmacologic and nonpharmacologic therapies to minimize acute postoperative pain
5. Optimizing the above "menu" to best meet the needs of young or older persons
6. Predicting which patients are most vulnerable to develop chronic postoperative pain, aided by the application of new predictive tools. The degree of hyperexcitability of specific pain mechanism seems to be a strong predictive factor
7. Setting up practical data capture to develop evidence that supports paradigm shifts in clinical pain practice

This expanded edition provides comprehensive information on the science and clinical practice of pain control after surgery. The present book will be of interest to scientists involved in pain research as well as for clinicians involved in perioperative care and management of chronic pain. Such a volume is still greatly needed. Existing publications concentrate on procedure-specific acute pain control or management of established individual chronic pain entities—e.g., neuropathic, visceral, or somatic—rather than the continuum from acute pain and its evolution into diverse chronic pain conditions. This monograph's relevance extends further than pain researchers, pain specialists, anesthesiologists, and surgeons managing surgical patients: we are convinced that it will also provide useful information to general practitioners, internists, neurologists, psychologists, and psychiatrists, who face the task of preventing and managing the short- and long-term consequences of pain after trauma, particularly surgical trauma.

– **Daniel B. Carr, Lars Arendt-Nielsen, and Kris C. P. Vissers**

CONTRIBUTORS

Eske Kvanner Aasvang, MD, DMSci
Associate Professor
Department of Anesthesiological Abdominal
Centre, Rigshospitalet
Copenhagen University
Copenhagen, Denmark

Ole Kæseler Andersen, Dr Scient, PhD
Professor
Center for Neuroplasticity and Pain, SMI
Department of Health Science and Technology
Aalborg University
Aalborg, Denmark

Lars Arendt-Nielsen, dr.med.sci., PhD
Professor
Center for Sensory-Motor Interaction (SMI)
Translation Pain Biomarkers
Department of Health Science and Technology
Aalborg University
Aalborg, Denmark

Dipika Bansal, MBBS, MD, DM
Assistant Professor
Clinical Research Unit, Department of
Pharmacy Practice
National Institute of Pharmaceutical
Education and Research (NIPER)
Punjab, India

Timothy J. Brennan, PhD, MD
Samir Gergis Professor and Vice Chair for Research
Department of Anesthesia
University of Iowa
Iowa City, IA, United States

Emanuel N. van den Broeke, MSc, PhD
Postdoctoral Researcher
Institute of Neuroscience
Catholic University of Louvain
Brussels, Belgium

Jacques E. Chelly, MD, PhD, MBA
Professor & Director of the Regional
Anesthesiology & Acute Pain Medicine
Department of Anesthesiology
University of Pittsburgh
Pittsburgh, PA, United States

Anthony H. Dickenson, BSc, PhD
Professor of Neuropharmacology
Department of Neuroscience, Physiology and
Pharmacology
University College London
London, United Kingdom

Asbjørn Mohr Drewes, MD, PhD, DMSc, EDPM
Professor
Clinical Medicine
Aalborg University
Aalborg, Denmark

G. Allen Finley, MD, FRCPC, FAAP
Professor of Anesthesia and Psychology
Dalhousie University
Halifax, NS, Canada

Lauren V. Friend, BSc, PhD
Postgraduate Student
Department of Neuroscience, Physiology and
Pharmacology
University College London
London, United Kingdom

Babita Ghai, MD, DNB, FAMS
Professor
Department of Anaesthesiology and
Intensive Care
Post Graduate Institute of Medical
Education and Research
Chandigarh, India

Debra B. Gordon, RN, DNP, FAAN
Teaching Associate
Department of Anesthesiology &
Pain Medicine
University of Washington
Seattle, Washington, United States

Thomas Graven-Nielsen, DMSc, PhD
Professor, Director
Center for Neuroplasticity and Pain (CNAP)
SMI, Department of Health Science and Technology
The Faculty of Medicine
Aalborg University
Aalborg, Denmark

Mary M. Heinricher, PhD
Professor
Departments of Neurological Surgery and Behavioral Neuroscience
Oregon Health & Science University
Portland, OR, United States

John Jarrell, MD, MSc, FRCSC
Professor
Department of Obstetrics and Gynecology
University of Calgary
Calgary, AB, Canada

Sinyoung Kang, MD, PhD
Assistant Professor
Department of Anesthesia
University of Iowa
Iowa City, IA, United States

Lee-Bareket Kisler, MA, PhD
Department of Medicine
Technion – Israel Institute of Technology
Haifa, Israel

Ronald J. Kulich, PhD
Professor
Department of Diagnostic Sciences
Tufts University School of Dental Medicine
Boston, MA, United States

Patricia Lavand'homme, MD, PhD
Professor
Department of Anesthesiology
Catholic University of Louvain
Brussels, Belgium

Dermot P. Maher, MD, MS
Assistant Professor
Division of Chronic Pain
Department of Anaesthesia and Critical Care Medicine
Johns Hopkins Hospital
Baltimore, MD, United States

Jeetinder Kaur Makkar, MD, DNB, MNAMS, FRCA
Additional Professor
Department of Anaesthesiology and Intensive Care
Post Graduate Institute of Medical Education & Research
Chandigarh, India

José Alberto Biurrun Manresa, MSc Biomed Eng, PhD
Associate Researcher
Institute for Research and Development in Bioengineering and Bioinformatics (IBB)
National Scientific and Technical Research Council (CONICET)
Oro Verde, Entre Ríos, Argentina

Renee C.B. Manworren, PhD, RN-BC, APRN, PCNS-BC, AP-PMN, FAAN
Associate Professor of Pediatrics
Feinberg School of Medicine
Northwestern University
Chicago, IL, United States

Winfried Meissner, MD
Head of Pain Management
Department of Anesthesiology and Intensive Care
Jena University Hospital
Jena, Germany

André Mouraux, MD, PhD
Professor
Institute of Neuroscience
Catholic University of Louvain
Brussels, Belgium

Kristian Kjær Petersen, Ph.D., M.Sc.
Associate Professor
Department of Health Science and Technology
Aalborg University
Aalborg, Denmark

Esther M. Pogatzki-Zahn, MD, PhD
Professor of Anesthesiology
Head of Acute Pain Service
Anesthesiologist, Pain Specialist
Department of Anesthesiology
Critical Care Medicine and Pain Therapy
University Hospital Muenster
Muenster, Germany

Stephan A. Schug, MD, FANZCA, FPMANZCA, EDPM
Professor and Chair of Anaesthesiology
Medical School
University of Western Australia
Perth, WA, Australia

Enrico Schulz, PhD
Postdoctoral Researcher
Department of Neurology
Ludwig-Maximilians-Universität
Munich, Germany

Guy Simonnet, PhD
Professor emeritus
Institut de Neurosciences Cognitive et Intégratives d'Aquitaine (INCIA)
Université de Bordeaux et CNRS
Bordeaux, France

Till Sprenger, PhD
Professor
Department of Neurology
DKD Helios Klinik Wiesbaden
Wiesbaden, Germany

Anne Stankewitz, PhD
Postdoctoral Researcher
Department of Neurology
Technische Universität München
Munich, Germany

Daisuke Sugiyama, MD, PhD
Postdoctoral Research Scholar
Department of Anesthesia
University of Iowa
Iowa City, IA, United States

Thomas R. Tölle, MD, PhD
Professor
Department of Neurology
Technische Universität München
München, Germany

Louisa D. Townson, BSc, PhD
Postgraduate Student
Department of Neuroscience, Physiology and Pharmacology
University College London
London, United Kingdom

Ana-Maria Vranceanu, PhD
Associate Professor
Department of Psychiatry
Harvard Medical School
Boston, MA, United States

Emily A. Walsh, BA
Research Assistant
Craniofacial Pain and Headache Center
Tufts University School of Dental Medicine
Boston, MA, United States

Oliver H.G. Wilder-Smith, MBChB, MD, PhD, DSc
Associate Professor
Department of Anesthesiology, Pain and Palliative Medicine, Pain and Nociception Research Group
Radboudumc Medical Center Nijmegen
Nijmegen, The Netherlands

David Yarnitsky, MD, PhD
Professor
The Ruth and Bruce Rappaport Faculty of Medicine
Technion – Israel Institute of Technology
Haifa, Israel

Ruth Zaslansky, DSc
Scientific Manager
Department of Anesthesiology and Intensive Care
Jena University Hospital
Jena, Germany

Min Zhuo, PhD
Professor
Neuroscience Platform
Department of Physiology
University of Toronto
Toronto, ON, Canada

ABOUT THE AUTHORS*

Eske Kvanner Aasvang has a decade-long interest and activity in pain research within the area of acute and chronic postoperative pain, focusing on identifying patient- and surgery-related risk factors for prediction, prevention, and surgical treatment, including the relative role of nerve injury, nociceptive function, genetics, and surgical trauma.

Ole Kæseler Andersen is professor at Department of Health Science and Technology, Aalborg University. He conducts research into the neural mechanisms underlying central sensitization in humans with a special focus on the use of electrophysiologic outcome measures.

Lars Arendt-Nielsen is full professor in translational pain research, founder and director of the International Center for Sensory-Motor Interaction (SMI), Aalborg University, Denmark, and founder and director of R&D at the clinical trial unit C4Pain. He has published more than 1006 peer-reviewed journal papers on experimental and clinical assessment of pain and on application of human pain biomarkers in drug development. He has delivered more than 250 keynote lectures at international conferences. He has served on the IASP Council, as cochair of the IASP Global Year Against Musculoskeletal Pain in 2010, as cochair of the IASP Global Year Against Joint Pain in 2016, as cochair for IASP's SIG on Musculoskeletal Pain, as head of the IASP Grant Committee, and as editor in chief of the IASP Press. In 2016, he was president-elect of IASP. In 2007, he was knighted by the Danish Queen for his contribution to science.

Dipika Bansal is assistant professor of Clinical Research Unit, Department of Pharmacy Practice, National Institute of Pharmaceutical Education and Research (NIPER). She has 14 years of experience in clinical pharmacology. She has founded and developed Clinical Research Unit at NIPER for research, teaching, and practice. Her major research interests are in pain management. She has conducted numerous clinical trials and outcomes research in pain-related field.

Timothy J. Brennan is the first investigator to model incision-induced pain to understand the etiology of postoperative pain. He pioneered work on plasticity caused by surgery and used postoperative models to aid the development of new analgesic drugs. Clinically, he practices on the acute pain service and in the operating rooms.

Emanuel N. van den Broeke is postdoctoral researcher at the Institute of Neuroscience of the Université catholique de Louvain (UCL) in Brussels, Belgium. His research focuses on pain- or nociception-induced CNS plasticity in humans and how this leads or contributes to hyperalgesia.

Daniel B. Carr holds appointments in Public Health, Anesthesiology and Medicine at Tufts Medical School, where he is the founding director of its program on pain research, education, and policy. An IASP member since 1988 and honorary member since 2018, his research spans bench (opioid peptide chemistry) to bedside (clinical analgesic trials). He inaugurated IASP's *Pain: Clinical Updates* and with Professor Harald Breivik convened the first WHO-IASP-EFIC Global Year Against Pain. He

---
*Biosketches are as provided by the authors or their institutional or society websites.

has contributed to IASP publications including monographs on pain and narrative, World Congress proceedings, and sickle cell pain. His non-IASP publications include two US federal clinical practice guidelines, the classic text on neural blockade first prepared by long-term collaborator Professor Michael Cousins, a text on postoperative pain by Professor George Shorten and other EFIC colleagues, and a monograph on evidence and outcomes with Professor Harriet Wittink. He participated in the formation of IASP SIGs including evidence-based medicine, building on his service as inaugural editor for acute pain trials in the Cochrane Collaboration, under Phil Wiffen. As chair of IASP's Acute Pain SIG, with Professors Treede, Arendt-Nielsen, Schug, and Pogatzki-Zahn of IASP, and EFIC President Professor Bart Morlion, he provided editorial and political support for the 2017 Global Year Against Pain After Surgery. He has served on multiple professional, advisory, and editorial boards including IASP Council, the US federal National Pain Strategy, and the Interagency Pain Research Coordinating Committee of the US National Institutes of Health. Many former students and trainees hold positions of prominence around the world.

Jacques E. Chelly received his MD degree and his anesthesiology and intensive care board certification from Paris, France, in 1976 and 1979, respectively. He completed the requirement for a PhD in pharmacology in 1985 and an MBA in 1992 from the University of Houston, Houston, Texas. In 2016, he obtained a diploma in scientific auriculotherapy from the University of Paris. He currently holds a position of professor at the University of Pittsburgh School of Medicine in the Department of Anesthesiology and Orthopedic Surgery, fellowship director of the accredited Regional Anesthesiology and Acute Pain Medicine Fellowship. He is an acute pain physician and chief and founder of the Acute Interventional Perioperative Pain Service at UPMC Presbyterian-Shadyside Hospitals, Department of Anesthesiology, University of Pittsburgh Medical Center, Pittsburgh, Pennsylvania. His research interest includes regional anesthesiology, acute pain, genetic of pain, pharmacology, addiction medicine, and more recently complementary medicine. He has published over 190 peer-reviewed articles, 45 editorial and letters to the editors, and 300 abstracts and presented his research at over 100 national and international meetings. He has authored three regional anesthesia textbooks.

Anthony H. Dickenson is professor of Neuropharmacology in the Department of Neuroscience, Physiology and Pharmacology at University College, London, United Kingdom. His work is on translational mechanisms of pain and its control.

Asbjørn Mohr Drewes is professor (chair) at the Department of Gastroenterology and Hepatology, Aalborg University Hospital in Denmark. He is also director of Mech-Sense (www.mech-sense.com) and Centre for Pancreatic Diseases. As author of nearly 500 publications, his research interests include diseases of the pancreas, visceral pain, motility, electrophysiology, imaging, pharmacologic studies, and technological development to understand gastrointestinal physiology and pathophysiology.

G. Allen Finley is a pediatric anesthesiologist who has worked for almost 30 years in pain research and management. He is professor of Anesthesia and Psychology at Dalhousie University and holds the inaugural Dr. Stewart Wenning Chair in Pediatric Pain Management at the IWK Health Centre in Halifax. He has published (http://tinyurl.com/gaf-cits) and lectured widely. He started the PEDIATRIC-PAIN e-mail discussion list in 1993, bringing together pain researchers and clinicians from more than 40 countries. His main interest is pain service development and advocacy for improved pain care for children around the world, and he is board chair of the ChildKind International Initiative (http://childkindinternational.org).

Lauren V. Friend completed her PhD at University College London under the supervision of Professor Anthony Dickenson. Her research investigated the neuropharmacologic mechanisms of pain, with a specific focus on the activity of reward-processing brain regions in persistent pain states. Over the past 2 years, Lauren has spent time working in the biotech industry and has since moved onto a role in life sciences strategy.

Babita Ghai is a professor of Anaesthesia and consultant in charge of Pain Clinic, Post Graduate Institute of Medical Education and Research (PGIMER), Chandigarh, India. She has 22 years of teaching and research experience. She is actively engaged in pain research, pain education, and pain policy. She holds national and international distinction, awards, and important positions in pain-related field. She is current editor of newsletter of *Acute Pain SIG* of IASP (2016 to 2020) and joint secretary of Indian Society for Study of Pain (2015 to 2018).

Debra B. Gordon is the codirector for the Harborview Integrated Pain Care Program and teaching associate with the Department of Anesthesiology & Pain Medicine at the University of Washington, Seattle. She works in conjunction with the inpatient and outpatient Pain Relief Services, clinics, and hospital staff to collaborate on improving systems of care and designing outcome evaluations that benefit patients and populations across the continuum of care. She is a coinvestigator for the UW's NIH-designated Center of Excellence in Pain Education. Deb has also been involved in a number of national and international projects focused on improving pain management.

Thomas Graven-Nielsen received an M.Sc.EE. degree within Biomedical Engineering from Aalborg University, Denmark in 1994 and acquired his Ph.D. within Biomedical Science and Engineering in 1997 (Aalborg University). In 2006 he obtained a doctoral degree in Medical Science (Copenhagen University). He is director at Center for Neuroplasticity and Pain (CNAP), SMI, Department of Health Science and Technology, Aalborg University, Denmark (since 2015), and full professor in Pain Neuroscience since 2008. The Danish National Research Foundation funds CNAP. He is adjunct professor at University at Western Sydney, Australia (since 2015), and adjunct professor at Curtin University of Technology, Perth, Australia (since 2004). The research focuses on translational studies of musculoskeletal pain bridging the gap between basic animal findings and clinical manifestations of pain. The scope is to identify and modulate key features of human pain neuroplasticity, leading to prevention of maladaptive neuroplasticity and promote advantageous neuroplasticity. Development of pain models, biomarkers, and assessment technologies are key biomedical tools for the translational studies. The core areas are muscle pain, joint pain, referred pain, localized and widespread deep tissue hyperalgesia, pharmacologic screening, and electrophysiologic techniques to assess muscle pain physiology and neuroplasticity. He has published 300+ papers and reviews (260+ peer-reviewed, H-factor: 54) and received several awards. He reviews papers on a regular basis for high-ranked journals, has presented as keynote speaker at several international conferences, and organized scientific workshops and symposia at international meetings. More than 10 national and international collaborations on translational pain research have been established including research groups in Sweden, United Kingdom, Japan, United States, and Australia. Several international guest professors have worked with Dr. Graven-Nielsen in his laboratory facilities.

Mary M. Heinricher is professor and vice-chair for research in the Department of Neurological Surgery and professor in the Department of Behavioral Neuroscience at Oregon Health & Science University. She obtained her Ph.D. in Behavioral Neuroscience at Northwestern University. She then moved to the University of California, San Francisco as a postdoctoral fellow, staying as a faculty member in the Department of Neurology until 1995, when she was recruited to the Oregon Health & Science University. Her work focuses on the physiologic and pharmacologic properties of brainstem neurons that modulate pain by enhancing or suppressing transmission of nociceptive information from the spinal cord up to the brain.

John Jarrell is professor of Obstetrics and Gynecology at the University of Calgary, Canada, and a member of the Calgary Chronic Pain Centre. His academic interests are related to the diagnosis and treatment of pain sensitization in women from pelvic visceral disease.

Sinyoung Kang is assistant professor of Anesthesia—Acute Pain and Regional Anesthesia at the University of Iowa Carver College of Medicine. She received her MD and PhD in Medical Science from Ewha Womans University College of Medicine in Seoul, South Korea, where she completed her residency, chief residency, and fellowship in Anesthesiology and Pain Medicine. She continued her research in Iowa in the laboratory of Professor Timothy Brennan. Her clinical work aims not only to optimize pain management but also to maximize functional recovery of patients after surgery. Her research interests lie in understanding the mechanisms of functional impairment after major surgery.

Lee-Bareket Kisler is a Ph.D. candidate in the lab for neurophysiology at the medical faculty in the Technion Israel Institute of Technology and will soon begin a post doctorate at the University Health Network in Toronto, Canada.

Ronald J. Kulich is a full professor and clinical psychologist at Tufts School of Dental Medicine and holds a lecturer appointment in Department of Anesthesia, Critical Care and Pain Medicine at Harvard-Massachusetts General Hospital (MGH). His responsibilities include development and management of opioid risk assessment protocols for the MGH Pain Center and Facial Pain/Headache Center at Tufts School of Dental Medicine. Other academic responsibilities include treatment guideline development for work injury with Massachusetts Department of Industrial Accidents, training committee for the Massachusetts Prescription Monitoring Program, multiple opioid risk guideline committees, and cochairing the Massachusetts Governor's Committee for the Curriculum on Substance Abuse Assessment for Dentistry. Fellowship training responsibilities include supervision of Anesthesia/Pain Medicine and Orofacial Pain Medicine Fellows (MGH), as well as contributing to the behavioral sciences curriculum for Tufts School of Dental Medicine, teaching graduate students enrolled in Tufts program on Pain Research, Education and Policy, and supervision of psychology graduate interns.

Patricia Lavand'homme is a professor of Anesthesiology and head of the Acute Pain Service and Transitional Pain unit. She is also a member of the IASP Task Force mandated by the WHO to develop a new classification of chronic pain to be included in the revised version of the *International Classification of Diseases* (ICD-11) (she is in charge of chronic postsurgical and posttraumatic pain).

Dermot P. Maher earned his first graduate degree in pharmacology and completed medical school at Georgetown University. He then completed an anesthesia residency at Cedars-Sinai Medical Center in Los Angeles, California, followed by a chronic pain fellowship at the Massachusetts General Hospital in Boston, Massachusetts. Dr. Maher joined the faculty at Johns Hopkins School of Medicine in the Department of Anesthesia and Critical Care Medicine. During his first year on faculty, Dr. Maher earned an additional graduate degree from the Johns Hopkins Bloomberg School of Public Health. He has authored over two-dozen peer-reviewed manuscripts and book chapters. He currently serves as the medical director of one of Johns Hopkins outpatient pain clinics and as the assistant fellowship director. Dr. Maher's work focuses on optimization of pain treatment strategies in oncology patients.

Jeetinder Kaur Makkar is additional professor of Anaesthesia & Intensive Care, Post Graduate Institute of Medical Education and Research (PGIMER), Chandigarh, India. She has 17 years of teaching and research experience. Dr. Makkar is actively involved in clinical and research activities involving acute pain, chronic pain, and posttrauma pain with several publications in international and national journals.

José Alberto Biurrun Manresa received his biomedical engineering degree from the National University of Entre Ríos (Argentina) in 2007 and his Ph.D. degree in Biomedical Science and Engineering from Aalborg University (Denmark) in 2011. He is currently associate researcher at the National Scientific and Technical Research Council (CONICET) in Argentina. His research is primarily focused on the neurophysiology of the sensory systems, with emphasis on nociceptive processing.

Renee C.B. Manworren received her bachelor's degree from Loyola University, her Master's in Pediatric Nursing from Rush University, and in 2010, her PhD in nursing research from the University of Texas at Arlington. Dr. Manworren is now the Posy and Fred Love Chair in Nursing Research and Director of Nursing Research and Professional Practice at Ann & Robert H. Lurie Children's Hospital of Chicago. She is also an associate professor of Pediatrics at Northwestern University's Feinberg School of Medicine. Dr. Manworren was the first pediatric health care provider and researcher elected to the board of the American Pain Society. She is also a member of the master faculty for the American Society for Pain Management Nursing. Dr. Manworren is a founding member and past president of the American Pediatric Surgical Nurses Association, and a fellow in the American Academy of Nursing. Dr. Manworren lectures nationally and internationally about pediatric post-surgical pain. Her current research focuses on identifying biopsychosocial and genetic risk factors for challenging-to-control postoperative pain, as well as interventions to reduce postoperative pain. Dr. Manworren provides direct patient consultation, assessment, and treatment for pediatric patients with acute pain, postoperative pain, and at risk for postoperative pain.

Winfried Meissner was appointed head of Jena University Hospital's Pain Unit in 1994 and head of the Palliative Care Department in 2009. His clinical work is focused on acute and chronic pain management. Meissner and his group have initiated and coordinated two large registries in the area of acute pain: QUIPS (quality improvement in postoperative pain management; in Germany) and its international counterpart PAIN OUT (improvement in postoperative pain outcome), which resulted so far in more than 40 publications. In addition, he was coordinator of the NeuroPAIN project (chronic pain and neurologic consequences in sepsis survivors) and has broad teaching experience. Meissner is a member of several national and international societies, including ESA and IASP.

André Mouraux is professor at the Faculty of Medicine and Institute of Neuroscience of the Université catholique de Louvain. Using noninvasive functional neuroimaging techniques such as electroencephalography and functional magnetic resonance imaging (fMRI), combined with novel techniques to selectively activate specific classes of nociceptive afferents, André Mouraux aims to understand how the human brain processes nociceptive sensory input and how this leads to the perception of pain. Furthermore, he aims to understand the plastic changes in nociceptive pathways that occur after inflammation, injury, or sustained nociceptive input that induce peripheral and central sensitization and may underlie the development of chronic pain in humans.

Kristian Kjær Petersen was initially trained as a biomedical engineer (2011), later finalized his Doctor of Philosophy thesis entitled "Chronic Pain after Total Knee Replacement" (2014), followed by a 2-year post-doc (2014 to 2015), and currently holds an assistant professor position at Aalborg University, Denmark. The basis of his research focuses on a biomedical engineering approach to develop pain biomarkers to study the underlying pain mechanisms for patients with chronic pain. This understanding is utilized to develop better diagnosis and treatments with special focus on predicting outcomes after surgery.

Esther M. Pogatzki-Zahn is an anesthesiologist, pain specialist and Full Professor in the Department of Anaesthesiology, Intensive Care and Pain Medicine, University Hospital Muenster, Germany. Her main clinical work is pain management (acute, chronic and palliative); she leads the acute pain service at the University Clinic. Furthermore, she leads a large pain research group at the University of Muenster. Her research goal is to bridge the gap between basic animal research and clinical practice. She was trained as a PhD in Neuroscience in 2 basic science laboratories in the US from 1998-2003 and in Muenster, she performs basic science studies aiming to provide insight into the neuropathology of incisional, chronic inflammatory, neuropathic and cancer-related pain. In addition, she is working with human surrogate models of postoperative and neuropathic pain and uses quantitative sensory testing and imaging techniques like fMRI to explore acute and chronic pain in humans. Clinically, she is involved as a Principal Investigator in international multicenter projects like PAIN OUT, a large acute international acute pain registry. She is member of the Prospect initiative (www.postoppain.org) and the German Research Network on Neuropathic Pain. She won a number of national and international research awards and is part of several advisory and society boards including the Acute Pain Special Interest Group of the IASP (Co-Chair since 2016) and the European Society of Anaesthesiologists (Chair of the Scientific Subcommittee 8, acute and chronic pain and palliative care). She is an active member of several international pain, anesthesia and neuroscience societies and on review boards of leading journals including Anesthesiology, Pain, NeuroImage, Journal of Neuroscience, and Anesthesia & Analgesia.

Stephan A. Schug is professor and chair of Anaesthesiology in the Medical School of the University of Western Australia, Perth, Australia, and director of Pain Medicine at Royal Perth Hospital, Australia. His principal research interests include the management of acute and chronic pain, cancer pain, regional anesthesia, the pharmacology of local anesthetics and analgesics, and quality improvement in health care.

Enrico Schulz received his Ph.D. at the University of Zurich. He worked as a post-doctoral researcher at the Technische Universität Munich and the University of Oxford before becoming a PI at Ludwig-Maximilians-Universität Munich.

Guy Simonnet is an emeritus professor of Cell Biology at the University of Bordeaux (France) and is working into the "Aquitaine Institute for Cognitive and Integrative Neuroscience" and the head of the research team "Homeostasie-Allostasie-Pathologie-Rehabilitation." His research activity is based on the "Opponent Process Theory" (Solomon, 1974), which leads him to propose the concept that acute or repeated exposures of the CNS to drugs that are "inhibitory," such as opioids, could result in adaptive changes, which are, in fact, "facilitatory." Based on both behavioral and cellular/molecular studies, he proposed the concept of "latent pain sensitization" in which it has been shown that prior pain experiences as surgery, associated with exogenous administration or endogenous opioid release (stress) in CNS of an individual, produce an increase in pain vulnerability leading to postoperative hyperalgesia. This "adaptive" neurobiologic process may explain some aspects of interindividual differences in pain sensitivity and how the pain becomes chronic in humans after surgery.

Till Sprenger was trained in neurology in Munich/Germany and later worked as postdoc and faculty at UCSF. He was then appointed as research professor at the University Hospital Basel and is now head of the Department of Neurology at the DKD Helios Klinik Wiesbaden/Germany. His research interests include clinical trials and structural/functional neuroimaging in headache disorders, neuropathic pain, and multiple sclerosis.

Anne Stankewitz received her PhD at the Department of Systems Neuroscience at the University Hospital in Hamburg before joining Prof. Tölle's working group as a postdoctoral researcher at the Technical University in Munich. Currently, she is working on the neurobiological mechanisms underlying migraine disease.

Daisuke Sugiyama is a postdoctoral research scholar at University of Iowa, where he studies the mechanisms of functional impairment, including pain and motor dysfunction, after major surgery using rodent models to develop new perioperative strategies and treatments.

Thomas R. Tölle is a professor of *Neurology* at the Technische Universität München, Germany. He is a neurologist and psychologist by training. He set up an interdisciplinary research group for clinical and experimental research into pain, focusing primarily on the neurobiologic mechanisms of neuronal plasticity, pharmacologic treatment, and central imaging with fMRI and positron emission tomography.

His research and clinical interests also include the prevention and treatment of chronic neuropathic pain and he is spokesman and runs the head office of the German Research Network for Neuropathic Pain (DFNS). Prof. Tölle has authored many peer-reviewed publications and lectures on many aspects of pain medicine all over the world, served as the president of the German IASP chapter, and chaired the scientific program committee for the EFIC European Pain Congress in 2017 in Copenhagen. He combines a basic and clinical research department with running a multidisciplinary pain clinic.

Louisa D. Townson works in the strategy group of at a top-tier pharmaceutical company, supporting the clinical development of assets for the treatment of a range of neurologic and rare diseases, including pain conditions. She completed her PhD in the laboratory of Prof. Anthony Dickenson, where her research focused on changes in brainstem contributions to pain in osteoarthritis.

Kris C. P. Vissers is an anesthesiologist, professor in Pain and Palliative Medicine, and chairman of the Radboud Expertise Center of Pain and Palliative Medicine of the Radboud University Nijmegen Medical Centre in the Netherlands. As a principal investigator, his research program is connected to the Health Care Improvement Science program of Radboud University. He obtained his graduation in Medical Sciences at the University of Antwerp (Belgium) and his graduation as an anesthesiologist at the University of Antwerp and the Catholic University of Leuven (Belgium). He specialized in pain medicine in Leuven and Nijmegen. As of 1995, he was staff member of the University-affiliated Hospital East-Limburg, Genk, Belgium, where he founded the Multidisciplinary Pain Center in 1995. He was visiting consultant for the palliative care unit and hospital team. He was responsible consultant for the home care organization in Palliative Care "Pallium." He obtained the degree of doctor in the medical sciences (PhD) in 2004 at Radboud University Nijmegen Medical Center, The Netherlands. He graduated as fellow in Interventional Pain Practice in 2004. Since 2005, he is full-time professor in Pain and Palliative Medicine at the Radboudumc University Nijmegen. He is ex officio board member of the Benelux Chapter of the World Institute of Pain and the first chairman of the Dutch Society of Multidisciplinary Palliative Care Professionals (Palliactief: Dutch Society of Multidisciplinary Professionals in Palliative Care), chapter of the European Association of Palliative Care (EAPC), and current president of the Pain Alliance in the Netherlands, chapter of the IASP. He is immediate past president of the World Institute of Pain. His main research interests are (1) translational approach and research on neuropathic pain, (2) practical and ethical application of palliative sedation, (3) proactive care and identification of patients in a palliative trajectory, (4) quality indicators of the organization and practice of pain and palliative medicine, (5) e-health and telemedicine in transmural care programs, (6) decision-making in palliative care and end-of-life care, and (7) the description of competences and performances for the education and training in pain and palliative medicine. He succeeded in getting external funding resources for major research projects in pain and palliative care (Europall, 7th framework, ZonMw, NWO, KWF). He is author of more than 200 publications in international peer-reviewed journals and contributed to more than 20 textbooks. He contributes to local and national education with regular articles in Belgian and Dutch journals for physicians and for the lay public. He is frequently asked as speaker during national and international congresses and teaching courses. He is promotor of 26 PhD students in his topics of interest. He organized 10 international congresses and workshops. He was member of several scientific committees of congresses.

Ana-Maria Vranceanu is an associate professor of Psychology at Harvard Medical School and the director of the Integrated Brain Health Clinical and Research Program within the Department of Psychiatry at Massachusetts General Hospital. Her clinical and research program is focused on preserving brain health through lifestyle changes, promoting recovery after surgery or injury, and optimizing health and well-being in individuals with chronic illness. She has over 100 publications, with more than half addressing psychosocial issues common in acute and chronic pain. She has been the principal investigator on over 10 foundation and federally funded grants, 4 of which directly addressed acute or chronic pain concerns.

Emily A. Walsh is a research assistant in the Craniofacial Pain Center at the Tufts University School of Dental Medicine. She also works a clinical research coordinator in the Cancer Outcomes Research Program at Massachusetts General Hospital.

Oliver H.G. Wilder-Smith has set up and published a large body of research (130+ publications in international peer-reviewed journals) in pain neuroscience during last 5 years. He has built an extensive international network of top pain research groups, particularly in Denmark (Aalborg), Israel (Haifa), and Germany (DFNS). He obtained a DSc title in Denmark in 2013. A main thrust of his research is altered sensory and cognitive function in patients with chronic pain and persisting pain after surgery using psychophysical testing, electroencephalography, and neuropsychological testing. He has developed these methods using experimental pain models in healthy volunteers and then clinically implemented them in patients in both cross-sectional and longitudinal studies. His group has published a collection of pioneering studies comprehensively documenting sensory and cognitive neuroplasticity in chronic pancreatitis pain using psychophysical and neuropsychological testing, electroencephalography, and MRI (morphology, connectivity). This body of research also involves studies covering drug therapy (ketamine, pregabalin, namisol), including indications for use, prediction of drug response, and monitoring of effect. He has also initiated several projects studying the association between altered sensory and cognitive processing and the development of chronic pain after surgery in both cross-sectional and longitudinal studies, publishing the first comprehensive, long-term account of altered sensory processing 6 months after surgery. This research reached significant clinical conclusions permitting the preoperative prediction and postoperative monitoring of risk for chronic pain development in surgical patients. Based on this research, his group has become the first worldwide to implement quantitative sensory testing into routine clinical practice, both for screening and diagnostic purposes.

David Yarnitsky is a neurologist interested in neuropathic pain, migraine, and neuromuscular disorders; his research focuses on pain processing in health and disease. As of past year he is editor in chief of IASP's new journal *PAIN Reports*.

Ruth Zaslansky trained as a pain neurophysiologist, is currently scientific director of PAIN OUT, an international quality improvement and research network working to improve management and outcomes of pain in patients undergoing surgery. PAIN OUT is coordinated from Jena, in Germany.

Min Zhuo is the Michael Smith Chair in Neuroscience and Mental Health, and the Canada Research Chair Tier I in Pain and Cognition. He is a full professor in University of Toronto, Department of Physiology.

INTRODUCTION

Pain After Surgery: Achievements and Future Challenges
Patricia Lavand'homme, Esther M. Pogatzki-Zahn, Stephan A. Schug, Daniel B. Carr

The IASP, in collaboration with the European Pain Federation, declared 2017 the Global Year Against Pain After Surgery. Almost 10 years earlier, an editorial titled "Management of acute postoperative pain: still a long way to go!" launched a wakeup-call to health care providers, reminding them that poorly managed postoperative pain is a major health care issue [8]. A decade before that wake-up call, the intensity of acute postoperative had been proposed as a risk factor for subsequent persistent postsurgical pain (PPSP) [24].

The present book addresses multiple aspects of postsurgical pain, from basic pathophysiology of acute and chronic pain to pain prevention, perioperative management, and long-term assessment and treatment. It summarizes achievements and future challenges in the field of pain after surgery.

Specific objectives of individual chapters include the following:

1. Highlighting the clinical and societal issues that pain persistence after surgery represents, and the context within which research on pain persistence needs to take place
2. Defining effects of surgical damage on relevant tissues and structures, including skin, muscles, bones, joints, nerves, and viscera, with emphasis on effects regarding sensory processing
3. Recognizing the impact of ongoing nociception on the various systems affected by noxious surgical inputs, how these effects are integrated, and the research challenges that this provides
4. Understanding methods available for making nociception effects visible in humans and recognizing the limitations/hurdles associated with application in clinical research and practice
5. Developing a comprehensive, integrated model of processes and factors involved in pain persistence and highlighting opportunities and challenges for research and clinical practice
6. Evaluating research to date into prevention and management of pain persistence, review the unmet research need, and identify priorities for research and implementation into clinical practice

Pain after surgery is the most common manifestation of acute pain in medically supervised settings. This is not surprising in view of the fact that more than 310 million operations were performed worldwide in 2012, a number that is increasing continuously [34]. Pain after surgery is often severe and its management remains suboptimal in many cases. Better management of acute postoperative pain is first and foremost required to reduce unnecessary suffering of patients in this setting because unrelieved pain after surgery has many adverse consequences [28]. These include unfavorable patient experiences such as fear, anxiety, impaired sleep and unnecessary stress, delayed postoperative recovery and rehabilitation and hence increased length of stay in hospital, and higher complication rates leading to increased health care costs. It is therefore not surprising that optimization of postoperative analgesia is a mandatory component of all fast-track surgical pathways such as those proposed by the enhanced recovery after surgery (ERAS) initiative [12].

A major reason for the ongoing poor quality of postoperative pain management is that anesthetists and surgeons have focused on the intraoperative period, in which improved surgical techniques and anesthetic approaches have made the outcome extremely successful and safe. In comparison, the postoperative period has for many years been relatively neglected [20]. The increased risk of morbidity and mortality in the postoperative period and the implications of poor management of this period with regard to complications, delayed or unsuccessful rehabilitation, and poor outcomes have been slow to be recognized. Growing awareness of the importance of optimal pain management and attention to other components of perioperative management, such as fluid and temperature management, has led to an increasing interest in the field of perioperative medicine. Driven to a large degree by the pioneering and relentless efforts of Henrik Kehlet [22], these efforts have resulted in a better understanding of the preclinical physiology of the postoperative period and translation of this knowledge into improved clinical management [27]. Differentiation between pain at rest versus during movement and the discovery of peripheral and central inflammation and sensitization after incision are elements of a distinct pathophysiology of postoperative pain [3,23,38]. Increasingly comprehensive yet precise knowledge enables identification of promising new targets for the development of innovative analgesics for postoperative pain [27,29,32].

Clinical research studies and their synthesis over the last 30 years have already generated a strong evidence base guiding the management of pain after surgery [31]. This evidence base has resulted in the implementation of a number of novel approaches to pain management in this setting. These include emphasis on techniques of regional analgesia as well as multimodal analgesia. In parallel with these findings, introduction of new routes of administration, such as peripheral nerve catheters, and new drug delivery concepts, such as patient-controlled analgesia, have revolutionized the management of pain after surgery. However, one of the major reasons for the insufficient pain control in many postoperative patients is the evidence/practice gap, as scientific evidence is not implemented in the day-to-day management of postoperative patients. In recent years, real-life data from acute pain registries have revealed persistently poor acute pain management after many (including relatively limited) operations. One analysis of more than 50,000 patients, divided into 179 surgical types, found that the majority of patients reporting moderate to severe pain are those undergoing minor- to medium-level procedures [13]. Possibly, randomized controlled trials (RCTs) are not generalizing well into clinical practice, and several reasons may explain this (narrow enrollment criteria for patients, high standards for routine patient care to which new interventions are added, etc.). We need to understand factors related to better postoperative pain control and pain-related outcomes in the clinical setting. In fact, we do not know yet the exact patient-reported outcomes (PROs) indicative of successful perioperative pain management; those used in clinical trials are often heterogeneous and maybe not that important to patients. Filling such knowledge gaps is a major challenge facing this area and would not only result in diminishing needless suffering but also has the potential to improve clinical outcomes after surgery, with the additional benefit of cost containment in this expensive and increasing component of health care. Tools to identify patients at risk of increased pain after surgery and impaired pain-related outcomes could be enormously helpful to optimally allocate resources and potentially reduce the evolution of acute pain after surgery into PPSP.

For almost 20 years, numerous single-center, multicenter, or nationwide studies have identified PPSP as an important negative outcome of otherwise successful operations, which may negatively affect daily life [21]. From clinical studies, we have learned that PPSP may occur after any surgical procedure although its incidence and severity vary substantially depending on the methods used to ascertain and estimate it. In this book, several aspects of the pathogenesis and possibilities for prevention/treatment are covered. Although there is general agreement about the clinical relevance of PPSP, several issues remain to be better evaluated to understand the relative role of *pre-*, *intra-* and *post*operative risk factors or, from another view, patient- versus surgery-related factors.

Advances include the crafting of a uniform working definition of PPSP to standardize future data collection and analysis. The initial definition proposed by Macrae [24] has been recently refined [35]. Also, as PPSP has become a health care priority, it is scheduled to be included in the upcoming revision of the *International Classification of Diseases (ICD-11)* with the aim to increase its visibility and to promote multidisciplinary research in the field [33].

Nevertheless challenges remain.

Persistent "pain" is one of the PROs after surgery. Beyond a number on a scale, individual consequences on patients' quality of life (including sleep and mood) and societal impact (e.g., new persisting opioid use observed after both minor and major surgical procedures) should be captured [9]. Much of the literature has historically been developed in the absence of a uniform assessment of acute postoperative pain or PPSP and its clinical consequences [19]. Most importantly, both acute postoperative pain and PPSP must be assessed during meaningful, well-defined function and probably also with greater frequency to discern spontaneous versus tonic pain patterns [6].

The need for "procedure-specific" assessment of PPSP extends to the consequences of PPSP on everyday functions of daily life[14]. To date, this has only been accomplished for a few surgical procedures (e.g., inguinal hernia repair, thoracotomy, or breast cancer surgery) [30]. The need for preoperative procedure-specific assessments has recently been questioned, taking knee replacement and breast cancer surgery as examples [25]. There is a growing interest in pain after orthopedic procedures, as the volume of arthroplasties is increasing with the aging of the population and arthroplasties generate intense nociception [13]. Further, pediatric PPSP has been studied only recently despite the major impact of pain in this vulnerable population [4]. It is also worth noting that routine outpatient electronic data capture allows the occurrence of PPSP to be examined in populations other than adult hospitalized patients.

A neuropathic component is observed in approximately 35% of patients with PPSP and is usually associated with worse pain [17]. Because a main question to be answered relates to the "neuropathic" versus the "inflammatory" component in PPSP [17,21], some type of neurophysiologic assessment is required, as the neuropathic component seems dominant. Although quantitative sensory testing (QST) is a well-documented technique to assess the neuropathic component of various chronic pain conditions, studies in PPSP have highlighted the wide range of normal variability in sensory functions [18]. Studies in patients with inguinal hernia [1], breast cancer [16], and thoracic surgery [36] have demonstrated that although "positive" QST phenomena may be more frequent in PPSP patients, many QST abnormalities are found in pain-free patients. The same applies to different "neuropathic" pain questionnaires [25]. Despite of these limitations, assessment of PPSP should be supplemented by adding the most relevant QST assessment and "neuropathic" pain questionnaires to improve our understanding of PPSP.

Despite the abovementioned limitations, assessment of PPSP should be supplemented by adding the most relevant QST assessment and "neuropathic" pain questionnaires to improve our understanding of PPSP. Finally, it must be described whether PPSP patients were pain-free preoperatively, whether the preoperative pain was the same character and localization or different from PPSP, or whether other chronic pain syndromes were apparent preoperatively (low back pain, migraine, fibromyalgia, etc.) [6]. These aspects are addressed in various chapters in this book.

For example, the presence of a neuropathic component in early postoperative pain is a risk factor for neuropathic PPSP [5].

Because prevention is better than treatment after a problem has emerged, predictive risk indices have been developed to identify patients in whom intensive efforts are warranted [2]. To date, however, they lack specificity or sensitivity. The preoperative function of the nociceptive system, e.g., preoperative hyperalgesia, may be important, and several studies have shown a degree of predictive value for various preoperative nociceptive tests [37]. The exact role of genetic testing remains to be established; clinical factors predict approximately 70% of PPSP risk [26].

In summary, preventive strategies for PPSP development can be classified as primary (e.g., avoid surgery when possible, modification of surgical technique leading to less tissue trauma), secondary (e.g., perioperative application of preventive strategies), and tertiary (e.g., rapid detection and early treatment of PPSP) [15]. Regarding perioperative preventive strategies, existing data are mostly inconclusive [10]. One explanation is that the analgesic interventions applied have been too selective and brief to influence later, more central nociceptive processing.

There is a clear need for better understanding of the mechanisms underlying the transition from acute postoperative pain to chronic pain after surgery [11]. On the positive side, fundamental research has provided many opportunities for advancing this field. For example, future studies should focus on novel targets such as neuroinflammatory and immune mechanisms for the generation of "neuropathic" pain [7,39] and the potential benefits of next-generation pharmacologic interventions to extend the therapeutic armamentarium.

REFERENCES

1. Aasvang EK, Brandsborg B, Jensen TS, Kehlet H. Heterogeneous sensory processing in persistent postherniotomy pain. Pain 2010;150:237–242
2. Althaus A, Hinrichs-Rocker A, Chapman R, Arranz Becker O, Lefering R, Simanski C, et al. Development of a risk index for the prediction of chronic post-surgical pain. Eur J Pain 2012;16(6):901–10.
3. Amirmohseni S, Segelcke D, Reichl S, Wachsmuth L, Gorlich D, Faber C, et al. Characterization of incisional and inflammatory pain in rats using functional tools of MRI. Neuroimage 2016;127:110–22.
4. Batoz H, Semjen F, Bordes-Demolis M, Benard A, Nouette-Gaulain K. Chronic postsurgical pain in children: prevalence and risk factors. A prospective observational study. Br J Anaesth 2016;117(4):489–96.
5. Beloeil H, Sion B, Rousseau C, Albaladejo P, Raux M, Aubrun F, et al. Early postoperative neuropathic pain assessed by the DN4 score predicts an increased risk of persistent postsurgical neuropathic pain. Eur J Anaesthesiol 2017;34(10):652–7.
6. Bennett GJ. What is spontaneous pain and who has it? J Pain 2012;13:921–929.
7. Borsook D, Kussman BD, George E, Becerra LR, Burke DW. Surgically induced neuropathic pain: understanding the perioperative process. Ann Surg 2013;257(3):403–12.
8. Breivik H, Stubhaug A. Management of acute postoperative pain: still a long way to go! Pain 2008;137(2):233–4.
9. Brummett CM, Waljee JF, Goesling J, Moser S, Lin P, Englesbe MJ, et al. New persistent opioid use after minor and major surgical procedures in US adults. JAMA Surg 2017:e170504.
10. Chaparro LE, Smith SA, Moore RA, Wiffen PJ, Gilron I. Pharmacotherapy for the prevention of chronic pain after surgery in adults. Cochrane Database Syst Rev 2013;7:CD008307.
11. Chapman CR, Vierck CJ. The transition of acute postoperative pain to chronic pain: an integrative overview of research on mechanisms. J Pain 2017;18(4):359 e1–e38.
12. ERAS©Society. The official ERAS Website. September 28, 2015. Available from: http://www.erassociety.org.
13. Gerbershagen HJ, Aduckathil S, van Wijck AJ, Peelen LM, Kalkman CJ, Meissner W. Pain intensity on the first day after surgery: a prospective cohort study comparing 179 surgical procedures. Anesthesiology 2013;118(4):934–44.
14. Gerbershagen HJ, Pogatzki-Zahn E, Aduckathil S, Peelen LM, Kappen TH, van Wijck AJ, et al. Procedure-specific risk factor analysis for the development of severe postoperative pain. Anesthesiology 2014;120(5):1237–45.
15. Gilron I, Kehlet H. Prevention of chronic pain after surgery: new insights for future research and patient care. Can J Anaesth 2014;61(2):101–11.
16. Gottrup H, Andersen J, Arendt-Nielsen L, Jensen TS. Psychophysical examination in patients with post-mastectomy pain. Pain 2000;87:275–284
17. Haroutiunian S, Nikolajsen L, Finnerup NB, Jensen TS. The neuropathic component in persistent postsurgical pain: a systematic literature review. Pain 2013;154(1):95–102.
18. Johansen A, Schirmer H, Nielsen CS, Stubhaug A. Persistent post-surgical pain and signs of nerve injury: the Tromso study. Acta Anaesthesiol Scand 2016;60(3):380–92.
19. Kehlet H, Bay-Nielsen M, Kingsnorth A. Chronic postherniorrhaphy pain – a call for uniform assessment. Hernia 2002;6:178–181.
20. Kehlet H, Dahl JB. Anaesthesia, surgery, and challenges in postoperative recovery. Lancet 2003;362(9399):1921–8.
21. Kehlet H, Jensen TS, Woolf CJ. Persistent postsurgical pain: risk factors and prevention. Lancet 2006;367(9522):1618–25.
22. Kehlet H. Surgical stress: the role of pain and analgesia. Br J Anaesth 1989;63(2):189–95.
23. Kido K, Gautam M, Benson CJ, Gu H, Brennan TJ. Effect of deep tissue incision on pH responses of afferent fibers and dorsal root ganglia innervating muscle. Anesthesiology 2013;119(5):1186–97.
24. Macrae WA, Davies HTO. Chronic postsurgical pain. In: Crombie IK, Linton S, Croft P, Von Korff M, LeResche L, editors. Epidemiology of pain. Seattle: IASP Press; 1999. p. 125–42.
25. Masselin-Dubois A, Attal N, Fletcher D, Jayr C, Albi A, Fermanian J, et al. Are psychological predictors of chronic postsurgical pain dependent on the surgical model? A comparison of total knee arthroplasty and breast surgery for cancer. J Pain 2013;14(8):854–64.

26. Montes A, Roca G, Sabate S, Lao JI, Navarro A, Cantillo J, et al. Genetic and clinical factors associated with chronic post-surgical pain after hernia repair, hysterectomy, and thoracotomy: a two-year multicenter cohort study. Anesthesiology 2015;122(5):1123–41.
27. Pogatzki-Zahn EM, Segelcke D, Schug SA. Postoperative pain—from mechanisms to treatment. Pain Rep 2017;2(2):e588.
28. Prabhakar A, Mancuso KF, Owen CP, Lissauer J, Merritt CK, Urman RD, et al. Perioperative analgesia outcomes and strategies. Best Pract Res Clin Anaesthesiol 2014;28(2):105–15.
29. Reichl S, Augustin M, Zahn PK, Pogatzki-Zahn EM. Peripheral and spinal GABAergic regulation of incisional pain in rats. Pain 2012;153(1):129–41.
30. Ringsted TK, Wildgaard K, Kreiner S, Kehlet H. Pain-related impairment of daily activities after thoracic surgery: a questionnaire validation. Clin J Pain 2013;29(9):791–9.
31. Schug SA, Palmer GM, Scott DA, Halliwell R, Trinca J; APM:SE Working Group of the Australian and New Zealand College of Anaesthetists and Faculty of Pain Medicine. Acute pain management: scientific evidence. 4th ed. Melbourne: ANZCA & FPM; 2015.
32. Spofford CM, Brennan TJ. Gene expression in skin, muscle, and dorsal root ganglion after plantar incision in the rat. Anesthesiology 2012;117(1):161–72.
33. Treede RD, Rief W, Barke A, Aziz Q, Bennett MI, Benoliel R, et al. A classification of chronic pain for ICD-11. Pain 2015;156(6):1003–07.
34. Weiser TG, Haynes AB, Molina G, Lipsitz SR, Esquivel MM, Uribe-Leitz T, et al. Estimate of the global volume of surgery in 2012: an assessment supporting improved health outcomes. Lancet 2015;385(Suppl. 2):S11.
35. Werner MU, Kongsgaard UE. I. Defining persistent post-surgical pain: is an update required? Br J Anaesth 2014;113(1):1–4.
36. Wildgaard K, Ringsted TK, Hansen HJ, Petersen RH, Werner MU, Kehlet H. Quantitative sensory testing of persistent pain after video-assisted thoracic surgery lobectomy. Br J Anaesth 2012;108:126–133
37. Yarnitsky D. Role of endogenous pain modulation in chronic pain mechanisms and treatment. Pain 2015;156(Suppl. 1):S24–31.
38. Zahn PK, Pogatzki-Zahn EM, Brennan TJ. Spinal administration of MK-801 and NBQX demonstrates NMDA-independent dorsal horn sensitization in incisional pain. Pain 2005;114(3):499–510.
39. Zhuo M, Wu G, Wu LJ. Neuronal and microglial mechanisms of neuropathic pain. Mol Brain 2011;4:31.

ACKNOWLEDGMENTS

We would like to acknowledge the enthusiastic, professional and dedicated support of Susanne Nielsen Lundis in coordinating the logistics of the book, writing and editing. We also thank the production teams at IASP Press and Wolters Kluwer for their careful management of each step in this book's production.

CONTENTS

Preface V

Contributors VII

About the Authors XI

Introduction XIX

Acknowledgments XXV

SECTION 1
Researching the Building Blocks: CNS Effects of Damage to Tissues and Structures

1. Effect of Deep Tissue Damage on Nociceptive Pathways 3
   Sinyoung Kang, Daisuke Sugiyama, and Timothy J. Brennan

2. The Nociceptive Capacity of Muscle, Skeletal, and Connective Tissue 15
   Thomas Graven-Nielsen and Lars Arendt-Nielsen

3. Attribution Bias in Gynecologic Laparoscopy 33
   John Jarrell and Lars Arendt-Nielsen

4. Central Nervous System Effects of Damage to Visceral Tissues in Humans 41
   Asbjørn Mohr Drewes

SECTION 2
Researching Integration: Systems Effects of Ongoing Nociception

5. Descending Control Mechanisms and Persistent Pain after Surgery 59
   Mary M. Heinricher

6. Neurotransmitters, Neuromodulators, and Ionophores in Mechanisms of Pain Persistence After Surgery: From Periphery to the Brain 71
   Lauren V. Friend, Louisa D. Townson, and Anthony H. Dickenson

7. Central Sensitization, Synaptic Potentiation, and Microglia 83
   Min Zhuo

SECTION 3
Research Methods: Quantifying Peripheral and CNS Responses

8. Mechanistic Pain Phenotyping in Pre- and Postoperative Settings 103
   Lars Arendt-Nielsen

9 Electrophysiologic Techniques: Assessment of Spinal Nociceptive Processing Using the Withdrawal Reflex 121
Ole Kæseler Andersen and José Alberto Biurrun Manresa

10 Electrophysiologic Techniques to Study the Supraspinal Responses to Nociceptive Input in Humans 133
André Mouraux

11 Contribution of Positron Emission Tomography (PET) for Understanding Neuronal Activation and Neurotransmission in Pain 153
Anne Stankewitz, Till Sprenger, Enrico Schulz, and Thomas R. Tölle

SECTION 4
Researching Mechanisms of Chronification of Acute Pain

12 Predicting Chronic Pain After Joint Surgery 167
Kristian Kjær Petersen and Lars Arendt-Nielsen

13 Altered Perioperative Pain Processing and Persistent Pain After Surgery 177
Oliver H.G. Wilder-Smith

14 Electroencephalography: A Potentially Valuable Tool for Measuring Central Neuroplasticity in the Context of Acute Postoperative Pain 187
Emanuel N. van den Broeke

15 Drug Effects and Altered Perioperative Pain Processing 195
David Yarnitsky and Lee-Bareket Kisler

SECTION 5
Researching Interventions to Inhibit or Prevent Chronification of Acute Pain

16 Pain Sensitization: A Critical Process in the Transition from Acute to Chronic Postsurgical Pain (CPSP) 207
Guy Simonnet

17 The Role of Intraoperative Nerve Injury in Persistent Postoperative Pain 223
Eske Kvanner Aasvang

18 Prevention of Pain Persistence: Anesthesiologic Aspects 233
Patricia Lavand'homme

SECTION 6
Translating Research into Clinical Practice

19 Multimodal Drug Therapies for Postoperative Pain Control in Adults 249
Stephan A. Schug

20 Regional Anesthesia and Analgesia for Postoperative Pain Control in Adults 259
Dermot P. Maher and Jacques E. Chelly

21 Pre- and Postsurgical Psychological Assessment and Management of Pain 271
Ronald J. Kulich, Emily A. Walsh, and Ana-Maria Vranceanu

22 Children's Pain After Surgery 281
Renee C.B. Manworren and G. Allen Finley

23 **Postoperative Pain Control for Older Persons** 289
   Babita Ghai, Jeetinder Kaur Makkar, and Dipika Bansal

24 **Methods and Measures to Improve the Quality of Pain After Surgery** 301
   Debra B. Gordon, Ruth Zaslansky, and Winfried Meissner

   Index 315

SECTION 1

Researching the Building Blocks: CNS Effects of Damage to Tissues and Structures

CHAPTER 1

Effect of Deep Tissue Damage on Nociceptive Pathways

Sinyoung Kang, Daisuke Sugiyama, and Timothy J. Brennan

Postoperative pain is a common cause of acute pain. Those working in postoperative pain management recognize that the etiology of incisional nociception may be different than that of inflammation, chemical irritation, and burn, and the responses to treatments may also differ [39]. Recognizing there was a gap between preclinical models of nociception and clinical postsurgical pain, we have been interested in better understanding the mechanisms of nociception caused by incisions. This chapter will review studies on a rat plantar hindpaw model for postoperative pain and propose mechanisms for enhanced excitability of sensory neurons caused by incisions. Presumably, if we learn more about the etiology of acute incisional nociception and the sensory processes that activate nociceptive pathways, new perioperative pain treatments can be advanced.

HISTORICAL PERSPECTIVE

Incisional-type injuries were studied by two other investigative groups interested in nociception. When Perl and colleagues were studying primary afferent nerve fibers and discovered nociceptors [3,5], they examined responses of C nociceptors to needle penetrations in the posterior femoral cutaneous nerve of the cat. Needle penetrations, even to mechanically insensitive afferents, elicited responses during the penetrations, but activation was not sustained. Except for an occasional postinjury afterdischarge for a few seconds after the penetration, no sustained activity could be produced by these needle penetrations. Evoked responses to various stimuli after injury were not tested.

In 1988, Campbell and colleagues examined the effects of a cut injury on the heat responsiveness of C nociceptors from the superficial radial nerve innervating hairy skin of the monkey [6]. Heat sensitivity of these C mechanoheat nociceptors was increased by a skin cut into the receptive field of the fiber but not by a cut adjacent to the receptive field. The heat threshold was reduced, and suprathreshold responses were increased after the cut injury. Effects of the cut on spontaneous activity and mechanical responsiveness were not reported. Together, these studies of injuries to cutaneous nociceptors demonstrated detection of tissue injury and heat sensitization. Spontaneous activity in these fibers was not demonstrated.

A Rat Model of Incisional Postoperative Pain

In 1993, we began studying the behavioral effects of the hindpaw incision. The incision was accomplished in rats using volatile general anesthesia and surgical conditions [4].

We avoided inflammatory irritation by closing the skin with nylon suture because we thought that there was an overreliance on inflammatory pain models in pain research at that time. Three nociceptive behaviors largely characterize the model: guarding behavior, heat sensitivity, and mechanical sensitivity [36]. Recently, conditioned place preference (CPP) has been utilized to examine spontaneous nociception [21,33]. Other behaviors have also been examined [23,30,38]. In this chapter, we will emphasize unprovoked, ongoing behaviors.

Guarding Behavior

At first we noted that, when rats were undisturbed and sitting quietly, they held their incised paw off the floor of the cage, tending not to rest it on the plastic mesh. We graded this guarding behavior by observing the position of the incised paw on the mesh for a 1-hour period and compared it with the contralateral unincised hindpaw [4]. Before surgery, there was little difference in the position of the hindpaws. However, immediately after surgery, the guarding behavior was greatest; this behavior gradually subsided over 3 to 4 days (Figure 1-1). This behavior has some similarities to the time course of pain at rest in surgical patients treated with patient-controlled analgesia [20]. Guarding was eliminated by hindpaw denervation [4], local anesthetic infiltration [24], and intrathecal morphine administration [37]. Guarding was reduced by parenteral morphine administration [26,37]; in fact, the weight-based dosages are similar to those used to treat pain at rest in patients after surgery [1]. This behavior was also decreased by anti–nerve growth factor [2,32], capsaicin infiltration [13,17], sciatic nerve application of capsaicin [13], and parenteral and locally administered ketoprofen [26].

To understand the role of deep tissue injury to guarding pain, we developed the method to incise skin only and limit the damage to the underlying fascia [34,36] and avoid muscle injury. The comparisons to skin incision only versus skin plus deep tissue injury could be evaluated. Very little guarding pain could be elicited in rats that underwent skin incision [36], even though it was difficult to limit the injury exclusively to the skin (Figure 1-1). Any guarding resolved by postoperative day 1 after skin incision, whereas those animals that had deep tissue injury (incision to skin, fascia, and muscle) had marked guarding for several

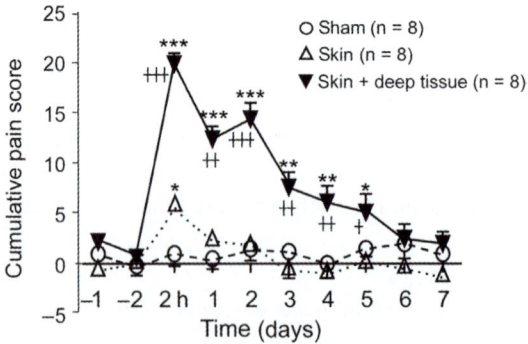

FIGURE 1-1 Guarding behaviors of rats after sham procedure, skin, or skin plus deep tissue incision. The guarding behavior was measured during a 60-min test period. The results are presented as mean and SEM. $*P < 0.05$, $**P < 0.01$, $***P < 0.001$ versus sham, $†P < 0.05$, $††P < 0.01$, $†††P < 0.001$ versus skin incision. (From Anesthesiology 112:153–64. http://anesthesiology.pubs.asahq.org/article.aspx?articleid=1932502. With permission from Lippincott Williams and Wilkins/Wolter Kluwer Health. Copyright 2010.)

days after incision. These results indicate that skin incision is insufficient to elicit unprovoked guarding pain in the plantar incision model, but after deep muscle injury, guarding was evident.

Conditioned Place Preference

Incisional pain-related behaviors have been studied using the novel technique of CPP [21,33]. Investigators utilized a pain-relieving treatment, local anesthetic administration into the popliteal fossa, to produce CPP in rats with hindpaw incision (Figure 1-2A and B). Thus, CPP has been used to demonstrate the presence of ongoing, unprovoked nociceptive behaviors after plantar incision. Two parenterally administered nonsteroidal anti-inflammatory drugs, ketorolac and naproxen, like local anesthetic administration, induced CPP. The data from these studies are in general agreement with the results of guarding pain. They also indicate that, early after incision, ongoing nociceptive behaviors are evident and there is a role for peripheral prostaglandins in this postoperative model.

In Vivo Neurophysiology and Spontaneous Activity After Incision

In several studies, we examined dorsal horn neurons for spontaneous activity before and immediately after plantar incision [24,29,40]. Incision increased spontaneous activity of approximately 40% to 50% of dorsal horn neurons that received input from the plantar region [24,29,40] (see the example in Figure 1-3). In general, the amount of spontaneous activity was low, averaging 1 to 2 imp/s 1 hour after incision. This small amount of activity occurs at a time when guarding nociception is greatest, and we hypothesized that spontaneous activity should be high. We suggested that examining the dorsal horn neurons in normal skin and then making an incision largely selects for neurons that receive predominately cutaneous primary afferent input [35]. Thus, only low levels of spontaneous activity would be expected after incision in normal skin.

Similarly, incision in normal skin did not increase spontaneous activity in nociceptive primary afferent fibers [12]. Our data, in addition to the work of Perl and colleagues [3,5] and that of Campbell and colleagues [6], support the notion that incision of skin produces very little spontaneous activity of primary afferent fibers innervating the skin.

Further electrophysiology experiments support the concept that cutaneous injury elicits a small amount of spontaneous activity in dorsal horn neurons and primary afferent fibers. We recorded dorsal horn neurons from rats that underwent sham incision and from rats that underwent skin incision only [34]. Of dorsal horn neurons, 30% had spontaneous activity in sham-operated animals, and approximately 50% had spontaneous activity 1 day after skin incision. There was no difference between sham and skin incision in the percentage of dorsal horn neurons innervating the plantar region with spontaneous activity and average rate of spontaneous activity. In contrast, a greater proportion, approximately 80%, of dorsal horn neurons from rats that had undergone an incision that included deep muscle tissue injury had spontaneous activity. The average rate of spontaneous activity tended to be greater in rats that underwent deep tissue incision. Thus marked spontaneous activity was elicited after plantar incision that included deep muscle tissue.

We also recorded primary afferent fibers from rats that underwent sham incision and from rats that underwent skin incision only (Figure 1-4A and B) [36]. Of nociceptive afferents, 13% had spontaneous activity in sham-operated animals, and approximately 17% of nociceptive fibers had spontaneous activity 1 day after skin incision (Figure 1-4B). There was no difference between sham and skin incision in the percentage of afferents with spontaneous activity and average rate of spontaneous activity. In contrast, a greater proportion,

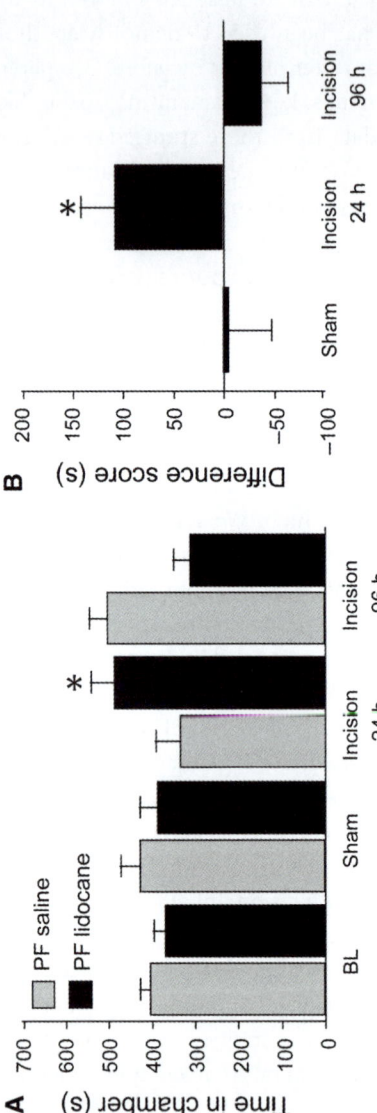

FIGURE 1-2 Peripheral nerve block in rats with incisional pain produced conditioned place preference (CPP). Peripheral nerve block in incised rats 24 h, but not 96 h, following incision of the hindpaw induced CPP as demonstrated by **(A)** increased time spent in chambers paired with popliteal fossa (PF) lidocaine and **(B)** difference scores. The results are presented as mean and SEM. *$P < 0.05$, Student paired t test. BL, baseline. (From Proc Natl Acad Sci USA 109(50):20709-13. http://www.pnas.org/content/109/50/20709.long. With permission from Proceedings of the National Academy of Sciences of the United States of America (PNAS). Copyright 2012.)

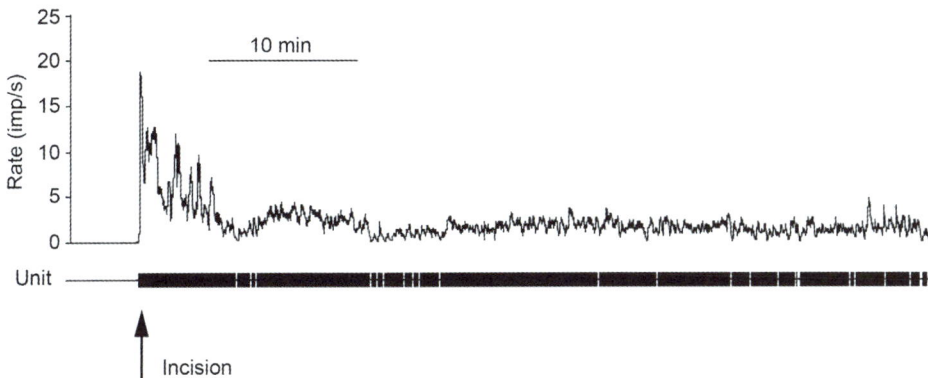

FIGURE 1-3 Example of increase in activity of a wide dynamic range neuron after incision. Each unit trace represents a single action potential. The neuron had no background activity before incision and sustained activity after incision. (From Pain 114:499–510. http://journals.lww.com/pain/Abstract/2005/04000/Spinal_administration_of_MK_801_and_NBQX.22.aspx. With permission from Lippincott Williams and Wilkins/Wolter Kluwer Health. Copyright 2005.)

approximately 80%, of nociceptors from rats that had undergone an incision that included deep tissue injury, had spontaneous activity. Although there was much variability, the average rate of spontaneous activity tended to be greater in afferents from rats that underwent deep tissue incision.

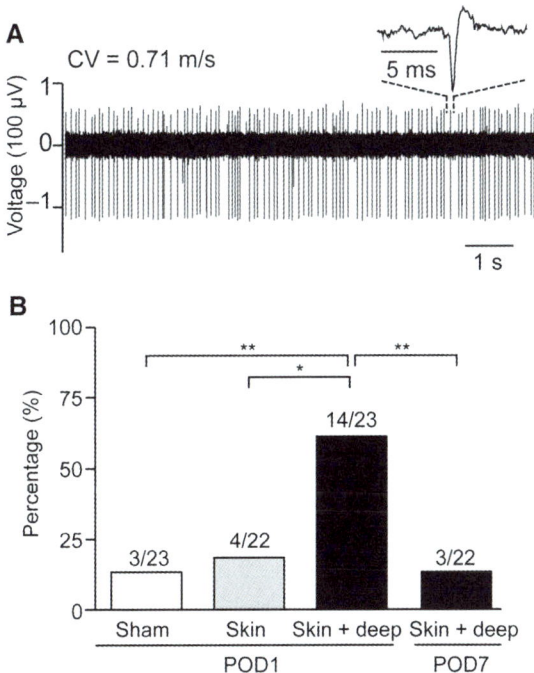

FIGURE 1-4 Spontaneous activity of nociceptors 1 day after sham procedure, skin, or skin plus deep tissue incision and 7 days after skin plus deep tissue incision. **A:** Digitized oscilloscope trace of spontaneous action potentials of a C nociceptor from a rat 1 day after skin plus deep tissue incision. Inset shows a representative single action potential. **B:** Percentage of nociceptors with spontaneous activity in each of the four groups. *$P < 0.05$, **$P < 0.01$. There was no difference in average rate among the groups. CV, conduction velocity; POD, postoperative day. (From Anesthesiology 112:153-64. http://anesthesiology.pubs.asahq.org/article.aspx?articleid=1932502. With permission from Lippincott Williams and Wilkins/Wolter Kluwer Health. Copyright 2010.)

Human Studies

Two human studies also indicate a very low amount of ongoing pain after skin incision. Kawamata et al. [18] made a forearm skin incision in human volunteers. Significant spontaneous pain was only present for 30 minutes after this incision. One hour later, there was no difference in spontaneous pain between a local anesthetic-treated, control group and the group that underwent forearm skin incision. Fimer et al. [9] also measured ongoing pain after a forearm incision. On a scale of 1 to 100, pain ratings were less than 1 for 2 minutes after the incision and pain ratings remained less than 1 for 3 hours and thereafter. Fimer et al. demonstrated that skin incision produces heat hyperalgesia in human volunteers as well [9]. The heat pain threshold decreased by 2°C and heat hyperalgesia was maintained throughout the day of incision. The heat hyperalgesia in humans was not as great as that produced by hindpaw incision in rats nor did it have the duration of enhanced heat responses observed in the rat model.

Clinical studies support a role for deep tissue injury as a key driver of pain after surgery and suggest a limited role for incised skin in clinical postoperative pain. In a clinical study comparing a mini-incision total hip arthroplasty with a standard-incision approach, two groups of patients were randomized to varying length of skin incision [22]. In the standard 16-cm length incision group, the subcutaneous tissues and fascia lata were divided. In the minimal skin incision group, skin incision was equal or less than 10 cm and only the proximal 1 cm of the fascia lata was incised. The remainder of the surgical approach in the deep tissue was the same between the two groups. Therefore, the only difference in surgical technique was the length of the skin incision, and the remainder of the surgical approach to the deep tissue was the same between the two groups. There was no difference in pain or opioid use between the two groups. In another similar study, two different surgical approaches for total hip arthroplasty were studied [8]. Both approaches used the same length of skin incision. The minimally invasive approach preserved the underlying muscles; however, muscles were incised and divided in the standard approach. The minimally invasive approach to the deep tissue resulted in less postoperative pain and opioid use than the conventional approach. Both studies indicate that deep tissue is a key driver of clinical postoperative pain, whereas the contribution of incised skin to postoperative pain after major surgeries is small.

Translational Aspects

In humans, nerve blockade with local anesthetics for particular surgeries produces profound postoperative analgesia, nearly eliminating postoperative pain. In two carefully performed studies [10,11], patients undergoing upper extremity surgery were randomized to receive nerve block or no nerve block. Pain scores and opioid utilization were recorded over the next 72 hours. Those patients that received the nerve blockade had little or no pain immediately after surgery; the patients that did not receive a nerve block required opioids and had clinically meaningful pain in the recovery room. However, on postoperative days 1 and 2, opioid use and pain scores were similar between the two groups. These data demonstrate that nearly eliminating pain with nerve blockade using local anesthetics produces early postoperative analgesia, but limited later effects, 24 to 48 hours afterward. Thus, in patients, peripheral primary afferent activation is predominant in the early postoperative period.

In the plantar incision model, local anesthetic infiltration and nerve block are effective immediately after plantar incision, eliminating guarding pain [24]. However, the next day guarding pain was not different between the group administered local anesthetic nerve blockade and the group administered saline. Further studies recording dorsal horn neuron activity in rats 1 day after plantar incision were undertaken [35]. Infiltration and nerve blockade with local anesthetics on postoperative day 1 decreased the magnitude of spontaneous activity and the percentage of neurons that had spontaneous activity back to that of the sham, unoperated group.

These results indicate that, early after plantar incision, peripheral sensitization is the primary driver of unprovoked pain behavior and dorsal horn neuron activity, and there is limited benefit to infiltration and nerve block beyond the expected duration of action of the local anesthetic. In patients, once the local anesthetic nerve block resolves, pain and opioid use are similar to the group that did not receive the nerve block. Together, these data point to peripheral nociceptor sensitization and incision-induced peripheral nociceptive mediators dominating the postoperative pain signal in the first few days.

One nociceptive signal that we have studied extensively is an ischemic-like signal (Figure 1-5) present immediately and continuing for several days after incision [14–16,19,28,31]. Concomitant hypoxemia [16], acidosis [31], and high lactate [19] are present in incisions of both skin and muscle. This ischemic-like signal resolves over 7 to 10 days after incision. Because data indicating nociceptive pathway activation by deep muscle incision is evident, we focused our studies on nociceptors from injured muscle. Enhanced responses of nociceptors to lactic acid in incised muscle tissue are present (Figure 1-6). In addition, we propose that hydrogen peroxide, which is increased in wounds [7,25] and increased after plantar incision [27], contributes to the early injury nociceptive signal in deep tissue (Figure 1-7). Chemosensitivity of nociceptors in deep tissue such as muscle is an understudied acute pain mechanism.

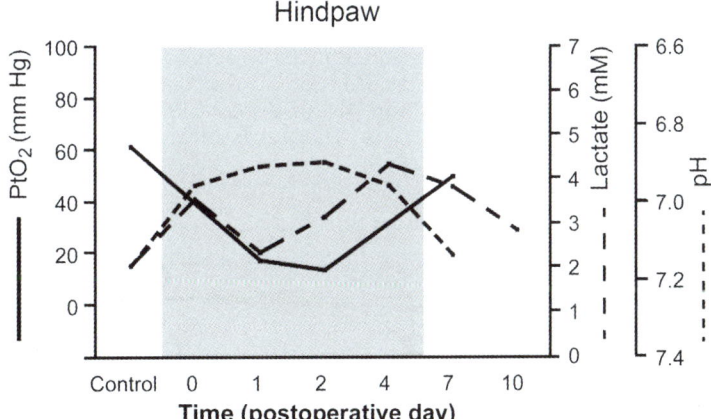

FIGURE 1-5 Schematic of time course changes in tissue pH, lactate concentration, and tissue oxygen tension (PtO_2) after plantar incision. A decrease in tissue oxygen tension occurs concurrently with a decrease in pH and an increase in lactate after incision. By postoperative day 10, tissue oxygen tension, lactate, and pH have returned to that of the control. The area shaded in gray represents the time after incision when pain-related behaviors are observed. Control is the value for the contralateral unincised site. (From Wound Repair Regen 21(5):730–9 http://onlinelibrary.wiley.com/doi/10.1111/wrr.12081/abstract;jsessionid=E38FDEC10F21D10A9107F91CA421BBB0.f03t01. John Wiley & Sons, Inc. Copyright 2013.)

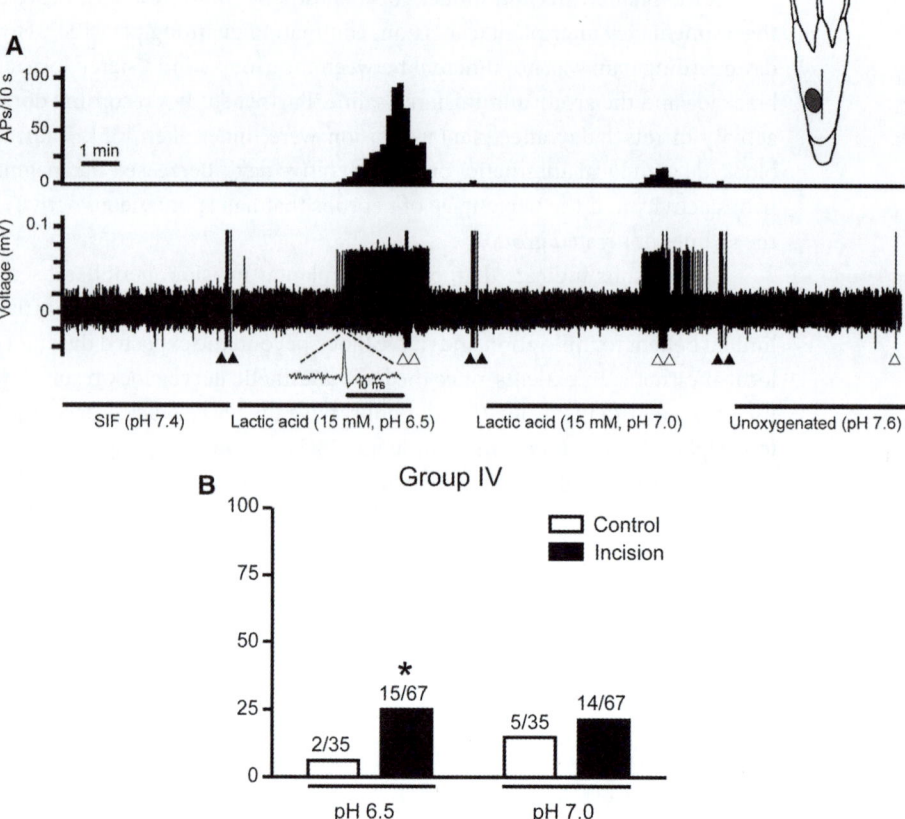

FIGURE 1-6 A: An example recording of the response of a mechanosensitive, group IV muscle afferent fiber from an incised muscle to 15 mM lactic acid with varying pH (pH 6.5 to 7.0) and unoxygenated synthetic interstitial fluid (SIF; pH 7.6). The upper panel shows a spike-density histogram (bin width = 10 s), and the lower panel shows the digitized oscilloscope tracing. Filled arrowheads mark artifacts generated by the addition of the acid solution; the open arrowheads mark artifacts created during removal of the solution. The receptive field is depicted in the inset. **B:** Percentage of group IV afferents activated by lactic acid at each pH level. More group IV afferents in the incision group responded to pH 6.5 than the control group (*$P = 0.022$, chi-square test). APs, action potentials. (From Anesthesiology: 119(5):1186–97. http://anesthesiology.pubs.asahq.org/article.aspx?articleid=1918103. Lippincott Williams and Wilkins/Wolter Kluwer Health. Copyright 2013.)

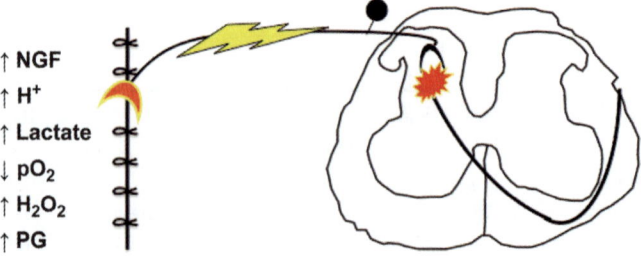

FIGURE 1-7 Schematic of peripheral and central sensitization early after incision. Nerve growth factor (NGF), hydrogen ion (H^+), lactate, and hydrogen peroxide (H_2O_2) are increased. Decreased oxygen tension (pO_2) and increased prostaglandins (PG) also contribute to incisional pain. Nociceptor activation and sensitization is evident and drives dorsal horn neurons that are also activated.

Other mediators appear to contribute to this incision-induced nociception in deep muscle tissue [2,32]. Reduced guarding pain by anti–nerve growth factor indicates that in the plantar incision model, nerve growth factor is an early mediator of the early postoperative pain signal. Nonsteroidal anti-inflammatory drugs reduce guarding [26] and CPP [21,33] after plantar incision, and these drugs also decrease opioid requirements in patients after surgery, suggesting that prostaglandins contribute to the nociceptive signal after deep tissue injury.

SUMMARY

In patients, surgery produces pain at rest. A correlate to pain at rest in animal models is unprovoked nociceptive behaviors and CPP in the plantar incision model for postoperative pain. Deep muscle injury is required to produce ongoing, spontaneous activity in primary afferent nociceptors and dorsal horn nociceptive neurons. Primary afferent nociceptor activation is predominant early after plantar incision and is required for dorsal horn neuron activation.

This model provides a physiologic basis for nearly eliminating postoperative pain with local anesthetic nerve blockade early after surgery, but postoperative pain largely recurs after the local anesthetic effect abates. Likely, nociceptive mediators, which contribute to multiple physiologic processes including wound healing, are involved in the generation of postoperative pain.

Acknowledgments

Source of Funding: The authors are grateful for the support by the Department of Anesthesia at the University of Iowa and by the National Institutes of Health, Bethesda, Maryland, grant GM067762 to T.J.B.

REFERENCES

1. Aubrun F, Langeron O, Quesnel C, Coriat P, Riou B. Relationships between measurement of pain using visual analog score and morphine requirements during postoperative intravenous morphine titration. Anesthesiology 2003;98:1415–21.
2. Banik RK, Subieta AR, Wu C, Brennan TJ. Increased nerve growth factor after rat plantar incision contributes to guarding behavior and heat hyperalgesia. Pain 2005;117:68–76.
3. Bessou P, Perl ER. Response of cutaneous sensory units with unmyelinated fibers to noxious stimuli. J Neurophysiol 1969;32:1025–43.
4. Brennan TJ, Vandermeulen EP, Gebhart GF. Characterization of a rat model of incisional pain. Pain 1996;64:493–501.
5. Burgess PR, Perl ER. Myelinated afferent fibres responding specifically to noxious stimulation of the skin. J Physiol 1967;190:541–62.
6. Campbell JN, Khan AA, Meyer RA, Raja SN. Responses to heat of C-fiber nociceptors in monkey are altered by injury in the receptive field but not by adjacent injury. Pain 1988;32:327–32.
7. Cho M, Hunt TK, Hussain MZ. Hydrogen peroxide stimulates macrophage vascular endothelial growth factor release. Am J Physiol Heart Circ Physiol 2001;280:H2357–63.
8. Dorr LD, Maheshwari AV, Long WT, Wan Z, Sirianni LE. Early pain relief and function after posterior minimally invasive and conventional total hip arthroplasty. A prospective, randomized, blinded study. J Bone Joint Surg Am 2007;89:1153–60.
9. Fimer I, Klein T, Magerl W, Treede RD, Zahn PK, Pogatzki-Zahn EM. Modality-specific somatosensory changes in a human surrogate model of postoperative pain. Anesthesiology 2011;115:387–97.

10. Hadzic A, Arliss J, Kerimoglu B, Karaca PE, Yufa M, Claudio RE, Vloka JD, Rosenquist R, Santos AC, Thys DM. A comparison of infraclavicular nerve block versus general anesthesia for hand and wrist day-case surgeries. Anesthesiology 2004;101:127–32.
11. Hadzic A, Williams BA, Karaca PE, Hobeika P, Unis G, Dermksian J, Yufa M, Thys DM, Santos AC. For outpatient rotator cuff surgery, nerve block anesthesia provides superior same-day recovery over general anesthesia. Anesthesiology 2005;102:1001–7.
12. Hamalainen MM, Gebhart GF, Brennan TJ. Acute effect of an incision on mechanosensitive afferents in the plantar rat hindpaw. J Neurophysiol 2002;87:712–20.
13. Hamalainen MM, Subieta A, Arpey C, Brennan TJ. Differential effect of capsaicin treatment on pain-related behaviors after plantar incision. J Pain 2009;10:637–45.
14. Hunt TK, Conolly WB, Aronson SB, Goldstein P. Anaerobic metabolism and wound healing: an hypothesis for the initiation and cessation of collagen synthesis in wounds. Am J Surg 1978;135:328–32.
15. Immke DC, McCleskey EW. Lactate enhances the acid-sensing Na+ channel on ischemia-sensing neurons. Nat Neurosci 2001;4:869–70.
16. Kang S, Lee D, Theusch BE, Arpey CJ, Brennan TJ. Wound hypoxia in deep tissue after incision in rats. Wound Repair Regen 2013;21:730–9.
17. Kang S, Wu C, Banik RK, Brennan TJ. Effect of capsaicin treatment on nociceptors in rat glabrous skin one day after plantar incision. Pain 2010;148:128–40.
18. Kawamata M, Watanabe H, Nishikawa K, Takahashi T, Kozuka Y, Kawamata T, Omote K, Namiki A. Different mechanisms of development and maintenance of experimental incision-induced hyperalgesia in human skin. Anesthesiology 2002;97:550–9.
19. Kim TJ, Freml L, Park SS, Brennan TJ. Lactate concentrations in incisions indicate ischemic-like conditions may contribute to postoperative pain. J Pain 2007;8:59–66.
20. Moiniche S, Dahl JB, Erichsen CJ, Jensen LM, Kehlet H. Time course of subjective pain ratings, and wound and leg tenderness after hysterectomy. Acta Anaesthesiol Scand 1997;41:785–9.
21. Navratilova E, Xie JY, Okun A, Qu C, Eyde N, Ci S, Ossipov MH, King T, Fields HL, Porreca F. Pain relief produces negative reinforcement through activation of mesolimbic reward-valuation circuitry. Proc Natl Acad Sci USA 2012;109:20709–13.
22. Ogonda L, Wilson R, Archbold P, Lawlor M, Humphreys P, O'Brien S, Beverland D. A minimal-incision technique in total hip arthroplasty does not improve early postoperative outcomes. A prospective, randomized, controlled trial. J Bone Joint Surg Am 2005;87:701–10.
23. Pogatzki EM, Niemeier JS, Brennan TJ. Persistent secondary hyperalgesia after gastrocnemius incision in the rat. Eur J Pain 2002;6:295–305.
24. Pogatzki EM, Vandermeulen EP, Brennan TJ. Effect of plantar local anesthetic injection on dorsal horn neuron activity and pain behaviors caused by incision. Pain 2002;97:151–61.
25. Roy S, Khanna S, Nallu K, Hunt TK, Sen CK. Dermal wound healing is subject to redox control. Mol Ther 2006;13:211–20.
26. Spofford CM, Ashmawi H, Subieta A, Buevich F, Moses A, Baker M, Brennan TJ. Ketoprofen produces modality-specific inhibition of pain behaviors in rats after plantar incision. Anesth Analg 2009;109:1992–9.
27. Sugiyama D, Kang S, Brennan TJ. Muscle reactive oxygen species (ROS) contribute to post-incisional guarding via the TRPA1 receptor. PLoS One 2017;12:e0170410.
28. Trabold O, Wagner S, Wicke C, Scheuenstuhl H, Hussain MZ, Rosen N, Seremetiev A, Becker HD, Hunt TK. Lactate and oxygen constitute a fundamental regulatory mechanism in wound healing. Wound Repair Regen 2003;11:504–9.
29. Vandermeulen EP, Brennan TJ. Alterations in ascending dorsal horn neurons by a surgical incision in the rat foot. Anesthesiology 2000;93:1294–302 [discussion 1296A].
30. Whiteside GT, Harrison J, Boulet J, Mark L, Pearson M, Gottshall S, Walker K. Pharmacological characterisation of a rat model of incisional pain. Br J Pharmacol 2004;141:85–91.
31. Woo YC, Park SS, Subieta AR, Brennan TJ. Changes in tissue pH and temperature after incision indicate acidosis may contribute to postoperative pain. Anesthesiology 2004;101:468–75.
32. Wu C, Erickson MA, Xu J, Wild KD, Brennan TJ. Expression profile of nerve growth factor after muscle incision in the rat. Anesthesiology 2009;110:140–9.
33. Xie JY, Qu C, Patwardhan A, Ossipov MH, Navratilova E, Becerra L, Borsook D, Porreca F. Activation of mesocorticolimbic reward circuits for assessment of relief of ongoing pain: a potential biomarker of efficacy. Pain 2014;155:1659–66.

34. Xu J, Brennan TJ. Comparison of skin incision vs. skin plus deep tissue incision on ongoing pain and spontaneous activity in dorsal horn neurons. Pain 2009;144:329–39.
35. Xu J, Richebe P, Brennan TJ. Separate groups of dorsal horn neurons transmit spontaneous activity and mechanosensitivity one day after plantar incision. Eur J Pain 2009;13:820–8.
36. Xu J, Brennan TJ. Guarding pain and spontaneous activity of nociceptors after skin versus skin plus deep tissue incision. Anesthesiology 2010;112:153–64.
37. Zahn PK, Gysbers D, Brennan TJ. Effect of systemic and intrathecal morphine in a rat model of postoperative pain. Anesthesiology 1997;86:1066–77.
38. Zahn PK, Brennan TJ. Primary and secondary hyperalgesia in a rat model for human postoperative pain. Anesthesiology 1999;90:863–72.
39. Zahn PK, Pogatzki EM, Brennan TJ. Mechanisms for pain caused by incisions. Reg Anesth Pain Med 2002;27:514–6.
40. Zahn PK, Pogatzki-Zahn EM, Brennan TJ. Spinal administration of MK-801 and NBQX demonstrates NMDA-independent dorsal horn sensitization in incisional pain. Pain 2005;114:499–510.

CHAPTER 2

The Nociceptive Capacity of Muscle, Skeletal, and Connective Tissue

Thomas Graven-Nielsen and Lars Arendt-Nielsen

Surgery most often involves deep somatic pain, which is known to play an important role for the manifestations of postoperative sensitization in animals [14]. Postoperative pain arising from deep structures being a particular entity has therefore recently received increased attention. In the daily pain clinic or at the GPs office, pain from joint, bone, muscle, and connective soft tissue is the most common clinical symptom causing patients to seek medical treatment and is a major cause of disability worldwide. Several conditions may cause musculoskeletal pain, such as osteoporosis, osteoarthritis (OA), rheumatoid arthritis, tendinopathies, low-back pain, bone fracture, bone metastases, and myofascial and muscle injury/overuse. Deep tissues have important capacities for initiating and maintaining sensitization in the periphery and central systems, which may be detrimental for the chronification of pain; e.g., deep somatic pain is known to cause more sensitization than cutaneous input [107]. Developing an understanding of the mechanisms driving persistent musculoskeletal pain and novel mechanism-based therapies to treat these unique pain states (including deep somatic postoperative pain) would address a major unmet clinical need and have significant clinical, economic, and societal benefits.

This chapter outlines the potency of muscle, joint, bone, and connective tissues to cause sensitization of mechanisms potentially responsible for spreading hypersensitivity. Likewise, the ability of musculoskeletal pain to evoke central integration (temporal summation) of pain and referred pain will be presented as examples of important central mechanisms, as these phenomena most likely contribute to postoperative pain. Although important for deep tissue nociception as well as postoperative pain, the descending pain control system will be covered in another chapter [80].

MUSCULOSKELETAL PAIN

Muscle

Excitation of polymodal muscle nociceptors related with group III and IV (Aδ and C) afferent nerve fibers by chemical or strong (noxious) mechanical stimulation is presumably associated with the perception of acute muscle pain [69]. The muscle nociceptors are free nerve endings located in connective tissue and around vascular structures. Animal studies have shown a robust excitation of group III and IV afferent muscle fibers by algesic substances such as hypertonic saline in contrast to the thick, fast afferent fibers [17]. Within group IV afferent fibers, hypertonic saline excites both low- and high-threshold mechanosensitive units, indicating the nonspecific excitation of hypertonic saline. The nonspecificity of hypertonic saline is well known for other animal models of muscle nociception; glutamate, capsaicin, acidic buffers, and bradykinin excite thin muscle afferent fibers with low and high mechanical thresholds (for references see Graven-Nielsen [37]). Receptor types such as the TRPV1, stretch-inactivated channel, P2X, TrkA, and ASIC have been identified and are, among many others, likely involved in the transduction process of chemically induced muscle pain.

Several methods exist for evoking standardized experimental muscle pain in humans. Endogenous methods use natural stimuli for the induction of pain (e.g., by ischemia or exercise), whereas exogenous techniques are methods using external interventions to induce pain, e.g., electrical stimulation of muscle afferents or injection of algesic substances. Pressure algometry is manually applied pressure stimulation used to induce pain from muscle structures and has been extensively applied and validated [57]; computer-controlled stimulation may reduce the variability, which also allows accurate construction of the stimulus–response function related to the somatosensory sensitivity [42]. A novel approach combining rotational movements or radial vibration with simultaneous pressure stimulation resulted in higher pain perception compared with plain pressure, suggesting that the multidirectional stimulations excited the nociceptors more robustly [1]. Pressure algometry stimulates a relatively small volume of tissue [31]. Instead, a larger volume can be assessed by computer-controlled cuff algometry technique [67], where the pain intensity related to inflation of a tourniquet applied around an extremity is used to establish stimulus–response curves between the pain perception and stimulus intensity [81]. Reliability of cuff algometry for pain sensitivity assessment has been demonstrated [43], and this technology has the advantage of being user-independent and causes a general activation of the deep structures [67]. Muscle pain can as well be induced by injection of a variety of algogenic substances, such as hypertonic saline, glutamate, capsaicin, and acidic saline [37]. This induces a more tonic pain stimulation and the option to assess local and referred pain patterns. Less used in clinical settings are ischemic exercise, powerful exercise, and nonmechanical external stimuli (e.g., thermal, electrical), which have been shown to induce muscle pain in humans [37].

Joint

The joint is innervated by afferent nerves including group II to IV fibers (Aβ-, Aδ-, and C-fibers) [86]. Corpuscular endings related to group II fibers are identified in ligaments and in the fibrous capsule, whereas all joint structures are innervated by free nerve endings (group III and IV) although not the cartilage. As articular cartilage and subchondral bone pathogenesis are key elements of OA, a variety of biochemical markers of tissue turnover have been developed targeting key proteins that are remodeled. The clinical presentation of OA is normally associated with joint pain, but at the individual patient level there is little or no correlation between the pain intensity and the degree of joint damage [29]. Intra-articular activation of joint nociceptors in humans can be carried out by pressure stimuli during an arthroscopic procedure [26], electrical needle stimulation [56], or focused ultrasound stimulation [109]. Intra-articular stimulation is, however, not a procedure that can be used in clinical trials because of the various risks such as inflammation and triggering of an autoimmune reaction. Therefore, attempts have been made to use external stimulation such as pressure pain thresholds for mapping joint pain sensitivity in volunteers and OA pain patients [8]. Electrical facet joint stimulation [76], intradiscal pressure

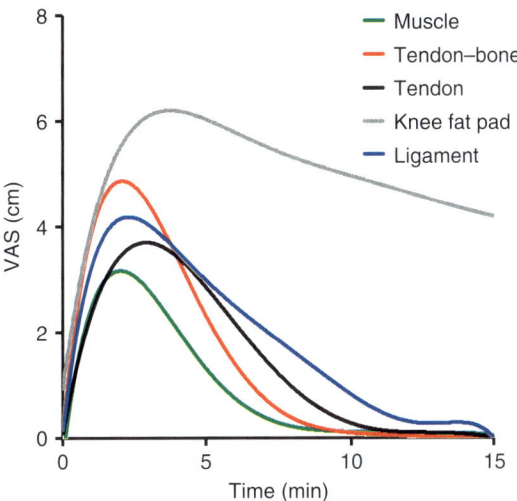

FIGURE 2-1 Typical visual analogue scale (VAS, 10 cm) scores of saline-induced pain in muscle, distal tendon, and proximal tendon–bone junction of the tibialis anterior muscle and in the joint (knee fat pad) and sacroiliac joint ligament. Hypertonic saline (5.8%, 0.5 to 1.0 mL) was injected in healthy subjects as bolus injections. (Based on data from Gibson W, Arendt-Nielsen L, Graven-Nielsen T. Referred pain and hyperalgesia in human tendon and muscle belly tissue. Pain 2006;120:113–23; Palsson TS, Graven-Nielsen T. Experimental pelvic pain facilitates pain provocation tests and causes regional hyperalgesia. Pain 2012;153:2233–40; and Joergensen TS, Henriksen M, Danneskiold-Samsoee B, Bliddal H, Graven-Nielsen T. Experimental knee pain evoke spreading hyperalgesia and facilitated temporal summation of pain. Pain Med 2013;14:874–83.)

provocation [87], external facet joint pressure stimulation [90], and periarticular injections of hypertonic saline (knee fat pad, Figure 2-1) have also been explored as potential models for inducing joint pain in humans.

Bone

Based on extensive studies from Mantyh and colleagues, basic mechanisms of bone pain have been discovered [68]. Mineralized bone, marrow, and periosteum receive significant innervations by thin afferent sensory fibers. The bone is innervated by calcitonin gene–related peptide (CGRP) and neurofilament 200 sensory receptors where many express TrkA receptors [68]. The periosteum is the most densely innervated tissue, while the bone marrow receives the greatest total number of sensory fibers followed by mineralized bone and then periosteum. However, it is not fully clarified which sensory neurons are excited in which skeletal pain conditions. Fracture pain has been suggested to initially involve the receptors located in the periosteum [13]. Cancer bone pain is probably promoted by nerve growth factor (NGF) produced by bone remodeling [68]. Tumor growth or bone fracture may result in nociceptive mechanical stimuli exciting the mechanosensitive receptors. Finally, the neuropathic pain component due to tumor-induced damage of sensory endings in bone adds to the complexity of potential mechanisms involved in bone cancer pain [68].

Mechanical stimulation of the periosteum in humans induces an immediate sharp arresting pain with the lowest threshold as compared with the ligaments, fascia, tendon, and muscle as the least sensitive [53]. Likewise, injecting hypertonic saline in the surface of the human periosteum elicits more pain than when injecting in muscle (Figure 2-1) [37]. Recently, a novel human experimental model of bone pain was developed based on standardized mechanical impact stimulation [30].

Connective Tissue

Connective soft tissues are supplied with nociceptive afferent fibers and are probably an important source of nociceptive afferent activity during clinical pain conditions. Slowly conducting afferent fibers (group III and IV) and nerve endings, presumably nociceptive, have been observed in animal connective tissue, such as tendon and fascia [6,103]. CGRP and substance P (SP) immunoreactivities have also been demonstrated in human tendon tissue [12], indicating a thin fiber sensory innervation most likely serving a nociceptive function. The nerve endings in tendon are mainly located in proximity to small arterioles and blood vessels in the tissue [12]. Histologically, small-fiber free nerve endings have been demonstrated in human fascial tissue [110]. A quantitative evaluation of CGRP- and SP-containing free nerve endings was performed in the thoracolumbar fascia illustrating that the fascia, especially the outer part, is densely innervated; in a pilot study, the human thoracolumbar fascia was further demonstrated to show similar properties [103] and may therefore be important in low-back pain conditions. Recently, single fiber recordings from thin myelinated and unmyelinated afferent fibers located in the fascia demonstrated nociceptive characteristics to mechanical, heat, and chemical modalities [102].

Human studies have used experimental pain induction techniques directed toward the fascia, ligaments, and tendon tissues [35,53,60]. Interestingly, the experimental tendon and ligament pain models based on injection of hypertonic saline report higher pain intensity and longer pain duration compared with muscle pain models [34,53]. There is also a marked difference in the pain response following hypertonic saline injected into the deep part of the muscle and the fascia where fascial injection induced more pain compared with muscle belly injections [36]. This is clinically relevant, as it implies that the contribution of connective tissues to the clinically prevalent entity "muscle pain" needs to be carefully considered. Recently, a study compared the pain sensitivity with injections of hypertonic saline into connective tissue around the hip and reported that the gluteus medius tendon injection caused higher pain intensities than injections into the adductor longus tendon and gluteus medius muscle [54]. Similarly, Gibson et al. [34] reported higher pain intensity following hypertonic saline injected into the tendon–bone junction of the tibialis anterior muscle compared with its tendon and muscle belly site (Figure 2-1). Injecting into the tendon–bone junction probably stimulates the periosteal tissue, which is known to be more sensitive than the muscle belly [53], thus contributing to the higher pain intensity at this site. Slater et al. [94] demonstrated a higher pain intensity following hypertonic saline injection into tendoachilles compared with the common extensor tendon. The different tendon pain profiles are likely explained by variation in nociceptor density and innervation patterns of individual tendons.

LOCALIZED HYPERSENSITIVITY

Localized Muscle Hypersensitivity

Sensitization of muscle nociceptors is normally evoked by overuse, trauma, or inflammation, causing release of substances from neural and muscular tissues. Damaged deep tissue releases, e.g., potassium ions, prostaglandin E2, bradykinin, and serotonin (5-HT), and the nerve ending releases, e.g., neuropeptides such as SP, CGRP, or somatostatin [71]. Most of the sensitizing substances released in muscles are similar to those released in other tissues, but adenosine triphosphate (ATP) is present in muscle cells in high concentration and may be more specific for muscles. During muscle inflammation, the density of nerve endings containing SP and NGF increases [83]. Moreover, the acid-sensing ion channel 3 (ASIC3) has been shown to be important for the mechanical hyperalgesia in an animal inflammatory muscle pain model [97].

Short-lasting muscle hyperalgesia in humans can be studied after intramuscular (IM) injections of capsaicin, glutamate, or combined IM injections of 5-HT and bradykinin. Ernberg et al. [27] found that IM coinjection of 5-HT and the 5-HT(3) receptor antagonist granisetron reduced the spontaneous pain evoked by injection of 5-HT and prevented hypersensitivity to mechanical pressure stimuli. Later it was demonstrated that IM injection of granisetron in patients with localized myalgia increased the pressure pain thresholds [20]. It is also known that the N-methyl-D-aspartate (NMDA) receptor is involved in glutamate-evoked muscle hypersensitivity because this can be reduced by coadministration of an NMDA antagonist [16].

Tonic muscle hyperalgesia may be induced if a muscle is eccentrically exercised; it will become sore after 1 to 2 days. This model of delayed onset muscle soreness (DOMS) shows hypersensitivity to pressure at different sites among subjects, and these localized spots of hyperalgesia might link to the initial mechanisms for hypersensitive trigger points in myofascial pain patients. The mechanism underlying DOMS is not clear but is probably related to ultrastructural overloading resulting in release of sensitizing substances such as bradykinin and NGF [72]. The hypersensitive component in DOMS has also been suggested to be mediated by the thick myelinated afferent fibers and not exclusively by the thin unmyelinated nociceptive afferent fibers [11].

A clinical example of muscle hyperalgesia is muscle sites located in taut bands of muscle fibers with a hard and hypersensitive locus, trigger points in myofascial pain patients [91]. A novel methodology has been proposed to visualize the taut band related to trigger points in muscles [19]. Trigger point assessment may involve pressure algometry to record pain thresholds [18,106], which is a more standardized approach than the manual palpation. Nonetheless, the overlap of sites with reduced pressure pain thresholds and sites palpated with tender points in healthy subjects is poor [5].

Localized Joint Hypersensitivity

In line with muscle nociceptors, the joint nociceptors have been demonstrated to be sensitized in inflammatory and degenerative animal joint models [86]. One particular example is the silent nociceptors, which do not respond to noxious mechanical stimuli under normal condition but are active in inflammatory conditions. Sluka demonstrated that muscle and joint tissues in rats show different sensory responses to experimental nociception with prolonged allodynia in joint compared with muscle tissue [95]. It would appear reasonable to presume that human muscle and other deep tissue (e.g., tendon) have a similar difference in sensory manifestations to experimental pain stimulation. The animal joint sensitization models cannot be translated into human models, but there are human studies focusing on pain sensitization related to perijoint structures. An example is experimentally induced pain in the fat pad of the knee by injections of hypertonic saline in asymptomatic subjects. In this model, hyperalgesia to pressure is found close to the injection site [59].

Recently there has been focus on the peripatellar hypersensitivity detected in OA patients compared with healthy control subjects [8,44]. Peripheral sensitization of the nociceptors is likely by, e.g., inflamed synovium and damaged subchondral bone. Proinflammatory cytokines (e.g., tumor necrosis factor α [TNF-α] and interleukin 1β [IL-1β]) influence the nociceptive system directly as well as by having a major role in the pathogenesis of joint diseases [86]. In an explorative study including OA patients, associations between pressure pain sensitivity and TNF-α, as well as IL-6 and IL-10, were found, which was correlated with the OA pain intensity and scores for rigidity [52]. Inhibiting IL-6 is a promising drug target for management of particular rheumatoid arthritis [15]. As a sensitive marker of low-grade systemic inflammation, high-sensitive C-reactive protein has been shown to correlate with pain severity in OA patients [101] although the specificity of this protein is low. Moreover, the most sensitive site around the OA knee was located on the medial side in the patients with the highest habitual pain intensity [8] in accord with the medial compartment structures being predominately involved in the osteoarthritic process [22]. The peripatellar hyperalgesia to pressure was mainly expressed in patients with severe knee pain, indicating a relationship between the tenderness in the encapsulated tissue and the intra-articular lesion in patients with knee OA [8]. Identifying different sensitization patterns in OA may pave the way for developing individualized pain management procedures in the future.

Localized Bone Hypersensitivity

In cancer bone pain, tumor cells and associated inflammatory cells include several inflammatory mediators that may sensitize the bone nociceptors [68]. In particular, NGF has been suggested as a major player in developing microneuromas and thereby sensitization in the vicinity of tumor cells. Therefore, in more recent years, there has been focus on the role of NGF for nerve sprouting and formation of microneuromas in animal bone cancer models, and hence, anti-NGF compounds may be an interesting target [66,68]. In addition to the sensitization process, tumor-induced injury to primary afferent nerve fibers may cause a neuropathic pain component [68]. It is expected that the nociceptors are sensitized by inflammatory mediators after bone damage such as fractures [13]. Following intramedullary nailing of tibial fractures, localized pressure hypersensitivity was detected compared with the contralateral leg and progressively normalized in the period from 6 weeks to 12 months [64]. A similar process although less intensive is probably also reflected in a human experimental model where impact stimuli were repeatedly applied to the tibia bone and after 1 day, hyperalgesia to pressure and impact stimulations were detected [30].

Localized Hypersensitivity in Connective Tissue

Tendon tissue has been shown to express sensory afferent NMDA receptors [2], and increased tissue glutamate level is associated with tendinopathy [3], implying glutamate may be important in tendon sensitization and pain. Gibson et al. [35] characterized the pain responses from asymptomatic tendons and found that glutamate and capsaicin injections to the tendon caused pain and hyperalgesia. Moreover, experimental tendon and ligament pain models based on hypertonic saline injections also include localized hyperalgesia [34,79,94].

The DOMS developing after eccentric contractions has been suggested to include sensitization of nociceptors in various tissues including epimysium/fascia rather than muscle tissue proper. Indeed, increased sensitivity of mechanoreceptors was found in animal fascial/epimysium tissue 2 days after eccentric contractions in rats [36]. In humans, hypertonic saline injected into fascia during DOMS resulted in higher pain intensities compared with pre-exercise, suggesting the relevance of sensitized fascia in DOMS [36].

This is in line with increased sensitivity to electrical stimulation in fascial tissue shown in humans following eccentric exercise [65]. Connective tissue may be exposed to excessive stress causing sensitization during eccentric contraction when the myofibrillar contractile mechanism becomes inefficient. Another interesting demonstration of localized sensitization in fascial tissue is seen after injection of NGF into the fascia of erector spinae muscle [23], which seems to be more sensitive than the same procedure applied for the tibialis anterior muscle [108].

SPREADING HYPERSENSITIVITY

As outlined below, musculoskeletal nociceptors are potential generators for central hyperexcitability. However, the dorsal horn neurons are also strongly controlled by the descending inhibitory pathways, and potential impairments of the descending control will give reason to similar manifestations as central hyperexcitability, e.g., reduced excitation threshold of spinal cord neurons to musculoskeletal nociceptive input, increased receptive fields, and increased ongoing discharges of neurons.

Muscle as the Source for Spreading Hypersensitivity

Animal experiments suggest that expansion of receptive fields may account for spreading hypersensitivity and is working through opening of "silent" (ineffective) synapses in the spinal cord by nociceptive input from muscle [46]. The contralateral spread of sensitization following repeated IM injections of low-pH saline [96] is another demonstration of the central hyperexcitability. Data suggest that different substances used for exciting muscle nociceptors have different influences on the dorsal horn neurons. In contrast to hypertonic saline, which gives a clear excitation of dorsal horn neurons, one injection of NGF mainly results in subthreshold potentials in the dorsal horn neurons but still leaves the central neurons sensitized [51]. Moreover, two IM NGF injections separated by 5 days resulted in dorsal horn neurons having more receptive fields in muscle and fascia [48], which also illustrates the central hyperexcitability.

Long-lasting muscle hypersensitivity can be induced in healthy subjects by IM injection of NGF. Interestingly, IM NGF injection in humans causes no pain, but a localized hypersensitivity develops after a few hours, and after 1 day the hypersensitivity has spread to a large portion of the muscle presumably because of central mechanisms [4]. Daily IM injections of NGF result in progressive increasing muscle soreness [45]. Therefore, the NGF model is an interesting model for muscle sensitization and spreading hypersensitivity in muscle tissue. If the original NGF injection site is anesthetized after one day, when the spreading hypersensitivity is present, there is no immediate effect on the spreading hypersensitivity [33]. This suggests that the spreading hypersensitivity is based on a robust central mechanism independent of the peripheral drive at least in the short time frame. In line, capsaicin-induced sensitization of the skin dermatome (C5, arm) evoked reduced pressure pain threshold (hyperalgesia) in the infraspinatus (C5-C6) muscle [99], illustrating the segmental interaction, which may be crucial for understanding comorbid symptoms.

Fibromyalgia or whiplash-associated pain is often categorized as widespread pain or hyperalgesic conditions. The more widespread a musculoskeletal pain problem becomes, the more quantitative sensory abnormalities occur [18], which may be another finding indicating central hyperexcitability. A detailed trigger point examination in fibromyalgia patients showed an increased number of trigger points in patients compared with controls [32], suggesting that more trigger points may be a result of facilitated central mechanisms.

Joint as the Source for Spreading Hypersensitivity

Intense and prolonged nociceptive input from the joint in animals may result in central hyperexcitability manifested as, e.g., expanded receptive fields [84]. Ongoing nociceptive activity from the joint capsule (stretching), the synovium (inflammation), and corroded subchondral bone [24] could be the peripheral generators leading to facilitated central pain mechanisms.

In the early stage of OA pain, this is recognized as a localized pain condition, but the persistent pain or hypersensitivity may result in a progression to more regional or even widespread symptoms. Hyperalgesia to pressure stimulation outside the symptomatic joint has been reported in patients with OA in either the carpometacarpal joints [28], knee [8], or hip [55,62]. Widespread hyperalgesia was also demonstrated in knee OA patients with increased pain thresholds after treatment by total knee replacement [44]. Generally, in postoperative joint pain conditions the widespread hyperalgesia is a key finding [80]. Spreading hypersensitivity to the contralateral knee has also been observed [8] and is most likely due to the fact that some knee OA patients have bilateral symptoms, and in addition, contralateral subclinical changes may exist in the patients only presenting with one symptomatic knee. In chronic diseases such as knee OA, it is also possible that the central neuronal systems are sensitized bilaterally. In such scenarios the clinical pain manifestations start to spread together with sensitization of central mechanisms; e.g., a joint pain patient begins complaining about pain in other regions, and the pain potentially develops into a widespread pain, and comorbid pain conditions may develop. In low-back pain (herniated disc) patients a similar widespread hyperalgesia to pressure has been detected with reduced pressure pain threshold in the shin muscle [77]. The spreading hyperalgesia seems to depend on tonic pain for some time, as 10 minutes of electrical stimulation on the lumbar facet joint (L3-L4) did not evoke hyperalgesia outside the stimulation area [76]. The use of cuff algometry in patients with arthritis has demonstrated the feasibility of using cuff algometry on the lower leg to measure hyperalgesia in knee OA patients [44]. Similar spreading hypersensitivity to those observed using a conventional pressure algometry on the tibialis anterior muscle was found with cuff pressure pain thresholds being significantly lower in OA patients than those in controls.

A higher frequency of latent myofascial trigger points was detected in the lower leg of OA patients compared with healthy controls [9], and such a comorbid condition might be explained by a generalized reduced threshold for eliciting a painful perception due to central hyperexcitability. The habitual OA pain areas do not consistently include the latent myofascial trigger points. Because the etiology of myofascial trigger points is not clear, peripheral factors contributing to the frequent development of trigger points cannot be excluded although it seems unlikely.

Bone as the Source for Spreading Hypersensitivity

Widespread hypersensitivity in nonmalignant bone pain such as fractures or malignant bone pain has not been extensively described. In an animal model with tumor induced in the femur bone, it was demonstrated that nonnoxious palpation of the tumor induced a nocifensive behavioral response that was not found in control animals and was correlated with the extent of bone destruction [89]. Similar responses were found after palpation of the knee, which may illustrate the spreading hypersensitivity. In animal bone tumor models, it has been demonstrated that wide dynamic range dorsal horn neurons become hyperexcitable and the receptive field enlarges [105]. So it is likely that spreading hypersensitivity may occur due to the peripheral sensitization such as tumor growth and/or in combination with central hyperexcitability. Some bone cancer patients present with widespread bone metastases and little pain, whereas others have minimal bone metastases and severe pain [78], indicating that the central mechanisms may be important.

Connective Tissue as the Source for Spreading Hypersensitivity

Excitation of nociceptors from ligaments and the fascia has demonstrated to drive hyperexcitability of dorsal horn neurons where more neurons are involved during hyperexcitability compared with control conditions [50,82]. Experimental pain induced in the human sacroiliac join ligament by hypertonic saline injections resulted in hyperalgesia distant from the injection site [79]. Likewise, capsaicin injection caused significant increases in mechanosensitivity at the tendon injection site and 2 cm proximally [35]. Clinical tendinopathy is associated with increased mechanical sensitivity in the affected tendons [63], but no studies have reported widespread hypersensitivity. If experimental muscle pain is evoked in the symptomatic arm of lateral epicondylalgia patients, the pressure thresholds decreased in the contralateral asymptomatic arm, indicating a facilitated central mechanism [93]. Using cuff algometry in lateral epicondylalgia patients compared with controls, hyperalgesia on the arm and lower leg was detected, demonstrating spreading hypersensitivity [58].

TEMPORAL SUMMATION OF PAIN

Repeated somatosensory stimuli with the same intensity evoke a pain perception that is progressively increasing. This phenomenon is defined as temporal summation of pain and probably parallels the initial phase of the neuronal windup process reported in animals. Short duration intervals between sequential stimuli at constant strength (e.g., 10 stimuli and 1 s interstimulus interval) are needed to evoke temporal summation of pain.

Temporal Summation of Muscle Pain

In clinical and experimental studies, electrical, chemical, pressure, and focused ultrasound repeated stimulation has been used to assess the temporal summation of muscle pain [40,98,109]. Computer-controlled sequential pressure stimulation on muscle evoked temporal summation that was more efficient compared with sequential stimulation on the skin only (Figure 2-2) [73]. The temporal summation of muscle pain is facilitated in musculoskeletal pain patients, and the involvement of central hyperexcitability has been proposed as an explanation for the findings [8,98,100]. Cuff algometry has also been used to assess temporal summation of cuff-induced pain from the calf muscles in knee OA patients with and without clinical pain after revision total knee replacement; the temporal summation of cuff pain was significantly facilitated in the group of patients with pain [92]. Facilitated temporal summation of continuous cuff-evoked pain has also been reported in lateral epicondylalgia [58].

In healthy subjects, experimental muscle soreness has been reported to facilitate the temporal summation of pressure-induced muscle pain [74], indicating that the time window with the nociceptive activity needed to cause the central hyperexcitability is relatively short. Facilitated temporal summation of the nociceptive withdrawal reflex elicited by repeated cutaneous electrical stimulation has also been used as an indicator for central hyperexcitability in fibromyalgia patients and whiplash pain patients [10]. In some patients, a minor nociceptive activity is plausible without confirmed tissue damage, and facilitated temporal summation is likely to explain the perceived pain in such cases. Moreover, facilitated preoperative temporal pain summation is an important factor associated with chronic postoperative pain as discussed in detail elsewhere in this book [80].

Temporal Summation of Joint Pain

In an experimental study, Joergensen et al. [59] demonstrated that temporal summation elicited by sequential pressure stimuli at the fat pad of the knee and knee-related muscles was facilitated during experimental fat pad pain. Temporal summation assessed by pressure stimulation on the knee was significantly facilitated in knee OA patients compared with controls [8]. Interestingly, patients with high-intensity habitual knee pain showed more temporal summation of muscle pain than OA patients less affected. The duration of OA pain was correlated with the degree of temporal summation of pain [8], suggesting that the involved plasticity is a progressive process. Interestingly, a serologic biomarker related with cartilage structure in knee OA patients was correlated with the degree of temporal pain summation [7]. An intriguing finding was facilitated temporal summation assessed contralaterally to the most affected knee [8] that may be due to the fact, however, that most knee OA patients have OA symptoms in the contralateral knee although less affected. An alternative or additional explanatory component is that the same neurons sensitized by the most affected knee contribute to enhanced temporal summation on the contralateral side because some neurons have bilateral receptive fields [85].

Temporal Summation of Bone Pain

A progressive pain response was found during 10 repeated pressure stimuli on the tibia (Figure 2-2), which was higher than the response from similar stimulation only on the

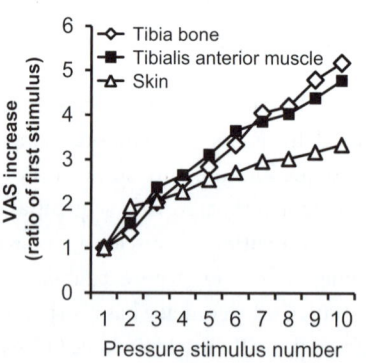
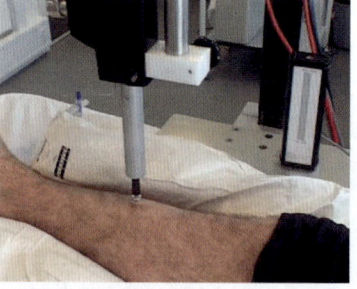

FIGURE 2-2 Temporal summation following repeated pressure stimuli to the muscle, tibia bone, and skin (web space). Ten pressure stimuli were delivered with 2-s intervals by the computer-controlled pressure algometer (right). The subject scored the pain intensity on a visual analogue scale (VAS), and the ratio of increase with respect to the first stimulus is illustrated. (Modified from data in Nie H, Arendt-Nielsen L, Andersen H, Graven-Nielsen T. Temporal summation of pain evoked by mechanical stimulation in deep and superficial tissue. J Pain 2005;6:348–55.)

skin [73], strongly suggesting the capacity of bone to elicit temporal summation of pain. Recently, similar observations have been established with mechanical impact stimulations [30].

Temporal Summation of Connective Tissue Pain

So far temporal summation of pain from the tendon, ligaments, and fascia has not been distinctly studied in humans. However, it is likely to exist in line with temporal summation of pain from the muscle, joint, and bone.

PAIN REFERRAL

Referred pain from a localized painful structure is often associated with musculoskeletal and visceral pain syndromes. Referred pain is defined as pain located in structures away from the source of nociception. The neurophysiologic mechanisms involved in referred pain are not fully described, although a central mechanism is highly likely because referred pain can be evoked in areas with an effective regional anesthetic block. The effect of sensory information from the referred pain area is not clarified because the intensity of referred pain is either not affected or reduced when the referred pain structures are anesthetized [37]. In many conditions, it is not possible to separate between spread of pain and fusion between referred and local pain areas. Common pain mechanisms might be involved in the spread of pain and referred pain.

Pain Referral from Muscle

Referred pain from myofascial trigger points in myofascial pain patients illustrates an extensive mapping of referred pain patterns from many skeletal muscles [91]. The size and location of referred pain may reflect sensitization of central neural mechanisms. Animal studies have shown that muscle nociception results in development of new receptive fields and expansion in receptive fields as components of the central hyperexcitability [47], which may be involved in the mechanism mediating referred pain [37]. Interestingly, more subjects develop referred pain after prolonged painful pressure stimulation on tibialis anterior muscle compared with brief pressure stimuli at the same intensity [34], suggesting that a critical time period of nociceptive input is required for eliciting referred pain or that temporal summation is a key component of the referred pain mechanism. Another finding suggesting the involvement of central hyperexcitability in the referred pain mechanism is the reduced number of healthy subjects developing referred pain by experimental muscle pain when treated with an NMDA antagonist (ketamine) compared with placebo [88].

In pain patients with, e.g., low-back pain, OA pain, tennis elbow pain, fibromyalgia, and whiplash enlarged experimentally induced referred pain areas are found when comparing with similar assessments in control subjects without pain (for review see Ref. [38]). The expanded referred pain areas in patients were found after inducing pain in the tibialis anterior muscle often not described with habitual ongoing pain. The referred pain from the tibialis anterior muscle is typically described as pain perceived in the ankle area in healthy subjects (Figure 2-3), but in some patients proximal referred pain has been reported. In line with the proximal spread of referred pain in pain patients, it has been demonstrated that myositis in animal causes sensitization of dorsal horn neurons, which spreads mainly proximally [49]. The expanded areas of referred pain suggest that that the central neuronal mechanisms are sensitized in chronic musculoskeletal pain patients. Accordingly, if the increased referred pain areas in pain patients are reassessed when antagonized by ketamine, reduced and partly normalized referred pain areas are found [41].

Pain Referral from Joint

Experimental electrical facet joint stimulation induces low-back pain and pain referral into the anterior leg, ipsilaterally, proximal to the knee, similar to what is observed clinically in facet joint pain [76]. In contrast, fairly localized pain is induced by stimulation of the fat pad of the knee (Figure 2-3) [59].

Clinically, OA in the hip joint is often accompanied by complaints of knee pain (and vice versa), which may in some cases be the only symptom. Interestingly, older age knee OA patients in contrast to younger patients were more likely to have pain spreading to larger regions than the most typical pattern of localized knee pain [104]. Pain patterns from joints have been extensively studied typically by joint provocation followed by recordings of the

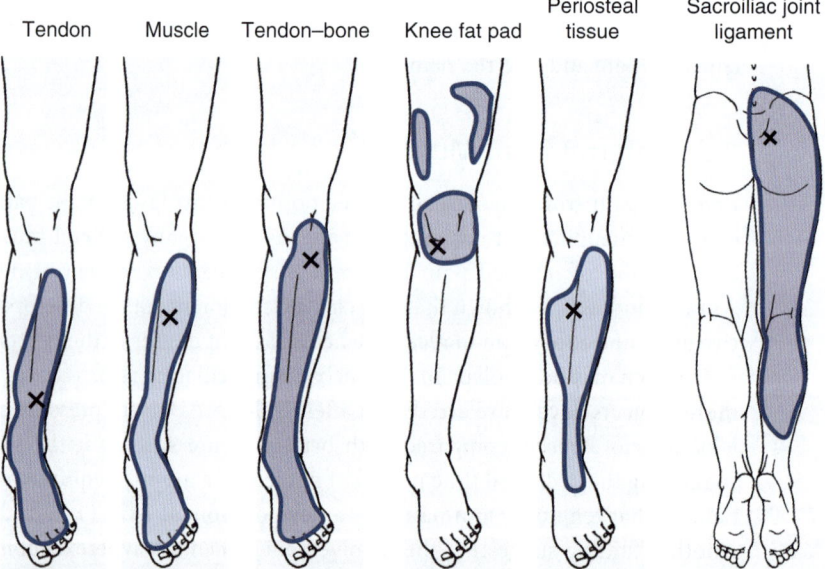

FIGURE 2-3 General pain distribution of saline-induced pain in muscle, distal tendon, and proximal tendon–bone junction of the tibialis anterior muscle and in the joint (knee fat pad), periosteal tissue on the tibia bone, and sacroiliac joint ligament. Hypertonic saline (5.8%, 0.2 to 1.0 mL) was injected in healthy subjects as bolus injections. (Based on data from Gibson W, Arendt-Nielsen L, Graven-Nielsen T. Referred pain and hyperalgesia in human tendon and muscle belly tissue. Pain 2006;120:113–23; Palsson TS, Graven-Nielsen T. Experimental pelvic pain facilitates pain provocation tests and causes regional hyperalgesia. Pain 2012;153:2233–40; Graven-Nielsen T, Arendt-Nielsen L, Svensson P, Jensen TS. Experimental muscle pain: a quantitative study of local and referred pain in humans following injection of hypertonic saline. J Musculoskel Pain 1997;5:49–69; and Joergensen TS, Henriksen M, Danneskiold-Samsoee B, Bliddal H, Graven-Nielsen T. Experimental knee pain evoke spreading hyperalgesia and facilitated temporal summation of pain. Pain Med 2013;14:874–83.)

referred pain areas. As an example, the pain patterns from the cervical zygapophysial joints were assessed by distending the joint capsule in healthy volunteers with injections of contrast medium under fluoroscopic control [25]. The opposite approach was used in patients where the referred pain areas from the zygapophysial joint pain were eliminated by selective nerve blocks [21]. The referred pain areas from zygapophysial joints show that these may coexist with pain areas typically considered as referred pain from myofascial trigger points, and regions of pain in the myofascial pain syndrome can actually originate from joints rather than from muscles. Despite the fact that this represents a diagnostic challenge for the identification of the source of pain, it also suggests the possibility of joint pain being comorbid with the myofascial pain syndrome.

In patients with discogenic pain, electrothermal stimulation of the lumbar intervertebral discs evoked pain that distributed from the low back to the buttocks, to the hip, and to the distal leg areas [75]. Progressively increasing heat stimulation intensities initially induced pain at the back and later developed pain distally to the leg. Low-back pain patients often report a similar manifestation with pain in the legs and feet especially with high-pain intensity. Unfortunately, it has not been possible to establish a uniform pain distribution for each individual disc. Nevertheless, the extensive referred pain areas from nociceptive disc structures may cause a diagnostic problem (e.g., separating the cause from nerve root compression) and facilitate other pain manifestations in the lower leg if accompanied by, e.g., referred hyperalgesia.

Pain Referral from Bone

In pioneer experiments by Kellgren [61], direct mechanical stimulation of the compact bone demonstrated only a vibration and pressure sensation. In contrast, stimulation of the deep periosteal tissue evoked localized pain and pain referral [53,61]. A later study demonstrated that injections of hypertonic saline into the periosteal tissue evoked localized and referred pain (Figure 2-3) [39]. Clinical reports of pain referral from bone metastases exist [70]: Bone destruction of the atlas C1 bone typically results in pain in the occipital or nuchal region, whereas destruction of the C7-T1 vertebrae gives pain referral to the interscapular region. Referred pain to the buttock or posterior thigh may arise from the sacral segments. Interestingly, pain in the sacroiliac joint or iliac crest may be due to bone destruction of the T12 or L1 segments. It is not fully understood, however, how much of the pain distribution relates to the central mechanism responsible for referred pain and how much is due to peripheral spread of bone destruction.

Pain Referral from Connective Tissue

Tendinous structures do exhibit referred pain with varying frequency after injection of algesic substances, but referred pain is generally associated with higher pain intensities [34,35]. The fascia has been shown to exhibit referred pain, however, despite significantly higher pain intensities not to the same extent as muscle tissue [36]. Experimental pelvic pain by injection of hypertonic saline into the long posterior sacroiliac ligament showed extensive pain referral (Figure 2-3) [31]. However, variations in the pain referral exist between different tendons; e.g., referred pain areas spread to a larger part of the leg after injections of hypertonic saline into the gluteus medius tendon compared with more regionalized pain pattern after adductor longus tendon injections [54].

CONCLUSION

Musculoskeletal structures hold a powerful nociceptive capacity to be sensitized locally and to evoke central changes that are highly relevant to development of persistent postoperative pain. Spreading hypersensitivity, facilitated temporal summation of pain, and extensive pain referral are some factors involved in the manifestation of chronic musculoskeletal pain including postoperative pain conditions. Muscle, joint, and connective tissue all seem to have these characteristics, whereas more data are needed to clarify the nonmalignant bone pain mechanisms. Acknowledging the deep tissue as a major source for generating widespread hypersensitivity is deemed for developing better diagnostics and new treatment targets.

REFERENCES

1. Adnadjevic D, Graven-Nielsen T. Vibration and rotation during biaxial pressure algometry is related with decreased and increased pain sensations. Pain Med 2014;15:2095–104.
2. Alfredson H, Forsgren S, Thorsen K, Fahlstrom M, Johansson H, Lorentzon R. Glutamate NMDAR1 receptors localised to nerves in human Achilles tendons. Implications for treatment? Knee Surg Sports Traumatol Arthrosc 2001;9:123–6.
3. Alfredson H, Ljung BO, Thorsen K, Lorentzon R. In vivo investigation of ECRB tendons with microdialysis technique–no signs of inflammation but high amounts of glutamate in tennis elbow. Acta Orthop Scand 2000;71:475–9.
4. Andersen H, Arendt-Nielsen L, Svensson P, Danneskiold-Samsoe B, Graven-Nielsen T. Spatial and temporal aspects of muscle hyperalgesia induced by nerve growth factor in humans. Exp Brain Res 2008;191:371–82.
5. Andersen H, Ge HY, Arendt-Nielsen L, Danneskiold-Samsoe B, Graven-Nielsen T. Increased trapezius pain sensitivity is not associated with increased tissue hardness. J Pain 2010;11:491–9.
6. Andres KH, von Düring M, Schmidt RF. Sensory innervation of the Achilles tendon by group III and IV afferent fibers. Anat Embryol (Berl) 1985;172:145–56.
7. Arendt-Nielsen L, Eskehave TN, Egsgaard LL, Petersen KK, Graven-Nielsen T, Hoeck HC, Simonsen O, Siebuhr AS, Karsdal M, Bay-Jensen AC. Association between experimental pain biomarkers and serologic markers in patients with different degrees of painful knee osteoarthritis. Arthritis Rheumatol 2014;66:3317–26.
8. Arendt-Nielsen L, Nie H, Laursen MB, Laursen BS, Madeleine P, Simonsen OH, Graven-Nielsen T. Sensitization in patients with painful knee osteoarthritis. Pain 2010;149:573–81.
9. Bajaj P, Graven-Nielsen T, Arendt-Nielsen L. Trigger points in patients with lower limb osteoarthritis. J Musculoskel Pain 2001;9:17–33.
10. Banic B, Petersen-Felix S, Andersen OK, Radanov BP, Villiger PM, Arendt-Nielsen L, Curatolo M. Evidence for spinal cord hypersensitivity in chronic pain after whiplash injury and in fibromyalgia. Pain 2004;107:7–15.
11. Barlas P, Walsh DM, Baxter GD, Allen JM. Delayed onset muscle soreness: effect of an ischaemic block upon mechanical allodynia in humans. Pain 2000;87:221–5.
12. Bjur D, Alfredson H, Forsgren S. The innervation pattern of the human Achilles tendon: studies of the normal and tendinosis tendon with markers for general and sensory innervation. Cell Tissue Res 2005;320:201–6.
13. Bove SE, Flatters SJ, Inglis JJ, Mantyh PW. New advances in musculoskeletal pain. Brain Res Rev 2009;60:187–201.
14. Brennan TJ. Pathophysiology of postoperative pain. Pain 2011;152:S33–40.
15. Burmester GR, Feist E, Kellner H, Braun J, Iking-Konert C, Rubbert-Roth A. Effectiveness and safety of the interleukin 6-receptor antagonist tocilizumab after 4 and 24 weeks in patients with active rheumatoid arthritis: the first phase IIIb real-life study (TAMARA). Ann Rheum Dis 2011;70:755–9.
16. Cairns BE, Svensson P, Wang K, Castrillon E, Hupfeld S, Sessle BJ, Arendt-Nielsen L. Ketamine attenuates glutamate-induced mechanical sensitization of the masseter muscle in human males. Exp Brain Res 2006;169:467–72.
17. Cairns BE, Svensson P, Wang K, Hupfeld S, Graven-Nielsen T, Sessle BJ, Berde CB, Arendt-Nielsen L. Activation of peripheral NMDA receptors contributes to human pain and rat afferent discharges evoked by injection of glutamate into the masseter muscle. J Neurophysiol 2003;90:2098–105.

18. Carli G, Suman AL, Biasi G, Marcolongo R. Reactivity to superficial and deep stimuli in patients with chronic musculoskeletal pain. Pain 2002;100:259–69.
19. Chen Q, Wang HJ, Gay RE, Thompson JM, Manduca A, An KN, Ehman RE, Basford JR. Quantification of myofascial taut bands. Arch Phys Med Rehabil 2016;97:67–73.
20. Christidis N, Nilsson A, Kopp S, Ernberg M. Intramuscular injection of granisetron into the masseter muscle increases the pressure pain threshold in healthy participants and patients with localized myalgia. Clin J Pain 2007;23:467–72.
21. Cooper G, Bailey B, Bogduk N. Cervical zygapophysial joint pain maps. Pain Med 2007;8:344–53.
22. Creamer P, Lethbridge-Cejku M, Hochberg MC. Where does it hurt? Pain localization in osteoarthritis of the knee. Osteoarthritis Cartilage 1998;6:318–23.
23. Deising S, Weinkauf B, Blunk J, Obreja O, Schmelz M, Rukwied R. NGF-evoked sensitization of muscle fascia nociceptors in humans. Pain 2012;153:1673–9.
24. Dieppe PA. Relationship between symptoms and structural change in osteoarthritis: what are the important targets for therapy? J Rheumatol 2005;32:1147–9.
25. Dwyer A, Aprill C, Bogduk N. Cervical zygapophyseal joint pain patterns. I: A study in normal volunteers. Spine 1990;15:453–7.
26. Dye SF, Vaupel GL, Dye CC. Conscious neurosensory mapping of the internal structures of the human knee without intraarticular anesthesia. Am J Sports Med 1998;26:773–7.
27. Ernberg M, Lundeberg T, Kopp S. Effect of propranolol and granisetron on experimentally induced pain and allodynia/hyperalgesia by intramuscular injection of serotonin into the human masseter muscle. Pain 2000;84:339–46.
28. Farrell M, Gibson S, McMeeken J, Helme R. Pain and hyperalgesia in osteoarthritis of the hands. J Rheumatol 2000;27:441–7.
29. Felson DT. The sources of pain in knee osteoarthritis. Curr Opin Rheumatol 2005;17:624–8.
30. Finocchietti S, Graven-Nielsen T, Arendt-Nielsen L. Bone hyperalgesia after mechanical impact stimulation: a human experimental pain model. Somatosens Mot Res 2014;31:178–85.
31. Finocchietti S, Nielsen M, Morch CD, Arendt-Nielsen L, Graven-Nielsen T. Pressure-induced muscle pain and tissue biomechanics: a computational and experimental study. Eur J Pain 2011;15:36–44.
32. Ge HY, Nie H, Madeleine P, Danneskiold-Samsoe B, Graven-Nielsen T, Arendt-Nielsen L. Contribution of the local and referred pain from active myofascial trigger points in fibromyalgia syndrome. Pain 2009;147:233–40.
33. Gerber RK, Nie H, Arendt-Nielsen L, Curatolo M, Graven-Nielsen T. Local pain and spreading hyperalgesia induced by intramuscular injection of nerve growth factor are not reduced by local anesthesia of the muscle. Clin J Pain 2011;27:240–7.
34. Gibson W, Arendt-Nielsen L, Graven-Nielsen T. Referred pain and hyperalgesia in human tendon and muscle belly tissue. Pain 2006;120:113–23.
35. Gibson W, Arendt-Nielsen L, Sessle BJ, Graven-Nielsen T. Glutamate and capsaicin-induced pain, hyperalgesia and modulatory interactions in human tendon tissue. Exp Brain Res 2009;194:173–82.
36. Gibson W, Arendt-Nielsen L, Taguchi T, Mizumura K, Graven-Nielsen T. Increased pain from muscle fascia following eccentric exercise: animal and human findings. Exp Brain Res 2009;194:299–308.
37. Graven-Nielsen T. Fundamentals of muscle pain, referred pain, and deep tissue hyperalgesia. Scand J Rheumatol 2006;35(suppl 122):1–43.
38. Graven-Nielsen T, Arendt-Nielsen L. Assessment of mechanisms in localized and widespread musculoskeletal pain. Nat Rev Rheumatol 2010;6:599–606.
39. Graven-Nielsen T, Arendt-Nielsen L, Svensson P, Jensen TS. Experimental muscle pain: a quantitative study of local and referred pain in humans following injection of hypertonic saline. J Musculoskel Pain 1997;5:49–69.
40. Graven-Nielsen T, Arendt-Nielsen L, Svensson P, Jensen TS. Quantification of local and referred muscle pain in humans after sequential i.m. injections of hypertonic saline. Pain 1997;69:111–7.
41. Graven-Nielsen T, Kendall SA, Henriksson KG, Bengtsson M, Sörensen J, Johnson A, Gerdle B, Arendt-Nielsen L. Ketamine reduces muscle pain, temporal summation, and referred pain in fibromyalgia patients. Pain 2000;85:483–91.
42. Graven-Nielsen T, Mense S, Arendt-Nielsen L. Painful and non-painful pressure sensations from human skeletal muscle. Exp Brain Res 2004;159:273–83.
43. Graven-Nielsen T, Vaegter HB, Finocchietti S, Handberg G, Arendt-Nielsen L. Assessment of musculoskeletal pain sensitivity and temporal summation by cuff pressure algometry: a reliability study. Pain 2015;156:2193–202.

44. Graven-Nielsen T, Wodehouse T, Langford RM, Arendt-Nielsen L, Kidd BL. Normalization of widespread hyperesthesia and facilitated spatial summation of deep-tissue pain in knee osteoarthritis patients after knee replacement. Arthritis Rheum 2012;64:2907–16.
45. Hayashi K, Shiozawa S, Ozaki N, Mizumura K, Graven-Nielsen T. Repeated intramuscular injections of nerve growth factor induced progressive muscle hyperalgesia, facilitated temporal summation, and expanded pain areas. Pain 2013;154:2344–52.
46. Hoheisel U, Koch K, Mense S. Functional reorganization in the rat dorsal horn during an experimental myositis. Pain 1994;59:111–8.
47. Hoheisel U, Mense S, Simons DG, Yu X-M. Appearance of new receptive fields in rat dorsal horn neurons following noxious stimulation of skeletal muscle: a model for referral of muscle pain? Neurosci Lett 1993;153:9–12.
48. Hoheisel U, Reuter R, de Freitas MF, Treede RD, Mense S. Injection of nerve growth factor into a low back muscle induces long-lasting latent hypersensitivity in rat dorsal horn neurons. Pain 2013;154(10):1953–60.
49. Hoheisel U, Sander B, Mense S. Myositis-induced functional reorganisation of the rat dorsal horn: effects of spinal superfusion with antagonists to neurokinin and glutamate receptors. Pain 1997;69:219–30.
50. Hoheisel U, Taguchi T, Treede RD, Mense S. Nociceptive input from the rat thoracolumbar fascia to lumbar dorsal horn neurones. Eur J Pain 2011;15:810–5.
51. Hoheisel U, Unger T, Mense S. Sensitization of rat dorsal horn neurons by NGF-induced subthreshold potentials and low-frequency activation. A study employing intracellular recordings in vivo. Brain Res 2007;1169:34–43.
52. Imamura M, Ezquerro F, Marcon AF, Vilas BL, Tozetto-Mendoza TR, Chen J, Ozcakar L, Arendt-Nielsen L, Rizzo BL. Serum levels of proinflammatory cytokines in painful knee osteoarthritis and sensitization. Int J Inflamm 2015;2015:329792.
53. Inman VT, Saunders JBCM. Referred pain from skeletal structures. J Nerv Ment Dis 1944;99:660–7.
54. Izumi M, Petersen KK, Arendt-Nielsen L, Graven-Nielsen T. Pain referral and regional deep tissue hyperalgesia in experimental human hip pain models. Pain 2014;155:792–800.
55. Izumi M, Petersen KK, Laursen MB, Arendt-Nielsen L, Graven-Nielsen T. Facilitated temporal summation of pain correlates with clinical pain intensity after hip arthroplasty. Pain 2017;158:323–32.
56. Jadidi F, Wang K, Arendt-Nielsen L, Svensson P. Effects of different stimulus locations on inhibitory responses in human jaw-closing muscles. J Oral Rehabil 2011;38:487–500.
57. Jensen K, Andersen HØ, Olesen J, Lindblom U. Pressure-pain threshold in human temporal region. Evaluation of a new pressure algometer. Pain 1986;25:313–23.
58. Jespersen A, Amris K, Graven-Nielsen T, Arendt-Nielsen L, Bartels EM, Torp-Pedersen S, Bliddal H, Danneskiold-Samsoe B. Assessment of pressure-pain thresholds and central sensitization of pain in lateral epicondylalgia. Pain Med 2013;14:297–304.
59. Joergensen TS, Henriksen M, Danneskiold-Samsoee B, Bliddal H, Graven-Nielsen T. Experimental knee pain evoke spreading hyperalgesia and facilitated temporal summation of pain. Pain Med 2013;14:874–83.
60. Kellgren JH. Observations on referred pain arising from muscle. Clin Sci 1938;3:175–90.
61. Kellgren JH. On the distribution of pain arising from deep somatic structures with charts of segmental pain areas. Clin Sci 1939;4:35–46.
62. Kosek E, Ordeberg G. Lack of pressure pain modulation by heterotopic noxious conditioning stimulation in patients with painful osteoarthritis before, but not following, surgical pain relief. Pain 2000;88:69–78.
63. Kregel J, van Wilgen CP, Zwerver J. Pain assessment in patellar tendinopathy using pain pressure threshold algometry: an observational study. Pain Med 2013;14(11):1769–75.
64. Larsen P, Elsoe R, Graven-Nielsen T, Laessoe U, Rasmussen S. Local and widespread hyperalgesia after isolated tibial shaft fractures treated with intramedullary nailing. Pain Med 2016;17:1174–80.
65. Lau WY, Blazevich AJ, Newton MJ, Wu SS, Nosaka K. Changes in electrical pain threshold of fascia and muscle after initial and secondary bouts of elbow flexor eccentric exercise. Eur J Appl Physiol 2015;115:959–68.
66. Majuta LA, Guedon JG, Mitchell SA, Ossipov MH, Mantyh PW. Anti-nerve growth factor therapy increases spontaneous day/night activity in mice with orthopedic surgery-induced pain. Pain 2017;158:605–17.
67. Manafi-Khanian B, Arendt-Nielsen L, Graven-Nielsen T. An MRI-based leg model used to simulate biomechanical phenomena during cuff algometry: a finite element study. Med Biol Eng Comput 2016;54:315–24.
68. Mantyh PW. Bone-related nociception. In: Graven-Nielsen T, Arendt-Nielsen L, editors. Musculoskeletal pain: basic mechanisms and implications. Washington: IASP Press; 2014. p. 205–22.
69. Mense S, Hoheisel U. Morphology and functional types of muscle nociceptors. In: Graven-Nielsen T, Arendt-Nielsen L, Mense S, editors. Fundamentals of musculoskeletal pain. Seattle: IASP Press; 2008. p. 3–17.

70. Middlemiss T, Laird BJ, Fallon MT. Mechanisms of cancer-induced bone pain. Clin Oncol (R Coll Radiol) 2011;23:387–92.
71. Molander C, Ygge J, Dalsgaard C-J. Substance P-, somatostatin- and calcitonin gene-related peptide-like immunoreactivity and fluoride resistant acid phosphatase-activity in relation to retrogradely labeled cutaneous, muscular and visceral primary sensory neurons in the rat. Neurosci Lett 1987;74:37–42.
72. Murase S, Terazawa E, Queme F, Ota H, Matsuda T, Hirate K, Kozaki Y, Katanosaka K, Taguchi T, Urai H, Mizumura K. Bradykinin and nerve growth factor play pivotal roles in muscular mechanical hyperalgesia after exercise (delayed-onset muscle soreness). J Neurosci 2010;30:3752–61.
73. Nie H, Arendt-Nielsen L, Andersen H, Graven-Nielsen T. Temporal summation of pain evoked by mechanical stimulation in deep and superficial tissue. J Pain 2005;6:348–55.
74. Nie H, Arendt-Nielsen L, Madeleine P, Graven-Nielsen T. Enhanced temporal summation of pressure pain in the trapezius muscle after delayed onset muscle soreness. Exp Brain Res 2006;170:182–90.
75. O'Neill CW, Kurgansky ME, Derby R, Ryan DP. Disc stimulation and patterns of referred pain. Spine 2002;27:2776–81.
76. O'Neill S, Graven-Nielsen T, Manniche C, Arendt-Nielsen L. Ultrasound guided, painful electrical stimulation of lumbar facet joint structures: an experimental model of acute low back pain. Pain 2009;144:76–83.
77. O'Neill S, Manniche C, Graven-Nielsen T, Arendt-Nielsen L. Generalized deep-tissue hyperalgesia in patients with chronic low-back pain. Eur J Pain 2007;11:415–20.
78. Oster MW, Vizel M, Turgeon LR. Pain of terminal cancer patients. Arch Intern Med 1978;138:1801–2.
79. Palsson TS, Graven-Nielsen T. Experimental pelvic pain facilitates pain provocation tests and causes regional hyperalgesia. Pain 2012;153:2233–40.
80. Petersen KK, Arendt-Nielsen L. Predicting chronic pain after joint surgery [this book!]. 2017. p. XX.
81. Polianskis R, Graven-Nielsen T, Arendt-Nielsen L. Spatial and temporal aspects of deep tissue pain assessed by cuff algometry. Pain 2002;100:19–26.
82. Quinn KP, Dong L, Golder FJ, Winkelstein BA. Neuronal hyperexcitability in the dorsal horn after painful facet joint injury. Pain 2010;151:414–21.
83. Reinert A, Kaske A, Mense S. Inflammation-induced increase in the density of neuropeptide-immunoreactive nerve endings in rat skeletal muscle. Exp Brain Res 1998;121:174–80.
84. Schaible HG. Spinal mechanisms contributing to joint pain. Novartis Found Symp 2004;260:4–22 [discussion 22–7, 100–4, 277–9].
85. Schaible H-G, Grubb BD. Afferent and spinal mechanisms of joint pain. Pain 1993;55:5–54.
86. Schaible H-G, Richter F. Receptors relevant for joint pain. In: Graven-Nielsen T, Arendt-Nielsen L, editors. Musculoskeletal pain: basic mechanisms and implications. Washington: IASP Press; 2014. p. 187–204.
87. Schliessbach J, Arendt-Nielsen L, Heini P, Curatolo M. The role of central hypersensitivity in the determination of intradiscal mechanical hyperalgesia in discogenic pain. Pain Med 2010;11:701–8.
88. Schulte H, Graven-Nielsen T, Sollevi A, Jansson Y, Arendt-Nielsen L, Segerdahl M. Pharmacological modulation of experimental phasic and tonic muscle pain by morphine, alfentanil and ketamine in healthy volunteers. Acta Anaesthesiol Scand 2003;47:1020–30.
89. Schwei MJ, Honore P, Rogers SD, Salak-Johnson JL, Finke MP, Ramnaraine ML, Clohisy DR, Mantyh PW. Neurochemical and cellular reorganization of the spinal cord in a murine model of bone cancer pain. J Neurosci 1999;19:10886–97.
90. Siegenthaler A, Eichenberger U, Schmidlin K, Arendt-Nielsen L, Curatolo M. What does local tenderness say about the origin of pain? An investigation of cervical zygapophysial joint pain. Anesth Analg 2010;110:923–7.
91. Simons DG, Travell JG, Simons L. Myofascial pain and dysfunction. The trigger point manual. Philadelphia, USA: Lippincott Williams & Wilkins; 1999.
92. Skou ST, Graven-Nielsen T, Rasmussen S, Simonsen OH, Laursen MB, Arendt-Nielsen L. Widespread sensitization in patients with chronic pain after revision total knee arthroplasty. Pain 2013;154:1588–94.
93. Slater H, Arendt-Nielsen L, Wright A, Graven-Nielsen T. Sensory and motor effects of experimental muscle pain in patients with lateral epicondylalgia and controls with delayed onset muscle soreness. Pain 2005;114:118–30.
94. Slater H, Gibson W, Graven-Nielsen T. Sensory responses to mechanically and chemically induced tendon pain in healthy subjects. Eur J Pain 2011;15:146–52.
95. Sluka KA. Stimulation of deep somatic tissue with capsaicin produces long-lasting mechanical allodynia and heat hypoalgesia that depends on early activation of the cAMP pathway. J Neurosci 2002;22:5687–93.
96. Sluka KA, Kalra A, Moore SA. Unilateral intramuscular injections of acidic saline produce a bilateral, long-lasting hyperalgesia. Muscle Nerve 2001;24:37–46.

97. Sluka KA, Radhakrishnan R, Benson CJ, Eshcol JO, Price MP, Babinski K, Audette KM, Yeomans DC, Wilson SP. ASIC3 in muscle mediates mechanical, but not heat, hyperalgesia associated with muscle inflammation. Pain 2007;129:102–12.
98. Sörensen J, Graven-Nielsen T, Henriksson KG, Bengtsson M, Arendt-Nielsen L. Hyperexcitability in fibromyalgia. J Rheumatol 1998;25:152–5.
99. Srbely JZ, Dickey JP, Bent LR, Lee D, Lowerison M. Capsaicin-induced central sensitization evokes segmental increases in trigger point sensitivity in humans. J Pain 2010;11:636–43.
100. Staud R, Cannon RC, Mauderli AP, Robinson ME, Price DD, Vierck Jr CJ. Temporal summation of pain from mechanical stimulation of muscle tissue in normal controls and subjects with fibromyalgia syndrome. Pain 2003;102:87–95.
101. Sturmer T, Brenner H, Koenig W, Gunther KP. Severity and extent of osteoarthritis and low grade systemic inflammation as assessed by high sensitivity C reactive protein. Ann Rheum Dis 2004;63:200–5.
102. Taguchi T, Yasui M, Kubo A, Abe M, Kiyama H, Yamanaka A, Mizumura K. Nociception originating from the crural fascia in rats. Pain 2013;154:1103–14.
103. Tesarz J, Hoheisel U, Wiedenhofer B, Mense S. Sensory innervation of the thoracolumbar fascia in rats and humans. Neuroscience 2011;194:302–8. doi:10.1016/j.neuroscience.2011.07.066.
104. Thompson LR, Boudreau R, Newman AB, Hannon MJ, Chu CR, Nevitt MC, Kent KC. The association of osteoarthritis risk factors with localized, regional and diffuse knee pain. Osteoarthritis Cartilage 2010;18:1244–9.
105. Urch CE, Donovan-Rodriguez T, Dickenson AH. Alterations in dorsal horn neurones in a rat model of cancer-induced bone pain. Pain 2003;106:347–56.
106. Vanderweeën L, Oostendorp RA, Vaes P, Duquet W. Pressure algometry in manual therapy. Man Ther 1996;1:258–65.
107. Wall PD, Woolf CJ. Muscle but not cutaneous C-afferent input produces prolonged increases in the excitability of the flexion reflex in the rat. J Physiol (Lond) 1984;356:443–58.
108. Weinkauf B, Deising S, Obreja O, Hoheisel U, Mense S, Schmelz M, Rukwied R. Comparison of nerve growth factor-induced sensitization pattern in lumbar and tibial muscle and fascia. Muscle Nerve 2015;52:265–72.
109. Wright A, Graven-Nielsen T, Davies II, Arendt-Nielsen L. Temporal summation of pain from skin, muscle and joint following nociceptive ultrasonic stimulation in humans. Exp Brain Res 2002;144:475–82.
110. Yahia L, Rhalmi S, Newman N, Isler M. Sensory innervation of human thoracolumbar fascia. An immunohistochemical study. Acta Orthop Scand 1992;63:195–7.

CHAPTER 3

Attribution Bias in Gynecologic Laparoscopy

John Jarrell and Lars Arendt-Nielsen

Operative laparoscopy for pelvic pain is a common procedure with significant improvement for some women. However, the procedure is commonly repeated with limited or no success. The fundamental attribution bias can be described as the tendency to place an undue emphasis on the "visible" findings at surgery rather than invisible factors. Such attribution of "visible" findings at surgery to no disease present may miss dysmenorrhea as the one of the actual causes of pain. Similarly, the attribution of the cause of pain to minimal regions of endometriosis may be made when the woman has actually developed central pain sensitization. The purpose of this study is to review the potential role that the recognition of dysmenorrhea and pain sensitization may play in the generation of the fundamental attribution bias.

PERSPECTIVE

The fundamental attribution bias may be present at the time of operative laparoscopy for pelvic pain. This chapter highlights that dysmenorrhea is a possible common contributor to chronic pelvic pain and, with no visible abnormality, the source of pain may be attributed to other "visible" lesions. Pain sensitization is another potential source of bias, as pain may be attributed to visible lesions when the problem is changes to the central nervous system with an increased gain to pain.

BACKGROUND

Attribution is the process of ascribing a quality or an inherent characteristic or right to a person or thing [30]. Attribution has been studied primarily in the psychological literature [8]. The process of attributing cause to a particular disease process is fundamental to clinical diagnosis but is vulnerable to error and bias [7]. The fundamental attribution error is defined as the tendency for people to place an undue emphasis on internal characteristics of the agent (character or intention), rather than external factors [6]. This chapter is directed to the possibility that the fundamental attribution error can be present in the determination of the cause of pelvic pain at the time of operative laparoscopy. If there is to be an attribution bias at the time of laparoscopy, it would then require a cognitive error in the determination of the specific cause of pain when an alternative explanation exists. This review will explore the possible reasons that an attribution bias may exist in the performance of an operative laparoscopy for chronic pelvic pain. The possible biases or alternative explanations for the source of pain include the finding that no abnormality is present in the pelvis when in fact there is a source of the pain and a determination that the pain is due to endometriosis when another explanation may be valid.

One of the most common procedures undertaken in the field of gynecology is operative laparoscopy in the diagnosis and management of acute and chronic pelvic pain. In the former situation, the diagnosis is usually apparent: hemorrhage emanating from an ectopic pregnancy or ruptured ovarian cyst, inflammation from pelvic infection or mechanical torsion of a visceral structure, etc. In chronic states, however, there is less specificity. Reports consistently demonstrate there is a "negative" rate of laparoscopy of 25% to 40% in cases of chronic pelvic pain [14,35]. Even when there is evidence of a lesion in the pelvis, the effect of surgery may not have any bearing on the change in pain postoperatively [11]. It is possible the cause of the pain is attributed to a visible lesion while in fact the cause of the pain is due to a nonvisible lesion, a perspective commonly seen in many other conditions, e.g., revision surgery after otherwise technically successful total knee replacement and revision back surgery [2].

It is the specific objective of this commentary to explore the evidence that attribution bias is possible in the determination of pain at the time of operative gynecologic laparoscopy.

IS ENDOMETRIOSIS THE ACTUAL CAUSE OF PAIN?

Diseases commonly identified as a cause of nonacute pelvic pain include endometriosis, chronic pelvic inflammatory disease, pelvic adhesions, and ovarian cyst development [13]. Prior surgery has been identified as a possible cause because of the development of pelvic adhesions [13]. Endometriosis, which is associated with the extrauterine location of endometrial tissue, is known to present in various forms at the time of laparoscopic surgery [43]. Much has been written concerning the varied appearance of the disease from nonvisible lesions to extensive and widespread invasion and nodularity [1,43,46]. The condition is classified as a cause to visceral pain mediated through the peripheral release of inflammatory mediators from the endometriotic lesions [12,27]. Once identified, it is the standard of care to undertake its removal. Although electrical monopolar or bipolar cauterization of surface disease is a common approach, the preferred method is the removal through excision from sharp dissection or laser therapy [33]. The benefits of the surgery can for some women be short-lived, and repeated operative laparoscopy is often undertaken over the course of the reproductive years [17,18]. The repeat rate of laparoscopy in individual women within a fiscal year has been proposed as a marker of medical quality [5,17]. However, at some point in the longitudinal history of a specific woman, the attribution of pain to endometriosis may in fact be an incomplete or inaccurate explanation. Endometriosis is assumed to be a major cause of chronic pelvic pain, and it is possible this emerges during the course of repeated surgical procedures. Several observations indicate the strength of benefit from repeated surgery in fact requires further evaluation.

Although some women have pain severe enough to have surgical intervention, there were no obvious lesions apparent at the time of laparoscopy in a substantial proportion of women randomly selected from a population study of interrater reliability of endometriosis staging, suggesting that another possibly nonvisible pain process is operational [36]. Furthermore, it has been long recognized that the severity of pain does not correlate with the extent of the pain experience. Many asymptomatic women having tubal ligations for sterilization purposes have been identified as having asymptomatic disease. Also, repeat surgical procedures are often associated with minimal to mild forms of the disease or pathologic specimens that are simply fibrotic tissue. One randomized controlled trial of sham surgery demonstrated improvement in pain [40,41]. However, another randomized controlled trial of sham excision versus excision of primarily stage 1 and 2 endometriosis compared the composite monthly daily pain scores of the abdomen, pelvis, back, chest, and legs for a month before surgery and quarterly after surgery for a year [25]. In this series, there was no difference in the pain between those observed and those with excision. These women were followed up for a 14-year period to determine the next operative procedure for pelvic pain [22]. There was no difference in the groups in the time to the next operative procedure for pain. Importantly, the pain rating in the month preceding the operative procedure (not the group or the stage of the disease) significantly predicted the time for the next operative procedure [22].

These observations permit a consideration of possible alternative and nonvisible explanations for pelvic pain at the time of operative laparoscopy.

WHAT ARE THE POSSIBLE ALTERNATIVES IF ENDOMETRIOSIS IS NOT THE CAUSE OF PAIN?

Dysmenorrhea—The Invisible Lesion

The basis for these observations relates to alternative explanations that may not be obvious through the laparoscope but can be detected at the bedside. A brief review of the three commonly used search engines indicates a much greater emphasis on the visible condition of endometriosis and a relative paucity of attention directed to a condition invisible at laparoscopy. The number of citations for endometriosis and chronic pelvic pain compared with that for dysmenorrhea and chronic pelvic pain when compared in association with or without laparoscopy differ significantly (Table 3-1).

The emphasis on endometriosis is understandable owing to its visibility in many forms [1]. There is extensive literature on the nociceptive features of the disease, and there are even reports of the benefits of treating occult endometriosis with surgical excision [3]. The surgical elimination of pain following excision of endometriosis can be successful in cases of invasive disease although the rates of persistent pain have been reported to

TABLE 3-1 Comparison of Rates of Citations Directed to Chronic Pelvic Pain by Endometriosis and Dysmenorrhea with and without Laparoscopy

Search Engine	With Laparoscopy	Endometriosis Chronic Pelvic Pain	Dysmenorrhea Chronic Pelvic Pain No Endometriosis	Chi Square (P Value)
PubMed	No	1018	146	22.6 (<0.001)
	Yes	438	21	
PMC	No	2044	715	165.9 (<0.001)
	Yes	884	45	
Google Scholar	No	40,500	11,200	250.8 (<0.001)
	Yes	20,400	1400	

be substantial [44]. Additionally, the effectiveness in early stages of the disease is not apparent [22,25]. The identification of the source of pain as the endometriotic spot on the peritoneum could be therefore an error. What then can be the cause of the pain and how can this be determined?

One of the causes may well be the presence of dysmenorrhea [19]. This condition is complex and as a self-reported pain state is particularly difficult in some instances to ascertain correctly. The condition is often complicated by the woman's prior upbringing and ignored by caregivers. Culturally, it is common for women who experience severe pain that cripples them for days each month to accept this as a normal state. This changes, however, when women with chronic pelvic pain are specifically interrogated regarding menstrual pain. Notably, in a review of a large population of women who have developed severe chronic pelvic pain, the rate of severe dysmenorrhea was 89% despite a much lower rate of clinical endometriosis [19].

Pain Sensitization—Detectable Preoperatively but Invisible at Laparoscopy

Another aspect that can contribute to the attribution bias of pain may be the presence of peripheral and centralized pain sensitization. Pain sensitization is defined as "increased responsiveness of nociceptive neurons to their normal input, and/or recruitment of a response to normally subthreshold inputs." Sensitization is only indirectly appreciated by testing that indicates hyperalgesia or allodynia. Sensitization is deemed peripheral when there is increased responsiveness and reduced threshold of stimulated nociceptive neurons in the periphery [16,28,42]. Central sensitization is increased responsiveness of nociceptive neurons in the central nervous system to their normal or subthreshold afferent input [28].

The history of pain sensitization is actually lengthy, but it was not recognized as such until relatively recently. It is instructive to review some of the comments of early gynecologists. Hugh L. Hodge's observations in 1860 are germane to the discussion of pain without obvious pathology: "…it may fairly be inferred that, under various names, the idea of a morbid irritability of the tissues without any inflammatory or other lesion, is a very common affectation. It often exists without any perceptible alteration in the condition of the parts; it is a morbid state of exaltation of the nerves, a state of hyperesthesia, frequently excited by mental and moral; causes as well as by physical disturbances, and yet involving almost exclusively the nervous system" [15]. Henry Head undertook a review of the referral patterns of visceral disease as part of his MD thesis [10]. Within the thesis, he also noted "*areas of tenderness with sharp borders*"—now an early recognition of the sharp borders of allodynia. Sir James Mackenzie, in his book *Symptoms and Their Interpretation*, has depicted a diagram of a man suffering from biliary colic with the description of an area of allodynia that importantly recognizes where a thoracic nerve penetrating the *rectus abdominus* muscle as a source of tenderness [29]. This same presentation of allodynia and tender regions of the T12 and L1 abdominal cutaneous nerves is present in cases of visceral pelvic pain and is thought to be a focus of the pain morbidity of chronic pelvic pain [21].

Pain sensitization has been associated with a large number of conditions such as osteoarthritis, fibromyalgia, rheumatoid arthritis, headache, neuropathic pain, temporomandibular pain, complex regional pain, musculoskeletal pain, postsurgical pain, and a variety of visceral pain syndromes [45]. It has been shown that repeated surgical procedures further enhance the sensitization [37].

One condition that closely mimics the issues related to visceral pelvic pain is that of the postcholecystectomy syndrome, where there is pain similar to that when the diseased gall bladder was present [9]. Pelvic disease causes visceral pain, and when it is severe, the pain system becomes sensitized usually with the development of noncyclic, persisting, and unrelenting pain and changes to the woman's emotional well-being [4,39]. Hyperalgesic priming is a process associated with the shift from acute episodic to persistent pain [34]. This may have a role in the shift from episodic to persistent pain as an evolutionary mismatch resulting from the dramatic increase in lifetime menstrual function over the millennia [20,38]. When sensitization occurs, there is activation of somatic nerves corresponding to the innervation of the pelvic organs (T12-L1 and S234). The sensitized state can be detected at the bedside using simple clinical tests of the assessment of allodynia or muscle hyperalgesia [23,32,47]. A dramatic representation of the identification of allodynia and corresponding tender areas that conform to the regions of the T9-T12 anterior cutaneous nerves is presented in Figure 3-1. Not only is allodynia expanded rapidly after testing, but new identifiable tender areas emerge rapidly as well, indicating dynamic spinal activity in the presence of chronic pain.

The detection of allodynia can be accomplished by drawing a cotton-tipped applicator down the midclavicular line along an imaginary line of the lateral border of the rectus muscle bilaterally toward the region where the T12 and L1 nerves would emerge from the anterior rectus sheath (Figure 3-1) [24]. In some instances, the allodynia must be provoked by placing pressure on these areas [23,31]. Also, the sensation in some instances is not initially painful but appears to be a paresthesia initially. However, repetitive testing will enhance the pain experience and commonly results in an expansion of the areas of allodynia, presumably from increasing activity in the corresponding segments of the spinal cord.

Within the area of allodynia, but the T12 and L1 nerves, pain pressure thresholds can detect hyperalgesia defined as excessive pain. The test can be carried out with an algometer

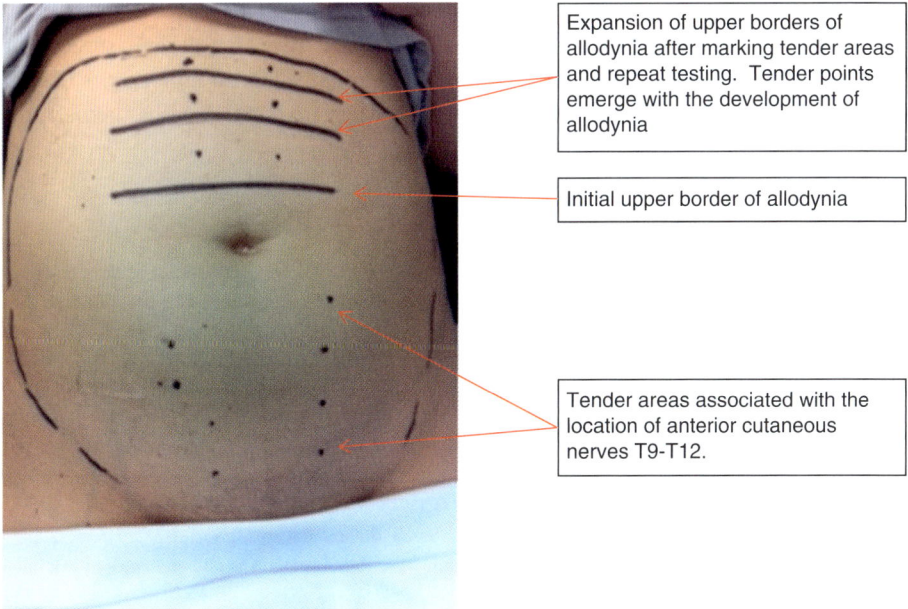

FIGURE 3-1 Examination of the abdomen of a woman with severe chronic pelvic pain demonstrating initial upper level of allodynia, expansion of allodynia, and tender areas associated with the anterior cutaneous nerves T9-T12 as they emerge from the rectus sheath. Tender points also emerge with the development of induced allodynia.

such as that provided by Somedic (Somedic Algometer, Solna, Sweden). Reduced pressure pain thresholds permit further objective confirmation of the presence and severity of central sensitization. Additionally, in a review of 185 women with chronic pelvic pain, the history of severe dysmenorrhea was significantly greater among women with allodynia (68% vs. 90%) [19]. In this cohort, as the years of severe dysmenorrhea increased, so too was there a significant increase in pain sensitization detected by pressure pain thresholds [26].

The benefit of these tests permits an ability to categorize chronic pain based on severity, appreciate the morbidity of the condition more fully, and have objective means to follow the effectiveness of treatment. The value of these clinical tests, the ease of bedside testing, and the ability to provide an alternative explanation for the pelvic pain can improve diagnostic accuracy at the time of laparoscopy.

CONCLUSION

There appears to be support for the presence of an attribution bias at the time of operative laparoscopy for nonacute pain, implicating severe dysmenorrhea and pain sensitization as instigators. There is a need for further exploration of the role of dysmenorrhea as one of the more prominent causes of nonacute and chronic pelvic pain alone and in the presence of early stages of endometriosis. The detection of pain sensitization with simple validated tests provides a broader understanding of the mechanisms involved in a woman's pain state and may provide an alternative explanation for a source of pain because of the facilitated central gain. Operative laparoscopy for the detection and excision of endometriosis is commonly associated with recurrent pain, usually at 6 months postoperatively. Although it is appropriate for a woman to assume that "endometriosis is back," there is an alternative explanation—the presence of pain sensitization as assessed by cutaneous allodynia and myofascial pain. In this circumstance, repeated surgery will only enhance the pain sensitization and alternative therapies directed to the chronic pain state are indicated.

It is possible that the success rate of operative laparoscopic surgery may be enhanced by the recognition that attributing the woman's pain to minor areas of endometriosis may misattribute the pain to these lesions when in actual fact the uterus and/or sensitization may be playing a greater role.

REFERENCES

1. Albee Jr RB, Sinervo K, Fisher DT. Laparoscopic excision of lesions suggestive of endometriosis or otherwise atypical in appearance: relationship between visual findings and final histologic diagnosis. J Minim Invasive Gynecol 2008;15(1):32–7.
2. Arendt-Nielsen L. Joint pain: more to it than just structural damage. Pain 2017;158(4):S66–73.
3. Audebert AJ. Occult and minimal forms of endometriosis: therapeutic strategies. Rev Fr Gynecol Obstet 1990;85(2):79–84.
4. Berkley KJ, Rapkin AJ, Papka RE. The pains of endometriosis. Science 2005;308(5728):1587–9.
5. Berlanda N, Vercellini P, Fedele L. The outcomes of repeat surgery for recurrent symptomatic endometriosis. Curr Opin Obstet Gynecol 2010;22(4):320–5.
6. Canadian Medical Protective Association. Fundamental attribution error. 2016.
7. Croskerry P. The importance of cognitive errors in diagnosis and strategies to minimize them. Acad Med 2003;78:775–80.
8. Funder DC. Errors and mistakes: evaluating the accuracy of social judgment. Psychol Bull 1987;101(1):75–90.
9. Giamberardino MA, Affaitati G, Lerza R, Lapenna D, Costantini R, Vecchiet L. Relationship between pain symptoms and referred sensory and trophic changes in patients with gallbladder pathology. Pain 2005;114(1–2):239–49.

10. Head H. On disturbances of sensation with especial reference to the pain of visceral disease. Brain 1893;16:1–133.
11. Howard FM. Chronic pelvic pain. Obstet Gynecol 2003;101(3):594–611.
12. Howard FM. Endometriosis and mechanisms of pelvic pain. J Minim Invasive Gynecol 2009;16(5):540–50.
13. Howard FM. The role of laparoscopy as a diagnostic tool in chronic pelvic pain. Baillieres Best Pract Res Clin Obstet Gynaecol 2000;14(3):467–94.
14. Howard FM, Sanchez R. A comparison of laparoscopically assisted vaginal hysterectomy and abdominal hysterectomy. J Gynecol Surg 1993;9(2):83–90.
15. Hodge HL. Diseases peculiar to women. 2nd ed. Pennsylvania; 1868.
16. IASP. Pain terms: a list with definitions and notes on usage. Recommended by the IASP Subcommittee on Taxonomy. Pain 1979;6(3):249.
17. Jarrell J. Annual repeat rates of laparoscopic surgery: a marker of practice variation. Am J Med Qual 2010;25(5):378–83.
18. Jarrell J. Diagnostic and operative laparoscopy in Alberta 1994–2006. J Obstet Gynaecol Can 2008;30:1039–45.
19. Jarrell J, Arendt-Nielsen L. Allodynia and dysmenorrhea. J Obstet Gynaecol Can 2016;38(3):270–4.
20. Jarrell J, Arendt-Nielsen L. Evolutionary considerations in the development of chronic pelvic pain. Am J Obstet Gynecol 2016;215(2):201–4.
21. Jarrell J, Arendt-Nielsen L. Quantitative sensory testing in gynaecology: improving preoperative and postoperative pain diagnosis. J Obstet Gynaecol Can 2013;35(6):531–5.
22. Jarrell J, Brant R, Leung W, Taenzer P. Women's pain experience predicts future surgery for pain associated with endometriosis. J Obstet Gynaecol Can 2007;29(12):988–91.
23. Jarrell J, Giamberardino MA, Robert M, Nasr-Esfahani M. Bedside testing for chronic pelvic pain: discriminating visceral from somatic pain. Pain Res Treat 2011;2011:692102.
24. Jarrell J, Malekzadeh L, Yang H, Arendt-Nielsen L. The significance of cutaneous allodynia in a woman with chronic pelvic pain. J Obstet Gynaecol Can 2015;37(7):628–32.
25. Jarrell J, Mohindra R, Ross S, Taenzer P, Brant R. Laparoscopy and reported pain among patients with endometriosis. J Obstet Gynaecol Can 2005;27(5):477–85.
26. Jarrell J, Ross S, Robert M, Wood S, Tang S, Stephanson K, et al. Prediction of postoperative pain after gynecologic laparoscopy for nonacute pelvic pain. Am J Obstet Gynecol 2014;211(4):360.
27. Kobayashi H, Yamada Y, Morioka S, Niiro E, Shigemitsu A, Ito F. Mechanism of pain generation for endometriosis-associated pelvic pain. Arch Gynecol Obstet 2013;289(1):13–21.
28. Loeser JD, Treede RD. The Kyoto protocol of IASP Basic Pain Terminology. Pain 2008;137(3):473–7.
29. Mackenzie J. Symptoms and their interpretation. 2nd ed. New York: Paul B Hoeber; 1913.
30. Merriam Webster Dictionary. Attribution; 2016. http://www.dictionary.com/browse/attribute. http://www.dictionary.com/browse/attribute?s=t.
31. Nasr-Esfahani M, Jarrell J. Cotton-tipped applicator test: validity and reliability in chronic pelvic pain. Am J Obstet Gynecol 2013;208(1):52–5.
32. Nourmoussavi M, Bodmer-Roy S, Mui J, Mawji N, Williams C, Allaire C, et al. Bladder base tenderness in the etiology of deep dyspareunia. J Sex Med 2014;11(12):3078–84.
33. Radosa MP, Bernardi TS, Georgiev I, Diebolder H, Camara O, Runnebaum IB. Coagulation versus excision of primary superficial endometriosis: a 2-year follow-up. Eur J Obstet Gynecol Reprod Biol 2010;150(2):195–8.
34. Reichling BD, Levine JD. Critical role of nociceptor plasticity in chronic pain. Trends Neurosci 2009;32:611–8.
35. Reiter RC. A profile of women with chronic pelvic pain. Clin Obstet Gynecol 1990;33(1):130–6.
36. Schliep K, Stanford JB, Chen Z, Zhang B, Dorais JK, Johnstone EB, et al. Interrater and intrarater reliability in the diagnosis and staging of endometriosis. Obstet Gynecol 2012;120(1):104–12.
37. Skou ST, Graven-Nielsen T, Rasmussen S, Simonsen OH, Laursen MB, Arendt-Nielsen L. Widespread sensitization in patients with chronic pain after revision total knee arthroplasty. Pain 2013;154(9):1588–94.
38. Stearns S, Nesse RM, Govindaraju DR, Ellison PT. Evolutionary perspectives on health and medicine. Proc Natl Acad Sci USA 2010;107(Suppl. 1):1691–5.
39. Stratton P, Berkley KJ. Chronic pelvic pain and endometriosis: translational evidence of the relationship and implications. Hum Reprod Update 2011;17(3):327–46.
40. Sutton CJ, Ewen SP, Whitelaw N, Haines P. Prospective, randomized, double-blind, controlled trial of laser laparoscopy in the treatment of pelvic pain associated with minimal, mild, and moderate endometriosis. Fertil Steril 1994;62(4):696–700.

41. Sutton CJ, Pooley AS, Ewen SP, Haines P. Follow-up report on a randomized controlled trial of laser laparoscopy in the treatment of pelvic pain associated with minimal to moderate endometriosis. Fertil Steril 1997;68(6):1070-4.
42. Turk DC, Rudy TE. IASP taxonomy of chronic pain syndromes: preliminary assessment of reliability. Pain 1987;30(2):177-89.
43. Vercellini P, Bocciolone L, Vendola N, Colombo A, Rognoni MT, Fedele L. Peritoneal endometriosis. Morphologic appearance in women with chronic pelvic pain. J Reprod Med 1991;36(7):533-6.
44. Vercellini P, Crosignani PG, Abbiati A, Somigliana E, Vigano P, Fedele L. The effect of surgery for symptomatic endometriosis: the other side of the story. Hum Reprod Update 2009;15(2):177-88.
45. Woolf CJ. Central sensitization: implications for the diagnosis and treatment of pain. Pain 2011;152(3 Suppl.):S2-15.
46. Wright JT. The diagnosis and management of infiltrating nodular recto-vaginal endometriosis. Curr Opin Obstet Gynecol 2000;12(4):283-7.
47. Yong PJ, Mui J, Allaire C, Williams C. Pelvic floor tenderness in the etiology of superficial dyspareunia. J Obstet Gynaecol Can 2014;36(11):1002-9.

CHAPTER 4

Central Nervous System Effects of Damage to Visceral Tissues in Humans

Asbjørn Mohr Drewes

Information from activities in the viscera does not normally reach the higher brain centers, except that from activities such as filling of the esophagus, stomach, and rectum. When the organs are potentially in danger, for example, due to diseases, symptoms such as discomfort and pain are sensed. These symptoms are typically vague and difficult to characterize and are often quite distinct from what is felt during noxious diseases of the somatic system. The difference in the anatomical structure of the nervous system (especially at the central level) explains to major degree symptoms in visceral pain disorders, and therefore, an understanding of the central processing of visceral pain in health and disease is of major importance. Most of our basic knowledge about visceral pain processing in the central nervous system (CNS) is taken from animal experiments. Where the first general section is mainly based on basic physiologic studies, the subsequent sections will focus on imaging and electrophysiologic studies in humans. As changes in the brain during and after visceral surgery are sparsely documented in the literature, this chapter will review the most important literature exploring changes in CNS following stimulation of visceral structures and diseases.

HOW INFORMATION FROM VISCERA IS PROCESSED IN THE CENTRAL NERVOUS SYSTEM

The scope of this section is not to give a complete overview of the visceral pain system but rather to give a brief introduction into the specific characteristics of visceral pain processing in the CNS necessary to understand the subsequent sections dealing with CNS changes to visceral pain and lesions (Figure 4-1).

Enteric Nervous System and Vagal Afferents

The viscera have a complex dual innervation with both intrinsic and extrinsic sensory neurons (the latter is referred to as visceral afferents). Intrinsic afferents mainly project locally in the wall of the gut and are involved in regulation of the visceral functions, such as secretion, motility, mucosal transport, and blood flow [16]. Extrinsic afferents project to the CNS via the vagal nerve to the brainstem or through splanchnic nerves to the spinal cord [75] (Figure 4-1). Most *afferent vagal fibers* are unmyelinated C-fibers that project viscerotopically to the medial division of the nucleus of the solitary tract. Second-order neurons project to sites in the brainstem, hypothalamus, and amygdala including the vagal motor nuclei, the rostral areas of the ventrolateral medulla, and the parabrachial nuclei [72]. Cortical

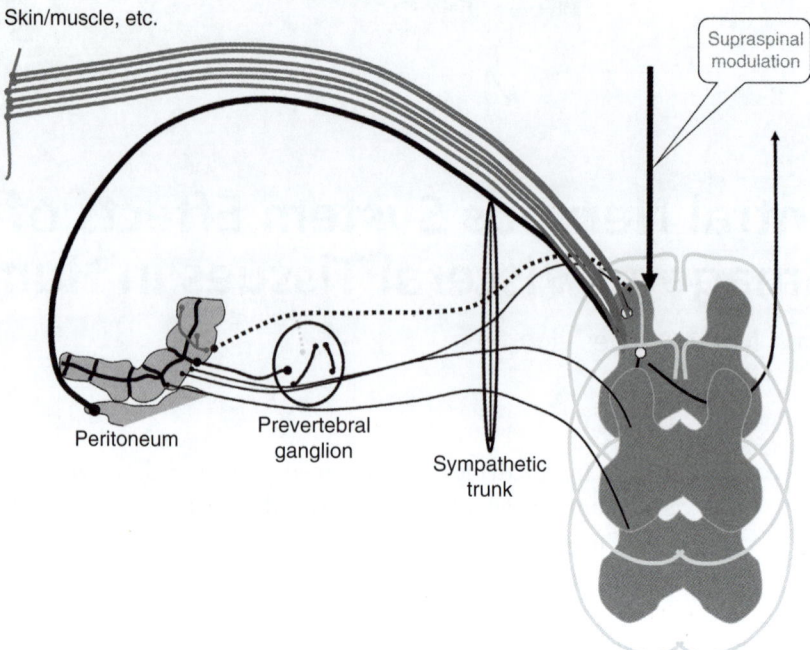

FIGURE 4-1 The afferent nerve supply of the gut. "True" visceral afferents (*thin, black*) innervate the gut, and most run temporarily together with either the sympathetic or parasympathetic nerves to enter the spinal cord. During inflammation, "silent afferents" (*dashed black line*) may become activated and contribute to the sensory response. The peritoneum and parietal serous membranes of the lungs and heart have their own parietal nerve supply (*thick, black*), which is organized like the somatic structures. The innervation of the viscera is very sparse compared with the somatic system. On the other hand, most visceral afferents converge with neurons that receive input from superficial and deep somatic tissue as well as other viscera. The diffuse and widespread innervation of the spinal cord may explain the unpleasant nature of visceral pain.

projections from these brainstem areas include the orbitofrontal cortex, infralimbic anterior cingulate cortex (ACC), and insula cortex, the latter having reciprocal connections with the secondary somatosensory cortex (SII). The vagal afferents are believed mainly to mediate nonnoxious physiologic sensations such as satiety and nausea (low-response thresholds) [3]. However, vagal afferents may be involved in the central inhibitory modulation of pain [65].

Spinal Afferents

Although other pathways such as vagus are involved, visceral pain is mainly conveyed to the spinal cord together with the sympathetic nerves. These are passing through the dorsal root ganglion and project to distinct laminae of the spinal cord dorsal horn (mainly laminae I and V and occasionally to laminae V and X). These afferent projections are organized in a somewhat segmental manner but distributed over several spinal segments in both rostral and caudal directions [44]. This diffuse spinal termination pattern may explain the poor localization of visceral sensations often seen in clinical practice [13]. From the spinal cord, pain transmits to the brain through diverse pathways. Most afferents travel in the spinothalamic tract to the thalamus. From the thalamus projections to the insula, hypothalamus, and amygdala as well as to higher cortical levels such as cingulate cortex and prefrontal cortex (PFC) have been described. Insula has an important function for integrating the visceral sensory and motor activity together with limbic integration and is particularly important in pain perception from the gut [53]. The ACC and PFC are a part of the medial pain system, which mediates the affective, emotional, and cognitive components of pain experience [83]. In addition to the spinothalamic tract, some afferents ascend in the spinoreticular tract, mediating arousal and autonomic responses through interaction with the reticular formation. Finally, a population of afferents ascends in the spinomesencephalic tract, which relates to a complex neuronal network including the periaqueductal gray, rostroventral medulla, and the dorsolateral pontine tegmentum. This network comprises the structural basis of descending pain control and possesses modulation of spinal pain processing through so-called ON- and OFF-cells in the rostroventral medulla, which are pronociceptive or antinociceptive, respectively [40].

Mechanisms Behind Referred Pain to Somatic and Visceral Structures

The fact that each segment in the spinal cord receives afferent fibers from visceral as well as somatic structures causes another phenomenon known as *referred pain*. Although simplified, referred pain originates because of convergence between visceral and somatic fibers on the same second-order neuron (for details see Refs. [4,48]). Because the brain cannot localize the precise origin of the visceral pain stimulus, it may therefore interpret the pain as originating from a somatic structure with the same segmental innervation.

Viscerovisceral hyperalgesia is a complex form of hypersensitivity probably explained by more than one mechanism. Because this phenomenon takes place between visceral organs sharing their central afferent termination, it is plausible that central sensitization play an important role [63]. Animal experiments as well as human experimental studies have shown that convergence to the same second-order neuron of afferents from different organs exists [36,69]. Also, our group has shown that after esophageal perfusion with acid and capsaicin, the referred pain areas to duodenal stimulation were increased [11,30]. Besides changes at the spinal level, changes in the cortical processing of pain may be involved in these mechanisms [68]. Viscerovisceral hyperalgesia may explain the epidemiologic findings that several clinical conditions with organic diseases show evidence of increased pain from other organs. This was recently investigated in patients suffering, among others, from coronary artery disease and gallbladder stones or inflammatory bowel disease and dysmenorrhea [6]. In these studies, coexisting visceral pain conditions with share of spinal projections between organs increased the symptoms generated from the other pain conditions. Besides, effective treatment of one condition significantly improved symptoms from the other.

Sensitization

Like in other tissues, visceral nerves are able to sensitize with major changes in the CNS. The *peripheral* nociceptor sensitization underlies the hyperalgesia that develops immediately around an injury site. Analogous to mechanisms documented in the somatic system, visceral afferent fibers may become sensitized by endogenous chemicals. This results in an increase in their responsiveness to a given stimulus and/or an increase in the spontaneous activity. In contrast to the cutaneous system, where only nociceptors sensitize, both low- and high-threshold fibers in the viscera can undergo sensitization [6,37]. This reduces the perception threshold of primary afferents and recruits previously silent nociceptors again leading to increased afferent activity to the spinal cord and exacerbation of the pain. Enhanced spinal input can activate intracellular signaling cascades within the *spinal dorsal horn neurons*. This results in an increased synaptic efficacy and is known as central sensitization. Visceral pain input to the spinal cord is more potent than cutaneous pain in the induction of central sensitization [1]. Simplified, the input leads to, e.g., activation of the *N*-methyl-D-aspartic acid (NMDA) receptor and results in changes of the resting potential of the second-order neuron. Blocking the NMDA receptor has been shown to prevent experimentally acid-induced central sensitization from esophageal afferents [82]. This effect is used clinically, where antagonism of the receptor during surgery leads to less postoperative pain [80]. Sensitization of the viscera also affects the brain processing of pain as discussed later in this chapter.

CENTRAL NERVOUS SYSTEM EFFECTS TO EXPERIMENTAL PAIN IN *HEALTHY VOLUNTEERS*

Our knowledge about human pain is, to a major degree, based on clinical studies. However, pain in patients is often blurred by other symptoms such as anxiety and cognitive consequences of the pain. Furthermore, sedative properties of some analgesics make evaluation difficult. Experimental methods to evoke and assess pain under controlled circumstances are advantageous, as they encompass many of these problems and offer a unique opportunity to investigate analgesic effects on different pain modalities arising from different tissues as well as peripheral and central pain mechanisms; for details see Refs. [5,19].

In human experimental pain models, the evoked sensations can be assessed with subjective methods quantitatively (e.g., by using a visual analogue scale) and qualitatively (e.g., by using the McGill Pain Questionnaire) and stimulus–response relationships can be investigated. Objective, physiologic responses for the pain can also be recorded with, e.g., the nociceptive reflex, cerebral evoked potentials, and imaging reflecting central changes.

Referred Pain and Viscerovisceral Hyperalgesia

Several studies have confirmed animal experiments showing that sensitization of the human gut such as with acid perfusion of the esophagus results in CNS alterations reflected in, e.g., an increase in the referred pain area as well as a lowering of the pain thresholds to stimulation of other organs. We previously showed that perfusion of the distal esophagus induced an increase in the referred pain to subsequent stimulations of the sensitized area [25]. Furthermore, Frøkjær et al. showed that acidification of the distal esophagus resulted in hypersensitivity to stimulation of very remote organs such as the rectum [30]. Such changes thought to be mainly spinal may be modality-specific and influenced by descending modulation. Hence, in a subsequent study where a more intense sensitization model was used (perfusion of the esophageal with *both* acid and capsaicin), there was rectal hyperalgesia to heat and mechanical stimulations, whereas there was hypoalgesia to electro-stimulation of both the esophagus and the sigmoid colon [11]. The sensitization may also lead to profound changes in the autonomic systems and thereby influence the brain's so-called pain matrix [77].

The Nociceptive Reflex

The connection from the primary afferents to the motor neurons is a polysynaptic *spinal pathway*, which can be modulated by other afferent input, spinal neuronal excitability, and activity in descending control systems. In the studies by Bouhassira et al. [8,9], tonic distension of the stomach and rectum resulted in inhibition of the reflex. In other studies of somatic tissues, however, painful stimuli resulted in either a decrease or an increase in reflex excitability depending on the conditioning site [2]. In a study where we distended the esophagus, no change in reflex size was present before sensitization was induced [24]. Therefore, the different stimulation sites and experimental situations may explain the discrepancies between the experiments. In our experiments of the esophagus sensitization to acid, perfusion resulted in a significant increase in the baseline reflex excitability followed by a gradual inhibition during the visceral stimulus. The initial increased excitability may be explained by the chemical stimulation resulting in increased visceral input to the spinal cord.

Imaging Studies (and Their Limitations)

Most previous reviews have focused on imaging methods, as these have many advantages. For example, functional magnetic resonance imaging (fMRI) has an excellent spatial resolution (2 to 5 mm), especially in the more superficial layers. However, as the temporal resolution ranges from a 300 ms theoretical value to a more realistic 1 to 3 seconds, there will invariably be many biases relating to nonspecific activation of centers and networks not related directly to pain. Therefore, in this chapter the focus will be on findings from electroencephalographic (EEG) studies although the most important imaging studies will also be highlighted. For a more comprehensive overview, the reader is referred to, e.g., Refs. [60,76]. Neuroimaging has mainly been based on tools such as positron emission tomography (PET), fMRI, and magnetoencephalography. Results of these studies are, despite some emerging consistencies, fairly heterogeneous. Differences are likely due to methodological differences in stimulation method (fixed stimulus intensity or titrated to individual perception threshold), imaging modality (PET vs. fMRI), and/or image processing and analysis [60]. Nevertheless, the studies have greatly improved our knowledge of the brain regions involved in visceral sensory processing by permitting the identification of the "visceral pain neuromatrix," including brainstem regions, thalamus, insular cortex, SI (primary somatosensory cortex) and SII, cingulate cortex subregions (mainly ACC and midcingulate cortex [MCC]), PFC subregions, and cerebellar areas.

Even in healthy volunteers, psychosocial context and normal psychological processes exert a profound influence on pain processing through complex reciprocal interactions between emotional and cognitive pain modulatory brain networks [60]. For example, in a study where the esophagus was distended, it was shown that a nonpainful visceral stimulus is associated with higher activation of the pain-processing areas in anterior MCC and insula when perceived in a negative emotional context [62]. In more recent studies, Coen et al. found that the reduction in pain ratings during distraction from a painful esophageal stimulus was paralleled by a reduction in neural activity in the right MCC and the PFC [14]. Experimentally induced sadness was also associated with higher activity in the right anterior MCC, insula, and PFC during painful esophageal distension but not with higher pain scores [15]. Apart from the discussion of pain specificity, the common interpretation that the signal reflects synaptic activity is also disputed. Critics refer to alternative neurobiologic accounts of the hemodynamic response, among these the removal of lactate, adjustment of the tissues acid–base or ionic balance, or temperature regulation. Furthermore, there are many technical limitations with fMRI that will not be discussed in the current chapter; for review, the reader is referred to [34,66,73]. Therefore, there is a constant search to improve the methods and try new modalities more specific for pain such as localizing networks with resting state MRI and arterial spin labeling. Structural assessment of the brain with cortex volumetric methods and diffusion tensor imaging has also improved our understanding of the pain system [34]. For example, a combination of diffusion tensor imaging and fMRI was used to investigate the anatomical relationships between areas involved in sensations to rectal distension in healthy subjects, giving insight into the neural network of visceral sensory perception with direct connections between insula and the ACC, thalamus, SI, SII, and PFC [54].

Electro- and Magnetoencephalography

Although EEG methods also have many limitations—some of them shared with fMRI—they are generally highly available, relatively easy to use, and of low cost [41,73]. The main advantage is the high temporal resolution, which allows assessment of the primary pain processing, including sequential activation and analysis of coherence and cross talk between brain centers. However, EEG has a relative poor spatial resolution even though various inverse modeling algorithms and signal decomposition procedures (see below) have overcome this limitation to some extent. Even though multichannel EEG, cerebral evoked potentials (EPs), and inverse modeling of the brain sources offer a noninvasive approach to study brain activity with time resolution on the millisecond scale, it must not be overlooked that the position of the calculated dipolar sources does not represent the accurate position but rather the "center of gravity" of brain activity. The resting EEG is typically used to study the pathophysiology of pain in chronic pain patients, whereas the EPs are used to study the nociceptive pain response including the sequential brain activation following visceral stimulations [22]. Taken together, spontaneous EEG and EPs provide complimentary information about the modulation of CNS after painful stimuli.

In spite of the chaotic nature of the signals, it has been shown that the resting stage EEG oscillates in certain frequency bands associated with specific brain functions such as pain perception and attention to pain. EEG changes to experimental pain have been described in several studies of somatic tissues, but no studies were carried out in volunteers to experimental visceral pain. In contrast to the spontaneous EEG, the EP presents the time-locked response to an external stimulus. As this response is highly influenced by the sequential activation of distinct brain centers, the morphology of the EP is different from the spontaneous EEG (Figure 4-2). The EP is characterized by several peaks of both negative and positive polarity and may be quantified by the peak amplitudes and latencies. Although simplified the amplitudes represent the number of synchronous activated neurons, whereas the latency represents the delay in activation due to corticocortical connections.

Multichannel EEG recordings combined with inverse modeling can determine the location of brain centers underlying EPs. This method possesses the opportunity to study pain-specific cortical activation dynamically, as it reflects the sequential activation of neuronal pain networks underlying the EPs. There are a number of commercial software and freeware packages available for inverse modeling (Figure 4-3). However, one of the major limitations with inverse modeling has been the instability of algorithms to model several

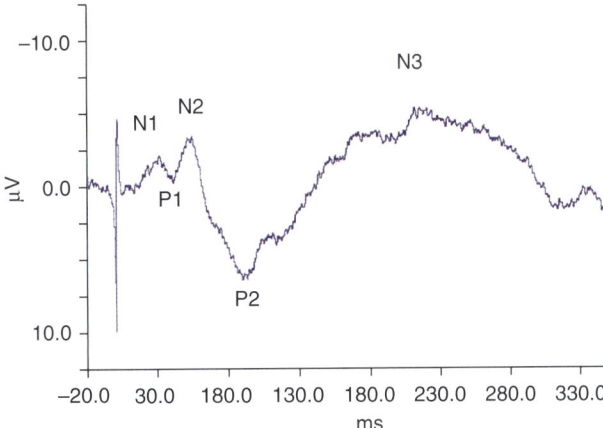

FIGURE 4-2 A typical evoked potential (vertex electrode, average of 40 electrical stimuli) recorded after stimulation of the rectosigmoid junction in a patient with chronic pancreatitis. The different peaks are denoted N1, P1, N2, and P2, each defined by latency (ms) and amplitude (μV).

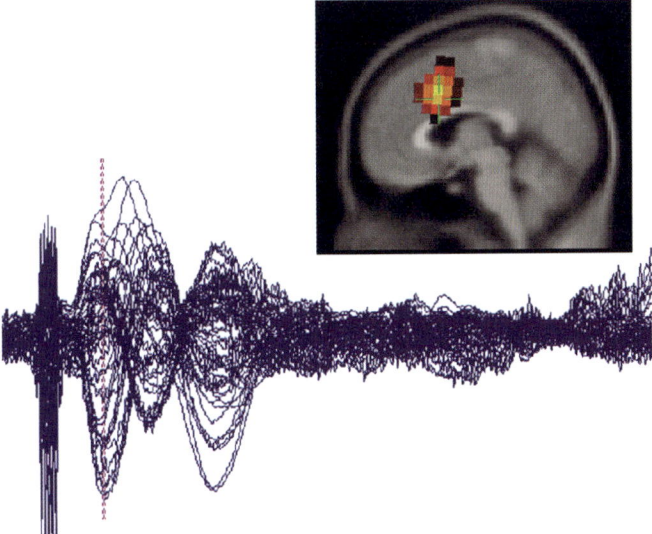

FIGURE 4-3 Source localization using a current density method called LORETA (low-resolution electromagnetic tomographic analysis). The volunteer studied in this figure was stimulated at the pain threshold 30 times at 5 Hz in the esophagus while EEG was recorded. Bottom of the figure represents the evoked potential signal of 62 electrodes superimposed on each other. The *red, dotted vertical line* represents the peak under analysis. Top of the figure: LORETA solution around cingulate cortex.

simultaneously active sources and sources in deep brain structures such as thalamus or brainstem. To bypass these problems, signal decomposition methods have been developed to separate the signal into a sum of waveforms, whereby signals corresponding to specific evoked brain activity can be separated from artifacts and noise. Some of the most common approaches for signal decomposition are blind source separation algorithms such as independent component analysis and second-order blind identification. We have successfully used signal decomposition with independent component analysis to study sequential brain activation and cross talk between brain centers following electrical stimulation of the esophagus in healthy controls [23]. Recently, multichannel matching pursuit was introduced, which decomposes the EP data into a sum of waveforms (usually termed atoms), each of them being defined in time, frequency, and space. Inverse modeling on these atoms is superior to inverse modeling on instantaneous EP data and other signal decomposition methods [52]. For a short review, the reader is referred to [34].

Evoked potentials have been used to explore the pain matrix following experimental visceral pain in healthy volunteers. For example, we modeled the brain sources of EPs to electrical stimulation of the upper gut and sigmoid colon, and these were explained by bilateral brain sources in the SII and insular cortices and a single dipole in the ACC [18]. Interestingly, a viscerotopic organization of the different gut segments was seen, thus revealing a "visceral homunculus" mimicking that seen for the somatic sensory system. Acid sensitization of the esophagus has been shown to cause neuroplastic changes at the spinal cord level reflected in increased referred pain areas and amplitude of the nociceptive withdrawal reflex [24,25]. Sarker et al. used stimulation of a proximal region of the esophagus in healthy volunteers (apart from the distal acid exposure) and found a decrease in latency of the N1 and P2 components in the vertex recordings [70]. In a subsequent experiment where we stimulated the acid perfused area in the lower esophagus, we also found a reduction of P2 latency, and using inverse modeling, a posterior shift and latency reduction of the ACC dipole was seen [68]. Short-term sensitization of the esophagus therefore results in central neuroplastic changes involving, e.g., the cingulate gyrus, which has in many studies in functional diseases of the gut shown pathologic activation, thus reflecting the importance of this region in visceral pain and hyperalgesia. Hence, experimental pain and sensitization in healthy volunteers are able to induce rather profound changes in the way pain is sequentially processed in the brain. The stability and temporal resolution of the EPs and source modeling validate their use in patient studies; however, advanced inverse modeling is still restricted to expert use.

Magnetoencephalography has been extensively used for investigation of the superficial brain areas where their neuronal columns result in equivalent current dipoles with a marked tangential direction, the magnetic fields of which are optimal for the measurement. In visceral pain the use of magnetoencephalography has been limited. Hobson et al. used the technique to determine the sequential brain activation following esophageal electrical stimulation in healthy volunteers [42]. They found the earliest cortical activities in the SI and SII cortices and posterior insula, followed by later activities in the anterior part of insula and cingulate cortex. The excellent spatial and temporal resolution warrants further studies in patients with visceral pain disorders, but the technically demanding technique is only available in few specialist centers.

CENTRAL NERVOUS SYSTEM EFFECTS TO SURGERY AND CLINICAL VISCERAL PAIN

Acute Clinical Pain

Several studies have explored the CNS effects following acute clinical pain. Giamberardino et al. investigated a series of patients with symptomatic renal/ureteral calculosis and found that pain thresholds to electrical stimulation were found to be significantly lower than normal in the referred pain area in the deep tissues. For overview, see Ref. [38]. Later they investigated patients treated with extracorporeal shock wave lithotripsy. They found that in the cutaneous, subcutaneous, and muscular tissue, the hyperalgesia in the lumbar region of the affected side decreased after treatment reflecting reversal of central sensitization [39]. We took this further to look at patients with acute appendicitis and acute cholecystitis and found hyperalgesia in the somatic referred pain area but not in the control area [78,79].

The central changes may also lead to trophic alterations in the deep tissues as shown by the Italian group [70]. However, in a recent study using both ultrasound and computerized tomography in patients with renal stones, we were not able to reproduce these findings, which therefore awaits further studies [61]. To the author's knowledge, no imaging or electrophysiologic studies have been performed in acute visceral pain patients.

Peri- and Postoperative Pain

It has been speculated whether CNS plasticity as reflected in changes in the referred pain areas is a permanent phenomenon or whether it can reverse. In a study from our group, 40 patients were tested with quantitative sensory testing in the referred pain area and in a control area on the contralateral side of the abdomen before and 2 to 7 years after laparoscopic cholecystectomy. The initial hypersensitivity returned to normal in the follow-up period, and also in the five patients with postcholecystectomy syndrome, there were no differences [47]. Hence, the neuroplastic changes seen before surgery [78] seem to disappear after successful surgery. Likely the minimal invasive procedures, etc., are responsible for the findings. Finally, Pedersen et al. [61] studying patients with painful stones in the renal pelvis found that after the operation, there was a tendency toward increase in the pain thresholds for both single and repeated electrical stimuli on the affected flank. On the other hand, the pain thresholds on the contralateral (control) site were unaltered after surgery. Although the studies only indirectly reflect CNS changes after surgery, they call for further direct studies of the brain to verify the changes.

The EEG is extensively used to follow the depth of anesthesia. Recently Lee et al. used the EEG during surgery to measure directional connectivity across frontal and parietal regions [50]. They found that diverse anesthetics disrupted the frontal–parietal communication despite major differences in the molecular composition of the drugs. Even though this study did not examine the effect of visceral pain during surgery, the methods may pave the road for studies of the gut–brain axis during surgery.

Chronic Clinical Pain

Several studies have reported findings compatible with central sensitization in patients with functional and organic disorders. As stated previously, patterns of *referred pain* can be examined to assess central sensitization, as viscerasomatic convergence between peripheral nerves occurs at the spinal cord and higher levels of the CNS. Increased and abnormal referred pain areas were seen in patients with functional chest pain and functional dyspepsia. Furthermore, patients with erosive esophagitis had increased referred pain areas selective to heat stimulation, a finding that likely reflects sensitization afferents with transient receptor potential cation channel receptors [20]. Similarly, in chronic pancreatitis patients, increased areas of referred pain to electrical stimulation of the esophagus, stomach, and duodenum were reported as compared with controls [17]. Other studies in these patients reported decreased pain thresholds to visceral stimulation of the rectosigmoid as well as somatic stimulation of muscle and bone [12,56]. Taken together, these findings characterize a generalized hyperalgesic state and likely mirrors widespread sensitization of the CNS.

A variety of studies have used *imaging techniques* to explore the brain in patients with chronic pain. Most of these have studied patients with functional visceral pain disorders such as irritable bowel syndrome (IBS). Only a few will be highlighted here. Kwan et al. identified abnormal event-related sensations in five brain regions following rectal distensions in IBS [49]. In the SI, urge-related responses to rectal distension in the IBS group were seen compared with the control group. This could be interpreted as upregulated afferent input underlying visceral hypersensitivity. In the IBS group pain-related responses were seen in the medial thalamus and hippocampus. However, pronounced urge- and pain-related activations were present in the right anterior insula and the right ACC in the control group but not the IBS group. Finally, lack of activation in right anterior insula was found in IBS patients, interpreted by the authors as either a ceiling effect or a dysfunction in interoceptive processing or control of visceromotor responses. In a similar study, Bonaz et al. demonstrated significant deactivations within the right insula, the right amygdala, and the right striatum following rectal stimulations in patients suffering from IBS [7]. Cortex volumetric studies further showed decreased gray matter density in IBS patients in widespread areas of the brain, including PFC, posterior parietal cortex, ventral striatum, and thalamus [74]. Furthermore, increased gray matter density was seen in IBS in the pregenual ACC and the orbitofrontal cortex. These changes in density of gray matter in regions involved in cognitive/evaluative functions are specifically observed in patients with IBS, indicating neuroplastic changes. fMRI can also be used to study dynamic changes. In an elegant study, Wilder-Smith et al. studied brain activation changes to distension of the rectum during heterotopic stimulation (to investigate descending control systems) and found that the brain areas in the limbic system and brainstem responded differently between control subjects and IBS patients with predominant diarrhea and constipation reflecting differences in endogenous pain inhibitory mechanisms [81].

The brain was also investigated in *organic visceral diseases* such as chronic pancreatitis. Using diffusion tensor imaging, we found structural changes in several regions of the "pain matrix," and these were related to the pain pattern [33]. In another study in this patient group, brain areas known to be essential in pain processing show reduced cortical thickness, with a positive correlation to diary pain scores [31] (Figure 4-4). It was concluded that the structural findings were likely a result of long-standing pain input to the neuromatrix as also seen in other diseases characterized by chronic pain. Finally, in patients with autonomic neuropathy and affection of the visceral nerves due to diabetes, we found several microstructural changes that were for some areas correlated to clinical parameters such as bloating and autonomic function based on electrocardiographic results [29] (Figure 4-4).

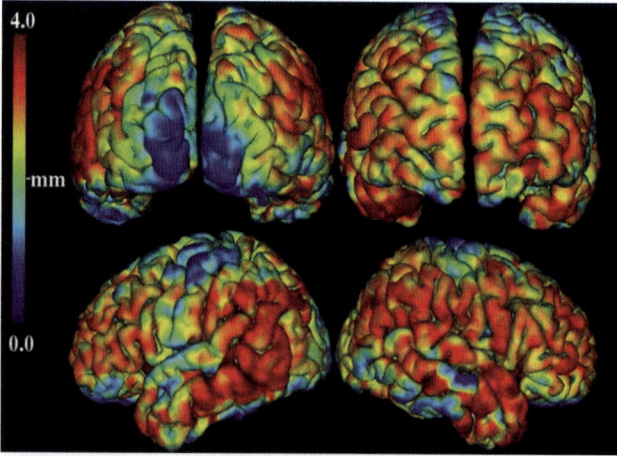

FIGURE 4-4 Example of cortical thickness distribution using Fast Accurate Cortical Extraction (FACE) in a patient with chronic pancreatitis. The *color bar* denotes the relative thickness. For details see Ref. [64].

Imaging can also be used to explore the *brain metabolism* in the brain at the metabolic level. A recent pilot study using PET looked at the binding of the neurokinin-1 receptor (the target for substance P) in the brain in nine patients with inflammatory bowel disease, nine with IBS, and nine healthy subjects [45]. Patients with inflammatory bowel disease had neurokinin-1 receptor deficits across a widespread network of cortical and subcortical regions, whereas patients with IBS had similar but less pronounced deficits. Interestingly, these deficits were related to different clinical parameters such as disease severity and duration as well as pain thresholds in each patient population.

Electrophysiology

The resting EEG is typically used to study the pathophysiology of pain in chronic pain patients, whereas the EPs are used to study the nociceptive pain response including the sequential brain activation following gastrointestinal (GI) stimulations [57]. The *resting EEG* frequency bands are typically defined as delta (up to 4 Hz), theta (4 to 8 Hz), alpha (8 to 12 Hz), beta (12 to 30 Hz), and gamma (above 30 Hz). Few studies have looked at resting EEG in visceral diseases. We showed that patients with chronic pancreatitis had slowed EEG rhythmicity (as evident in the theta and alpha bands) [71]. This has previously been observed in patients with neuropathic pain of mixed origin and possibly mirrors abnormal central pain processing. The present method could be used to assist clinicians in establishing optimal pain treatment indications in patients with pain due to chronic pancreatitis. The resting EEG has recently also been evaluated in patients with functional chest pain of presumed esophageal origin [43]. However, in this study of very well characterized patients, no differences were seen in comparison with controls.

Evoked brain potentials can be analyzed either as single sweeps or after an average process. The single-sweep analysis enables an evaluation of both synchronized and unsynchronized brain activity relative to the stimulus, which may provide additional information on abnormal pain processing in some patients. The average process is performed over multiple stimuli, which improve the signal-to-noise ratio, thereby revealing less prominent peaks. Several studies have explored the EPs in functional and organic diseases. Patients with functional chest pain have also been extensively evaluated. For example, in patients with IBS, we found decreased latency and reduced amplitude of the first positive peak of the EPs to painful stimuli of the gut [67]. EPs were also used to investigate patients with functional chest pain where reduced latencies to painful electrical stimuli in the esophagus and the sternal skin were found [28]. Hobson and Aziz were later able to demonstrate that the EP response may subdivide patients with functional chest burn into those with either sensitization or hypervigilance [41]. However, in a recent study, we were not able to confirm these findings [43].

Patients with organic diseases have also been investigated with EPs. In painful chronic pancreatitis, decreased latencies of the early EP components were found, which is thought to reflect changes in exogenous pain processing [17]. Finally, in diabetes patients with autonomic neuropathy and GI symptoms, there were increased latencies and reduced amplitudes of most peaks in the EP in response to esophageal stimulations [35]. Overall these patient studies indicate differences in pain processing, which could be explained by a possible functional reorganization of the central nervous pathways.

Inverse Modeling of the Electrical Sources

The location of brain centers have been investigated more specifically in visceral pain disorders. In IBS patients, the ACC dipole following painful electrical stimulation of the sigmoid colon showed a more posterior position in patients than in control subjects [21]. This finding suggests that the cortical representations of painful stimuli are altered in IBS patients possibly because of reorganization of the cortical areas involved in visceral pain processing that mimics the reorganization seen in healthy volunteers after experimental sensitization [68]. Along this line, patients with chronic pancreatitis show reorganization of the brain areas involved in visceral pain processing including the insula, SII, and cingulate cortex following upper gut stimulations [17]. Interestingly, in a subsequent investigation the insular reorganization was associated with clinical pain intensity [57]. As the upper gut and pancreas share afferent neuronal pathways, these findings likely represent a reorganization of the visceral cortical projections induced by recurrent pain attacks due to pancreatitis. This parallels findings from somatic neuropathic pain studies where reorganization of the cortical pain matrix has been commonly reported [26]. In addition to reorganization of the brain areas involved in visceral pain processing, the excitability of these neural networks is abnormal in patients with chronic pancreatitis with evidence of impaired habituation to noxious stimuli, possibly reflecting a neuronal hyperexcitability (i.e., cortical sensitization) [59]. In favor of the latter, a recent pilot project documented generalized hyperalgesia (a clinical measurable proxy of central sensitization) to be associated with failure of thoracoscopic splanchnic denervation [10]. The authors concluded that in patients with hyperalgesia and failure to denervation, the disease has advanced and the generation of pain becomes self-perpetuating and independent of the initial peripheral nociceptive drive. However, these findings need confirmation in larger and longitudinal studies. Finally, in a study of diabetes patients with autonomic neuropathy and GI symptoms, patients had a posterior shift of the ACC dipole and additional sources close to the posterior insula and medial frontal gyrus, indicating that central neuronal reorganization may contribute to our understanding of the symptoms in these patients [32].

As stated previously, one of the major limitations with inverse modeling has been the instability of algorithms to model several simultaneously active sources and sources in deep brain structures such as thalamus or brainstem. Recently, we used multichannel matching pursuit to identify functional networks associated with brain reorganization following diabetes with GI symptoms [51], but the methods need to be used in patients with restricted visceral disorders.

THE CENTRAL NERVOUS SYSTEM RESPONSE TO TREATMENT OF VISCERAL DISEASES

Finally, imaging and electrophysiologic studies have also been used to explore the neural response to treatment with analgesics, and this may lead to increased understanding on how the brain responds to medical treatment and in selection of treatment responders. This is a very important aspect to understand as the brains response to surgery and diseases of the internal organs may be changed in a similar way, but word limitations of this chapter do not allow further discussion, and the reader is referred to, e.g., Refs. [55–58]. Neuromodulation such as with spinal cord stimulation and transcranial magnetic stimulation has been also been used successfully in treatment of visceral pain [27,46]. This also shows that the central changes as outlined earlier may be modified with proper treatment directed at the brain.

CONCLUSION

Even though there has been a tremendous development in the methods for electrophysiological assessment and imaging the CNS effects following damage to visceral tissues in humans, it should be kept in mind that all of these methods are not direct measures of brain activity and will never be able to assess the true neuronal activity and pathophysiologic mechanisms. However, as outlined in this chapter, development in hardware, computer power, and postprocessing is still ongoing. This allows high-quality data and new ways to interpret the results. Furthermore, the multimodal combinations of methods using the advantages of each single technique will likely in the future bring us closer to true events in the brain in visceral diseases. The future aims are to identify still better and more specific biomarkers for abnormal processing of sensory input underlying the pain and suffering in patients groups, eventually to identify different subgroups with different etiology, and to give directions for the development and testing of new treatment options with benefit for individuals and society.

REFERENCES

1. Anand P, Aziz Q, Willert R, et al. Peripheral and central mechanisms of visceral sensitization in man. Neuro Gastroenterol Motil 2007;19:29–46.
2. Andersen OK, Graven-Nielsen T, Matre D, et al. Interaction between cutaneous and muscle afferent activity in polysynaptic reflex pathways: a human experimental study. Pain 2000;84:29–36.
3. Andrews PL, Sanger GJ. Abdominal vagal afferent neurons: an important target for the treatment of gastrointestinal dysfunction. Curr Opin Pharmacol 2002;2:650–6.
4. Arendt-Nielsen L, Laursen RJ, Drewes AM. Referred pain as an indicator for neural plasticity. Prog Brain Res 2000;129:343–56.
5. Arendt-Nielsen L, Yarnitsky D. Experimental and clinical applications of quantitative sensory testing applied to skin, muscles and viscera. J Pain 2009;10:556–72.
6. Bielefeldt K, Christianson JA, Davis BM. Basic and clinical aspects of visceral sensation: transmission in the CNS. Neuro Gastroenterol Motil 2005;17:488–99.
7. Bonaz B, Baciu M, Papillon E, et al. Central processing of rectal pain in patients with irritable bowel syndrome: an fMRI study. Am J Gastroenterol 2002;97:654–61.
8. Bouhassira D, Chollet R, Coffin B, et al. Inhibition of a somatic nociceptive reflex by gastric distention in humans. Gastroenterology 1994;107:985–92.
9. Bouhassira D, Sabate JM, Coffin B, et al. Effects of rectal distensions on nociceptive flexion reflexes in humans. Am J Physiol 1998:275:G410–7.
10. Bouwense SA, Buscher HC, van Goor H, Wilder-Smith OH. Has central sensitization become independent of nociceptive input in chronic pancreatitis patients who fail thoracoscopic splanchnicectomy? Reg Anesth Pain Med 2011;36:531–6.
11. Brock C, Andresen T, Frokjaer JB, et al. Central pain mechanisms following combined acid and capsaicin perfusion of the human oesophagus. Eur J Pain 2010;14:273–81.
12. Buscher HC, Wilder-Smith OH, van Goor H. Chronic pancreatitis patients show hyperalgesia of central origin: a pilot study. Eur J Pain 2006;10:363–70.
13. Cervero F, Connell LA, Lawson SN. Somatic and visceral primary afferents in the lower thoracic dorsal root ganglia of the cat. J Comp Neurol 1984;228:422–31.
14. Coen SJ, Aziz Q, Yaguez L, et al. Effects of attention on visceral stimulus intensity encoding in the male human brain. Gastroenterology 2008;135:2065–74.
15. Coen SJ, Yaguez L, Aziz Q, et al. Negative mood affects brain processing of visceral sensation. Gastroenterology 2009;137:253–61.
16. Costa M, Brookes SJ. The enteric nervous system. Am J Gastroenterol 1994;89(8 Suppl.):129–37.
17. Dimcevski G, Sami SA, Funch-Jensen P, et al. Pain in chronic pancreatitis: the role of reorganization in the central nervous system. Gastroenterology 2007;132:1546–56.
18. Drewes AM, Dimcevski G, Sami SA, et al. The "human visceral homunculus" to pain evoked in the oesophagus, stomach, duodenum and sigmoid colon. Exp Brain Res 2006;174:443–52.

19. Drewes AM, Gregersen H, Arendt-Nielsen L. Experimental pain in gastroenterology: a reappraisal of human studies. Scand J Gastroenterol 2003;38:1115–30.
20. Drewes AM, Reddy H, Pedersen J, et al. Multimodal pain stimulations in patients with grade B oesophagitis. Gut 2006;55:926–32.
21. Drewes AM, Rossel P, Le Pera D, et al. Cortical neuroplastic changes to painful colon stimulation in patients with irritable bowel syndrome. Neurosci Lett 2005;375:157–61.
22. Drewes AM, Rossel P, Le PD, et al. Dipolar source modelling of brain potentials evoked by painful electrical stimulation of the human sigmoid colon. Neurosci Lett 2004;358:45–8.
23. Drewes AM, Sami SA, Dimcevski G, et al. Cerebral processing of painful oesophageal stimulation: a study based on independent component analysis of the EEG. Gut 2006;55:619–29.
24. Drewes AM, Schipper KP, Dimcevski G, et al. Multimodal assessment of pain in the esophagus: a new experimental model. Am J Physiol Gastrointest Liver Physiol 2002;283:G95103.
25. Drewes AM, Schipper KP, Dimcevski G, et al. Multi-modal induction and assessment of allodynia and hyperalgesia in the human oesophagus. Eur J Pain 2003;7:81–91.
26. Flor H, Elbert T, Knecht S, et al. Phantom-limb pain as a perceptual correlate of cortical reorganization following arm amputation. Nature 1995;375:482–4.
27. Fregni F, Potvin K, Dasilva D, et al. Clinical effects and brain metabolic correlates in non-invasive cortical neuromodulation for visceral pain. Eur J Pain 2011;15:53–60.
28. Frøbert O, Arendt-Nielsen L, Bak P, et al. Pain perception and brain evoked potentials in patients with angina despite normal coronary angiograms. Heart 1996;75:436–41.
29. Frøkjær JB, Andersen LW, Brock C, et al. Altered brain microstructure assessed by diffusion tensor imaging in patients with diabetes mellitus and gastrointestinal symptoms. Diabetes Care 2013;36(3):662–8.
30. Frøkjaer JB, Andersen SD, Gale J, et al. An experimental study of viscero-visceral hyperalgesia using an ultrasound-based multimodal sensory testing approach. Pain 2005;119:191–200.
31. Frøkjær JB, Bouwense SAW, Olesen SS, et al. Reduce cortical thickness of brain areas involved in pain processing in patients with chronic pancreatitis. Clin Gastroenterol Hepatol 2012;10:434–8.
32. Frøkjaer JB, Egsgaard LL, Graversen C, et al. Gastrointestinal symptoms in type-1 diabetes: is it all about brain plasticity? Eur J Pain. 2011;5:249–57.
33. Frøkjær JB, Olesen SS, Gram M, et al. Altered brain microstructure assessed by diffusion tensor imaging in patients with chronic pancreatitis. Gut 2011;6011:1554–62.
34. Frøkjær JB, Olesen SS, Graversen C, et al. Neuroimaging of the human visceral pain system – a methodological review. Scand J Pain 2011;2:95–104.
35. Frøkjaer JB, Softeland E, Graversen C, et al. Central processing of gut pain in diabetic patients with gastrointestinal symptoms. Diabetes Care 2009;32:1274–7.
36. Garrison DW, Chandler MJ, Foreman RD. Viscerosomatic convergence onto feline spinal neurons from esophagus, heart and somatic fields: effects of inflammation. Pain 1992;49:373–82.
37. Gebhart GF. Visceral pain-peripheral sensitisation. Gut 2000;47(Suppl. 4):iv54–5.
38. Giamberardino MA. Recent and forgotten aspects of visceral pain. Eur J Pain 1999;3:77–92.
39. Giamberardino MA, Bigontina P, Martegiani C, Vecchiet L. Effects of extracorporeal shock-wave lithotripsy on referred hyperalgesia from renal/ureteral calculosis. Pain 1994;56:77–83.
40. Heinricher MM, Tavares I, Leith JL, Lumb BM. Descending control of nociception: specificity, recruitment and plasticity. Brain Res Rev 2009;60:214–25.
41. Hobson AR, Furlong PL, Sarkar S, et al. Neurophysiologic assessment of esophageal sensory processing in noncardiac chest pain. Gastroenterology 2006;130:80–8.
42. Hobson AR, Furlong PL, Worthen SF, et al. Real-time imaging of human cortical activity evoked by painful esophageal stimulation. Gastroenterology 2005;128:610–9.
43. Hoff DA, Krarup AL, Lelic D, et al. Central response to painful electrical esophageal stimulation in well-defined patients suffering from functional chest pain. Neuro Gastroenterol Motil 2013;25:(11)e718–27.
44. Janig W. Neurobiology of visceral afferent neurons: neuroanatomy, functions, organ regulations and sensations. Biol Psychol 1996;42:29–51.
45. Jarcho JM, Feier NA, Bert A, et al. Diminished neurokinin-1 receptor availability in patients with two forms of chronic visceral pain. Pain 2013;154;987–96.
46. Kapural L, Cywinski JB, Sparks DA. Spinal cord stimulation for visceral pain from chronic pancreatitis. Neuromodulation 2011;14:423–6.
47. Kjær DW, Stawowy M, Arendt-Nielsen L, et al. Reversibility of central neuronal changes in patients recovering from gallbladder stones or acute cholecystitis. World J Gastroenterol 2006;12:7522–6.
48. Knowles CH, Aziz Q. Basic and clinical aspects of gastrointestinal pain. Pain 2009;141:191–209.

49. Kwan CL, Diamant NE, Mikula K, Davis KD. Characteristics of rectal perception are altered in irritable bowel syndrome. Pain 2005;113:160–71.
50. Lee U, Ku S, Noh G, et al. Disruption of frontal–parietal communication by ketamine, propofol, and sevoflurane. Anaesthesiology 2013;118:1264–75.
51. Lelic D, Brock C, Simrén M, et al. Brain networks encoding rectal sensation in type 1 diabetes. Neuroscience 2013;237:96–105.
52. Lelic D, Gratkowski M, Valeriani M, et al. Inverse modeling on decomposed electroencephalographic data: a way forward? J Clin Neurophysiol 2009;26:227–35.
53. Mayer EA, Aziz Q, Coen S, et al. Brain imaging approaches to the study of functional GI disorders: a Rome working team report. Neuro Gastroenterol Motil 2009;21:579–96.
54. Moisset X, Bouhassira D, Denis D, et al. Anatomical connections between brain areas activated during rectal distension in healthy volunteers: a visceral pain network. Eur J Pain 2010;14:142–8.
55. Morgan V, Pickens D, Gautam S, et al. Amitriptyline reduces rectal pain related activation of the anterior cingulate cortex in patients with irritable bowel syndrome. Gut 2005;54:601–7.
56. Olesen SS, Brock C, Krarup AL, et al. Descending inhibitory pain modulation is impaired in patients with chronic pancreatitis. Clin Gastroenterol Hepatol 2010;8:724–30.
57. Olesen SS, Frøkjær JB, Lelic D, et al. Adaptive cortical reorganization to pain in chronic pancreatitis. Pancreatology 2011;10:742–51.
58. Olesen SS, Graversen C, Olesen AE, et al. Randomized clinical trial: pregabalin attenuates experimental visceral pain through sub-cortical mechanisms in patients with painful chronic pancreatitis. Aliment Pharmacol Ther 2011;34:878–87.
59. Olesen SS, Hansen TM, Graversen C, et al. Cerebral excitability is abnormal in patients with painful chronic pancreatitis. Eur J Pain 2013;17:46–54.
60. Oudenhove LV. Understanding gut-brain interactions in gastrointestinal pain by neuroimaging: lessons from somatic pain studies. Neuro Gastroenterol Motil 2011;23:292–302.
61. Pedersen KV, Drewes AM, Graumann O, et al. Somatosensory and trophic findings in the referred pain area in Patients with kidney stone disease. Scand J Pain 2013;4(3):165–70.
62. Phillips M, Gregory L, Cullen S, et al. The effect of negative emotional context on neural and behavioural responses to oesophageal stimulation. Brain 2003;126:669–84.
63. Qin C, Malykhina AP, Akbarali HI, et al. Cross-organ sensitization of lumbosacral spinal neurons receiving urinary bladder input in rats with inflamed colon. Gastroenterology 2005;129:1967–78.
64. Randich A, Ren K, Gebhart GF. Electrical stimulation of cervical vagal afferents. II. Central relays for behavioral antinociception and arterial blood pressure decreases. J Neurophysiol 1990;64:1115–24.
65. Ren K, Randich A, Gebhart GF. Effects of electrical stimulation of vagal afferents on spinothalamic tract cells in the rat. Pain 1991;44:311–9.
66. Robinson ME, Staud R, Price DD. Pain measurement and brain activity: will neuroimages replace pain ratings? J Pain 2013;14:323–7.
67. Rossel P, Pedersen P, Niddam D, et al. Cerebral response to electric stimulation of the colon and abdominal skin in healthy subjects and patients with irritable bowel syndrome. Scand J Gastroenterol 2001;36:1259–66.
68. Sami SA, Rossel P, Dimcevski G, et al. Cortical changes to experimental sensitization of the human esophagus. Neuroscience 2006;140:269–79.
69. Sarkar S, Aziz Q, Woolf CJ, et al. Contribution of central sensitisation to the development of non-cardiac chest pain. Lancet 2000;356:1154–9.
70. Sarkar S, Hobson AR, Furlong PL, et al. Central neural mechanisms mediating human visceral hypersensitivity. Am J Physiol Gastrointest Liver Physiol 2001;281:G1196–202.
71. Sarnthein J, Stern J, Aufenberg C, et al. Increased EEG power and slowed dominant frequency in patients with neurogenic pain. Brain 2006;129:55–64.
72. Sawchenko PE. Central connections of the sensory and motor nuclei of the vagus nerve. J Auton Nerv Syst 1983;9:13–26.
73. Schleim S, Roiser JP. fMRI in translation: the challenges facing real-world applications. Front Hum Neurosci 2009;63:1–7.
74. Seminowicz DA, Labus JS, Bueller JA, et al. Regional gray matter density changes in brains of patients with irritable bowel syndrome. Gastroenterology 2010;139:48–57.
75. Sengupta JN, Gebhart GF. Gastrointestinal afferent fibers and sensation. In: Johnson L, editor. Physiology of the gastrointestinal tract. New York: Raven Press; 1994. p. 483–519.
76. Sharma A, Lelic D, Brock C, et al. New technologies to investigate the brain-gut axis. World J Gastroenterol 2009;15:182–91.

77. Sharma A, Paine P, Rhodes S, et al. The autonomic response to human esophageal acidification and the development of hyperalgesia. Neuro Gastroenterol Motil 2012;24:285–93.
78. Stawowy M, Bluhme C, Arendt-Nielsen L, et al. Somatosensory changes in the referred pain area in patients with acute cholecystitis before and after treatment with laparoscopic or open cholecystectomy. Scand J Gastroenterol 2004;39:988–93.
79. Stawowy M, Rössel P, Bluhme C, et al. Somatosensory changes in the referred pain area following acute inflammation of the appendix. Eur J Gastroenterol Hepatol 2002;14:1–6.
80. Vadivelu N, Mitra S, Narayan D. Recent advances in postoperative pain management. Yale J Biol Med 2010;83:11–25.
81. Wilder-Smith CH, Schindler D, Lovblad K, et al. Brain functional magnetic resonance imaging of rectal pain and activation of endogenous inhibitory mechanisms in irritable bowel syndrome patient subgroups and healthy controls. Gut 2004;53:1595–601.
82. Willert RP, Woolf CJ, Hobson AR, et al. The development and maintenance of human visceral pain hypersensitivity is dependent on the N-methyl-D-aspartate receptor. Gastroenterology 2004;126:683–92.
83. Willis WD, Westlund KN. Neuroanatomy of the pain system and of the pathways that modulate pain. J Clin Neurophysiol 1997;14:2–31.

SECTION 2

Researching Integration: Systems Effects of Ongoing Nociception

CHAPTER 5

Descending Control Mechanisms and Persistent Pain after Surgery

Mary M. Heinricher

The attention of investigators interested in the neural basis of postoperative pain has been focused primarily on understanding the responses of primary afferent neurons to a surgical insult and how the responsiveness of those neurons changes over time after surgery. This line of investigation provides critical information about the sensory information that is reaching the central nervous system, which is an important component of acute and persistent postsurgical pain. However, sensory input cannot be the whole story. The thesis of the present chapter is that changes in intrinsic *brainstem modulatory systems* also contribute to persistent pain after surgery. There is now overwhelming evidence from studies in preclinical models of inflammatory and neuropathic pain that persistent pain states are driven, at least in part, by changes in modulatory systems [23,29]. Descending modulatory pathways are known to mediate top-down regulation of nociceptive processing, conveying cortical and limbic influences to the dorsal horn. They are also intimately intertwined with ascending transmission pathways in control loops that exert both positive and negative feedback. Any model of persistent pain that fails to include descending modulatory pathways is thus incomplete. The present chapter will consider the role of these systems in descending control and specifically how that might apply in the context of pain after surgery.

A host of studies have attempted to identify predictors of postoperative pain and whether acute postoperative pain is likely to persist [2,3,14,34,39,45,46,49,58,71]. One set of predictors, which might be described as "bottom-up" factors, centers around acute pain sensitivity and can include the response to painful test stimuli, preexisting pain, or severe pain in the early postoperative period. However, "top-down" cognitive and emotional factors appear to be equally or even more important. For example, anxiety and other psychological constructs, such as hypervigilance and pain catastrophizing, have been shown to predict a significant proportion of persistent pain, as do measures of "conditioned pain modulation" [46,55,88].

How are these predictors instantiated in the nervous system? Although the well-documented plasticity in nociceptive primary afferents and ascending transmission pathways likely explains some of the influence of acute pain severity on the development of persistent pain [10,83], this cannot account for the contribution of cognitive and emotional factors. One place where bottom-up and top-down influences converge is within the descending modulatory system, which has critical links in the midbrain periaqueductal gray and rostral ventromedial medulla (RVM, Figure 5-1). The physiology and function of the RVM are much better understood than those of the periaqueductal gray, particularly in the context of facilitated pain. The RVM is also the final output of a complex supraspinal network, of which the periaqueductal gray is one component. The focus of this chapter will therefore be on the RVM.

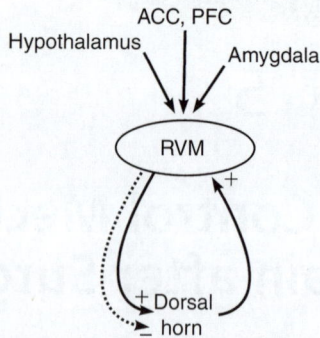

FIGURE 5-1 Convergence of bottom-up and top-down factors at the rostral ventromedial medulla (RVM). The RVM receives information from the dorsal horn about peripheral input and from higher structures such as hypothalamus, amygdala, and anterior cingulate cortex (ACC) and prefrontal cortex (PFC), through direct and indirect (e.g., via the periaqueductal gray) pathways. It is thus a central node in a network that allows noxious input and cognitive and emotional factors to influence pain processing and sensation. Activation of ON-cells with suppression of OFF-cell firing during noxious stimulation forms a positive feedback loop.

DESCENDING CONTROL IS BIDIRECTIONAL AND MEDIATED BY DISTINCT CLASSES OF NEURONS

The idea of a supraspinal system that specifically modulates pain grew out of an observation first made over 40 years ago that electrical stimulation in the periaqueductal gray of the rat produces potent antinociception [63]. This revolutionary finding inspired work in a number of different laboratories and ultimately led to the definition of a "pain-modulating network," with links in the periaqueductal gray and RVM. Stimulation at either site produces antinociception and inhibition of dorsal horn neurons. This network receives significant inputs from higher centers, including amygdala, hypothalamic nuclei, insula, and prefrontal cortex, providing a circuit through which nociceptive responsiveness can be influenced by cognitive and emotional factors and matched to behavioral context [3,48,74]. This network also receives ascending nociceptive information from the dorsal horn, with direct and indirect input to both the periaqueductal gray and RVM [72,89]. Nociceptive input to RVM is relayed primarily through the parabrachial complex [7,68]. Although the main output from this system is the RVM projection to the dorsal horn, the RVM also has ascending projections, with targets including amygdala and hypothalamus [31]. Although the function or functions of ascending RVM projections are at present unknown, it is interesting to speculate that they provide an anatomical substrate through which brainstem systems could influence pain processing at higher levels, including cortex.

The periaqueductal gray–RVM circuit was long viewed as an endogenous "analgesia system," and for several decades attention was focused on these areas as sources of descending inhibitory control. This system was implicated in both endogenous analgesia (for example, "stress-induced" analgesia) and in the actions of opioid analgesic drugs [24,73,85]. However, it subsequently became clear that descending control mediated by the RVM can be facilitatory as well as inhibitory [29]. The RVM modulates nociceptive tone on an ongoing basis, but the balance between inhibition and facilitation is dynamic and can be altered in different behavioral, emotional, and pathologic states. A facilitatory influence from the RVM is now known to be necessary for behavioral hypersensitivity in preclinical models of inflammatory and neuropathic pain [29,60,62]. A facilitatory role for the RVM has now been extended to incisional pain. Although an earlier study suggested that the RVM made no contribution to hyperalgesia induced by plantar incision [59], subsequent studies have reported that inactivation of the RVM reduces hyperalgesia in this model of postoperative pain [40,66].

Importantly, the influence of the RVM on nociception is not limited to control of nocifensor reflexes but extends to the affective aspect of pain [11,32,42,79]. This includes ongoing pain after incision, where RVM block supports a conditioned place preference [12]. This finding indicates that the RVM contributes not only to enhanced intraspinal processing but also to a state of aversion in animals subjected to surgery.

The physiology of RVM neurons is now reasonably well understood. RVM neurons can be divided into three classes based on changes in firing associated with noxious-evoked withdrawal responses [15]. "OFF-cells" are defined by a pause in firing associated with nociceptive withdrawal, and "ON-cells," by a withdrawal-related activation. The remaining RVM neurons, those without behavior-related changes in firing, are classified as "NEUTRAL-cells." The validity of this physiologic characterization of RVM neurons has been repeatedly confirmed in the distinct pharmacologic profiles exhibited by the different cell classes [23]. None of the three cell classes expresses a unique neurotransmitter. Indeed, a significant proportion of both OFF-cells and ON-cells is GABAergic [82]. Although serotonin was long argued to be restricted to NEUTRAL-cells [51], further study has suggested that it may be found in ON- and OFF-cells as well [8,16].

The significance of the ON/OFF/NEUTRAL categorization of RVM neurons is that it ties neuronal activity directly to a behavioral index of pain, the withdrawal response, rather than to the noxious stimulus. That is, the behavior-related changes in firing that define ON- and OFF-cells are related not to the stimulus intensity *per se* but to the decision to respond to the stimulus [6,36]. The implication is that the pause in OFF-cell firing and activation of ON-cells at the time of withdrawal are more closely related to the pain experienced than to the physical characteristics of the evoking stimulus.

The differentiation of these distinct cell classes has also allowed the pain-facilitating and pain-inhibiting output from the RVM to be dissected out. This is important because a change in pain measured behaviorally could reflect altered facilitation, changed inhibition, or a combination of both. That is, hyperalgesia could be due to increased descending facilitation and/or reduced descending inhibition. The fact that ON-cells are activated in association with the withdrawal reflex suggested early on that these neurons had a facilitatory role, and the reflex-related pause in OFF-cell firing pointed to an antinociceptive role for this class [15]. Both proposals were confirmed in subsequent work that went beyond mere correlation, using a combined microinjection/single-cell recording approach in which a behaviorally relevant dose of various pharmacologic agents was microinjected in lightly anesthetized, behaving animals while recording activity of an identified RVM neuron. In a series of studies, selective pharmacologic activation of the ON-cell population was shown to be sufficient to produce behaviorally measurable hyperalgesia, whereas activation of OFF-cells led to hypoalgesia [23,28,56].

"BOTTOM-UP" RECRUITMENT OF THE RVM IN NORMAL AND POTENTIATED PAIN STATES

What do ON- and OFF-cells contribute to basal pain sensitivity? In naïve animals, both ON- and OFF-cell populations display fluctuating ongoing activity [1]. Selective block of ON-cell activity under these conditions has no measurable effect on nociceptive *threshold* but reduces the *magnitude* of responses to noxious stimuli [27,37]. Presumed block of OFF-cells has at most a small hyperalgesic effect, indicating that the ongoing or "tonic" firing of OFF-cells has a modest influence on nociception under basal conditions [22,25,32]. This should not be surprising because ongoing firing, if present, can be inhibited by the nociceptive GABAergic input that causes the OFF-cells to pause, thus permitting a behavioral response to the stimulus. The antinociception action of opioids and some other analgesic drugs is explained not by their effects on the ongoing discharge of OFF-cells but by the fact that they act presynaptically to block this inhibitory input to OFF-cells, so that the neurons remain active [24,26]. This concept, first proposed in the early 1980s, was recently restated and confirmed in awake, head-restrained mice [30].

Acute Insult

Severe pain, either pre-existing or resulting from the surgical procedure itself, is a strong risk factor for development of persistent pain [14,39]. In rodents, significant surgical insult, acute inflammation, and cutaneous administration of capsaicin all drive substantial increases in ongoing activity of the ON-cells (which, it should be noted, can mask any response to additional noxious stimulation). Additionally, OFF-cell firing is suppressed [5,9,41,47,69]. The increase in ON-cell discharge is mediated by NMDA and neurokinin-1 receptors [5,84]. This increase can be blocked selectively using pharmacologic tools. When this is done experimentally, behavioral hypersensitivity is reversed [41,84]. Thus, acute inflammation leads to a shift in the balance between ON- and OFF-cell outputs such that ON-cells dominate (Figure 5-2, *Acute pain/inflammation*), functioning as a positive feedback element that reinforces increased nociceptive processing at the level of the dorsal horn (Figure 5-1). In essence, the increase in the ongoing activity of the ON-cells means that any primary afferent input enters a dorsal horn that is under a continuing pronociceptive modulatory influence [41,61]. Normally subthreshold inputs may therefore exceed the nociceptive threshold.

It is worth noting that a similar shift in the balance toward ON-cell output can be seen in acute opioid withdrawal [38]. In this state, increased ON-cell excitability presumably reflects an opponent-process, compensatory response to the activation of OFF-cells and analgesia produced by the opioid. Thus, a shift towards ON-cell dominance can be triggered by analgesia, as well as by tissue damage and nociception. This shift is thought to contribute to "opioid-induced hyperalgesia" [76] and very likely plays a role in the long-lasting state of latent hypersensitivity observed in animals after opioid exposure [52,65]. Because the great majority of surgical patients receive an opioid analgesic at some point, consideration of how noxious insult and analgesic drugs interact to drive descending facilitation is an important topic for further study.

The shift in overall balance with acute injury so that ON-cells dominate the output of the RVM appears to be self-limiting in many cases. For example, after a localized injection of complete Freund adjuvant, the *ongoing* activity of ON-cells returns toward normal levels within hours and is not maintained throughout the period of behavioral hyperalgesia [9,53]. Although the mechanisms underlying the apparent restoration of a "normal" ongoing balance between ON- and OFF-cells in the RVM are so far unknown, this is a critical question for future study because normalization of descending control likely limits the development of chronic pain after insult.

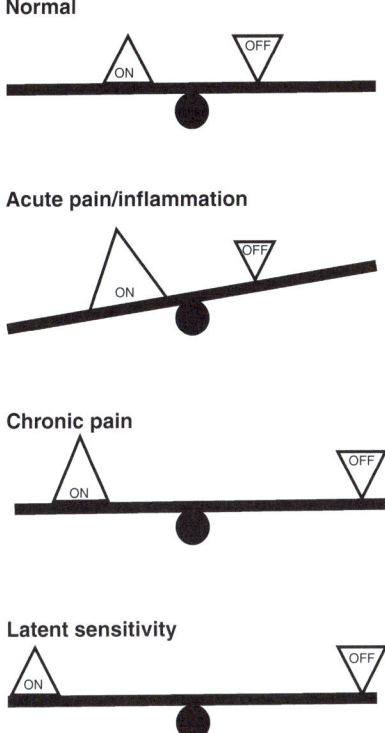

FIGURE 5-2 "Balance" of facilitatory and inhibitory outputs from the rostral ventromedial medulla in acute and chronic pain states. Using a seesaw analogy, we suggest that ON- and OFF-cells are essentially in balance under normal conditions. Both cell classes exhibit fluctuating activity, and neither output is dominant. During acute pain or inflammation, ON-cells are driven by noxious input while OFF-cell firing is inhibited. The facilitating output, the ON-cells, dominates. In chronic pain, potentiated inputs driven by sensitized primary afferents and dorsal horn circuitry are to some extent balanced by the inhibitory output. However, the system is less stable, as sensory inputs have moved further from the fulcrum. A smaller input is thus needed to trigger the behavior-related ON-cell burst and OFF-cell pause. Finally, in latent sensitization, the system returns to balance but remains less stable.

Chronic State

The transition from acute to chronic pain is linked to significant physiologic and molecular plasticity in the RVM. As inflammation becomes chronic, expression and function of NMDA, AMPA, neurokinin 1, opioid, nicotinic, and trkB receptors are modified over a period of days [19–21,33,35,44,70], and glial cells are activated [67].

The physiology of ON- and OFF-cells in chronic pain states is quite distinct from that seen immediately after an acute insult or early in the course of inflammation. As noted earlier, the *ongoing* activity of both ON- and OFF-cell classes in chronic pain states is not different from that seen in uninjured animals, so the system superficially appears to be more or less "in balance." However, both ON- and OFF-cells are sensitized and respond to stimuli normally considered innocuous. This sensitization parallels the lowered behavioral threshold and is seen in both inflammation and nerve injury [6,9]. Thus, in chronic pain states, the RVM system is rebalanced but unstable. Using the seesaw analogy of Figure 5-2, augmented nociceptive inputs from sensitized primary afferents and dorsal horn circuits are balanced by moving a compensatory OFF-cell output further from the fulcrum. In this situation, minor changes in input magnitude could drastically disturb the equilibrium of the system (Figure 5-2, *Chronic pain*).

In the chronic phase, the system is essentially "hypervigilant" for any potentially damaging input, with both ON- and OFF-cells more responsive. This may be maintained even after afferent drive returns to normal. This situation is likely to underlie the "latent hypersensitivity" demonstrated by Laboureyras, Simonnet, and colleagues [43], who showed that animals subjected to incisional pain displayed a potentiated hyperalgesia to inflammation of a different body part several weeks later, after hypersensitivity to stimulation of the area around the surgical wound had resolved (Figure 5-2, *Latent sensitivity*). However, while both ON- and OFF-cells are more responsive to stimulation, the apparently normal *ongoing* activity of the OFF-cells limits hyperalgesia and to some extent keeps abnormal dorsal horn processes in check [9]. This is what would be expected given the known, but fairly small, antinociceptive effect of ongoing activity of these neurons [22,25,32]. Moreover, De Felice and colleagues [13] suggest that variations in the efficacy of descending inhibition help explain why some individuals are less susceptible to development of neuropathic pain. Viewed collectively, these lines of evidence suggest that a restored balance between descending inhibition and facilitation limits persistent pain after surgery or other insult, and, conversely, that continued imbalance contributes to persistent pain.

"TOP-DOWN" ENGAGEMENT OF THE RVM

One of the biggest mysteries about pain, and possibly the most frustrating from the point of view of pain management, is the significant contribution of cognitive and emotional variables to the experience of pain. Psychological constructs including anxiety, hypervigilance, and pain catastrophizing are important risk factors for both acute and persisting pain after surgery [34,45,46,49,57]. While this is at least in part a manifestation of altered processing at higher levels, there is also strong evidence that psychological variables can modify dorsal horn nociceptive processing via descending control systems. Evidence that this is the case comes from functional imaging of the cord and changes in nociceptive reflexes induced by psychological manipulations such as viewing pictures with emotional content [4,17,18,64,81].

Although the aforementioned evidence from humans does not point directly to the RVM, animal studies suggest that this region is at the interface between psychological variables and pain. The strongest argument that the RVM makes a "top-down" contribution to persistent or abnormal pain comes from studies of "stress-induced hyperalgesia." Mild stress can sometimes produce hyperalgesia, and this response can be "primed" by prior incisional pain [52]. Opioid exposure has a similar effect, predisposing animals to stress-induced hyperalgesia for a period of days to weeks [65]. The latter observation has important implications for management of postsurgical pain because most patients receive at least some opioids as part of standard care. Since ON-cells are known to mediate hyperalgesia induced by mild stress [50,78], it seems reasonable to conclude that these neurons are the reason that stress could predispose a given patient to develop persistent postoperative pain.

THE RVM AND "CONDITIONED PAIN MODULATION"

In patients, an important predictor of subsequent persistent postoperative pain is the efficacy of "conditioned pain modulation (CPM)" [87] in which the response to a "test" painful stimulus is modulated by a remote, painful stimulus called the "conditioning" stimulus [88]. Individuals who demonstrated less effective CPM were found to be more likely to complain of continuing pain, weeks to months after surgery. Current evidence suggests that individuals have different capacities for CPM and that those with a greater capacity are less likely to develop persistent pain [75,80,86]. Unfortunately, the neural basis for the "conditioned pain modulation" phenomenon measured in humans is unclear. The animal analogue, "diffuse noxious inhibitory control (DNIC)," is mediated by the subnucleus reticularis dorsalis, which is not part of the periaqueductal gray/RVM system [54,77]. The extent to which CPM and DNIC reflect the same phenomenon and share underlying mechanisms remains to be determined. The evidence reviewed earlier suggests that RVM-mediated processes contribute to postoperative pain and very likely reflect some component of CPM. However, parallel circuits, including the subnucleus reticularis dorsalis and other regions identified as mediating DNIC, may also play a role.

CONCLUSION

There is now compelling evidence that descending modulatory systems are an important piece in the puzzle of persistent postsurgical pain [86]. Animal studies point to the RVM as the primary output of descending control, and this is a site where bottom-up and top-down factors can converge to influence pain. Understanding this system can be complicated by the fact that it includes facilitatory and inhibitory outputs, but it is nevertheless clear that strong descending inhibition, accomplished by the OFF-cells, militates against development of chronic pain. There is also no doubt that the facilitatory output from the RVM, the ON-cells, contributes to a host of persistent pain states. The RVM might most usefully be viewed as an essential node in a neural network that can limit or promote hypersensitivity to pain under different conditions. Understanding how this system responds to surgical insult and opioids and how it is engaged by emotional and cognitive factors is a necessary step in addressing persistent postoperative pain.

Acknowledgment

M.M.H. is supported by grants from NINDS (NS066159, NS098660).

REFERENCES

1. Barbaro NM, Heinricher MM, Fields HL. Putative nociceptive modulatory neurons in the rostral ventromedial medulla of the rat display highly correlated firing patterns. Somatosens Mot Res 1989;6:413–25.
2. Bayman EO, Brennan TJ. Incidence and severity of chronic pain at 3 and 6 months after thoracotomy: meta-analysis. J Pain 2014;15:887–97.
3. Bayman EO, Parekh KR, Keech J, Selte A, Brennan TJ. A prospective study of chronic pain after thoracic surgery. Anesthesiology 2017;126:938–51.
4. Bjerre L, Andersen AT, Hagelskjaer MT, Ge N, Morch CD, Andersen OK. Dynamic tuning of human withdrawal reflex receptive fields during cognitive attention and distraction tasks. Eur J Pain 2011;15:816–21.
5. Brink TS, Pacharinsak C, Khasabov SG, Beitz AJ, Simone DA. Differential modulation of neurons in the rostral ventromedial medulla by neurokinin-1 receptors. J Neurophysiol 2012;107:1210–21.
6. Carlson JD, Maire JJ, Martenson ME, Heinricher MM. Sensitization of pain-modulating neurons in the rostral ventromedial medulla after peripheral nerve injury. J Neurosci 2007;27:13222–31.
7. Chen Q, Roeder Z, Li M-H, Zhang Y, Ingram SL, Heinricher MM. Optogenetic evidence for a direct circuit linking nociceptive transmisison through the parabrachial complex with pain-modulating neurons of the rostral ventromedial medulla (RVM). eNeuro 2017;4(3).
8. Chen T, Wang XL, Qu J, Wang W, Zhang T, Yanagawa Y, Wu SX, Li YQ. Neurokinin-1 receptor-expressing neurons that contain serotonin and gamma-aminobutyric acid in the rat rostroventromedial medulla are involved in pain processing. J Pain 2013;14:778–92.

9. Cleary DR, Heinricher MM. Adaptations in responsiveness of brainstem pain-modulating neurons in acute compared with chronic inflammation. Pain 2013;154:845–55.
10. D'Mello R, Dickenson AH. Spinal cord mechanisms of pain. Br J Anaesth 2008;101:8–16.
11. da Silva LF, Coutinho MR, Menescal-de-Oliveira L. Opioidergic and GABAergic mechanisms in the rostral ventromedial medulla modulate the nociceptive response of vocalization in guinea pigs. Brain Res Bull 2010;82:177–83.
12. De Felice M, Eyde N, Dodick D, Dussor GO, Ossipov MH, Fields HL, Porreca F. Capturing the aversive state of cephalic pain preclinically. Ann Neurol 2013;74:257–65.
13. De Felice M, Sanoja R, Wang R, Vera-Portocarrero L, Oyarzo J, King T, Ossipov MH, Vanderah TW, Lai J, Dussor GO, Fields HL, Price TJ, Porreca F. Engagement of descending inhibition from the rostral ventromedial medulla protects against chronic neuropathic pain. Pain 2011;152:2701–9.
14. Eisenach JC, Pan PH, Smiley R, Lavand'homme P, Landau R, Houle TT. Severity of acute pain after childbirth, but not type of delivery, predicts persistent pain and postpartum depression. Pain 2008;140:87–94.
15. Fields HL, Heinricher MM. Anatomy and physiology of a nociceptive modulatory system. Philos Trans R Soc Lond B Biol Sci 1985;308:361–74.
16. Gau R, Sevoz-Couche C, Hamon M, Bernard JF. Noxious stimulation excites serotonergic neurons: a comparison between the lateral paragigantocellular reticular and the raphe magnus nuclei. Pain 2013;154:647–59.
17. Geuter S, Büchel C. Facilitation of pain in the human spinal cord by nocebo treatment. J Neurosci 2013;33:13784–90.
18. Goffaux P, Redmond WJ, Rainville P, Marchand S. Descending analgesia - when the spine echoes what the brain expects. Pain 2007;130:137–43.
19. Guan Y, Guo W, Robbins MT, Dubner R, Ren K. Changes in AMPA receptor phosphorylation in the rostral ventromedial medulla after inflammatory hyperalgesia in rats. Neurosci Lett 2004;366:201–5.
20. Guan Y, Guo W, Zou S-P, Dubner R, Ren K. Inflammation-induced upregulation of AMPA receptor subunit expression in brain stem pain modulatory circuitry. Pain 2003;104:401–13.
21. Guo W, Robbins MT, Wei F, Zou S, Dubner R, Ren K. Supraspinal brain-derived neurotrophic factor signaling: a novel mechanism for descending pain facilitation. J Neurosci 2006;26:126–37.
22. Heinricher MM, Barbaro NM, Fields HL. Putative nociceptive modulating neurons in the rostral ventromedial medulla of the rat: firing of on- and off-cells is related to nociceptive responsiveness. Somatosens Mot Res 1989;6:427–39.
23. Heinricher MM, Fields HL. Central nervous system mechanisms of pain modulation. In: McMahon S, Koltzenburg M, Tracey I, Turk DC, editors. Wall and Melzack's textbook of pain. 6th ed. London: Elsevier; 2013. p. 129–42.
24. Heinricher MM, Ingram SL. The brainstem and nociceptive modulation. In: Bushnell MC, Basbaum AI, editors. The science of pain. San Diego: Academic Press; 2008. p. 593–626.
25. Heinricher MM, Kaplan HJ. GABA-mediated inhibition in rostral ventromedial medulla: role in nociceptive modulation in the lightly anesthetized rat. Pain 1991;47:105–13.
26. Heinricher MM, Maire JJ, Lee D, Nalwalk JW, Hough LB. Physiological basis for inhibition of morphine and improgan antinociception by CC12, a P450 epoxygenase inhibitor. J Neurophysiol 2010;104:3222–30.
27. Heinricher MM, McGaraughty S. Analysis of excitatory amino acid transmission within the rostral ventromedial medulla: implications for circuitry. Pain 1998;75:247–55.
28. Heinricher MM, Neubert MJ. Neural basis for the hyperalgesic action of cholecystokinin in the rostral ventromedial medulla. J Neurophysiol 2004;92:1982–9.
29. Heinricher MM, Tavares I, Leith JL, Lumb BM. Descending control of nociception: specificity, recruitment and plasticity. Brain Res Rev 2009;60:214–25.
30. Hellman KM, Mason P. Opioids disrupt pro-nociceptive modulation mediated by raphe magnus. J Neurosci 2012;32:13668–78.
31. Hermann DM, Luppi PH, Peyron C, Hinckel P, Jouvet M. Forebrain projections of the rostral nucleus raphe magnus shown by iontophoretic application of choleratoxin B in rats. Neurosci Lett 1996;216:151–4.
32. Hirakawa N, Tershner SA, Fields HL, Manning BH. Bi-directional changes in affective state elicited by manipulation of medullary pain-modulatory circuitry. Neuroscience 2000;100:861–71.
33. Hurley RW, Hammond DL. The analgesic effects of supraspinal μ and δ opioid receptor agonists are potentiated during persistent inflammation. J Neurosci 2000;20:1249–59.
34. Ip HY, Abrishami A, Peng PW, Wong J, Chung F. Predictors of postoperative pain and analgesic consumption: a qualitative systematic review. Anesthesiology 2009;111:657–77.
35. Jareczek FJ, White SR, Hammond DL. Plasticity in brainstem mechanisms of pain modulation by nicotinic acetylcholine receptors in the rat. eNeuro 2017:4. doi:10.1523/ENEURO.0364-16.2017.

36. Jinks SL, Carstens E, Antognini JF. Isoflurane differentially modulates medullary on and off neurons while suppressing hind-limb motor withdrawals. Anesthesiology 2004;100:1224–34.
37. Jinks SL, Carstens EE, Antognini JF. Glutamate receptor blockade in the rostral ventromedial medulla reduces the force of multisegmental motor responses to supramaximal noxious stimuli. Neurosci Lett 2007;426:175–80.
38. Kaplan H, Fields HL. Hyperalgesia during acute opioid abstinence: evidence for a nociceptive facilitating function of the rostral ventromedial medulla. J Neurosci 1991;11:1433–9.
39. Kehlet H, Jensen TS, Woolf CJ. Persistent postsurgical pain: risk factors and prevention. Lancet 2006;367:1618–25.
40. Khasabov SG, Wang JC, Simone DA, Strichartz GR. A role for neurokinin-1 receptor neurons in the rostral ventromedial medulla in the development of chronic postthoracotomy pain. Pain 2017;158:1332–41.
41. Kincaid W, Neubert MJ, Xu M, Kim CJ, Heinricher MM. Role for medullary pain facilitating neurons in secondary thermal hyperalgesia. J Neurophysiol 2006;95:33–41.
42. King T, Vera-Portocarrero L, Gutierrez T, Vanderah TW, Dussor G, Lai J, Fields HL, Porreca F. Unmasking the tonic-aversive state in neuropathic pain. Nat Neurosci 2009;12:1364–6.
43. Laboureyras E, Chateauraynaud J, Richebe P, Simonnet G. Long-term pain vulnerability after surgery in rats: prevention by nefopam, an analgesic with antihyperalgesic properties. Anesth Analg 2009;109:623–31.
44. LaGraize SC, Guo W, Yang K, Wei F, Ren K, Dubner R. Spinal cord mechanisms mediating behavioral hyperalgesia induced by neurokinin-1 tachykinin receptor activation in the rostral ventromedial medulla. Neuroscience 2010;171:1341–56.
45. Lautenbacher S, Huber C, Kunz M, Parthum A, Weber PG, Griessinger N, Sittl R. Hypervigilance as predictor of postoperative acute pain: its predictive potency compared with experimental pain sensitivity, cortisol reactivity, and affective state. Clin J Pain 2009;25:92–100.
46. Lautenbacher S, Huber C, Schofer D, Kunz M, Parthum A, Weber PG, Roman C, Griessinger N, Sittl R. Attentional and emotional mechanisms related to pain as predictors of chronic postoperative pain: a comparison with other psychological and physiological predictors. Pain 2010;151:722–31.
47. Li HS, Monhemius R, Simpson BA, Roberts MH. Supraspinal inhibition of nociceptive dorsal horn neurones in the anaesthetized rat: tonic or dynamic? J Physiol 1998;506:459–69.
48. Lovick TA, Li P. Integrated function of neurones in the rostral ventrolateral medulla. Prog Brain Res 1989;81:223–32.
49. Lunn TH, Gaarn-Larsen L, Kehlet H. Prediction of postoperative pain by preoperative pain response to heat stimulation in total knee arthroplasty. Pain 2013;154:1878–85.
50. Martenson ME, Cetas JS, Heinricher MM. A possible neural basis for stress-induced hyperalgesia. Pain 2009;142:236–44.
51. Mason P. Physiological identification of pontomedullary serotonergic neurons in the rat. J Neurophysiol 1997;77:1087–98.
52. Meleine M, Rivat C, Laboureyras E, Cahana A, Richebe P. Sciatic nerve block fails in preventing the development of late stress-induced hyperalgesia when high-dose fentanyl is administered perioperatively in rats. Reg Anesth Pain Med 2012;37:448–54.
53. Montagne-Clavel J, Oliveras JL. Are ventromedial medulla neuronal properties modified by chronic peripheral inflammation? A single-unit study in the awake, freely moving polyarthritic rat. Brain Res 1994;657:92–104.
54. Morgan MM, Fields HL. Pronounced changes in the activity of nociceptive modulatory neurons in the rostral ventromedial medulla in response to prolonged thermal noxious stimuli. J Neurophysiol 1994;72:1161–70.
55. Nahman-Averbuch H, Nir RR, Sprecher E, Yarnitsky D. Psychological factors and conditioned pain modulation: a meta-analysis. Clin J Pain 2016;32:541–54.
56. Neubert MJ, Kincaid W, Heinricher MM. Nociceptive facilitating neurons in the rostral ventromedial medulla. Pain 2004;110:158–65.
57. Pan PH, Coghill R, Houle TT, Seid MH, Lindel WM, Parker RL, Washburn SA, Harris L, Eisenach JC. Multifactorial preoperative predictors for postcesarean section pain and analgesic requirement. Anesthesiology 2006;104:417–25.
58. Pan PH, Tonidandel AM, Aschenbrenner CA, Houle TT, Harris LC, Eisenach JC. Predicting acute pain after cesarean delivery using three simple questions. Anesthesiology 2013;118:1170–9.
59. Pogatzki EM, Urban MO, Brennan TJ, Gebhart GF. Role of the rostral medial medulla in the development of primary and secondary hyperalgesia after incision in the rat. Anesthesiology 2002;96:1153–60.
60. Porreca F, Ossipov MH, Gebhart GF. Chronic pain and medullary descending facilitation. Trends Neurosci 2002;25:319–25.
61. Ramirez F, Vanegas H. Tooth pulp stimulation advances both medullary off-cell pause and tail flick. Neurosci Lett 1989;100:153–6.

62. Ren K, Dubner R. Descending modulation in persistent pain: an update. Pain 2002;100:1–6.
63. Reynolds DV. Surgery in the rat during electrical analgesia induced by focal brain stimulation. Science 1969;154:444–5.
64. Rhudy JL, Williams AE, McCabe KM, Nguyen MA, Rambo P. Affective modulation of nociception at spinal and supraspinal levels. Psychophysiology 2005;42:579–87.
65. Rivat C, Laboureyras E, Laulin JP, Le Roy C, Richebe P, Simonnet G. Non-nociceptive environmental stress induces hyperalgesia, not analgesia, in pain and opioid-experienced rats. Neuropsychopharmacology 2007;32:2217–28.
66. Rivat C, Vera-Portocarrero LP, Ibrahim MM, Mata HP, Stagg NJ, De Felice M, Porreca F, Malan TP. Spinal NK-1 receptor-expressing neurons and descending pathways support fentanyl-induced pain hypersensitivity in a rat model of postoperative pain. Eur J Neurosci 2009;29:727–37.
67. Roberts J, Ossipov MH, Porreca F. Glial activation in the rostroventromedial medulla promotes descending facilitation to mediate inflammatory hypersensitivity. Eur J Neurosci 2009;30:229–41.
68. Roeder Z, Chen Q, Davis S, Carlson JD, Tupone D, Heinricher MM. The parabrachial complex links pain transmission to descending pain modulation. Pain 2016;157:2697–708.
69. Sanoja R, Tortorici V, Fernandez C, Price TJ, Cervero F. Role of RVM neurons in capsaicin-evoked visceral nociception and referred hyperalgesia. Eur J Pain 2010;14:120–9.
70. Schepers RJ, Mahoney JL, Shippenberg TS. Inflammation-induced changes in rostral ventromedial medulla mu and kappa opioid receptor mediated antinociception. Pain 2008;136:320–30.
71. Sommer M, de Rijke JM, van Kleef M, Kessels AG, Peters ML, Geurts JW, Patijn J, Gramke HF, Marcus MA. Predictors of acute postoperative pain after elective surgery. Clin J Pain 2010;26:87–94.
72. Sugiyo S, Takemura M, Dubner R, Ren K. Trigeminal transition zone/rostral ventromedial medulla connections and facilitation of orofacial hyperalgesia after masseter inflammation in rats. J Comp Neurol 2005;493:510–23.
73. Terman GW, Shavit Y, Lewis JW, Cannon JT, Liebeskind JC. Intrinsic mechanisms of pain inhibition: activation by stress. Science 1984;226:1270–7.
74. Tracey I, Mantyh PW. The cerebral signature for pain perception and its modulation. Neuron 2007;55:377–91.
75. van Wijk G, Veldhuijzen DS. Perspective on diffuse noxious inhibitory controls as a model of endogenous pain modulation in clinical pain syndromes. J Pain 2010;11:408–19.
76. Vanderah TW, Suenaga NM, Ossipov MH, Mala Jr TP, Lai J, Porreca F. Tonic descending facilitation from the rostral ventromedial medulla mediates opioid-induced abnormal pain and antinociceptive tolerance. J Neurosci 2001;21:279–86.
77. Villanueva L. Diffuse noxious inhibitory control (DNIC) as a tool for exploring dysfunction of endogenous pain modulatory systems. Pain 2009;143:161–2.
78. Wagner KM, Roeder Z, Desrochers K, Buhler AV, Heinricher MM, Cleary DR. The dorsomedial hypothalamus mediates stress-induced hyperalgesia and is the source of the pronociceptive peptide cholecystokinin in the rostral ventromedial medulla. Neuroscience 2013;238:29–38.
79. Wang R, King T, De Felice M, Guo W, Ossipov MH, Porreca F. Descending facilitation maintains long-term spontaneous neuropathic pain. J Pain 2013;14:845–53.
80. Wilder-Smith OH, Schreyer T, Scheffer GJ, Arendt-Nielsen L. Patients with chronic pain after abdominal surgery show less preoperative endogenous pain inhibition and more postoperative hyperalgesia: a pilot study. J Pain Palliat Care Pharmacother 2010;24:119–28.
81. Willer JC, Boureau F, Albe-Fessard D. Supraspinal influences on nociceptive flexion reflex and pain sensation in man. Brain Res 1979;179:61–8.
82. Winkler CW, Hermes SM, Chavkin CI, Drake CT, Morrison SF, Aicher SA. Kappa opioid receptor (kor) and gad67 immunoreactivity are found in off and neutral cells in the rostral ventromedial medulla. J Neurophysiol 2006;96:3465–73.
83. Woolf CJ. Central sensitization: implications for the diagnosis and treatment of pain. Pain 2011;152:S2–15.
84. Xu M, Kim CJ, Neubert MJ, Heinricher MM. NMDA receptor-mediated activation of medullary pro-nociceptive neurons is required for secondary thermal hyperalgesia. Pain 2007;127:253–62.
85. Yaksh TL, Rudy TA. Narcotic analgestics: CNS sites and mechanisms of action as revealed by intracerebral injection techniques. Pain 1978;4:299–359.
86. Yarnitsky D. Conditioned pain modulation (the diffuse noxious inhibitory control-like effect): its relevance for acute and chronic pain states. Curr Opin Anaesthesiol 2010;23:611–5.

87. Yarnitsky D, Arendt-Nielsen L, Bouhassira D, Edwards RR, Fillingim RB, Granot M, Hansson P, Lautenbacher S, Marchand S, Wilder-Smith O. Recommendations on terminology and practice of psychophysical DNIC testing. Eur J Pain 2010;14:339.
88. Yarnitsky D, Crispel Y, Eisenberg E, Granovsky Y, Ben-Nun A, Sprecher E, Best LA, Granot M. Prediction of chronic post-operative pain: pre-operative DNIC testing identifies patients at risk. Pain 2008;138:22–8.
89. Yezierski RP, Mendez CM. Spinal distribution and collateral projections of rat spinomesencephalic tract cells. Neuroscience 1991;44:113–30.

CHAPTER 6

Neurotransmitters, Neuromodulators, and Ionophores in Mechanisms of Pain Persistence After Surgery: From Periphery to the Brain

Lauren V. Friend, Louisa D. Townson, and Anthony H. Dickenson

Surgery, however necessary, invariably involves incision, retraction, and compression of somatic and neuronal tissue. The subsequent persistent pain is an entirely variable and individual experience, the intensity and duration of which depends on the balance of inflammatory and neuropathic pain to which a patient is exposed and variable mechanisms from the periphery to the brain. While this damage to nonneuronal tissue should heal, eliminating peripheral sensitized inflammatory drives to the pain state [42], by contrast neuronal damage generates ongoing activity that is likely to persist because healing is much less probable. This accordingly drives changes in spinal cord and brain processing of pain messages. Even small levels of peripheral activity deriving from inflammatory and/or neuropathic processes, arriving on an already sensitized CNS, may lead to abnormal pain perception, provoking allodynia and hyperalgesia. Patients who develop persistent pain are similarly more likely to develop secondary symptoms such as anxiety and depression, comorbidities that can both decrease quality of life and participate in the enhancement of the pain state. A range of individual differences, not least genetic susceptibilities, similarly influences the persistence of pain after surgery.

Postsurgical pathophysiology can be categorized into a number of broad themes. At one level, it is simplest to partition information between the periphery, the spinal cord, and the brain. However, alterations in pain processing should also be viewed in terms of overall changes to the neurotransmitters, neuromodulators, and ionophore systems to truly understand the pathophysiology behind the different sensory components of persistent pain.

AFFERENT DRIVE FROM THE PERIPHERY

The Importance of the Ionophore

As the conduction machinery of the lipid membrane, ionophores are crucial components of the transduction and transmission of sensory information. Both inflammation and nerve injury elicit plasticity in the function and expression of these ionophores, the result of which is the enhanced and spontaneous afferent drive of central excitability and maladaptive processing.

Transducers

At the site of incision, ionophores are crucial, producing depolarizing currents known as generator potentials, which may elicit action potentials or simply increase the membrane potential to sensitize afferents. Some of these ionophores, such as the acid-sensing ion channels (ASICs) that detect the drop in tissue pH that accompanies tissue damage, are critical to the initial nociception and sensitization after surgery [13]. There is also notable upregulation of ASIC3 expression in incision models of postoperative pain [13], which may contribute to the further sensitization of primary afferents.

Similarly transient receptor potential vanilloid 1 (TRPV1), the heat and acid-sensing cation channel, has a role not only in the initial detection of tissue damage but also in afferent sensitization, having been shown to mediate spontaneous firing and heat sensitization in postoperative pain [3]. These changes in afferent sensitivity and activity are brought about by both a functional upregulation and enhancement of TRPV1-depolarizing currents by mediators such as nerve growth factor (NGF) following incision [4,7]. Anti- NGF therapy in this model of postoperative pain significantly reduces guarding and heat hyperalgesia [4], revealing the significance of posttranslational modification and upregulation of these ionophores.

The transient receptor potential ankyrin 1 (TRPA1) ion channel has also come under scrutiny for a role in the generation of postoperative pain. This polymodal receptor, described as the "gatekeeper for inflammation" [11], has previously been shown to have roles in both inflammatory and neuropathic mechanical hyperalgesia [7]. It is speculated that TRPA1 similarly contributes to the generation of both mechanical hypersensitivity and spontaneous pain following deep incision [53]. However, cutaneous incision models in TRPA1 knockout mice contradict these findings [7]. It may be the case that TRPA1 plays a role exclusive to deep tissue procedures. In general, we have little data on how deep pains are generated and modulated. This will be a key area for future research on postsurgical pains.

As a consequence of the role these ionophores play in generating the afferent drive, these channels and their afferent subpopulations are attractive peripheral targets for pharmacologic interventions, both peri- and postoperative. One approach currently entering clinical trial is the use of the high-dose capsaicin patch [37], which causes the desensitization and eventual reversible degeneration of the peripheral terminals of TRPV1 primary afferents. The use of capsaicin in this manner has already proved to be successful in animal models of incision pain [29].

Sodium Channels

Ionophores similarly control the electrophysiologic properties of the primary afferents, not least the threshold for action potential generation, interspike intervals, and burst duration. Of particular importance to the transmission of pain signals are the voltage-gated sodium channels (VGSCs) Nav1.3, 1.7, 1.8, and 1.9. Directly after surgery and while inflammation is ongoing, the activation of signaling cascades by inflammatory messengers leads to the phosphorylation of VGSCs. Alteration in the threshold, current magnitude and kinetics of Nav1.7, 1.8, and 1.9 currents follow, increasing membrane excitability and thus the likelihood that a given stimulus will evoke an action potential [32]. This peripheral sensitization can be limited by the use of cyclooxygenase (COX) inhibitors, but the effects of these interventions are narrow should the postsurgical pain be largely neuropathic in nature.

In addition to these posttranslational changes to ionophore proteins evoked by the inflammatory milieu, there is dynamic regulation of sodium channels' expression, both in their distribution and population. Transcriptional regulation, triggered by both inflammatory cascades and nerve damage, leads to both upregulation and downregulation of VGSC populations. Crucially, following nerve damage there appears to be renewed expression of Nav1.3, despite restricted expression in normal adult rat dorsal root ganglion (DRG) [14]. It is suggested that this novel expression of Nav1.3 in adult sensory afferents results in ectopic firing and consequently spontaneous pain, symptoms which can be reversed by the application of glial cell–derived neurotrophic factor (GDNF), which normalizes Nav1.3 expression [14,32].

Similarly, the usually abundant Nav1.8 and 1.9 have been shown to be downregulated following nerve injury [14,32]. However, results are contradictory given alternate studies exhibiting a role for Nav1.8 in spontaneous activity in sensory afferents [43]. Gold et al. argue that while Nav1.8 is downregulated in the injured neurons, expression is redistributed to uninjured counterparts to produce aberrant activity [20], which consequently maintains an afferent drive. However, antisense for Nav1.8 fails to attenuate incision pain, suggesting that the role of this sodium channel may be greater in persistent postoperative pain involving nerve injury [28].

Consideration must also be made to the enhanced action of sodium channel populations within sympathetic neurons. Nav1.7 containing sympathetic and sensory neuron populations has been shown to work in concert to enhance pain sensation [34]. Although the exact mechanism of a sympathetic drive in acute and neuropathic pain is not yet clear, this system is already being targeted for analgesia in postoperative pain [33]. Future pharmacotherapy may prove more successful in preventing and treating persistent postoperative pain by blocking both sensory and sympathetic systems.

The importance of sodium channels is demonstrated in patients carrying the single nucleotide polymorphism (SNP) SCN9A 3312T allele. These individuals exhibit reduced postoperative pain and likelihood of developing inadequate analgesia after pancreatectomy [16]. This SNP occurs in the gene encoding Nav1.7, the VGSC which regulates release of peptide transmitters from central terminals, and consequently winds up, as well as exerting a key role in ectopic firing in neuromas [14,34]. The pain protection provided by this SNP, which alters the gating properties of Nav1.7, demonstrates the importance of ionophores in dictating the postoperative pain experience of patients.

In controlling the excitability and output of sensory afferents, and thus the input to the spinal cord, the VGSCs present as an attractive target for the prevention of activity-dependent changes in central processing after surgery. By the interruption of the sensory barrage, sodium channel blockers such as lidocaine provide proven short-term pain relief, but their long-term application may also hold the key to quenching the development of maladaptive central changes [30,57]. In the future, selective blockers of particular sodium channels could be the key to prevention of peripheral electrical drives.

Processing of Afferent Activity by the Spinal Cord

In inflammation, peripheral sensitization will produce higher levels of activity arriving in the spinal cord. The paradox between coexistent gain and loss of symptoms in neuropathic pain is associated with what appears to be compensations in the CNS for the loss of normal inputs; the sensory system adapts to loss of input due to nerve damage by opening circuits to amplify the signals from remaining intact pain fibers or to ectopic activity in afferent fibers. As a consequence nonnoxious inputs effectively synapse onto pain signaling systems.

Calcium Channels

The first synapse between the peripheral nerve and spinal neurons provides a good example of these sorts of changes. In inflammation, the calcium channel populations (N, P/Q, R, and T) appear to be driven harder by the enhanced peripheral inputs. Shifts in dose–response curves of calcium channel blockers are seen [52]. After neuropathy, the loss of afferents results in an upregulation of N-type channels, with an especially marked increase in the auxillary protein, the α2δ-1. This protein, associated with trafficking of the channels, is the target for gabapentin and pregabalin [10]. Neurons in the spinal cord of animals with overexpression of this subunit exhibit abnormal patterns of firing in the absence of nerve injury, notably increased and prolonged responses to peripheral stimuli [31]. It is believed that this upregulation is the key to the ability of these drugs to modulate neuropathic pains but not some inflammatory conditions where there is minor upregulation. Thus, in an animal model of osteoarthritis, where there are additional neuropathic components, pregabalin can be effective but fails when neuropathy is lacking [50]. There are additional permissive factors that allow the gabapentinoids to work, and these are discussed later in descending controls. Issues such as these need consideration in the use of α2δ ligands in the perioperative setting [41]. Whatever the case, the spinal neurons with projections to sensory and affective brain areas are highly likely to receive greater amounts of transmitter from the afferent fibers. This is the first stage in the induction of central sensitization (CS).

Central Inhibitory Transmission

Pain messages can be enhanced by increases in peripheral or central excitatory mechanisms but equally, by a loss in inhibition. 30% to 40% of spinal neurons are inhibitory interneurons, and their tonic activity is an important regulator of sensory tone in the spinal cord [49]. Prevention of local spinal cord inhibition in normal animals with $GABA_A$ receptor antagonists or glycine receptor antagonists mimics behavioral hypersensitivities to low-threshold stimuli, similar to that seen in animal models of chronic pain [58]. Thus, there is a dorsal horn pathway capable of mediating allodynia and hyperalgesia that is normally under strict inhibitory control that becomes pathologically disrupted in situations of chronic pain [51].

Central Excitatory Transmission

Alongside inhibitory controls, there are powerful excitatory systems within spinal circuits. The co-release of peptides and glutamate from incoming active peripheral nerves is likely to be enhanced in a number of pain states by the changes in calcium channel functions. These transmitters activate neurokinin and N-methyl-D-aspartate (NMDA) receptors for substance P and glutamate, which in turn generate CS or spinal hypersensitivity [12]. Key events in these processes are windup (when small fiber stimulation rapidly induces higher levels of spinal neuronal firing even though the peripheral drive remains constant) and long-term potentiation (LTP), where the frequency of stimulation to induce is very high [12,44]. In humans, the counterpart of windup is temporal summation [25]. These mechanisms are plausible candidates of the induction of CS, and although the original study on CS did describe bilateral changes, using motor reflexes most subsequent studies report local changes confined to the areas of tissue or nerve damage, in both animals and humans [25,56]. A number of analgesics can modulate CS, but the most direct is ketamine that directly blocks the NMDA receptor channel, effectively reducing postsurgical pain [9]; however, no drug that lacks the side effects of ketamine, due to other CNS functions of the receptor, has been developed [12].

It is important to note that if the input continues, the enhanced spinal responses remain, but if the peripheral input declines or is blocked, there is a slow return in neuronal responses back to baseline. In animal studies, CS can be attenuated by peripheral lidocaine acting on the afferent input. This clearly reinforces that once CS is induced, a degree of peripheral input is needed to maintain it [15]. In human psychophysical studies, temporal summation is induced in volunteers and is altered in some patient groups. In addition, pharmacologic block of the NMDA receptor reduces this in both healthy subjects and in patients, such as those with postsurgical pains [47].

Because spinal neurons project to higher centers where the final pain experience is generated, CS is a likely initiating substrate for the allodynia, hyperalgesia, and spontaneous pain these patients experience.

Descending Controls

Brain Circuitry Controlling Spinal Transmission

Changes in excitability at spinal levels have consequences for the brain through ascending pathways. In turn, descending controls from the brain to the spinal cord can further modulate spinal outputs in parallel with the peripheral drives and modulation of sensory signals within the dorsal horn. Altered pain processing in a number of higher centers, of both the ongoing and evoked activities after nerve injury, has been reported. These areas include the amygdala and cingulate cortex, implicated in fear, emotional memories, and aversion, where increases in ongoing activity in the former after nerve injury have been reported in animal models [21]. In addition, altering central affective processes, the amygdala in particular has access back to the spinal cord via pathways from lamina I of the spinal cord that project to this area and then loop back down through brainstem areas to the dorsal horn to either increase or decrease nociceptive transmission [5,48]. Pathways such as these are a likely route by which the brain, under the influence of motivational, cognitive, and affective systems, can influence nociception and pain at spinal levels and link mood with pain. Indeed, lamina I neurons of the spinal cord, responsible for the processes that lead to windup, are also at the origins of spinal GABA controls and both descending facilitations (through 5-HT) and inhibitions (through noradrenaline) [40].

Failure of Descending Inhibition

Thus, descending facilitatory influences from the midbrain and brainstem, or a decline in descending inhibitions, can increase spinal excitability in parallel with LTP [44]. In fact, a loss of diffuse noxious inhibitory controls (DNIC), one form of descending inhibition, has been reported in many patient groups [59]. DNIC appears to have reduced efficiency in a number of pains and may furthermore be predictive of other pain problems, including the likelihood of developing acute and chronic postoperative pain [54].

A loss of descending noradrenergic controls has been reported in animal models of neuropathy, inhibitions through the α2-adrenoceptor that normally hold down the low to medium intensity mechanical responses of spinal neurons [39]. This loss will thus result in a greater proportion of lower level mechanical stimuli signaling to the brain and so may contribute to static allodynias. Furthermore, despite identical DRG and spinal consequences of peripheral nerve damage, animals that have recruited this descending noradrenergic system do not develop mechanical hypersensitivities [17]. Thus, the spinal cord can determine the level of messages sent to the brain, but the brain can also adjust the level of spinal excitability through descending controls, both inhibitory and excitatory [5], and in some cases do this independently of the periphery [6]. The TCA, SNRI, tapentadol, dexmedetomidine, and related drugs act on these monoamine systems and presumably shift them back to more normal functions.

Brain Mechanisms

Although changes in the periphery and dorsal horn undoubtedly go a long way toward explaining the symptoms of chronic pain syndromes such as postsurgical pain, the story does not end at the brainstem: There is now strong evidence supporting a crucial role for dramatic alterations in cortical and subcortical processing. The "pain matrix" is a term frequently used to describe the set of brain structures thought to contribute to nociceptive processing and the subjective pain experience, including the anterior cingulate, insula, somatosensory, frontal and prefrontal cortices, thalamus, basal ganglia, cerebellum, and amygdala. Given that several brain regions are implicated in any one aspect of the pain experience, it makes sense not to focus on regions in isolation but instead on how they communicate, for disruption in communication will undoubtedly lead to pathologic pain sensations.

Neurochemical Alterations in Patients with Chronic Pain

Glutamate

Patients with fibromyalgia have been shown to have a higher concentration of the universal excitatory neurotransmitter glutamate in their cerebrospinal fluid (CSF) [45], associating enhanced glutamate signaling with this condition. In support of this, glutamate levels in the insula cortex are reduced following successful treatment of fibromyalgia [24]. The finding that fMRI-measured insula activity is increased in fibromyalgia patients together with that of a positive correlation between insula activity and glutamate levels during changes in perceived pain [24] further implicates altered/enhanced insula glutamate signaling in the pathology of clinical pain.

Dopamine

The dopamine (DA) neurotransmitter system in the brain, including projections terminating in the striatum (nigrostriatal) and those from the ventral tegmental area (VTA) to limbic regions such as the nucleus accumbens (mesolimbic), is thought to play a crucial role in pain modulation. Unsurprisingly, evidence for dopaminergic disruption contributing to the pathology of chronic pain is building. Positron emission tomography (PET) using 6-[^{18}F]fluorodopa shows a reduction in presynaptic dopaminergic signaling in the basal ganglia of patients with idiopathic burning mouth syndrome [26], suggesting decreased activity of nigrostriatal nociceptive projection neurons. In a separate investigation, fibromyalgia patients were found to lack the basal ganglia DA response to tonic noxious stimulation as well as the correlation between pain severity and DA release seen in healthy controls (as measured by PET imaging of DA receptor binding [55]). This evidence points toward an attenuation of dopaminergic signaling being implicated in chronic pain. Coming from a different angle, DA's involvement is highlighted in patients with Parkinson disease, where loss of dopaminergic innervation of the striatum is frequently associated with chronic pain [19].

Opioids

Also key to healthy modulation of nociceptive signaling, harboring a tight relationship with the DA system, are the endogenous opioids. In response to painful stimulation, acute or tonic, release of endogenous opioids occurs both spinally and supraspinally. There is very strong evidence that this contributes to a reduction in the perceived pain (antinociception), the basis behind morphine's efficacy as an analgesic. There is now some progress toward understanding the opioids' behavior in pathologic chronic pain conditions.

PET imaging has shown a reduction in the binding of opioid tracers in key brain areas such as the amygdala, cingulate cortex, and nucleus accumbens in patients with a variety of chronic pain conditions including fibromyalgia [23] and rheumatoid arthritis [27]. Reduction of chronic inflammatory pain through treatment is accompanied by an increase of the opioidergic binding toward normal levels, reinforcing this association [27]. Uncertainty in the interpretation of tracer binding results can be largely dismissed given that opioid immunoreactivity in the CSF is greater in chronic pain patients, suggesting an increase in opioid release leading to fewer available receptors is responsible for reduced binding [8].

At present, little is known about changes in these central transmitter systems in postoperative pain.

Rodent Models of Chronic Pain: Investigation of Affective Aspects of Pain with CPP

As informative as human investigations into the mechanisms behind chronic pain have proved, there are fundamental limitations associated with clinical research that can be overcome with the use of animal models. These include standardization of pain syndrome characteristics and all other factors that might influence outcome measures, which is unachievable in patient cohorts. Importantly, animal models of chronic pain can be manipulated in ways that are unethical in humans, allowing causal links to be made, for example, between neurotransmitter systems and specific aspects of pain processing.

Consequently the contribution of animal models of chronic pain conditions, including a model specific for postsurgical pain, to our understanding of the neurobiology of persistent pain is vast. Given the significant burden of the affective component, i.e., the aversiveness, is to patients with chronic pain [18], it is important to investigate the cerebral processing involved. Ongoing pain, alongside evoked hypersensitivity, is significant in persistent postoperative pain and is often reported as the most debilitating component for patients [2].

A behavioral paradigm that can give an indirect measure of the aversiveness of ongoing pain in rat models of chronic pain is conditioned place preference (CPP) [35]. This measure not only unmasks the presence of ongoing pain by demonstrating that its removal is rewarding but also allows measurement of the efficacy of an analgesic agent. By interfering with neurotransmitter and neuromodulator systems in rodent models of chronic pain and evaluating effects on ongoing pain using CPP, one can begin to unpick the mechanisms behind the complex pathology involved.

The Mesolimbic DA System and Motivational Aspects of Ongoing Pain

The surmounting clinical evidence suggesting disruption of DA in chronic pain, together with its role on positive reinforcement/reward, makes the mesolimbic dopaminergic system an attractive target for investigations using CPP into pain relief reward. In a rodent model of chronic postsurgical pain, pain relief by peripheral nerve block (PNB) elicited CPP [36]. Immunohistochemistry of the VTA indicates that PNB resulted in increased activity of mesolimbic DA neurons. Crucially, targeting lesions of these neurons with baclofen and disruption of DA signaling in the nucleus accumbens reduced or blocked expression of CPP, suggesting that activation of dopaminergic neurons of the VTA resulting in DA release in the nucleus accumbens is essential for negative reinforcement by pain relief [36].

The Anterior Cingulate Cortex Mediates Aversive Aspects of Pain

Another key finding resulting from CPP experiments is the role of the anterior cingulate cortex (ACC) in ongoing pain, a region previously implicated in the processing of acute and chronic pain in humans. In the rat SNL (spinal nerve ligation) model of neuropathic pain, CPP elicited by blockage of the descending pain facilitation (see previously) is prevented by bilateral lesions of the rostral ACC [38]. These findings suggest that activity in the ACC is required for the tonic aversive state induced by peripheral nerve injury. Direct and indirect projections from the rostral ACC to the mesolimbic DA neurons present a route through which the aversive consequences of chronic pain can motivate behavior. These insights hint an important direction for future research for development of targeted therapies in chronic pain aversiveness.

Long-Term Consequences of the Neurochemical Changes

Many neuroimaging studies have shown differences in brain structure between chronic pain patients and controls, providing evidence that prolonged pain is associated with structural brain alterations. Gray matter volume is typically found to have decreased in components of the "pain matrix", and the greater the decreases, the longer the pain duration [1]. This evidence, together with time course data from animal models [46] and the demonstration that gray matter measurements normalize when pain is resolved [22], suggests that structural changes are a consequence of the prolonged pain. It is possible that the neurochemical changes observed in both animal and human chronic pain contribute to the development of these structural changes, which in turn make successful treatment outcomes less likely over time. If this is the case, the sooner neurochemical alterations are rectified once chronic postsurgical pain is recognized, the better the outlook of intervention.

The periphery drives sensitization of the spinal cord, which in turn changes brain processing in terms of both sensory and affective function. To conclude, better understanding of the pharmacologic processes underlying these events is the key to better treatments or even the prevention of postsurgical pains. But there are many issues, not least which agents to use, predicting efficacy in patient groups and the duration of treatments that could be for months after the surgery to block slowly developing neuropathic pain states. But these are questions that can be answered by cooperation between the preclinical and clinical domains.

Acknowledgments

This work was funded by the Medical Research Council and Wellcome Trust London Pain Consortium through UCL studentships to L.V.F. and L.D.T.

REFERENCES

1. Apkarian AV, Sosa Y, Sonty S, Levy RM, Harden RN, Parrish TB, Gitelman DR. Chronic back pain is associated with decreased prefrontal and thalamic gray matter density. J Neurosci 2004;24:10410–5.
2. Backonja M-M, Stacey B. Neuropathic pain symptoms relative to overall pain rating. J Pain 2004;5:491–7.
3. Banik RK, Brennan TJ. Trpv1 mediates spontaneous firing and heat sensitization of cutaneous primary afferents after plantar incision. Pain 2009;141:41–51.
4. Banik RK, Subieta AR, Wu C, Brennan TJ. Increased nerve growth factor after rat plantar incision contributes to guarding behavior and heat hyperalgesia. Pain 2005;117:68–76.
5. Bannister K, Bee LA, Dickenson AH. Preclinical and early clinical investigations related to monoaminergic pain modulation. Neurotherapeutics 2009;6:703–12.
6. Bannister K, Dickenson AH. Opioid hyperalgesia. Curr Opin Support Palliat Care 2010;4:1–5.
7. Barabas ME, Stucky CL. TRPV1, but not TRPA1, in primary sensory neurons contributes to cutaneous incision-mediated hypersensitivity. Mol Pain 2013;9:9.
8. Baraniuk JN, Whalen G, Cunningham J, Clauw DJ. Cerebrospinal fluid levels of opioid peptides in fibromyalgia and chronic low back pain. BMC Musculoskelet Disord 2004;5:48.
9. Barreveld AM, Correll DJ, Liu X, Max B, McGowan JA, Shovel L, Wasan AD, Nedeljkovic SS. Ketamine decreases postoperative pain scores in patients taking opioids for chronic pain: results of a prospective, randomized, double-blind study. Pain Med 2013;14:925–34.
10. Bauer CS, Nieto-Rostro M, Rahman W, Tran-Van-Minh A, Ferron L, Douglas L, Kadurin I, Sri Ranjan Y, Fernandez-Alacid L, Millar NS, Dickenson AH, Lujan R, Dolphin AC. The increased trafficking of the calcium channel subunit $\alpha_2\delta$-1 to presynaptic terminals in neuropathic pain is inhibited by the $\alpha_2\delta$ ligand pregabalin. J Neurosci 2009;29:4076–88.
11. Bautista DM, Pellegrino M, Tsunozaki M. TRPA1: a gatekeeper for inflammation. Annu Rev Physiol 2013;75:181–200.
12. D'Mello R, Dickenson AH. Spinal cord mechanisms of pain. Br J Anaesth 2008;101:8–16.
13. Deval E, Noël J, Gasull X, Delaunay A, Alloui A, Friend V, Eschalier A, Lazdunski M, Lingueglia E. Acid-sensing ion channels in postoperative pain. J Neurosci 2011;31:6059–66.
14. Dib-Hajj SD, Cummins TR, Black JA, Waxman SG. Sodium channels in normal and pathological pain. Annu Rev Neurosci 2010;33:325–47.
15. Dickenson AH, Sullivan AF. Peripheral origins and central modulation of subcutaneous formalin-induced activity of rat dorsal horn neurones. Neurosci Lett 1987;83:207–11.
16. Duan G, Xiang G, Zhang X, Yuan R, Zhan H, Qi D. A single-nucleotide polymorphism in SCN9A may decrease postoperative paon sensitivity in the general population. Anesthesiology 2013;118:436–42.
17. De Felice M, Sanoja R, Wang R, Vera-Portocarrero L, Oyarzo J, King T, Ossipov MH, Vanderah TW, Lai J, Dussor GO, Fields HL, Price TJ, Porreca F. Engagement of descending inhibition from the rostral ventromedial medulla protects against chronic neuropathic pain. Pain 2011;152:2701–9.
18. Fields HL. Pain: an unpleasant topic. Pain 1999;(Suppl. 6):S61–9.
19. Ford B. Pain in Parkinson's disease. Mov Disord 2010;25(Suppl. 1):S98–103.
20. Gold MS, Weinreich D, Kim C-S, Wang R, Treanor J, Porreca F, Lai J. Redistribution of NaV1.8 in uninjured axons enables neuropathic pain. J Neurosci 2003;23:158–66.
21. Gonçalves L, Dickenson AH. Asymmetric time-dependent activation of right central amygdala neurones in rats with peripheral neuropathy and pregabalin modulation. Eur J Neurosci 2012;36:3204–13.
22. Gwilym SE, Filippini N, Douaud G, Carr AJ, Tracey I. Thalamic atrophy associated with painful osteoarthritis of the hip is reversible after arthroplasty: a longitudinal voxel-based morphometric study. Arthritis Rheum 2010;62:2930–40.
23. Harris RE, Clauw DJ, Scott DJ, McLean SA, Gracely RH, Zubieta J-K. Decreased central mu-opioid receptor availability in fibromyalgia. J Neurosci 2007;27:10000–6.
24. Harris RE, Sundgren PC, Pang Y, Hsu M, Petrou M, Kim S-H, McLean SA, Gracely RH, Clauw DJ. Dynamic levels of glutamate within the insula are associated with improvements in multiple pain domains in fibromyalgia. Arthritis Rheum 2008;58:903–7.

25. Herrero JF, Laird JM, López-García JA. Wind-up of spinal cord neurones and pain sensation: much ado about something? Prog Neurobiol 2000;61:169–203.
26. Jääskeläinen SK, Rinne JO, Forssell H, Tenovuo O, Kaasinen V, Sonninen P, Bergman J. Role of the dopaminergic system in chronic pain – a fluorodopa-PET study. Pain 2001;90:257–60.
27. Jones AK, Cunningham VJ, Ha-Kawa S, Fujiwara T, Luthra SK, Silva S, Derbyshire S, Jones T. Changes in central opioid receptor binding in relation to inflammation and pain in patients with rheumatoid arthritis. Br J Rheumatol 1994;33:909–16.
28. Joshi SK, Mikusa JP, Hernandez G, Baker S, Shieh C-C, Neelands T, Zhang X-F, Niforatos W, Kage K, Han P, Krafte D, Faltynek C, Sullivan JP, Jarvis MF, Honore P. Involvement of the TTX-resistant sodium channel Nav 1.8 in inflammatory and neuropathic, but not post-operative, pain states. Pain 2006;123:75–82.
29. Kang S, Wu C, Banik RK, Brennan TJ. Effect of capsaicin treatment on nociceptors in rat glabrous skin one day after plantar incision. Pain 2010;148:128–40.
30. Kehlet H, Jensen TS, Woolf CJ. Persistent postsurgical pain: risk factors and prevention. Lancet 2006;367:1618–25.
31. Li C-Y, Zhang X-L, Matthews EA, Li K-W, Kurwa A, Boroujerdi A, Gross J, Gold MS, Dickenson AH, Feng G, Luo ZD. Calcium channel $\alpha_2\delta_1$ subunit mediates spinal hyperexcitability in pain modulation. Pain 2006;125:20–34.
32. Liu M, Wood JN. The roles of sodium channels in nociception: implications for mechanisms of neuropathic pain. Pain Med 2011;12(Suppl. 3):S93–9.
33. McDonnell JG, Finnerty O, Laffey JG. Stellate ganglion blockade for analgesia following upper limb surgery. Anaesthesia 2011;66:611–4.
34. Minett MS, Nassar MA, Clark AK, Passmore G, Dickenson AH, Wang F, Malcangio M, Wood JN. Distinct Nav1.7-dependent pain sensations require different sets of sensory and sympathetic neurons. Nat Commun 2012;3:791.
35. Navratilova E, Xie JY, King T, Porreca F. Evaluation of reward from pain relief. Ann N Y Acad Sci 2013;1282:1–11.
36. Navratilova E, Xie JY, Okun A, Qu C, Eyde N, Ci S, Ossipov MH, King T, Fields HL, Porreca F. Pain relief produces negative reinforcement through activation of mesolimbic reward-valuation circuitry. Proc Natl Acad Sci USA 2012:6–10.
37. O'Neill J, Brock C, Olesen AE, Andresen T, Nilsson M, Dickenson AH. Unravelling the mystery of capsaicin: a tool to understand and treat pain. Pharmacol Rev 2012;64:939–71.
38. Qu C, King T, Okun A, Lai J, Fields HL, Porreca F. Lesion of the rostral anterior cingulate cortex eliminates the aversiveness of spontaneous neuropathic pain following partial or complete axotomy. Pain 2011;152:1641–8.
39. Rahman W, D'Mello R, Dickenson AH. Peripheral nerve injury-induced changes in spinal α_2-adrenoceptor-mediated modulation of mechanically evoked dorsal horn neuronal responses. J Pain 2008;9:350–9.
40. Rahman W, Suzuki R, Hunt SP, Dickenson AH. Selective ablation of dorsal horn NK1 expressing cells reveals a modulation of spinal α_2-adrenergic inhibition of dorsal horn neurones. Neuropharmacology 2008;54:1208–14.
41. Ramaswamy S, Wilson JA, Colvin L. Non-opioid-based adjuvant analgesia in perioperative care. Contin Educ Anaesth Crit Care Pain 2013;13(5):152–7.
42. Ringkamp M, Raja S, Campbell J, Meyer R. Peripheral mechanisms of cutaneous nociception. In: McMahon S, Koltzenburg M, Tracey I, Turk DC, editors. Wall & Melzack's textbook of pain. Philadelphia, PA: Elsevier Health Sciences; 2013. p. 1–30.
43. Roza C, Laird JMA, Souslova V, Wood JN, Cervero F. The tetrodotoxin-resistant Na$^+$ channel Nav1.8 is essential for the expression of spontaneous activity in damaged sensory axons of mice. J Physiol 2003;550:921–6.
44. Rygh LJ, Svendsen F, Hole K, Tjølsen A. Natural noxious stimulation can induce long-term increase of spinal nociceptive responses. Pain 1999;82:305–10.
45. Sarchielli P, Mancini ML, Floridi A, Coppola F, Rossi C, Nardi K, Acciarresi M, Pini LA, Calabresi P. Increased levels of neurotrophins are not specific for chronic migraine: evidence from primary fibromyalgia syndrome. J Pain 2007;8:737–45.
46. Seminowicz DA, Laferriere AL, Millecamps M, Yu JSC, Coderre TJ, Bushnell MC. MRI structural brain changes associated with sensory and emotional function in a rat model of long-term neuropathic pain. Neuroimage 2009;47:1007–14.
47. Stubhaug A, Breivik H, Eide PK, Kreunen M, Foss A. Mapping of punctuate hyperalgesia around a surgical incision demonstrates that ketamine is a powerful suppressor of central sensitization to pain following surgery. Acta Anaesthesiol Scand 1997;41:1124–32.
48. Suzuki R, Morcuende S, Webber M, Hunt SP, Dickenson AH. Superficial NK1-expressing neurons control spinal excitability through activation of descending pathways. Nat Neurosci 2002;5:1319–26.

49. Takahashi A, Mashimo T, Uchida I. GABAergic tonic inhibition of substantia gelatinosa neurons in mouse spinal cord. Neuroreport 2006;17:1331–5.
50. Thakur M, Rahman W, Hobbs C, Dickenson AH, Bennett DLH. Characterisation of a peripheral neuropathic component of the rat monoiodoacetate model of osteoarthritis. PLoS One 2012;7:e33730.
51. Torsney C, MacDermott AB. Disinhibition opens the gate to pathological pain signaling in superficial neurokinin 1 receptor-expressing neurons in rat spinal cord. J Neurosci 2006;26:1833–43.
52. Vanegas H, Schaible H-G. Effects of antagonists to high-threshold calcium channels upon spinal mechanisms of pain, hyperalgesia and allodynia. Pain 2000;85:9–18.
53. Wei H, Karimaa M, Korjamo T, Koivisto A, Pertovaara A. Transient receptor potential ankyrin 1 ion channel contributes to guarding pain and mechanical hypersensitivity in a rat model of postoperative pain. Anesthesiology 2012;117:137–48.
54. Van Wijk G, Veldhuijzen DS. Perspective on diffuse noxious inhibitory controls as a model of endogenous pain modulation in clinical pain syndromes. J Pain 2010;11:408–19.
55. Wood PB, Schweinhardt P, Jaeger E, Dagher A, Hakyemez H, Rabiner EA, Bushnell MC, Chizh BA. Fibromyalgia patients show an abnormal dopamine response to pain. Eur J Neurosci 2007;25:3576–82.
56. Woolf CJ. Evidence for a central component of post-injury pain hypersensitivity. Nature 1983;306:686–8.
57. Xie W, Strong JA, Meij JTA, Zhang J-M, Yu L. Neuropathic pain: early spontaneous afferent activity is the trigger. Pain 2005;116:243–56.
58. Yaksh TL. Behavioral and autonomic correlates of the tactile evoked allodynia produced by spinal glycine inhibition: effects of modulatory receptor systems and excitatory amino acid antagonists. Pain 1989;37:111–23.
59. Yarnitsky D. Conditioned pain modulation (the diffuse noxious inhibitory control-like effect): its relevance for acute and chronic pain states. Curr Opin Anaesthesiol 2010;23:611–5.

CHAPTER 7

Central Sensitization, Synaptic Potentiation, and Microglia

Min Zhuo

INTRODUCTION

Pain is an unpleasant sensory experience induced by noxious stimuli or described in such terms. There are at least two major forms of pain: physiologic pain and pathologic pain. Physiologic pain is important for animals to avoid potential injury, whereas pathologic pain is unpleasant and lasts for an extended period of time after injury. Pathologic pain is often caused by inflammation (called inflammatory pain) or nerve injury (neuropathic pain) and is often accompanied by a heightened responsiveness to noxious (called hyperalgesia) and nonnoxious stimuli (called allodynia). Neuropathic pain is defined as a chronic pain state resulting from peripheral or central nerve injury either due to acute events or systemic disease. Chronic pain costs approximately $600 billion annually in health care and lost productivity in the United States. Currently available treatments for neuropathic pain, including tricyclic antidepressants and the current "gold standard" gabapentin, typically show limited efficacy in most patients and frequently produce central side effects. The major aim of this review is to review recent progress in synaptic plasticity using animal models of neuropathic and inflammatory pain. I will focus on the roles of cortical long-term potentiation (LTP) in chronic pain.

CENTRAL SENSITIZATION VERSUS LONG-TERM POTENTIATION (LTP)

It is generally agreed that peripheral injury triggers long-term changes in the peripheral and central nervous systems (CNS). Central sensitization is first revealed in in vivo study and is the enhanced neuronal spike response to sensory stimuli after the injury [8,18,29]. Cumulative experimental data from animal studies suggest that central sensitization is unlikely mediated by one unique mechanism. It may be caused by different mechanisms at synaptic, cellular, and network levels. At the synaptic level, changes in excitatory or inhibitory transmission may contribute to sensitization. At the cellular level, alteration in spike properties or any ion channel properties affecting membrane potentials may affect central sensitization. Finally, changes in the local spinal circuits or descending inhibitory or facilitatory modulation [2,42–44] may affect central sensitization. Although the original discovery of central sensitization was made at the level of spinal cord, it is possible that similar sensitization may happen at higher brain structures that are involved in pain transmission and modulation such as the cortex.

Unlike central sensitization, which is a rather complex neuronal response, synaptic LTP presents an accessible cellular model for studying molecular mechanisms of pain-related plasticity [35]. Recently, progress has been made in understanding basic mechanisms of synaptic LTP. Glutamatergic synapses in the spinal cord dorsal horn undergo long-term enhancement in an activity-dependent manner, a situation that may mimic conditions after peripheral injuries. Indeed, in vivo studies have provided direct evidence that excitatory synaptic transmission is significantly enhanced in dorsal horn neurons after peripheral inflammation or nerve injury [16,40].

LTP AS A MAJOR FORM OF SYNAPTIC PLASTICITY IN THE CNS

LTP was first reported by Bliss and Lomo that excitatory transmission in the hippocampal dentate gyrus undergoes LTP after tetanic stimulation [1]. The original observations were reported in the anesthetized rabbit. Because of the unique anatomic structures of hippocampus, the circuits can be easily preserved in brain slice preparation in vitro. Much of the basic mechanisms for LTP come from in vitro studies using slice preparation. It is found that LTP can be induced by different induction protocols and molecular mechanisms underlying them may vary. According to the stimulation protocol and duration of LTP, it can be divided into at least two major forms: early LTP (E-LTP) and late-phase LTP (L-LTP). E-LTP is induced by one or two trains of stimuli, usually last for 1 to 3 hours, and does not require new protein synthesis. L-LTP is induced by multiple trains of stimuli delivered at 3 to 5 minutes' intervals and lasts from hours to days. It requires both translation and transcription [4]. In the anterior cingulate cortex (ACC) and insular cortex (IC), both E-LTP and L-LTP have been reported (see Figure 7-1) [14]. More importantly, the induction of ACC L-LTP is occluded by nerve injury [12]. As compared with central sensitization and hippocampal LTP, thus, according to the time phase, E-LTP is likely to parallel with central sensitization in the spinal cord. L-LTP, however, may cause other changes and may contribute to persistent or chronic pain. Future studies of L-LTP in pain-related cortex will provide key information for our understanding of basic mechanisms of chronic pain.

EVIDENCE OF LTP IN THE SPINAL CORD DORSAL HORN

Homosynaptic LTP

The spinal cord dorsal horn is the first relay for pain transmission in the CNS. Glutamate is the principal fast excitatory transmitter, and the corresponding postsynaptic responses are mediated by α-amino-3-hydroxy-5-methyl-4-isoxazole propionate (AMPA) and kainate receptors with a smaller contribution of N-methyl-D-aspartate (NMDA) receptors [10]. NMDA receptors serve as a key coincidence detector and are important for synaptic plasticity in central synapses. Therefore, it is believed that NMDA receptors play a critical role in injury-related synaptic plasticity in dorsal horn neurons, such as LTP. In in vitro spinal slices, LTP in the spinal dorsal horn neurons could be induced by several different protocols, including high-frequency stimulation, low-frequency stimulation, or a pairing protocol [16,26]. The mechanism of LTP induction involves the activation of NMDA receptors, neurokinin-1 receptors, and the downstream mitogen-activated protein (MAP) kinase pathway. In addition, in vivo LTP of C-fiber–evoked responses could also be induced by

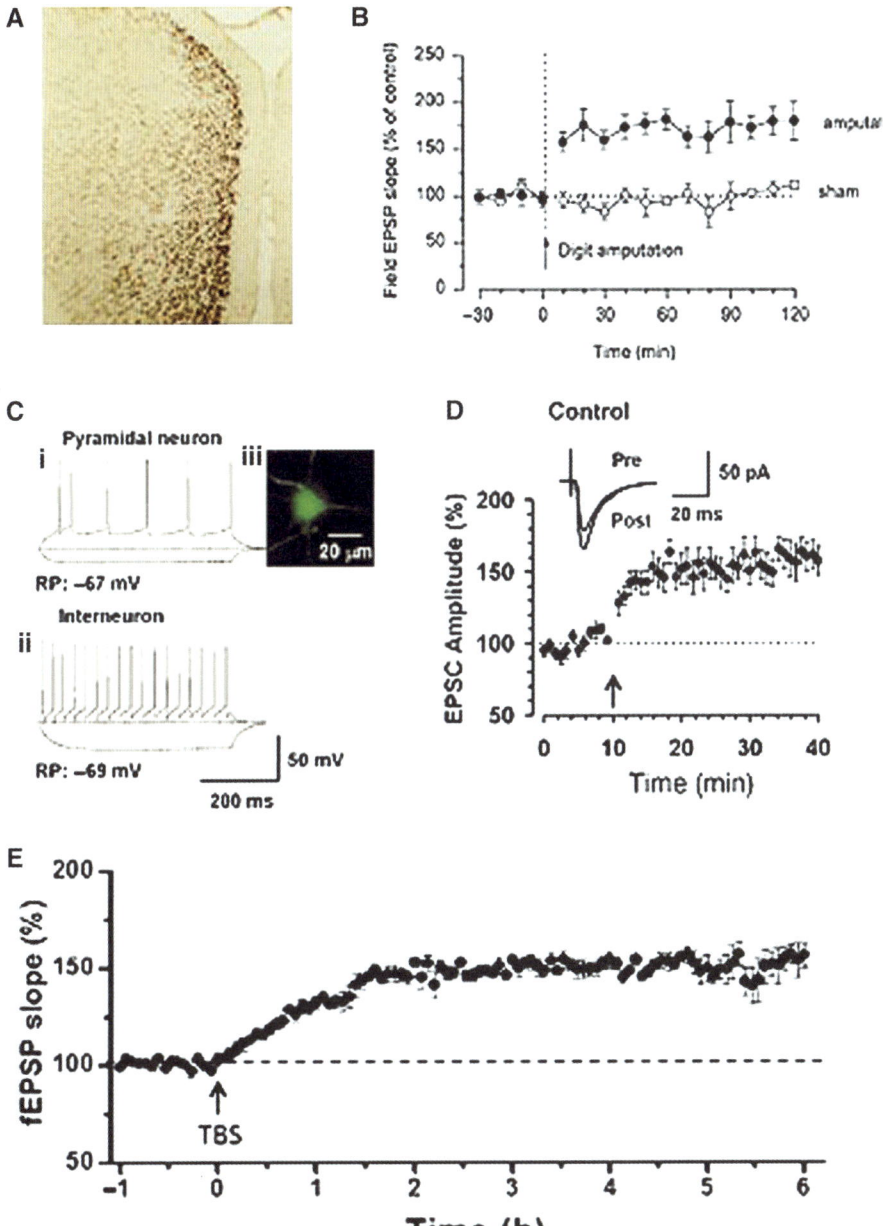

FIGURE 7-1 Long-term potentiation (LTP) as a cellular model for chronic pain in the anterior cingulate cortex (ACC). **A:** Activation of immediate early genes in ACC neurons of an adult rat after peripheral injury. **B:** In vivo recording of ACC LTP in adult rats after amputation of a single digit in the hind paw under anesthesia. **C:** Current-clamp recordings to identify pyramidal neurons (i) and interneurons (ii) of adult mice by current injections of -100, 0, and 100 pA. A labeled pyramid-like neuron is shown in (iii). RP, resting membrane potential. **D:** LTP was induced in pyramidal neurons in adult mouse ACC by the pairing training protocol (indicated by an *arrow*). The inset shows averages of six excitatory postsynaptic currents (EPSCs) 5 min before and 25 min after the pairing training (*arrow*). The *broken line* indicates the mean basal synaptic responses. **E:** Field recording of late-phase LTP in adult mouse ACC slices. fEPSP, field excitatory postsynaptic potential. (Adapted from Zhuo M. Targeting neuronal adenylyl cyclase for the treatment of chronic pain. Drug Discov Today 2012;17:573–82.)

low- or high-frequency stimulation of sensory nerve fibers. Recent studies showed that NR2B-containing NMDA receptors are required for spinal LTP induction. More importantly, in animals with the spinal cord and descending pathways intact, intraplantar injections of formalin or sciatic nerve jury induced LTP in the dorsal horn that was dependent on NMDA receptor activation.

Heterosynaptic LTP

In addition to homosynaptic LTP, heterosynaptic LTP has been also reported. 5-hydroxytryptamine (5-HT), an important neurotransmitter of the raphe–spinal projection pathway, transforms silent glutamatergic synapses into functional ones [9,11,20]. The mechanism underlying this conversion involves 5-HT–induced protein kinase C (PKC) activation, AMPA receptor–PDZ interactions, and the recruitment of AMPA receptors. Silent synapses are likely involved in synaptic potentiation in the spinal dorsal horn, considering that the recruitment of silent synapses could significantly enhance spinal sensory transmission, including nociceptive transmission. Another potential function of silent synapses is to contribute to a descending facilitatory modulatory network within the spinal cord [38]. The recruitment by 5-HT could strengthen spinal sensory synapses receiving innervation from descending 5-HT projection fibers, which most likely originate from the rostral ventromedial medulla (RVM) [39].

LTP IN PAIN-RELATED CORTEX

ACC and IC

Human and animal studies are consistent with the suggestion that the ACC, IC, and related areas are important for pain perception [7,19,40]. Both ACC and IC neurons respond to nociceptive stimuli, and activity within the ACC is related to the unpleasantness or discomfort of noxious stimuli. Peripheral injury caused bilateral increases in the expression of activity-dependent immediate early genes such as *c-fos*, egr1 (early growth response gene 1), and CREB (cAMP response element–binding protein) and increased electrophysiologic responses. Electrophysiologic experiments in cortical slices have shown that excitatory synaptic transmission in the ACC and IC is primarily glutamatergic [40].

It is commonly thought that mature cortical synapses are less plastic. In certain cortical areas, LTP is found to be age-dependent under experimental conditions. The disappearance of cortical LTP is related to the disappearance of glutamate silent synapses or maturation of cortical synapses. However, we found that the ability of cortical synapses to undergo LTP is mostly dependent on induction protocol. In both ACC and IC synapses, theta burst stimulation (TBS) can induce LTP in synapses of young and adult animals (Figure 7-1). Peripheral noxious foot shocks induced TBS-like neuronal activities of ACC neurons by in vivo recordings of freely moving mice [17]. In addition, LTP also can be induced using two other protocols, including the pairing training protocol and the spike-EPSP (excitatory postsynaptic potential) pairing protocol [37].

Pharmacologic studies using selective receptor antagonists reveal that ACC LTP exists in at least four different forms: NMDA receptor dependent, L-type voltage-gated calcium channel (L-VGCC) dependent, L-LTP, and presynaptic LTP (pre-LTP) under experimental in vitro brain slice conditions.

NMDA Receptor–Dependent LTP

In ACC synapses, LTP induced by different protocols is sensitive to the inhibition of NMDA receptors [37,40]. Application of an NMDA receptor antagonist AP-5 blocked the induction of LTP. NMDA receptor containing GluN2A (or called NR2A) or GluN2B (NR2B) subunits contribute to most of NMDA receptor currents, and application of a GluN2A antagonist NVP-AAM077 and GluN2B antagonist ifenprodil or Ro 25-6981 produce an almost complete blockade of NMDA receptor–mediated EPSCs. Application of GluN2A or GluN2B antagonist also reduces LTP, without complete abolishment of LTP. LTP only is abolished after the coapplication of both inhibitors.

Calcium Channel–Dependent LTP

L-VGCCs are also required for the induction of LTP by TBS in the field recording condition [13]. Unlike LTP recorded using field recording, LTP recorded using whole-cell patch clamp does not respond to the inhibition of L-VGCCs [37].

Protein Synthesis–Dependent L-LTP

Recent studies using a 64-channel multielectrode array (MED64) show that ACC LTP induced by multiple TBSs can last more than 5 hours. This form of potentiation is sensitive to inhibition of protein synthesis [3,14], indicating that protein synthesis–dependent L-LTP exists in the ACC. It is likely that L-LTP may contribute to long-term changes in the cortical circuits that are triggered by peripheral injury. Future investigations of basic mechanisms are clearly needed for ACC L-LTP.

MOLECULAR MECHANISMS FOR CORTICAL LTP

Recent genetic, pharmacologic and electrophysiologic approaches have been used to investigate the basic mechanisms for LTP in the ACC synapses [21,40,41]. Activation of NMDA receptors leads to an increase in postsynaptic Ca^{2+} in dendritic spines. Ca^{2+} serves as an important intracellular signal for triggering a series of biochemical events that contribute to the expression of LTP. Ca^{2+} binds to calmodulin (CaM) and leads to activation of calcium-stimulated signaling pathways. Furthermore, postsynaptic injection of BAPTA completely blocked the induction of LTP, indicating the importance of elevated postsynaptic Ca^{2+} concentrations. A work using electroporation of mutant CaM in the ACC neurons suggests that calcium binding sites of CaM are critical for the induction of ACC LTP. Ca^{2+}-stimulated, neuron-specific adenylyl cyclase subtype 1 (AC1) is highly expressed in the ACC neuron, and LTP induced by TBS or pairing stimulation is abolished in AC1 knockout (KO) mice. Several other signaling proteins or protein kinases are found to be involved in ACC LTP, including Ca^{2+}-CaM–dependent protein kinase IV (CaMKIV), early growth response gene 1 (egr1), MAP kinase, and fragile X mental retardation protein (FMRP).

At least four different synaptic mechanisms may contribute to the expression of LTP: (1) presynaptic enhancement of the release of glutamate; (2) postsynaptic enhancement of glutamate AMPA receptor–mediated responses; (3) recruitment of previously "silent" synapses or synaptic trafficking or insertion of AMPA receptors; and (4) structural changes in synapses. We have recently investigated the roles of GluR1 and GluR2/3 using genetic and pharmacologic approaches. We found that GluR1 subunit C-terminal peptide analogue, Pep1-TGL, blocked the induction of ACC LTP [40]. Thus, in the ACC, the interaction between the C-terminus of GluR1 and PDZ domain proteins is required for the induction of LTP. Synaptic delivery of the GluR1 subunit from extrasynaptic sites is the key mechanism underlying synaptic plasticity, and GluR1-PDZ interactions play a critical role in this type of plasticity. Application of philanthotoxin-433 (PhTx) 5 minutes after LTP induction reduced synaptic potentiation, whereas PhTx had no effect on basal AMPA receptor–mediated responses, suggesting that Ca^{2+}-permeable GluR2-lacking receptors contribute to the maintenance of ACC LTP. Our recent studies found that ACC LTP is absent in GluR1 KO mice [18]. We also examined the role of GluR2-related peptides in synaptic potentiation in the ACC and found that the GluR2/3-PDZ interaction had no effect on ACC LTP and the same interfering peptides inhibited ACC LTP.

Intracellular Signaling Pathways Required for Synaptic Potentiation

Ca-CaM

Activation of glutamate NMDA receptors leads to an increase in postsynaptic Ca^{2+} in dendritic spines. Ca^{2+} serves as an important intracellular signal for triggering a series of biochemical events that contribute to the expression of LTP. Ca^{2+} binds to CaM and leads to activation of calcium-stimulated signaling pathways [27]. Furthermore, postsynaptic injection of BAPTA completely blocked the induction of LTP, indicating the importance of elevated postsynaptic Ca^{2+} concentrations [37]. A recent study using electroporation of mutant CaM in the ACC suggests that calcium binding sites of CaM is critical for the induction of cingulate LTP [27].

Adenylyl Cyclases: AC1, AC8

cAMP signaling pathways are widely distributed in biologic systems. Among more than 10 subunits, AC1 and AC8 are two AC subtypes that respond positively to calcium-CaM, including in pain-related spinal and cortical neurons [40,41]. As compared with AC8, AC1 is more sensitive to calcium increase. In the ACC, AC1 is highly expressed in cingulate neurons located in most layers [25]. AC1 is selective for plastic changes; gene deletion of AC1 does not affect basal glutamate transmission in the ACC. By contrast, LTP induced by TBS or pairing stimulation is abolished in cingulate pyramidal cells [13]. AC1 is also contributing to synaptic potentiation induced by forskolin, an AC activator that is nonselective for AC isoform. Gene deletion of AC8 subunit partially contributes to forskolin-induced potentiation. Whole-cell patch-clamp recording also revealed that AC1 activity is required for the induction of LTP in ACC pyramidal cells. By using chemical design and biochemical screening, several selective inhibitors of AC1 have been identified. Consistently, pharmacologic inhibition of AC1 in ACC neurons abolished LTP induced by pairing training [22].

CaMKIV

A major neuronal signaling pathway by which Ca^{2+} activates CREB involves the CaMKIV. CaMKIV is a member of a group of multifunctional CaMKs, so-called because of their broad substrate specificity, which also includes CaMKI and CaMKII. CaMKIV is distinguished among the CaM kinases in its capacity to activate CREB-dependent transcription both by virtue of its nuclear localization and catalysis of CREB phosphorylation on serine 133. CaMKIV also promotes CREB function by activating the transcriptional coactivator CREB binding protein (CBP). CaMKIV is enriched in the ACC [24]. CaMKIV is required for CaM translocation triggered by neural activity into the nuclei of ACC neurons. Previous studies have shown that CaM translocation reflects the trapping of Ca^{2+}-CaM complexes by nuclear CaM binding proteins. The abolishment of CaM translocation in CaMKIV KO mice identifies CaMKIV as the critical sink that traps Ca^{2+}-CaM complexes in neuronal nuclei. This trapping leads to CaMKIV activation and subsequent CREB phosphorylation and activation. Consistently, we found in both in vitro and in vivo conditions that activation of CREB was significantly reduced or abolished in CaMKIV KO mice. Considering the important roles of CREB in LTP, we found that synaptic potentiation induced by TBS was reduced or abolished in the same areas [24].

Gene Expression and Synaptic Potentiation

Although the involvement of different protein kinases and second messengers in the ACC LTP is predicted, recent data of the requirement for several immediate early genes and gene-related proteins in ACC LTP are surprising. Potentiation induced in ACC synapses within 10 to 30 minutes is affected by the gene deletion of egr1 and FMRP. These effects are unlikely due to indirect inhibition of NMDA receptors, as NMDA receptor–mediated currents are not affected.

FMRP

FMRP is a ubiquitously expressed mRNA binding protein associated with polyribosomes and is thought to be involved in the translational efficiency and trafficking of certain mRNAs. FMRP is predominantly a cytoplasmatic protein, but it does shuttle between the nucleus and cytoplasm, perhaps transporting selective mRNA molecules to their final destination within the cell. In neurons, FMRP is found in the dendrite spine head, thereby playing a role in local protein synthesis. FMRP was shown to function as a translational repressor for some synaptic proteins, such as Arc, α-CaMKII, and the dendritic microtubule–associated protein 1b. Protein synthesis has been considered a necessary and important component of synaptic morphology and plasticity. The pairing training produced a significant, long-lasting potentiation of synaptic responses in wild-type mice. However, synaptic potentiation in slices of FMR1 KO mice was completely blocked. This finding provides the first evidence that FMRP may contribute to synaptic potentiation in the ACC neurons [36].

Egr1

The zinc finger transcription factor Egr1 (also called NGFI-A, Krox24, or zif/268) is critical for coupling extracellular signals to changes in cellular gene expression. The upstream promoter region of the Egr1 contains binding sites for cyclic AMP response elements (CRE), suggesting that Egr1 may act downstream from the CREB pathway. In the ACC neurons, Egr1 activity is activated by injury including amputation [23]. One possible role of Egr1 is to contribute to synaptic potentiation. KO mice with deleted egr1 indeed show defect in ACC LTP,

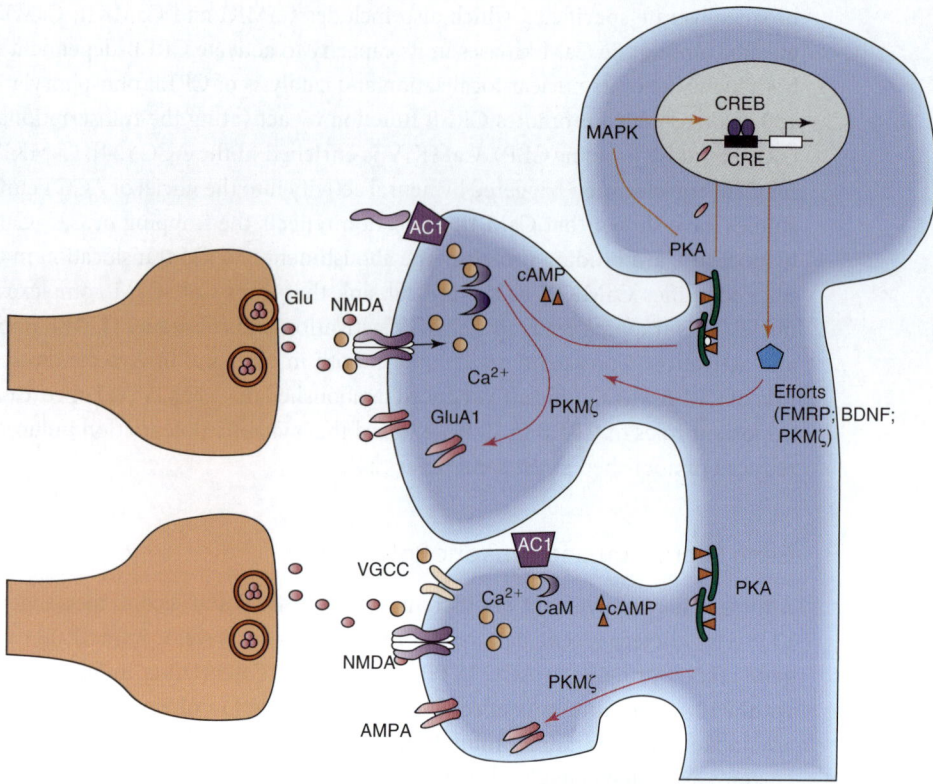

FIGURE 7-2 Model of anterior cingulate cortex (ACC) long-term potentiation (LTP). Neuronal activity triggers the release of glutamate (Glu: *pink circles*). Subsequent activation of glutamate *N*-methyl-D-aspartate (NMDA) receptors results in increases of postsynaptic Ca^{2+} in dendritic spines. Ca^{2+} is an important intracellular signal that triggers a series of biochemical events that contribute to the expression of ACC LTP. Intracellular Ca^{2+} binds to calmodulin (CaM) and leads to the activation of calcium-stimulated adenylyl cyclases (ACs), including AC1, and calcium-CaM–dependent protein kinases (e.g., protein kinase C [PKC], CaM-dependent protein kinase II and IV [CaMKII and CaMKIV]). In turn, calcium-CaMKs phosphorylate glutamate α-amino-3-hydroxy-5-methyl-4-isoxazole propionate (AMPA) receptors, increasing the sensitivity to extracellular glutamate. Trafficking of additional AMPA GluA1 receptors might also contribute to synaptic potentiation. CRE, cAMP response elements; CREB, cAMP response element–binding protein; MAPK, mitogen-activated protein kinase; VGCC, voltage-gated calcium channel; FMRP, fragile X mental retardation protein; BDNF, brain-derived neurotrophic factor.

whereas normal synaptic transmission is observed. Furthermore, NMDA receptor–mediated responses, a key component for the induction of cingulate LTP, are unaffected. Consistent with synaptic potentiation by Egr1, KO mice lacking Egr1 display significant reductions in behaviors associated with long-term fear memory, anxiety and persistent inflammatory pain [5,6].

Based on progress made as described earlier, a proposed synaptic model for the molecular mechanism of LTP in the ACC based on these studies is shown in Figure 7-2. Neural activity triggered by injury increases the release of glutamate at the ACC synapse. The activation of NMDA receptors by glutamate leads to an increase in postsynaptic calcium in dendritic spines. Calcium binds to CaM, leading to the activation of calcium-stimulated signaling pathways. CaM-stimulated ACs, including AC1 and AC8, and CaM-dependent protein kinases, PKC and CaMKII, can all phosphorylate glutamate AMPA receptors, boosting their sensitivity to glutamate or increasing the number of synaptic receptors. Activation of

CaMKIV, which is predominantly expressed in the nucleus, triggers CaMKIV-dependent CREB. In addition, activation of AC1 and AC8 leads to the activation of PKA and subsequently CREB. CREB, as well as other immediate early genes, activates targets that are thought to cause long-lasting changes in synaptic structure and function. Future studies are needed to map signaling pathways that contribute to the maintenance of LTP, including L-LTP, in the ACC.

MEASURING POTENTIATED SYNAPTIC RESPONSES AFTER INJURY

In brain slices, cingulate synapses can undergo LTP after experimentally designed training protocols. One key question regarding ACC plasticity is whether or not injury causes long-term changes in synaptic transmission in the ACC in intact animals. To test this, we performed experiments in anesthetized rats. We measured synaptic responses to peripheral electrical shocks by placing a recording electrode in the ACC of anesthetized rats 1 (5). At high intensities of stimulation, sufficient to activate nociceptive Aδ and C fibers, evoked field EPSPs were recorded in the ACC. Digit amputation at the contralateral hind paw causes a rapid and long-lasting enhancement (more than 120 minutes) of sensory responses. Potentiated sensory responses do not require persistent activity from the injured hind paw [28]. These findings indicate that plastic changes are likely occurring within the ACC synapses. Furthermore, in vivo intracellular recordings from anesthetized rats have confirmed similar findings.

Although in vivo electrophysiology provides direct evidence for pathologic relevance of LTP in the ACC, it is less helpful for studying cellular and molecular mechanisms. Detecting synaptic changes in brain slices of animals with chronic pain will provide opportunities to study the basic mechanisms of chronic pain. In fact, both postsynaptic and presynaptic changes are reported in brain slices of animals with inflammatory or neuropathic pain. Furthermore, in addition to changes in glutamate AMPA receptors, NMDA GluN2B receptors are found to undergo LTP as well.

AMPA Receptors

To detect possible changes in synaptic transmission within the ACC after nerve injury, AMPA receptor–mediated EPSCs in pyramidal neurons in the layer II/III of the ACC are measured in mice with peripheral nerve ligation [33]. The input (stimulation intensity)–output (EPSC amplitude) curve of AMPA receptor–mediated current is significantly shifted to the left after peripheral nerve injury, compared with that in control group. These results suggest that excitatory synaptic transmission is increased in the ACC after peripheral nerve injury. Similar changes are found in ACC neurons in animal models of inflammation induced by complete Freund adjuvant (CFA) [35]. Enhanced synaptic transmission is also found in rats with inflammation. These results demonstrate that AMPA receptor in ACC neurons has an inward rectification property in neuropathic pain. Similar rectification of the AMPA receptor–mediated responses in ACC neurons of rats has been reported after peripheral inflammation with hind paw CFA injection.

Biochemical and anatomic evidence further supports the involvement of postsynaptic AMPA receptors [33]. The membrane AMPA GluA1 receptors are significantly increased, whereas GluA2/3 receptors are not significantly affected. Such increases are dependent of

PKA phosphorylation of GluR1 receptors. Recent electron microscopic data further support that postsynaptic membrane GluA1 receptors are significantly increased after peripheral injury [3].

NMDA GluN2B Receptors

In addition to AMPA receptors, electrophysiologic and biochemical studies consistently indicate that peripheral injuries indeed cause the increases of NMDA GluN2B receptors in the ACC (as well as the insular cortex). After nerve injury or inflammation, cortical NMDA GluN2B receptors are significantly enhanced [15,30]. Furthermore, the upregulation of NMDA GluN2B receptors in the ACC or IC contributes to inflammation-related or nerve injury–related persistent pain [15]. In cases of persistent inflammation, the expression of NMDA GluN2B receptors in the ACC is upregulated, thereby increasing the GluN2B component in NMDA-mediated responses [30]. Consistently, microinjection into the ACC or systemic administration of GluN2B receptor–selective antagonists inhibits behavioral responses to peripheral inflammation. Recent studies in the insular cortex reveal that nerve injury also triggers the upregulation of NMDA GluN2B receptors. Thus, the central NMDA GluN2B receptor is a potential drug target for controlling chronic pain [39].

Presynaptic Release

In addition to postsynaptic enhancement, recent studies indicate that presynaptic neurotransmitter release is also enhanced in the ACC [33]. Paired-pulse facilitation (PPF) is a transient form of plasticity commonly used as a measure of presynaptic function, in which the response to the second stimulus is enhanced as a result of residual calcium in the presynaptic terminal after the first stimulus. After nerve ligation, there was a significant reduction in PPF in ACC neurons compared with those from control mice. These results indicate the presynaptic enhancement of the excitatory synaptic transmission in the ACC after nerve injury [33]. Similar changes in PPF ratio are found in ACC neurons of animals with CFA inflammation [35], indicating that presynaptic enhancement of glutamate release is also shared by peripheral inflammation.

In addition to the use of PPF in the ACC after peripheral nerve injury, AMPA receptor–mediated miniature EPSCs (mEPSCs) in ACC neurons in the presence of 0.5 μM tetrodotoxin (TTX) were also found to be affected. After peripheral nerve injury, there was an obvious increase of mEPSC frequency in ACC neurons compared with that of control groups. Considering that most LTPs studied in the ACC are postsynaptically expressed, it is important to develop an experimentally induced presynaptic LTP model to mimic presynaptic changes of glutamate release in the ACC after peripheral injury.

INHIBITING LTP REDUCES CHRONIC PAIN

Owing to important roles of NMDA receptors, in particular NMDA NR2B receptor in synaptic potentiation, it has been demonstrated that NR2B inhibitors indeed produce analgesic effects in animal models of chronic pain. However, due to their critical roles in cognition and other high-order brain functions, their potential usage for treating chronic pain is limited by their possible central cognitive side effects. Among several key second messengers that contribute to ACC LTP, AC1 is unique for LTP in this region. Unlike NMDA NR2B receptors, AC1 is not necessary for learning-related LTP in the hippocampus and learning behavioral responses in various memory tests. In contract, AC1 plays a critical role in pain-related LTP in both the spinal cord dorsal horn and ACC [41]. Behaviorally, AC1 KO mice show reduced inflammatory, deep muscle pain, and neuropathic pain [24], whereas other physiologic functions remain intact in AC1 KO mice, including acute pain, Morris water maze performance, and anxiety-like behaviors and motor functions. Considering that AC1 is mainly expressed in the CNS, AC1 is proposed to be a suitable neuron-specific drug target for treating neuropathic pain. Through rational drug design and chemical screening, we have identified a lead candidate AC1 inhibitor, NB001, which is relatively selective for AC1 over all other AC isoforms. Using a variety of behavioral tests and toxicity studies, we have found that NB001, when administered intraperitoneally or orally, has an analgesic effect in animal models of neuropathic pain, without any apparent side effects [21]. These findings show that AC1 could be a productive therapeutic target for neuropathic pain and chronic inflammatory pain. Considering the fact that many signaling molecules that are important for ACC LTP overlap with those for hippocampal LTP, it is important to note that AC1 is a unique one playing essential roles in different forms of ACC LTP but not hippocampal LTP. Future investigations of LTP mechanisms in these two regions may provide new drug targets for treating chronic pain with less cognitive side effects.

In addition to producing analgesic effects by inhibiting the upregulation of AMPA receptors in chronic pain conditions, our recent studies found that AC1 activity is also critical for the upregulation of NMDA GluN2B receptors in the insular cortex [15]. These findings provide strong evidence that AC1 plays dual roles in the chronic pain related to the upregulation of AMPA and NMDA receptors, further supporting AC1 as a novel target for treating chronic pain in the future. Finally, previous reports found that presynaptic enhancement after nerve injury or inflammation is also blocked in mice lacking AC1, indicating that presynaptic AC1 is important for presynaptic changes as well. Future studies are needed to examine the mechanism for presynaptic changes.

ACTIVATION OF SPINAL MICROGLIA IN NEUROPATHIC PAIN

Neuronal mechanisms for neuropathic pain and other forms of chronic pain have been mostly investigated. Recent studies, however, indicate that microglia and other glial cells may contribute to physiology- or pathology-related changes in the CNS. Microglia are the resident macrophages and principal immune response cells in the CNS. They comprise 5% to 10% of the glial cell population and are quite evenly distributed in the brain. Little is known about the function of resting microglia under normal conditions in the brain. It was found that resting microglia have highly dynamic processes and survey the microenvironment in the brain in vivo [45] or in acute brain slices in vitro. Under pathologic conditions, these cells are activated and exhibit chemotactic, phagocytoxic, and secretory responses to various stimuli. Immunostaining for microglia-specific antigens, such as Iba1, OX-42, CD11b, CD4, ED1, or major histocompatibility complex (MHC) II is commonly used for microglial identification in situ.

Under neuropathic pain conditions, microglial activation in the spinal dorsal horn has been demonstrated by different labeling methods. The activation of microglia by activity-dependent manner gains more attention, as it has been reported that microglial cells may also express glutamate receptors [45]. Furthermore, it is well known that they express ATP receptors, and ATP has thought to be released as a transmitter or cotransmitter in some reported studies [11]. These mechanisms provide evidence that microglial cells may be activated or recruited by release of glutamate or ATP in an activity-dependent manner.

ACTIVATION OF MICROGLIA BY GLUTAMATE OR ATP?

Spinal microglia are activated in the setting of neuropathic pain. However, signals that mediate microglial activation are still poorly understood. In the setting of neuropathic pain, peripheral neurons transmit signals to spinal dorsal horn neurons, releasing neurotransmitters such as calcitonin gene–related protein (CGRP), substance P, glutamate, and ATP. Locally in the dorsal horn, there are also other neurotransmitters involved, such as GABA, glycine, and serotonin. Therefore, it is plausible to suggest that these neurotransmitters may initiate microglial activation associated with neuropathic pain. However, by using whole-cell patch-clamp recordings, we found that resting microglia did not show any observable current using electric stimulation, exogenous glutamate, or GABA (Figure 7-3) [31,32]. Consistently, local applications of neurotransmitters such as glutamate, GABA, and substance P, neuromodulators, and chemokines such as serotonin, noradrenaline, carbachol, CX3CL1 (fractalkine), MCP-1, and interleukins (ILs) or electric stimulation of dorsal root fibers with noxious intensity did not induce microglial chemotaxis in the spinal cord dorsal horn (see Figure 7-5) [3]. Therefore, it seems that resting microglia do not have fast electrical or chemotactic responses to these neurotransmitters or cytokines. Nevertheless, microglia may still sense these neuronal signals via other means.

MICROGLIA ARE UNLIKELY TO BE ACTIVATED BY ACTIVITY

Activity-dependent synaptic plasticity is associated with the release of various neuromodulators, such as ATP, brain-derived neurotrophic factor (BDNF), and tissue plasminogen activator (tPA), which may affect microglia. However, we have found that high- or low-frequency stimulation of dorsal roots, which could induce long-term plasticity in the spinal dorsal, did not affect microglial motilities. Similarly, microglial motility is independent of LTP in brain slices. These results indicate that microglia are unlikely activated under physiologic condition in an activity-dependent manner. Furthermore, in the ACC, despite enhanced excitatory transmission between neurons, no microgliosis was found after peripheral nerve injury (Figure 7-4). It is thus likely that microglial motility plays a key role in injury-related changes in the ACC.

CORTICAL GLIAL CELLS ARE NOT ACTIVATED AFTER NEUROPATHIC PAIN

Finally, using transgenic mice in which microglia are selectively labeled with green fluorescent protein (GFP), we have recently performed systematic mapping of microglia in major pain-related brain areas in mice following nerve injury [34]. Although we have

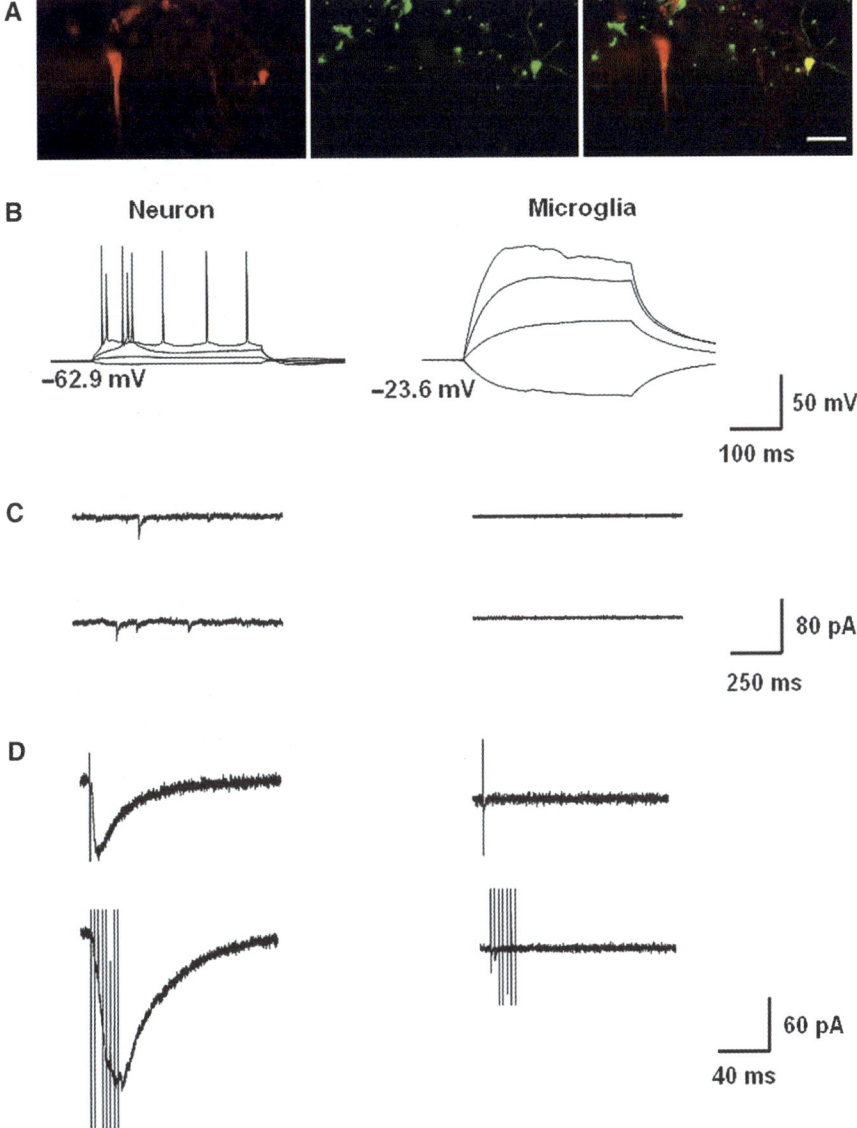

FIGURE 7-3 No synaptic response was observed in resting microglia in the hippocampus. **A:** Representative images showing whole-cell recording in CA1 pyramidal neurons and nearby microglia. Recording cells were labeled in red color by intracellular infusion of Alexa fluor 633 (left) Microglia were labeled by green fluorescent protein (GFP) and shown in green (middle). Merged image confirmed the recording in GFP-labeled microglia (right). Scale bar = 22 μm. **B:** Sample traces showing action potential were generated in CA1 pyramidal neurons but not in microglia. Under current-clamp configuration, currents were injected (400-ms, 40-pA step) from -20 to 100 pA into neuron (left) or microglia (right). Action potentials were fired in neurons but not in microglia. However, microglia showed larger changes in membrane potentials responding to current injections. **C:** Sample traces showing spontaneous synaptic currents were observed in neurons (left) but not in microglia (right). **D:** Synaptic currents were evoked in neurons (left) but not in microglia (right). Stimulation of Schaffer collateral induced inward current in neurons (top left) and high-frequency stimulation (HFS; 100 Hz, seven pulses) facilitated the current (bottom left). However, neither single stimulation nor HFS evoked any current in microglia. (Reused from Wu LJ, Zhuo M. Resting microglial motility is independent of synaptic plasticity in mammalian brain. J Neurophysiol 2008;28:7445–53, with permission.)

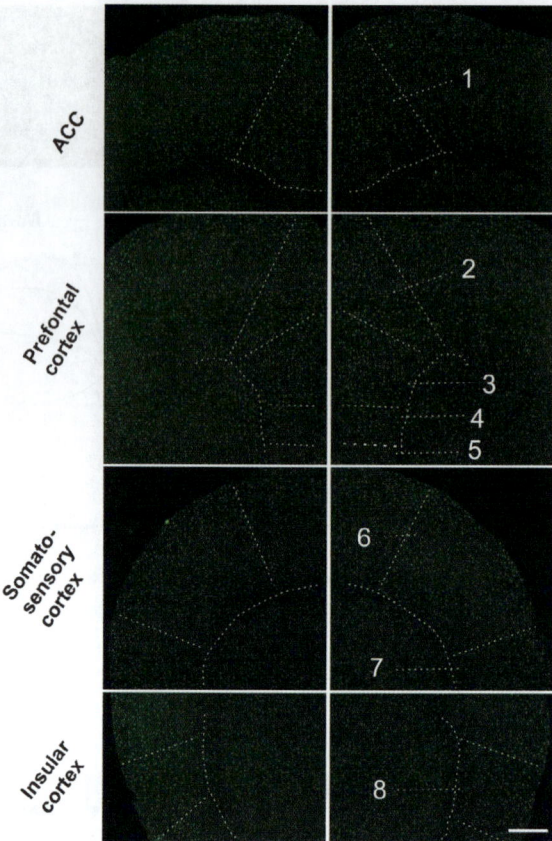

FIGURE 7-4 Microglia in pain-related cortices of control mice. Left column, sham-operated; right column, CPN (common peroneal nerve) ligated. The structures are enclosed by *dashed line*. 1, ACC (anterior cingulate cortex); 2, cingulate cortex, area 1; 3, prelimbic 16 cortex; 4, infralimbic cortex; 5, dorsal peduncular cortex; 6, S1 (primary somatosensory cortex); 7, S2 (secondary somatosensory cortex); 8, insular cortex. Bar = 400 μm.

confirmed the activation of spinal microglial cells after nerve injury, we did not find any microgliosis in supraspinal structures, including the somatosensory cortex and the ACC [34]. These findings are consistent with our recent study demonstrating that microglial motility was not altered by neuronal activity or LTP induction in the aforementioned brain regions.

In summary, the contribution of glia or astrocytes to neuronal plasticity during chronic pain remains to be investigated. It is well known that nociceptive information has to be conveyed to supraspinal structures including cortical areas to be perceived as pain. There is no evidence that spinal glial cells project to the brain. Thus, the influence of glial changes may act through ascending neuronal transmission. Future studies of any possible microglial influences on ascending projection cells are critical for confirming the roles of spinal microglia in pain.

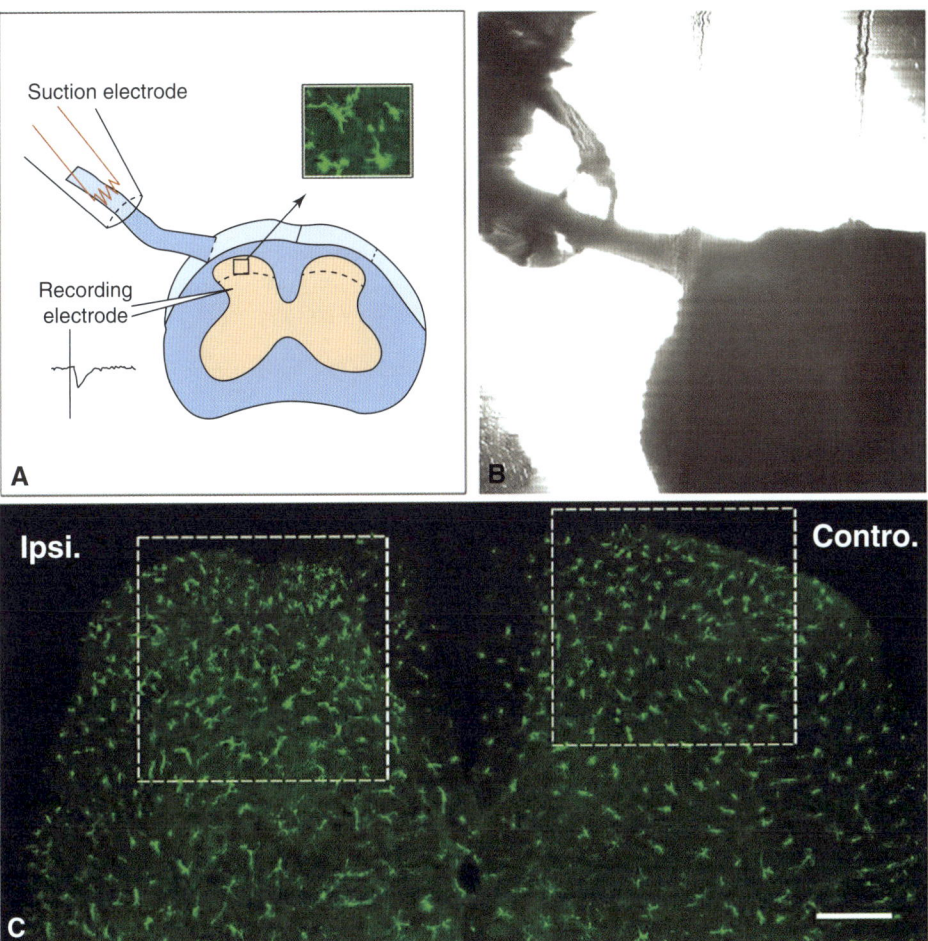

FIGURE 7-5 Histologic results of dorsal root stimuli on the motility of microglia in spinal dorsal horn. **A:** Schematic representation of the confocal imaging and field potential recording accompanying with dorsal root stimuli. **B:** Digitized photomicrographs of the dorsal root stimuli model in a transverse spinal cord section. **C:** Observation of microglia in one fixed section of spinal cord after low-frequency dorsal root stimuli. Ipsi., ipsilateral part of dorsal root; Contro., controlateral part of dorsal root. Bar = 100 μm. (Adapted from Chen T, Koga K, Li XY, Zhou M. Spinal microglial motility is independent of neuronal activity and plasticity in adult mice. Mol Pain 2010;6:19.)

Acknowledgments

This work was supported by grants from the EJLB-CIHR Michael Smith Chair in Neurosciences and Mental Health, Canada Research Chair, NSEC discovery grant 402555, and CIHR operating grants (M. Z.).

REFERENCES

1. Bliss TV, Cooke SF. Long-term potentiation and long-term depression: a clinical perspective. Clinics 2011;66(Suppl. 1):3–17.
2. Calejesan AA, Kim SJ, Zhuo M. Descending facilitatory modulation of a behavioral nociceptive response by stimulation in the adult rat anterior cingulate cortex. Eur J Pain 2000;4:83–96.

3. Chen T, Koga K, Li XY, Zhuo M. Spinal microglial motility is independent of neuronal activity and plasticity in adult mice. Mol Pain 2010;6:19.
4. Kandel ER. The molecular biology of memory storage: a dialogue between genes and synapses. Science 2001;294:1030–8.
5. Ko SW, Ao HS, Mendel AG, et al. Transcription factor Egr-1 is required for long-term fear memory and anxiety. Sheng Li Xue Bao 2005;57:421–32.
6. Ko SW, Vadakkan KI, Ao H, et al. Selective contribution of Egr1 (zif/268) to persistent inflammatory pain. J Pain 2005;6:12–20.
7. Koga K, Li X, Chen T, et al. In vivo whole-cell patch-clamp recording of sensory synaptic responses of cingulate pyramidal neurons to noxious mechanical stimuli in adult mice. Mol Pain 2010;6:62.
8. Latremoliere A, Woolf CJ. Central sensitization: a generator of pain hypersensitivity by central neural plasticity. J Pain 2009;10:895–926.
9. Li P, Kerchner GA, Sala C, et al. AMPA receptor-PDZ interactions in facilitation of spinal sensory synapses. Nat Neurosci 1999;2:972–7.
10. Li P, Wilding TJ, Kim SJ, et al. Kainate-receptor-mediated sensory synaptic transmission in mammalian spinal cord. Nature 1999;397:161–4.
11. Li P, Zhuo M. Silent glutamatergic synapses and nociception in mammalian spinal cord. Nature 1998;393:695–8.
12. Li XY, Ko HG, Chen T, et al. Alleviating neuropathic pain hypersensitivity by inhibiting PKMzeta in the anterior cingulate cortex. Science 2010;330:1400–4.
13. Liauw J, Wu LJ, Zhuo M. Calcium-stimulated adenylyl cyclases required for long-term potentiation in the anterior cingulate cortex. J Neurophysiol 2005;94:878–82.
14. Liu MG, Kang SJ, Shi TY, et al. Long-term potentiation of synaptic transmission in the adult mouse insular cortex: multielectrode array recordings. J Neurophysiol 2013;110:505–21.
15. Qiu S, Chen T, Koga K, et al. An increase in synaptic NMDA receptors in the insular cortex contributes to neuropathic pain. Sci Signal 2013;6:ra34.
16. Sandkuhler J. Understanding LTP in pain pathways. Mol Pain 2007;3:9.
17. Steenland HW, Li XY, Zhuo M. Predicting aversive events and terminating fear in the mouse anterior cingulate cortex during trace fear conditioning. J Neurosci 2012;32:1082–95.
18. Toyoda H, Zhao MG, Ulzhofer B, et al. Roles of the AMPA receptor subunit GluA1 but not GluA2 in synaptic potentiation and activation of ERK in the anterior cingulate cortex. Mol Pain 2009;5:46.
19. Vogt BA. Pain and emotion interactions in subregions of the cingulate gyrus. Nat Rev Neurosci 2005;6:533–44.
20. Wang GD, Zhuo M. Synergistic enhancement of glutamate-mediated responses by serotonin and forskolin in adult mouse spinal dorsal horn neurons. J Neurophysiol 2002;87:732–9.
21. Wang H, Xu H, Wu LJ, et al. Identification of an adenylyl cyclase inhibitor for treating neuropathic and inflammatory pain. Sci Transl Med 2011;3:65ra3.
22. Wang H, Zhang M. The role of Ca^{2+}-stimulated adenylyl cyclases in bidirectional synaptic plasticity and brain function. Rev Neurosci 2012;23:67–78.
23. Wei F, Li P, Zhuo M. Loss of synaptic depression in mammalian anterior cingulate cortex after amputation. J Neurosci 1999;19:9346–54.
24. Wei F, Qiu CS, Kim SJ, et al. Genetic elimination of behavioral sensitization in mice lacking calmodulin-stimulated adenylyl cyclases. Neuron 2002;36:713–26.
25. Wei F, Qiu CS, Liauw J, et al. Calcium calmodulin-dependent protein kinase IV is required for fear memory. Nat Neurosci 2002;5:573–9.
26. Wei F, Vadakkan KI, Toyoda H, et al. Calcium calmodulin-stimulated adenylyl cyclases contribute to activation of extracellular signal-regulated kinase in spinal dorsal horn neurons in adult rats and mice. J Neurosci 2006;26:851–61.
27. Wei F, Xia XM, Tang J, et al. Calmodulin regulates synaptic plasticity in the anterior cingulate cortex and behavioral responses: a microelectroporation study in adult rodents. J Neurosci 2003;23:8402–9.
28. Wei F, Zhuo M. Potentiation of sensory responses in the anterior cingulate cortex following digit amputation in the anaesthetised rat. J Physiol 2001;532:823–33.
29. Woolf CJ. Evidence for a central component of post-injury pain hypersensitivity. Nature 1983;306:686–8.
30. Wu LJ, Toyoda H, Zhao MG, et al. Upregulation of forebrain NMDA NR2B receptors contributes to behavioral sensitization after inflammation. J Neurosci 2005;25:11107–16.
31. Wu LJ, Vadakkan KI, Zhuo M. ATP-induced chemotaxis of microglial processes requires P2Y receptor-activated initiation of outward potassium currents. Glia 2007;55:810–21.
32. Wu LJ, Zhuo M. Resting microglial motility is independent of synaptic plasticity in mammalian brain. J Neurophysiol 2008;99:2026–32.

33. Xu H, Wu LJ, Wang H, et al. Presynaptic and postsynaptic amplifications of neuropathic pain in the anterior cingulate cortex. J Neurosci 2008;28:7445–53.
34. Zhang F, Vadakkan KI, Kim SS, et al. Selective activation of microglia in spinal cord but not higher cortical regions following nerve injury in adult mouse. Mol Pain 2008;4:15.
35. Zhao MG, Ko SW, Wu LJ, et al. Enhanced presynaptic neurotransmitter release in the anterior cingulate cortex of mice with chronic pain. J Neurosci 2006;26:8923–30.
36. Zhao MG, Toyoda H, Ko SW, et al. Deficits in trace fear memory and long-term potentiation in a mouse model for fragile X syndrome. J Neurosci 2005;25:7385–92.
37. Zhao MG, Toyoda H, Lee YS, et al. Roles of NMDA NR2B subtype receptor in prefrontal long-term potentiation and contextual fear memory. Neuron 2005;47:859–72.
38. Zhuo M. Silent glutamatergic synapses and long-term facilitation in spinal dorsal horn neurons. Prog Brain Res 2000;129:101–13.
39. Zhuo M. Glutamate receptors and persistent pain: targeting forebrain NR2B subunits. Drug Discov Today 2002;7:259–67.
40. Zhuo M. Cortical excitation and chronic pain. Trends Neurosci 2008;31:199–207.
41. Zhuo M. Targeting neuronal adenylyl cyclase for the treatment of chronic pain. Drug Discov Today 2012;17:573–82.
42. Zhuo M, Gebhart GF. Characterization of descending facilitation and inhibition of spinal nociceptive transmission from the nuclei reticularis gigantocellularis and gigantocellularis pars alpha in the rat. J Neurophysiol 1992;67:1599–614.
43. Zhuo M, Gebhart GF. Biphasic modulation of spinal nociceptive transmission from the medullary raphe nuclei in the rat. J Neurophysiol 1997;78:746–58.
44. Zhuo M, Sengupta JN, Gebhart GF. Biphasic modulation of spinal visceral nociceptive transmission from the rostroventral medial medulla in the rat. J Neurophysiol 2002;87:2225–36.
45. Zhuo M, Wu G, Wu LJ. Neuronal and microglial mechanisms of neuropathic pain. Mol Brain 2011;4:31.

SECTION 3

Research Methods: Quantifying Peripheral and CNS Responses

CHAPTER 8

Mechanistic Pain Phenotyping in Pre- and Postoperative Settings

Lars Arendt-Nielsen

Studies in animals or healthy volunteers have been somehow successful in providing mechanistic understanding of the clinical signs and symptoms and thus in suggesting a more rational use of available pain management regimes. Although part of this knowledge has been translated into benefits to the patients, the prevention of acute and chronic postoperative pain is still generally unsatisfactory. One reason can be the lack of adequate diagnostic tools and efficient analgesics providing the opportunity of developing targeted individualized treatment regimes. However, to date very few studies phenotyping patients based on mechanistic pain assessments have been able to predict which patients will respond to a given pain medication and which patients will have a beneficial outcome of the surgery seen from a pain perspective.

In pre-, peri-, and postoperative pain management, it would be important to have tools available to move the management from symptom-based to mechanism-based approaches in the attempt to achieve significant improvements in pain management and prevention of chronic postoperative pain.

However, despite increased theoretical understanding and major efforts to improve clinical practice, postoperative surveys continue to indicate major challenges. A meta-analysis from 2002 covering some 20,000 patients and 800 publications concluded that 41% of all postoperative patients still suffer moderate to severe acute pain and that 24% experience inadequate pain relief [40]. As outlined in this book, many attempts have been tried in recent years for pre- and perioperative pain control, but acute postoperative pain management still remains a challenge with new caveats (e.g., extensive use of opioids in some countries).

The picture is even more unsatisfactory with regard to preventing undesirable chronic postoperative pain as a direct consequence of surgical intervention or as a result of the patient's preoperative pain status (particularly aspects of centralized sensitization). Chronic pain after surgery demonstrates that this problem is very common with some types of surgery (e.g., thoracotomy, mastectomy, limb amputation), being associated with chronic pain incidences of up to 50% [86,108].

This chapter will focus on some translational, mechanistic pain assessment tools (quantitative sensory testing [QST]) to be used for pre- and postoperative phenotyping of patients and possibly for predicting the patients most vulnerable to develop chronic postoperative pain.

The aims of this chapter are (1) to describe how QST can provide information related to specific pain mechanisms (volunteers, patients) assumed important for development and maintenance of pain and (2) to give examples of how QST can be used for profiling patients with different pain conditions and can be used in preoperative as well as postoperative settings.

This chapter will not describe in detail the individual QST technologies for assessing pain from the different structures, as this is covered in many other reviews [17,23,41,59]. Furthermore, the chapter will not address how QST can be used in drug profiling and drug development, as this has also recently been thoroughly addressed [12,15,19,36,103].

THE BASIC CONCEPT OF QST

QST involves a large variety of stimulus modalities (such as thermal, mechanical, chemical, and electrical), assessment methods (such as psychophysics, electrophysiology, imaging, and microdialysis), and target structures (such as skin, musculoskeletal, and viscera).

A number of fundamental pain mechanisms observed in animals have had important implications for the development of human QST techniques and how to apply these techniques in human basic, clinical, and drug profiling studies. The fundamental aspects covered in this chapter are QST methods developed to assess more the dynamic aspects of the pain system by probing peripheral sensitization, central spreading sensitization, expansion of receptive fields, temporal summation (windup), after-discharge, spatial integration, and descending inhibition, as those factors are starting to prove their role as predictive mechanistic features for the acute postoperative period and for the development of chronic postoperative pain.

A number of factors need to be taken into consideration when performing QST. QST can provide an understanding of the mechanisms involved in pain transduction, transmission, modulation, and perception under normal and pathophysiologic conditions and as such may contribute to the development of mechanism-based diagnosis, prevention, and management of pain in future [74,152].

The first choice when selecting a QST tool is the selection of endpoint ("response"), usually threshold determination (e.g., pain detection or tolerance threshold) or pain magnitude rating for a given stimulus (e.g., by visual analogue scale [VAS]). More indicative of the basal state of the system, threshold determination has the advantage of involving an easily defined and taught endpoint that is stable and reproducible in practice. Pain magnitude rating necessitates more training of the subject but has the advantage of permitting investigation of suprathreshold nociceptive processing more strongly reflecting dynamic and supratentorial aspects of nociceptive hyperexcitability.

The second factor concerns the stimulus to be applied, which can be varied by type, characteristics, location, and tissue stimulated. The type of stimulus chosen determines the nociceptive system modalities being tested. Thus "physiologic" stimuli (e.g., pressure, temperature, chemical) will include peripheral nociceptors in the analysis of the nervous system processing, whereas electrical stimulation largely bypasses peripheral nociceptors. Regarding stimulus characteristics, QST can involve single or multiple stimuli. Stimulation summated either in time or space informs on aspects of nociceptive processing such as windup and centrally facilitated gain of great relevance to clinical pain states including postoperative pain. The location of stimulation provides further information on the underlying nociceptive neuroplasticity. Thus, QST close to and distant from the site of surgery can be used to differentiate between generalized (e.g., supraspinal) and segmental (e.g., spinal) neuroplasticity [156]. The different mechanisms underlying primary and secondary hyperalgesia surrounding a surgical wound are one aspect of postoperative pain, with the former reflecting mainly local and peripheral nociceptive mechanisms and the latter, more central mechanisms. With good preoperative instructions, QST measures can be obtained after surgery as soon as the patient is awake and cooperative: in practice, 1 to 2 hours postoperatively.

A number of QST studies have concentrated on this important early postoperative period and have successfully demonstrated the presence of pain hyperexcitability [156]. One of these studies investigated the impact of intra- and postoperative opioid analgesia on generalized and segmental hyperexcitability in the early postoperative period [156]. In the absence of intraoperative opioid supplementation for volatile anesthesia, postoperative patient-controlled analgesia (PCA) morphine inhibited generalized hyperexcitability only during the period of its use with significant hyperalgesia after discontinuation persisting until day 5 postoperatively. Moreover, significant segmental hyperalgesia (as revealed by dividing thresholds close to surgery by thresholds distant from surgery) was present during the entire 5 postoperative days studied, even during the period of morphine PCA. Both generalized and segmental postoperative hyperalgesia were depressed by intraoperative fentanyl supplementation. However, clinical measures of the pain experience (VAS scores, morphine PCA use) did not reflect this difference in neuroplasticity, being similar in both groups. Similar results have been found in other studies [148,155].

QST as a Mechanistic Tool for Assessing Pain Neuroplasticity

Many studies have repeatedly suggested this mechanism-based management approach over the last 2 decades, but not much has been achieved using QST so there is a need for a paradigm shift to move the field to the next level [37], and some suggestions will be provided in this chapter.

Different QST protocols have been suggested for profiling patients, and the QST battery developed by the German Research Network on Neuropathic Pain is the one applied in many studies [52,87,88]. Briefly, the protocol assesses the function of small (thermal thresholds) and large (tactile and vibration thresholds) nerve fiber pathways and increased/decreased pain sensitivity (hyperalgesia, allodynia, hyperpathia, windup like pain, etc.). The battery consists predominantly of cutaneous stimulus modalities developed for neuropathic pain and therefore is less adequate for profiling inflammatory, musculoskeletal, or visceral pain conditions. Furthermore, the battery does not include comprehensive assessment of, e.g., central summation or pain modulation. In addition, the future challenges are to develop QST platforms adequate also for children or elderly, possibly demented patients, and to establish normative values for those groups.

An important aspect is that most of the techniques applied in the past have been based on short, static, phasic, modality-specific stimuli and most often applied cutaneously [151,152]. In more recent years dynamic, mechanism-based approaches have been developed and applied clinically for phenotyping patients with respect to central temporal summation and conditioning pain modulation (CPM) [44]. The later has now started to show promising evidence as having predictive value for development of chronic postoperative pain [110,111,158]. In addition, the focus has been on developing and applying techniques that assess the excitability of the deeper somatic tissues, as musculoskeletal pain conditions compose the majority of chronic pain conditions [16].

In QST studies, the focus and mind set is often directed toward hyperexcitable responses, but it is important to focus both on "gain-of-function" and on "loss-of-function" as both increased and decreased pain sensitivity can be a prominent signs in, e.g., neuropathic pain [64,74].

Peripheral and Central Spreading Sensitization

When a peripheral nociceptor is sensitized, the firing to a given stimulus is increased and prolonged and the threshold for firing is lowered often as a consequence of recruitment of silent nerve branches. In psychophysical testing, this may result in localized lowering of the pain threshold to a given stimulus modality or an increased response to a fixed stimulus intensity (Figure 8-1). In the clinical setting, particularly for phasic, static stimulus modalities have been applied as electrical [155], thermal [151], tactile [33], and pressure [24] stimuli, as those tests are easy to apply in clinical settings even though they may not be the most optimal techniques, as they do not represent specific sensitization processes.

QST applied to different structures requires specific stimulators/activators. For cutaneous stimulation, controlled heat is easy, whereas activation of deep structures such as muscles, tendons, bones, joins, or viscera is more challenging. In recent years, the development has predominantly focused on ways to stimulate these latter structures because of their clinical relevance (for recent reviews see Refs. [23,41]), whereas for cutaneous stimulators

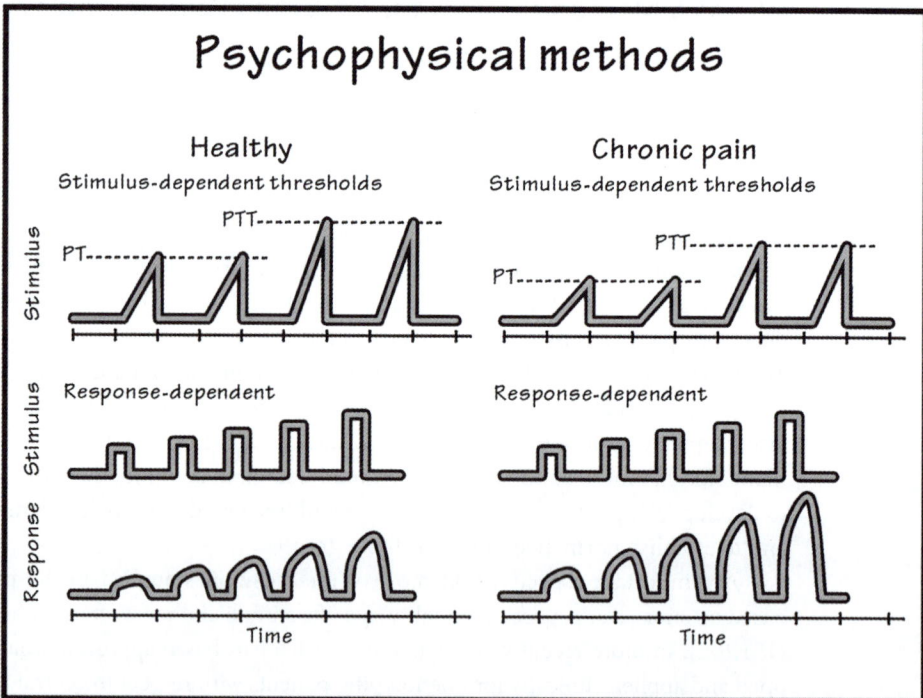

FIGURE 8-1 The fundamental principles of psychophysical assessment applied within the area of quantitative sensory testing. A given stimulus is increased in intensity until a pain threshold (PT) or a pain tolerance threshold (PTT) is reached. Alternatively, a well-defined stimulus intensity is delivered, and the pain intensity is rated on a visual analogue scale (discrete or continuous). If the thresholds or pain ratings are obtained from a pain patient with different degrees of sensitization, the thresholds are lower and the ratings, higher.

the focus has been on establishing normative values [87]. For preoperative monitoring, it is mandatory to have normative datasets for determining if patients are in a high- or low-sensitization group and thereby in a high- or low-risk group for developing chronic postoperative pain [157] or are in a high-sensitization postoperative group [153].

The most recent development in the area has been to quantify specific regions of the nerve territories [49], muscles [28], or joints [20] in which sensitization is most prominent. This pain mapping technique using, e.g., pressure pain [48], heat pain [124], or intraoral painful mechanical [85] stimulation has opened new opportunities for quantifying the extent and spreading of sensitization and the development over time.

As indicated, it is important to develop assessment technologies suitable for probing the deep somatic structures as such structures are inevitably involved in surgery and may be in a sensitized stage before as well as after surgery [113].

Specifically for pressure stimulation, design of probes to obtain stimulation of selected structures has been in focus. Finocchietti et al. [51] demonstrated that mainly the superficial structures of the muscle tissue are mechanically strained by pressure applications, suggesting that especially the fascia is efficiently stimulated by pressure algometry and that the procedure may be optimized by using a rounded probe instead of a flat probe for stimulation. Pressure stimulation can obviously also excite cutaneous receptors, and in a study applying cutaneous anesthesia, it was demonstrated that a mechanically elicited pain sensation originates from deep tissue and only to a minor degree from the skin when adequate probes are used [62].

One area, which has recently been developed, is selective stimulation of bone structures [6,50] and assessing periosteal sensitization [7]. This is important for obtaining better information about periosteal pain mechanisms in humans, as this is clinically a challenging area given that many cancer patients experience significant pain in relation to bone metastases.

Intradiscal pressure provocation [131] and external facet joint pressure stimulation [135] have been explored as potential models related to spine pain. Direct intra-articular activation of the knee joint nociceptors has been conducted by pressure stimulation that activates joint receptors during an arthroscopic procedure [43], which cannot be achieved by pressure applied externally to the joint [20]. Pressure algometry assesses a relatively small volume of tissue. In contrast, a larger volume can be assessed by the computer-controlled cuff algometry technique: The pain intensity related to the inflation of a tourniquet applied around an extremity is used to establish stimulus–response curves, and by this the deep tissue pain sensitivity can be assessed [114]. The cuff is wrapped around the leg or arm and inflated in a standardized way, and the volunteer/patient stops the inflation when the pain threshold is reached or rates the pain intensity to a given standardized stimulation. The pressure applied is distributed throughout the underlying tissues, activating a variety of deep somatic receptors and nociceptors (Figure 8-2). Finite element analysis of the cuff-applied pressure has shown that muscular as well as periosteal structures can be activated using this technique [90].

It has become more and more evident that a localized nociceptive focus (such as a neuroma or a painful joint) can drive central processes and cause contralateral or even extrasegmental widespread sensitization. There is ample experimental and clinical evidence that in neuropathic conditions the signs and symptoms extend into regions beyond those directly innervated by the injured nerve [79,89]. After chronic constriction injury of the sciatic nerve in rats, tactile allodynia in the hind paw territories of both the injured sciatic nerve and the uninjured saphenous nerve has been shown [146]. Similar contralateral sensitization is found in localized neuropathic pain conditions [79].

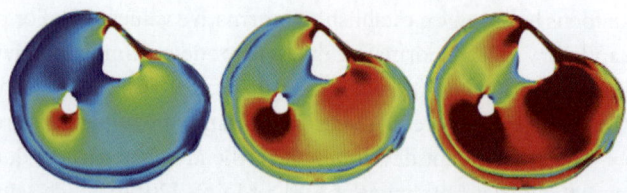

FIGURE 8-2 An example of a finite element estimation of the von Mises stress (a combination of the stress in all three dimensions) when the calf is stimulated with a cuff, where the applied pressure is increased from low (left) to high (right) intensity. The combined stress intensity is highest around a bony structure.

A simple procedure such as a 2-week cast immobilization causes widespread hyperalgesia [104]. This resembles other models where localized inflammation of one craniofacial muscle evoked mechanical allodynia in the hind paws [1] or inflammation in one hind limb caused contralateral spreading sensitization [138]. Conditions such as migraine and chronic tension-type headache also lead to spreading sensitization [47,48], and animal models have confirmed that chemical stimulation of the cranial dura elicited long-lasting hyperexcitability to innocuous (brush, pressure) and noxious (pinch, heat) stimulation of the paws [35]. Somatic pain cannot only cause widespread sensitization but also visceral hyperalgesia [92] and vice versa [53].

This widespread sensitization in otherwise localized pain problems offers a challenge in QST, as a separation between the two manifestations (peripheral and central) can be difficult. It has been found that generalized hyperalgesia is present in 17.5% to 35.3% of the chronic pain population [132]. An example could be pressure pain assessment over the knee joint in patients with osteoarthritis (OA) where localized joint sensitization is detected. In the same patient, the pressure pain thresholds are also reduced as compared with control subjects when assessed from, e.g., the arm [20]. Similar widespread sensory manifestations of sensitization are found in, e.g., unilateral epicondylitis [45,46]. This widespread pressure pain hyperalgesia has shown to be predictive of the patients developing chronic postoperative pain after total knee replacement [22].

This raises the issue that a true control site is most likely nonexisting in patients with chronic pain as consistently shown in neuropathic [79], musculoskeletal [38], visceral [34], and gynecologic [71] pain.

The only way to overcome this lack of a control site in pain patients is to use normative databases for all the tests applied [97] and to use statistical techniques such as z-scores to judge when an individual patient is outside the normative range [120,121]. This approach has not yet been widely implemented in preoperative settings but will be the only way to determine if a given patient is in a highly sensitized risk group for developing chronic postoperative pain after, e.g., joint replacement [9] or respond to a given treatment [14].

Another aspect of spreading sensitization is that the QST platform should include sets of normally nonnociceptive stimuli, as the sensitization processes may cause allodynia to, e.g., thermal or mechanical stimuli and as such cold/warmth, brush, or slight pressure.

Expansion of Receptive Fields

In many animal studies, expansion of receptive fields of dorsal horn neurons has been documented in neuropathic as well as inflammatory (cutaneous, muscle, and viscera) models. Expansion of receptive fields has been a challenging mechanism to assess in humans. A nerve ligation [27] or a paw inflammation [68] led to a significant increase in the size of convergent, cutaneous receptive fields of dorsal horn neurons. Similar findings have been reported after experimental myositis [66], joint inflammation [129], or sensitization of the colon [94].

In animals, an alternative method for assessment of receptive field expansion of dorsal horn neurons has been developed. This involves quantification of the so-called reflex receptive field [133,134], which was found to expand in the presence of sensitization [65,76]. This method based on assessment of the nociceptive withdrawal method has been translated to humans [4], and the reflex receptive field is found to be expanded in spinal cord injury patients [3], in chronic visceral pain patients [96], and in musculoskeletal pain patients [30]. Such an electrophysiologic method requires advanced laboratories as compared with simple psychophysical tests but may provide valuable information in clinical studies [96] or in the profiling of new centrally acting compounds. This technique has not yet been implemented and applied in pre- and postoperative settings, but the technology has now been refined and could start to be applied [29,73], as normative datasets have been established [95].

Windup, Temporal Summation, and After-Discharge

An important and potent mechanism in dorsal horn neurons is the temporal summation mechanisms termed windup. Repeated strong C-fiber stimulation of nociceptive fibers causes a frequency-dependent increase in the neuronal excitability, which outlasts the stimuli [91]. The resulting response of spinal cord neurons to successive stimuli of this type is a progressive increase in the magnitude of the nociceptive input and is often followed by persistent after-discharge. Windup has been used as a model of neural plasticity and central sensitization in the spinal cord. It has been shown to be sensitive to NMDA receptor antagonists and implicated in a number of nociceptive responses [118]. This windup process as assessed by neuronal recordings from dorsal horn neurons or as nociceptive withdrawal reflex is strongly facilitated in conditions of sensitization [165].

In humans, the initial phase of the windup process translates into temporal summation [11]. If a painful stimulus is repeated 1 to 3 times per second, the pain will integrate and become more painful with a summation dependent on intensity and stimulus frequency [11] (Figure 8-3). Temporal summation can be elicited using electrical, mechanical, or thermal stimulation modalities and is elicited from the skin, musculoskeletal structures, and viscera [8,23].

In many clinical conditions such as neuropathic, musculoskeletal, and visceral pain, patients show a significant facilitation of temporal summation [13,60,101].

In clinical bedside testing, simple devices are used for assessing temporal summation such as tapping the skin with a nylon filament [101]. However, when more standardization is required, automated user-independent methods are needed such as thermal [78], mechanical [98], or electrical stimulation techniques of the skin [11], muscles [18], or viscera [42]. Recently, a new user-independent technique has been developed based on a tourniquet cuff (Figures 8-2 and 8-3), which is automatically and repeatedly inflated, and the volunteer/patient rates the provoked pain intensity [84,136].

There is evidence of gender differences in temporal summation [127] that must be taken into consideration when comparing groups.

For heat stimulation, there is a difference in the temporal summation assessment protocol. For heat pulses with relatively slow rise times, summation is predominantly seen for second pain (C-fiber mediated) [5,100,117], whereas heat stimuli with rapid rise times, e.g., laser stimulation, summation of first pain (Aδ-fibers) can also be assessed [10].

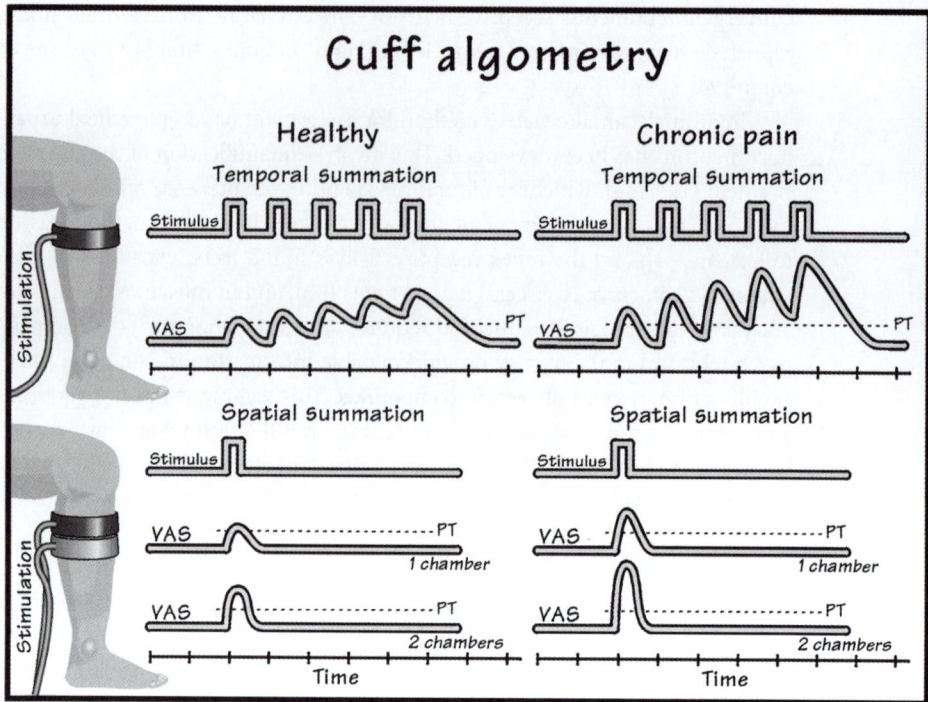

FIGURE 8-3 An example of how cuff algometry (inflating a cuff) can be used to assess temporal (stimuli delivered repeatedly over time) or spatial (stimuli delivered simultaneously to different areas) summation. If the time between individual stimuli is sufficiently short, temporal summation will occur. If two cuffs are activated simultaneously, stronger pain intensity will be provoked compared with single cuff stimulation. In pain patients, temporal and spatial summation can be facilitated as a result of sensitization. PT, pain threshold; VAS, visual analogue scale.

When repeated stimuli are delivered to assess temporal summation, sometimes pain patients experience an after-sensation (pain after the stimulus has stopped) [119]. This has been observed in patients with neuropathic [57] and musculoskeletal pain [140,141]. An exclusive facilitation of the after-sensation alone has been proposed to be of diagnostic value [128] and supports the basic finding that the summation and the after-sensation are mediated by different underlying mechanisms [116,163]. There seem to be some gender differences in the experience of the after-sensation phenomenon [126].

Recent studies have shown that preoperative monitoring of temporal summation reliably shows to predict chronic postoperative pain after, e.g., joint replacement [70,110,111,150]. In addition, temporal summation seems to be even further facilitated in patients suffering from chronic postoperative pain [136,137], and as such it is an important tool in clinical settings [150].

Spatial Integration

Spatial integration is another mechanism that relies on central networks and the general sensitization status [31]. In humans, spatial summation can be assessed in different ways where the stimulus is applied using different stimulation areas, e.g., using thermodes [99], pressure probes [98], or cuffs [114]. The cuff technology is the most recent where one or two cuffs can be automatically inflated in a standardized way and the volunteer/patient rates the provoked pain intensity [114] (Figure 8-3).

Spatial summation is facilitated in various pain conditions such as fibromyalgia [141,142], OA [63], and lateral epicondylitis [75]. A specific assessment of spatial summation has not yet been systematically implemented in pre- and postoperative settings, as in more recent studies it has been difficult to show the differences between chronic musculoskeletal pain patients and controls [58]. Recently a simple bedside test has been developed for assessing the degree of sensitization in chronic pain [93].

Descending Modulation of Neuronal Excitability

One manifestation of inhibitory influences is that associated with diffuse noxious inhibitory controls (DNIC), expressed as an inhibition of dorsal horn neurons produced by a noxious stimulus applied to a body region remote from the receptive field of the neurons [96], a phenomenon recently retermed as conditioning pain modulation [159].

In the past, the main focus has been on descending inhibition. However, emerging evidence indicates that descending facilitation contributes to the maintenance of neuropathic [149], inflammatory [2], and postoperative pain [154]. The descending facilitatory influences are manifested via pathways that originate in the midbrain and brainstem structures (e.g., the periaqueductal gray, raphe, and rostral ventromedial medulla). Descending controls allow a "top–down" influence on spinal processing and form a link between higher functions such as cognition, memory, and emotions and the level of pain transmission.

There is strong evidence that the balance between the descending inhibition and facilitation may be disturbed in chronic pain and that this phenomenon has a role in maintaining hypersensitivity [164] alongside mechanisms of central sensitization [115,145]. In addition, it may provide relevant information in relation to pain management strategies [161].

In humans, status assessment of the descending pathways has recently undergone a revival and the original DNIC terminology has been renamed to conditioning pain modulation [159]. The "pain-inhibits-pain" paradigm (the heterotopic conditioning tonic stimuli—thermal, mechanical, electrical, or chemical) is manifested as a decrease in the pain perception evoked by a painful test stimulus presented elsewhere on the body.

Less efficient descending pain control has been reported in musculoskeletal pain conditions such as patients with, e.g., myofascial temporomandibular joint pain [32], chronic low-back pain [109], fibromyalgia [80], painful OA [20], chronic tension-type headaches [125], and chronic pancreatitis [105]. OA patients with a deficient, descending pain inhibition show normalization to a pain-free state after surgery [63,81], suggesting that the chronic pain maintained the CPM dysfunction and that the chronic pain saturated the CPM mechanism so the conditioning pain stimulus is less efficient. The mechanism of CPM seems modulated differently in short- and long-term rheumatoid arthritis patients compared with that in control subjects [82]. A dysfunction of descending pain modulation mechanisms in, e.g., fibromyalgia reduced activation of the rostral anterior cingulate cortex [72], which may contribute to the clinical manifestations of widespread pain. Evidently, an alteration in the descending pain modulation could be a promising target for pharmacologic intervention [23] and may thereby add important mode-of-action information, increasing the understanding of how interventions work in pain [162].

An impaired CPM response can be interpreted as reduced inhibition, but alternatively it could also be the result of increased facilitation. At this stage, no diagnostic technique has been developed to separate those two competing pathways. Because impaired CPM may appear as spreading hypersensitivity, which may also link to sensitization of central mechanisms, it is important to combine assessments of different mechanisms, e.g., temporal summation of pain (as a signal of pain facilitation) along with assessment of CPM. Unfortunately, the CPM paradigms currently used show high variability [106] but has recently been refined and may start to be applied more routinely for diagnostics [61,69,112] or in the pre-/postoperative setting. However, studies have already shown that impaired CPM may predict chronic postoperative pain [111,160] and was shown to be normalized in patients surgically and successfully treated for their chronic pain [63]. A simple, reliable bedside test for CPM needs to be developed.

Projection of Pain Areas as a Sign of Central Pain Hyperexcitability

True referred pain is a phenomenon predominantly related to pain from deep somatic and visceral structures. Referred pain can occur as a result of a given pathology (e.g., ureteral calculosis, dysmenorrhea) or by provocation of a given structure (e.g., active myofascial trigger points). Referred pain is the result of a central mechanism, and when experimentally evoked, it can be facilitated in patients with, e.g., fibromyalgia [139], whiplash syndrome [77], OA [25], chronic low-back pain [102], or chronic pancreatitis [39]. In addition, it has been shown that referred pain areas evoked from muscle enlarge in visceral pain conditions [26] as a result of convergence between deep somatic and visceral structures.

The sensory convergence and synaptic mechanisms underlying referred pain are not entirely understood, but animal studies have consistently shown expansion or development of new receptive fields after muscle or joint sensitization [67,130], which most likely resembles the development of expanded referred pain in patients.

Referred pain is normally quantified subjectively by pain drawings [122], and some volunteers have large areas, whereas others tend to have small areas [123]. However, there is evidence of altered superficial blood flow and temperature changes in the referred muscle pain areas, which may be assessed objectively [83]. Referred pain in clinical viscera pain conditions has been suggested to cause trophic cutaneous changes [54] although this has not been shown in other studies [107]. It has also been put forward that cutaneous blood flow and temperature can increase in referred pain areas provoked by visceral stimulation [21].

QST assessment in patients with musculoskeletal or visceral pain introduces a complication, as specific sensory changes may occur in the referred pain areas defined as referred hyperalgesia. Such mechanisms are manifested as viscerovisceral and viscerosomatic sensitization [55]. In patients with, e.g., urinary calculosis, pain thresholds to electrical muscular stimulation in the referred pain areas show significant and long-lasting hyperalgesia [56], where patients suffering from a large number of colics show more hyperalgesia than those experiencing a limited number of colics. Similar somatic hyperalgesia is found in referred pain areas in acute appendicitis [144] and cholecystolithiasis [143].

In patients with chronic pain and increased centralized sensitization, the pain projection areas gradually increase [16,59] and the pain quality becomes more diffuse and more difficult to localize [147]. In the clinical preoperative setting, assessing the pain projection areas and quality (diffuse vs. localized) seems to be an indicator of the degree of centralized facilitated gain of pain and hence could serve as a simple clinical screening tool.

CONCLUSIONS AND FUTURE PERSPECTIVES

Basic pain research has led to significant improvements in the understanding of the mechanisms underlying chronic pain. Human experimental pain research and mechanistic QST tools have confirmed that some mechanisms described in animals can be translated into pain patients in a pre- and postoperative setting. QST is an important and integrated part of many basic and clinical studies and a tool in proof-of-mechanism studies related to new analgesics under development. Despite the significant developments in this filed over the last two decades, we have not yet been able to find the right treatment to the right patients to prevent development of chronic postoperative pain. However, more and more studies indicate that the pain assessment techniques reflecting different stages of the dynamic pain sensitization processes may be capable of predicting the outcome after surgery. The future perspectives are to translate such studies into the search for procedures that may interact with such processes in an attempt to better prevent the development of chronic postoperative pain using individualized, mechanism-based pain management regimes.

REFERENCES

1. Ambalavanar R, Moutanni A, Dessem D. Inflammation of craniofacial muscle induces widespread mechanical allodynia. Neurosci Lett 2006;399:249–54.
2. Ambriz-Tututi M, Cruz SL, Urquiza-Marin H, Granados-Soto V. Formalin-induced long-term secondary allodynia and hyperalgesia are maintained by descending facilitation. Pharmacol Biochem Behav 2011;98:417–24.
3. Andersen OK, Finnerup NB, Spaich EG, Jensen TS, Arendt-Nielsen L. Expansion of nociceptive withdrawal reflex receptive fields in spinal cord injured humans. Clin Neurophysiol 2004;115:2798–810.
4. Andersen OK, Sonnenborg FA, Arendt-Nielsen L. Reflex receptive fields for human withdrawal reflexes elicited by non-painful and painful electrical stimulation of the foot sole. Clin Neurophysiol 2001;112:641–9.
5. Anderson RJ, Craggs JG, Bialosky JE, Bishop MD, George SZ, Staud R, Robinson ME. Temporal summation of second pain: variability in responses to a fixed protocol. Eur J Pain 2013;17:67–74.
6. Andresen T, Pfeiffer-Jensen M, Brock C, Drewes AM, Arendt-Nielsen L. A human experimental bone pain model. Basic Clin Pharmacol Toxicol 2013;112:116–23.
7. Andresen T, Staahl C, Oksche A, Mansikka H, Arendt-Nielsen L, Drewes AM. Effect of transdermal opioids in experimentally induced superficial, deep and hyperalgesic pain. Br J Pharmacol 2011;164:934–45.
8. Arendt-Nielsen L. Induction and assessment of experimental pain from human skin, muscle and viscera. In: Jensen TS, Turner JA, Wiesenfeld-Hallin Z, editors. Proceedings of the 8th world congress on pain, vol. 8. Seattle: IASP Press; 1997. p. 393–425.
9. Arendt-Nielsen L. Joint pain: more to it than just structural damage? Pain 2017;158(Suppl. 1):S66–73.
10. Arendt-Nielsen L, Andersen OK, Jensen TS. Brief, prolonged, and repeated stimuli applied to hyperalgesic skin areas: a psychophysical study. Brain Res 1996;712:165–7.
11. Arendt-Nielsen L, Brennum J, Sindrup S, Bak P. Electrophysiological and psychophysical quantification of temporal summation in the human nociceptive system. Eur J Appl Physiol 1994;68:266–73.
12. Arendt-Nielsen L, Curatolo M. Mechanistic, translational, quantitative pain assessment tools in profiling of pain patients and for development of new analgesic compounds. Scand J Pain 2013;4:226–30.
13. Arendt-Nielsen L, Drewes AM, Hansen JB, Tage-Jensen U. Gut pain reactions in man: an experimental investigation using short and long duration transmucosal electrical stimulation. Pain 1997;69:255–62.
14. Arendt-Nielsen L, Egsgaard LL, Petersen KK. Evidence for a central mode of action for etoricoxib (COX-2 inhibitor) in patients with painful knee osteoarthritis. Pain 2016;157:1634–44.
15. Arendt-Nielsen L, Gazerani P. Human pain models in analgesic drug development. In: Handwerker H, Arendt-Nielsen L, editors. Pain models: translational relevance and applications. Washington, DC: International Association for the Study of Pain, IASP Press; 2013. p. 281–97.
16. Arendt-Nielsen L, Graven-Nielsen T. Muscle pain: sensory implications and interaction with motor control. Clin J Pain 2008;24:291–8.
17. Arendt-Nielsen L, Graven-Nielsen T. Translational musculoskeletal pain research. Best Pract Res Clin Rheumatol 2011;25:209–26.

18. Arendt-Nielsen L, Graven-Nielsen T, Svensson P, Jensen TS. Temporal summation in muscles and referred pain areas: an experimental human study. Muscle Nerve 1997;20:1311–3.
19. Arendt-Nielsen L, Hoeck HC. Optimizing the early phase development of new analgesics by human pain biomarkers. Expert Rev Neurother 2011;11:1631–51.
20. Arendt-Nielsen L, Nie H, Laursen MB, Laursen BS, Madeleine P, Simonsen OH, Graven-Nielsen T. Sensitization in patients with painful knee osteoarthritis. Pain 2010;149:573–81.
21. Arendt-Nielsen L, Schipper KP, Dimcevski G, Sumikura H, Krarup AL, Giamberardino MA, Drewes AM. Viscero-somatic reflexes in referred pain areas evoked by capsaicin stimulation of the human gut. Eur J Pain 2008;12:544–51.
22. Arendt-Nielsen L, Skou ST, Nielsen TA, Petersen KK. Altered central sensitization and pain modulation in the CNS in chronic joint pain. Curr Osteoporos Rep 2015;13:225–34.
23. Arendt-Nielsen L, Yarnitsky D. Experimental and clinical applications of quantitative sensory testing applied to skin, muscles and viscera. J Pain 2009;10:556–72.
24. Baad-Hansen L, Arima T, Arendt-Nielsen L, Neumann-Jensen B, Svensson P. Quantitative sensory tests before and 1(1/2) years after orthognathic surgery: a cross-sectional study. J Oral Rehabil 2010;37:313–21.
25. Bajaj P, Bajaj P, Graven-Nielsen T, Arendt-Nielsen L. Osteoarthritis and its association with muscle hyperalgesia: an experimental controlled study. Pain 2001;93:107–14.
26. Bajaj P, Bajaj P, Madsen H, Arendt-Nielsen L. Endometriosis is associated with central sensitization: a psychophysical controlled study. J Pain 2003;4:372–80.
27. Behbehani MM, Dollberg-Stolik O. Partial sciatic nerve ligation results in an enlargement of the receptive field and enhancement of the response of dorsal horn neurons to noxious stimulation by an adenosine agonist. Pain 1994;58:421–8.
28. Binderup AT, Arendt-Nielsen L, Madeleine P. Pressure pain threshold mapping of the trapezius muscle reveals heterogeneity in the distribution of muscular hyperalgesia after eccentric exercise. Eur J Pain 2010;14:705–12.
29. Biurrun Manresa JA, Hansen J, Andersen OK. Development of a data acquisition and analysis system for nociceptive withdrawal reflex and reflex receptive fields in humans. Conf Proc IEEE Eng Med Biol Soc 2010;1:6619–24.
30. Biurrun Manresa JA, Neziri AY, Curatolo M, Arendt-Nielsen L, Andersen OK. Reflex receptive fields are enlarged in patients with musculoskeletal low back and neck pain. Pain 2013;154:1318–24.
31. Bouhassira D, Gall O, Chitour D, Le Bars D. Dorsal horn convergent neurones: negative feedback triggered by spatial summation of nociceptive afferents. Pain 1995;62:195–200.
32. Bragdon EE, Light KC, Costello NL, Sigurdsson A, Bunting S, Bhalang K, Maixner W. Group differences in pain modulation: pain-free women compared to pain-free men and to women with TMD. Pain 2002;96:227–37.
33. Brandsborg B, Dueholm M, Kehlet H, Jensen TS, Nikolajsen L. Mechanosensitivity before and after hysterectomy: a prospective study on the prediction of acute and chronic postoperative pain. Br J Anaesth 2011;107:940–7.
34. Brock C, Arendt-Nielsen L, Wilder-Smith O, Drewes AM. Sensory testing of the human gastrointestinal tract. World J Gastroenterol 2009;15:151–9.
35. Burstein R, Jakubowski M, Garcia-Nicas E, Kainz V, Bajwa Z, Hargreaves R, Becerra L, Borsook D. Thalamic sensitization transforms localized pain into widespread allodynia. Ann Neurol 2010;68:81–91.
36. Chizh BA, Sang CN. Use of sensory methods for detecting target engagement in clinical trials of new analgesics. Neurotherapeutics 2009;6:749–54.
37. Cruz-Almeida Y, Fillingim RB. Can quantitative sensory testing move us closer to mechanism-based pain management? Pain Med 2014;15:61–72.
38. Curatolo M, Arendt-Nielsen L. Central hypersensitivity in chronic musculoskeletal pain. Phys Med Rehabil Clin N Am 2015;26:175–84.
39. Dimcevski G, Staahl C, Andersen SD, Thorsgaard N, Funch-Jensen P, Arendt-Nielsen L, Drewes AM. Assessment of experimental pain from skin, muscle, and esophagus in patients with chronic pancreatitis. Pancreas 2007;35:22–9.
40. Dolin SJ, Cashman JN, Bland JM. Effectiveness of acute postoperative pain management: I. Evidence from published data. Br J Anaesth 2002;89:409–23.
41. Drewes AM, Gregersen H, Arendt-Nielsen L. Experimental pain in gastroenterology: a reappraisal of human studies. Scand J Gastroenterol 2003;38:1115–30.
42. Drewes AM, Petersen P, Qvist P, Nielsen J, Arendt-Nielsen L. An experimental pain model based on electric stimulations of the colon mucosa. Scand J Gastroenterol 1999;34:765–71.

43. Dye SF, Vaupel GL, Dye CC. Conscious neurosensory mapping of the internal structures of the human knee without intraarticular anesthesia. Am J Sports Med 1998;26:773–7.
44. Edwards RR, Dworkin RH, Turk DC, Angst MS, Dionne R, Freeman R, Hansson P, Haroutounian S, Arendt-Nielsen L, Attal N, Baron R, Brell J, Bujanover S, Burke LB, Carr D, Chappell AS, Cowan P, Etropolski M, Fillingim RB, Gewandter JS, Katz NP, Kopecky EA, Markman JD, Nomikos G, Porter L, Rappaport BA, Rice AS, Scavone JM, Scholz J, Simon LS, Smith SM, Tobias J, Tockarshewsky T, Veasley C, Versavel M, Wasan AD, Wen W, Yarnitsky D. Patient phenotyping in clinical trials of chronic pain treatments: IMMPACT recommendations. Pain 2016;157:1851–71.
45. Fernandez-Carnero J, Fernandez-de-Las-Penas C, de la Llave-Rincon AI, Ge HY, Arendt-Nielsen L. Widespread mechanical pain hypersensitivity as sign of central sensitization in unilateral epicondylalgia: a blinded, controlled study. Clin J Pain 2009;25:555–61.
46. Fernandez-Carnero J, Fernandez-de-Las-Penas C, Sterling M, Souvlis T, Arendt-Nielsen L, Vicenzino B. Exploration of the extent of somato-sensory impairment in patients with unilateral lateral epicondylalgia. J Pain 2009;10:1179–85.
47. Fernandez-de-Las-Penas C, Madeleine P, Caminero AB, Cuadrado ML, Arendt-Nielsen L, Pareja JA. Generalized neck-shoulder hyperalgesia in chronic tension-type headache and unilateral migraine assessed by pressure pain sensitivity topographical maps of the trapezius muscle. Cephalalgia 2010;30:77–86.
48. Fernandez-de-Las-Penas C, Madeleine P, Cuadrado ML, Ge HY, Arendt-Nielsen L, Pareja JA. Pressure pain sensitivity mapping of the temporalis muscle revealed bilateral pressure hyperalgesia in patients with strictly unilateral migraine. Cephalalgia 2009;29:670–6.
49. Fernandez-de-Las-Penas C, Madeleine P, Martinez-Perez A, Arendt-Nielsen L, Jimenez-Garcia R, Pareja JA. Pressure pain sensitivity topographical maps reveal bilateral hyperalgesia of the hands in patients with unilateral carpal tunnel syndrome. Arthritis Care Res (Hoboken) 2010;62:1055–64.
50. Finocchietti S, Andresen T, Arendt-Nielsen L, Graven-Nielsen T. Pain evoked by pressure stimulation on the tibia bone – influence of probe diameter on tissue stress and strain. Eur J Pain 2012;16:534–42.
51. Finocchietti S, Nielsen M, Morch CD, Arendt-Nielsen L, Graven-Nielsen T. Pressure-induced muscle pain and tissue biomechanics: a computational and experimental study. Eur J Pain 2011;15:36–44.
52. Geber C, Klein T, Azad S, Birklein F, Gierthmuhlen J, Huge V, Lauchart M, Nitzsche D, Stengel M, Valet M, Baron R, Maier C, Tolle T, Treede RD. Test-retest and interobserver reliability of quantitative sensory testing according to the protocol of the German Research Network on Neuropathic Pain (DFNS): a multi-centre study. Pain 2011;152:548–56.
53. Giamberardino MA. Referred muscle pain/hyperalgesia and central sensitisation. J Rehabil Med 2003;41(Suppl.):85–8.
54. Giamberardino MA, Affaitati G, Lerza R, Lapenna D, Costantini R, Vecchiet L. Relationship between pain symptoms and referred sensory and trophic changes in patients with gallbladder pathology. Pain 2005;114:239–49.
55. Giamberardino MA, Costantini R, Affaitati G, Fabrizio A, Lapenna D, Tafuri E, Mezzetti A. Viscero-visceral hyperalgesia: characterization in different clinical models. Pain 2010;151:307–22.
56. Giamberardino MA, de BP, Martegiani C, Vecchiet L. Effects of extracorporeal shock-wave lithotripsy on referred hyperalgesia from renal/ureteral calculosis. Pain 1994;56:77–83.
57. Gottrup H, Kristensen AD, Bach FW, Jensen TS. Aftersensations in experimental and clinical hypersensitivity. Pain 2003;103:57–64.
58. Goubert D, Danneels L, Graven-Nielsen T, Descheemaeker F, Meeus M. Differences in pain processing between patients with chronic low back pain, recurrent low back pain, and fibromyalgia. Pain Physician 2017;20:307–18.
59. Graven-Nielsen T, Arendt-Nielsen L. Assessment of mechanisms in localized and widespread musculoskeletal pain. Nat Rev Rheumatol 2010;6:599–606.
60. Graven-Nielsen T, Aspegren KS, Henriksson KG, Bengtsson M, Sorensen J, Johnson A, Gerdle B, Arendt-Nielsen L. Ketamine reduces muscle pain, temporal summation, and referred pain in fibromyalgia patients. Pain 2000;85:483–91.
61. Graven-Nielsen T, Izumi M, Petersen KK, Arendt-Nielsen L. User-independent assessment of conditioning pain modulation by cuff pressure algometry. Eur J Pain 2017;21:552–61.
62. Graven-Nielsen T, Mense S, Arendt-Nielsen L. Painful and non-painful pressure sensations from human skeletal muscle. Exp Brain Res 2004;159:273–83.
63. Graven-Nielsen T, Wodehouse T, Langford RM, Arendt-Nielsen L, Kidd BL. Normalization of widespread hyperesthesia and facilitated spatial summation of deep-tissue pain in knee osteoarthritis patients after knee replacement. Arthritis Rheum 2012;64:2907–16.

64. Haanpaa M, Attal N, Backonja M, Baron R, Bennett M, Bouhassira D, Cruccu G, Hansson P, Haythornthwaite JA, Iannetti GD, Jensen TS, Kauppila T, Nurmikko TJ, Rice AS, Rowbotham M, Serra J, Sommer C, Smith BH, Treede RD. NeuPSIG guidelines on neuropathic pain assessment. Pain 2011;152:14–27.
65. Harris J, Clarke RW. Organisation of sensitisation of hind limb withdrawal reflexes from acute noxious stimuli in the rabbit. J Physiol 2003;546:251–65.
66. Hoheisel U, Koch K, Mense S. Functional reorganization in the rat dorsal horn during an experimental myositis. Pain 1994;59:111–8.
67. Hoheisel U, Mense S, Simons DG, Yu X-M. Appearance of new receptive fields in rat dorsal horn neurons following noxious stimulation of skeletal muscle: a model for referral of muscle pain? Neurosci Lett 1993;153:9–12.
68. Hylden JL, Nahin RL, Traub RJ, Dubner R. Expansion of receptive fields of spinal lamina I projection neurons in rats with unilateral adjuvant-induced inflammation: the contribution of dorsal horn mechanisms. Pain 1989;37:229–43.
69. Imai Y, Petersen KK, Morch CD, Arendt-Nielsen L. Comparing test-retest reliability and magnitude of conditioned pain modulation using different combinations of test and conditioning stimuli. Somatosens Mot Res 2016;33:169–77.
70. Izumi M, Petersen KK, Laursen MB, Arendt-Nielsen L, Graven-Nielsen T. Facilitated temporal summation of pain correlates with clinical pain intensity after hip arthroplasty. Pain 2017;158:323–32.
71. Jarrell J, Arendt-Nielsen L. Quantitative sensory testing in gynaecology: improving preoperative and postoperative pain diagnosis. J Obstet Gynaecol Can 2013;35:531–5.
72. Jensen KB, Kosek E, Petzke F, Carville S, Fransson P, Marcus H, Williams SC, Choy E, Giesecke T, Mainguy Y, Gracely R, Ingvar M. Evidence of dysfunctional pain inhibition in Fibromyalgia reflected in rACC during provoked pain. Pain 2009;144:95–100.
73. Jensen MB, Manresa JB, Andersen OK. A new objective method for acquisition and quantification of reflex receptive fields. Pain 2015;156:555–64.
74. Jensen TS, Baron R. Translation of symptoms and signs into mechanisms in neuropathic pain. Pain 2003;102:1–8.
75. Jespersen A, Amris K, Graven-Nielsen T, Arendt-Nielsen L, Bartels EM, Torp-Pedersen S, Bliddal H, Danneskiold-Samsoe B. Assessment of pressure-pain thresholds and central sensitization of pain in lateral epicondylalgia. Pain Med 2013;14:297–304.
76. Kelly S, Dobson KL, Harris J. Spinal nociceptive reflexes are sensitized in the monosodium iodoacetate model of osteoarthritis pain in the rat. Osteoarthritis Cartilage 2013;21:1327–35.
77. Koelbaek JM, Graven-Nielsen T, Schou OA, Arendt-Nielsen L. Generalised muscular hyperalgesia in chronic whiplash syndrome. Pain 1999;83:229–34.
78. Kong JT, Johnson KA, Balise RR, Mackey S. Test-retest reliability of thermal temporal summation using an individualized protocol. J Pain 2013;14:79–88.
79. Konopka KH, Harbers M, Houghton A, Kortekaas R, van VA, Timmerman W, den Boer JA, Struys MM, van Wijhe M. Bilateral sensory abnormalities in patients with unilateral neuropathic pain; a quantitative sensory testing (QST) study. PLoS One 2012;7:e37524.
80. Kosek E, Hansson P. Modulatory influence on somatosensory perception from vibration and heterotopic noxious conditioning stimulation (HNCS) in fibromyalgia patients and healthy subjects. Pain 1997;70:41–51.
81. Kosek E, Ordeberg G. Lack of pressure pain modulation by heterotopic noxious conditioning stimulation in patients with painful osteoarthritis before, but not following, surgical pain relief. Pain 2000;88:69–78.
82. Leffler AS, Kosek E, Lerndal T, Nordmark B, Hansson P. Somatosensory perception and function of diffuse noxious inhibitory controls (DNIC) in patients suffering from rheumatoid arthritis. Eur J Pain 2002;6:161–76.
83. Lei J, You HJ, Andersen OK, Graven-Nielsen T, Arendt-Nielsen L. Homotopic and heterotopic variation in skin blood flow and temperature following experimental muscle pain in humans. Brain Res 2008;1232:85–93.
84. Lemming D, Graven-Nielsen T, Sorensen J, Arendt-Nielsen L, Gerdle B. Widespread pain hypersensitivity and facilitated temporal summation of deep tissue pain in whiplash associated disorder: an explorative study of women. J Rehabil Med 2012;44:648–57.
85. Lu S, Baad-Hansen L, Zhang Z, Svensson P. Reliability of a new technique for intraoral mapping of somatosensory sensitivity. Somatosens Mot Res 2013;30:30–6.
86. Macrae WA. Chronic pain after surgery. Br J Anaesth 2001;87:88–98.
87. Magerl W, Krumova EK, Baron R, Tolle T, Treede RD, Maier C. Reference data for quantitative sensory testing (QST): refined stratification for age and a novel method for statistical comparison of group data. Pain 2010;151:598–605.

88. Maier C, Baron R, Tolle TR, Binder A, Birbaumer N, Birklein F, Gierthmuhlen J, Flor H, Geber C, Huge V, Krumova EK, Landwehrmeyer GB, Magerl W, Maihofner C, Richter H, Rolke R, Scherens A, Schwarz A, Sommer C, Tronnier V, Uceyler N, Valet M, Wasner G, Treede RD. Quantitative sensory testing in the German Research Network on Neuropathic Pain (DFNS): somatosensory abnormalities in 1236 patients with different neuropathic pain syndromes. Pain 2010;150:439–50.
89. Malan TP, Ossipov MH, Gardell LR, Ibrahim M, Bian D, Lai J, Porreca F. Extraterritorial neuropathic pain correlates with multisegmental elevation of spinal dynorphin in nerve-injured rats. Pain 2000;86:185–94.
90. Manafi-Khanian B, Arendt-Nielsen L, Frokjaer JB, Graven-Nielsen T. Deformation and pressure propagation in deep somatic tissue during painful cuff algometry. Eur J Pain 2015;19:1456–66.
91. Mendell LM. Physiological properties of unmyelinated fiber projection to the spinal cord. Exp Neurol 1966;16:316–32.
92. Miranda A, Peles S, Rudolph C, Shaker R, Sengupta JN. Altered visceral sensation in response to somatic pain in the rat. Gastroenterology 2004;126:1082–9.
93. Neogi T, Guermazi A, Roemer F, Nevitt MC, Scholz J, Arendt-Nielsen L, Woolf C, Niu J, Bradley LA, Quinn E, Law LF. Association of joint inflammation with pain sensitization in knee osteoarthritis: the multicenter osteoarthritis study. Arthritis Rheumatol 2016;68:654–61.
94. Ness TJ, Gebhart GF. Characterization of neurons responsive to noxious colorectal distension in the T13-L2 spinal cord of the rat. J Neurophysiol 1988;60:1419–38.
95. Neziri AY, Andersen OK, Petersen-Felix S, Radanov B, Dickenson AH, Scaramozzino P, Arendt-Nielsen L, Curatolo M. The nociceptive withdrawal reflex: normative values of thresholds and reflex receptive fields. Eur J Pain 2010;14:134–41.
96. Neziri AY, Haesler S, Petersen-Felix S, Muller M, Arendt-Nielsen L, Manresa JB, Andersen OK, Curatolo M. Generalized expansion of nociceptive reflex receptive fields in chronic pain patients. Pain 2010;151:798–805.
97. Neziri AY, Scaramozzino P, Andersen OK, Dickenson AH, Arendt-Nielsen L, Curatolo M. Reference values of mechanical and thermal pain tests in a pain-free population. Eur J Pain 2011;15:376–83.
98. Nie H, Graven-Nielsen T, Arendt-Nielsen L. Spatial and temporal summation of pain evoked by mechanical pressure stimulation. Eur J Pain 2009;13:592–9.
99. Nielsen J, Arendt-Nielsen L. Spatial summation of heat induced pain within and between dermatomes. Somatosens Mot Res 1997;14:119–25.
100. Nielsen J, Arendt-Nielsen L. The importance of stimulus configuration for temporal summation of first and second pain to repeated heat stimuli. Eur J Pain 1998;2:329–41.
101. Nikolajsen L, Hansen CL, Nielsen J, Keller J, Arendt-Nielsen L, Jensen TS. The effect of ketamine on phantom pain: a central neuropathic disorder maintained by peripheral input. Pain 1996;67:69–77.
102. O'Neill S, Manniche C, Graven-Nielsen T, Arendt-Nielsen L. Generalized deep-tissue hyperalgesia in patients with chronic low-back pain. Eur J Pain 2007;11:415–20.
103. Oertel BG, Lotsch J. Clinical pharmacology of analgesics assessed with human experimental pain models: bridging basic and clinical research. Br J Pharmacol 2013;168:534–53.
104. Ohmichi Y, Sato J, Ohmichi M, Sakurai H, Yoshimoto T, Morimoto A, Hashimoto T, Eguchi K, Nishihara M, Arai YC, Ohishi H, Asamoto K, Ushida T, Nakano T, Kumazawa T. Two-week cast immobilization induced chronic widespread hyperalgesia in rats. Eur J Pain 2012;16:338–48.
105. Olesen SS, Brock C, Krarup AL, Funch-Jensen P, Arendt-Nielsen L, Wilder-Smith OH, Drewes AM. Descending inhibitory pain modulation is impaired in patients with chronic pancreatitis. Clin Gastroenterol Hepatol 2010;8:724–30.
106. Oono Y, Matos RVL, Wang K, Arendt-Nielsen L. The inter- and intra-individual variance in descending pain modulation evoked by different conditioning stimuli in healthy men. Scand J Pain 2011;2:162–9.
107. Pedersen KV, Drewes AM, Graumann O, Osther SS, Olesen AE, Arendt-Nielsen L, Osther PJ. Somatosensory and trophic findings in the referred pain area in patients with kidney stone disease. Scand J Pain 2013;4:165–70.
108. Perkins FM, Kehlet H. Chronic pain as an outcome of surgery. A review of predictive factors. Anesthesiology 2000;93:1123–33.
109. Peters ML, Schmidt AJ, Van den Hout MA, Koopmans R, Sluijter ME. Chronic back pain, acute postoperative pain and the activation of diffuse noxious inhibitory controls (DNIC). Pain 1992;50:177–87.
110. Petersen KK, Arendt-Nielsen L, Simonsen O, Wilder-Smith O, Laursen MB. Presurgical assessment of temporal summation of pain predicts the development of chronic postoperative pain 12 months after total knee replacement. Pain 2015;156:55–61.
111. Petersen KK, Graven-Nielsen T, Simonsen O, Laursen MB, Arendt-Nielsen L. Preoperative pain mechanisms assessed by cuff algometry are associated with chronic postoperative pain relief after total knee replacement. Pain 2016;157:1400–6.

112. Petersen KK, Vaegter HB, Arendt-Nielsen L. An updated view on the reliability of different protocols for the assessment of conditioned pain modulation. Pain 2017;158:988.
113. Pogatzki EM, Niemeier JS, Brennan TJ. Persistent secondary hyperalgesia after gastrocnemius incision in the rat. Eur J Pain 2002;6:295–305.
114. Polianskis R, Graven-Nielsen T, Arendt-Nielsen L. Spatial and temporal aspects of deep tissue pain assessed by cuff algometry. Pain 2002;100:19–26.
115. Porreca F, Ossipov MH, Gebhart GF. Chronic pain and medullary descending facilitation. Trends Neurosci 2002;25:319–25.
116. Price DD, Hayes RL, Ruda M, Dubner R. Neural representation of cutaneous aftersensations by spinothalamic tract neurons. Fed Proc 1978;37:2237–9.
117. Price DD, Hu JW, Dubner R, Gracely RH. Peripheral suppresion of first pain and central summation of second pain evoked by noxious heat pulses. Pain 1977;3:57–68.
118. Ren K. Wind-up and the NMDA receptor: from animal studies to humans. Pain 1994;59:157–8.
119. Robinson ME, Bialosky JE, Bishop MD, Price DD, George SZ. Supra-threshold scaling, temporal summation, and after-sensation: relationships to each other and anxiety/fear. J Pain Res 2010;3:25–32.
120. Rolke R, Baron R, Maier C, Tolle TR, Treede RD, Beyer A, Binder A, Birbaumer N, Birklein F, Botefur IC, Braune S, Flor H, Huge V, Klug R, Landwehrmeyer GB, Magerl W, Maihofner C, Rolko C, Schaub C, Scherens A, Sprenger T, Valet M, Wasserka B. Quantitative sensory testing in the German Research Network on Neuropathic Pain (DFNS): standardized protocol and reference values. Pain 2006;123:231–43.
121. Rolke R, Magerl W, Campbell KA, Schalber C, Caspari S, Birklein F, Treede RD. Quantitative sensory testing: a comprehensive protocol for clinical trials. Eur J Pain 2006;10:77–88.
122. Rubin TK, Henderson LA, Macefield VG. Changes in the spatiotemporal expression of local and referred pain following repeated intramuscular injections of hypertonic saline: a longitudinal study. J Pain 2010;11:737–45.
123. Rubin TK, Lake S, van der Kooi S, Lucas NP, Mahns DA, Henderson LA, Macefield VG. Predicting the spatiotemporal expression of local and referred acute muscle pain in individual subjects. Exp Brain Res 2012;223:11–8.
124. Ruiz-Ruiz B, Fernandez-de-Las-Penas C, Ortega-Santiago R, Arendt-Nielsen L, Madeleine P. Topographical pressure and thermal pain sensitivity mapping in patients with unilateral lateral epicondylalgia. J Pain 2011;12:1040–8.
125. Sandrini G, Rossi P, Milanov I, Serrao M, Cecchini AP, Nappi G. Abnormal modulatory influence of diffuse noxious inhibitory controls in migraine and chronic tension-type headache patients. Cephalalgia 2006;26:782–9.
126. Sarlani E, Grace EG, Reynolds MA, Greenspan JD. Sex differences in temporal summation of pain and aftersensations following repetitive noxious mechanical stimulation. Pain 2004;109:115–23.
127. Sarlani E, Greenspan JD. Gender differences in temporal summation of mechanically evoked pain. Pain 2002;97:163–9.
128. Sato H, Saisu H, Muraoka W, Nakagawa T, Svensson P, Wajima K. Lack of temporal summation but distinct aftersensations to thermal stimulation in patients with combined tension-type headache and myofascial temporomandibular disorder. J Orofac Pain 2012;26:288–95.
129. Schaible HG. Spinal mechanisms contributing to joint pain. Novartis Found Symp 2004;260:4–22.
130. Schaible HG, Richter F, Ebersberger A, Boettger MK, Vanegas H, Natura G, Vazquez E, Segond von BG. Joint pain. Exp Brain Res 2009;196:153–62.
131. Schliessbach J, Arendt-Nielsen L, Heini P, Curatolo M. The role of central hypersensitivity in the determination of intradiscal mechanical hyperalgesia in discogenic pain. Pain Med 2010;11:701–8.
132. Schliessbach J, Siegenthaler A, Streitberger K, Eichenberger U, Nuesch E, Juni P, Arendt-Nielsen L, Curatolo M. The prevalence of widespread central hypersensitivity in chronic pain patients. Eur J Pain 2013;17:1502–10.
133. Schouenborg J, Weng H-R, Holmberg H. Modular organization of spinal reflexes: a new hypothesis. NIPS 1994;9:261–5.
134. Schouenborg J, Weng H-R, Kalliomäki J, Holmberg H. A survey of spinal dorsal horn neurones encoding the spinal organization of withdrawal reflexes in the rat. Exp Brain Res 1995;106:19–27.
135. Siegenthaler A, Eichenberger U, Schmidlin K, Arendt-Nielsen L, Curatolo M. What does local tenderness say about the origin of pain? An investigation of cervical zygapophysial joint pain. Anesth Analg 2010;110:923–27.
136. Skou ST, Graven-Nielsen T, Rasmussen S, Simonsen OH, Laursen MB, Arendt-Nielsen L. Widespread sensitization in patients with chronic pain after revision total knee arthroplasty. Pain 2013;154:1588–94.
137. Skou ST, Graven-Nielsen T, Rasmussen S, Simonsen OH, Laursen MB, Arendt-Nielsen L. Facilitation of pain sensitization in knee osteoarthritis and persistent post-operative pain: a cross-sectional study. Eur J Pain 2014;18:1024–31.

138. Sluka KA, Kalra A, Moore SA. Unilateral intramuscular injections of acidic saline produce a bilateral, long-lasting hyperalgesia. Muscle Nerve 2001;24:37–46.
139. Sorensen J, Graven-Nielsen T, Henriksson KG, Bengtsson M, Arendt-Nielsen L. Hyperexcitability in fibromyalgia. J Rheumatol 1998;25:152–5.
140. Staud R, Cannon RC, Mauderli AP, Robinson ME, Price DD, Vierck Jr CJ. Temporal summation of pain from mechanical stimulation of muscle tissue in normal controls and subjects with fibromyalgia syndrome. Pain 2003;102:87–95.
141. Staud R, Koo E, Robinson ME, Price DD. Spatial summation of mechanically evoked muscle pain and painful aftersensations in normal subjects and fibromyalgia patients. Pain 2007;130:177–87.
142. Staud R, Vierck CJ, Robinson ME, Price DD. Spatial summation of heat pain within and across dermatomes in fibromyalgia patients and pain-free subjects. Pain 2004;111:342–50.
143. Stawowy M, Funch-Jensen P, Arendt-Nielsen L, Drewes AM. Somatosensory changes in the referred pain area in patients with cholecystolithiasis. Eur J Gastroenterol Hepatol 2005;17:865–70.
144. Stawowy M, Rossel P, Bluhme C, Funch-Jensen P, Arendt-Nielsen L, Drewes AM. Somatosensory changes in the referred pain area following acute inflammation of the appendix. Eur J Gastroenterol Hepatol 2002;14:1079–84.
145. Suzuki R, Rygh LJ, Dickenson AH. Bad news from the brain: descending 5-HT pathways that control spinal pain processing. Trends Pharmacol Sci 2004;25:613–7.
146. Tal M, Bennett GJ. Extra-territorial pain in rats with a peripheral mononeuropathy: mechano-hyperalgesia and mechano-allodynia in the territory of an uninjured nerve. Pain 1994;57:375–82.
147. Thompson LR, Boudreau R, Newman AB, Hannon MJ, Chu CR, Nevitt MC, Kent KC. The association of osteoarthritis risk factors with localized, regional and diffuse knee pain. Osteoarthritis Cartilage 2010;18:1244–9.
148. Tverskoy M, Oz Y, Isakson A, Finger J, Bradley Jr EL, Kissin I. Preemptive effect of fentanyl and ketamine on postoperative pain and wound hyperalgesia. Anesth Analg 1994;78:205–9.
149. Wang R, King T, De FM, Guo W, Ossipov MH, Porreca F. Descending facilitation maintains long-term spontaneous neuropathic pain. J Pain 2013;14:845–53.
150. Weissman-Fogel I, Granovsky Y, Crispel Y, Ben-Nun A, Best LA, Yarnitsky D, Granot M. Enhanced presurgical pain temporal summation response predicts post-thoracotomy pain intensity during the acute postoperative phase. J Pain 2009;10:628–36.
151. Werner MU, Duun P, Kehlet H. Prediction of postoperative pain by preoperative nociceptive responses to heat stimulation. Anesthesiology 2004;100:115–9.
152. Wilder-Smith OH. Chronic pain and surgery: a review of new insights from sensory testing. J Pain Palliat Care Pharmacother 2011;25:146–59.
153. Wilder-Smith OH, Arendt-Nielsen L. Postoperative hyperalgesia: its clinical importance and relevance. Anesthesiology 2006;104:601–7.
154. Wilder-Smith OH, Schreyer T, Scheffer GJ, Arendt-Nielsen L. Patients with chronic pain after abdominal surgery show less preoperative endogenous pain inhibition and more postoperative hyperalgesia: a pilot study. J Pain Palliat Care Pharmacother 2010;24:119–28.
155. Wilder-Smith OH, Tassonyi E, Crul BJ, Arendt-Nielsen L. Quantitative sensory testing and human surgery: effects of analgesic management on postoperative neuroplasticity. Anesthesiology 2003;98:1214–22.
156. Wilder-Smith OH, Tassonyi E, Senly C, Otten P, Arendt-Nielsen L. Surgical pain is followed not only by spinal sensitization but also by supraspinal antinociception. Br J Anaesth 1996;76:816–21.
157. Wylde V, Palmer S, Learmonth ID, Dieppe P. The association between pre-operative pain sensitisation and chronic pain after knee replacement: an exploratory study. Osteoarthritis Cartilage 2013;21:1253–6.
158. Yarnitsky D. Conditioned pain modulation (the diffuse noxious inhibitory control-like effect): its relevance for acute and chronic pain states. Curr Opin Anaesthesiol 2010;23:611–5.
159. Yarnitsky D, Arendt-Nielsen L, Bouhassira D, Edwards RR, Fillingim RB, Granot M, Hansson P, Lautenbacher S, Marchand S, Wilder-Smith O. Recommendations on terminology and practice of psychophysical DNIC testing. Eur J Pain 2010;14:339.
160. Yarnitsky D, Crispel Y, Eisenberg E, Granovsky Y, Ben-Nun A, Sprecher E, Best LA, Granot M. Prediction of chronic post-operative pain: pre-operative DNIC testing identifies patients at risk. Pain 2008;138:22–8.
161. Yarnitsky D, Granot M, Granovsky Y. Pain modulation profile and pain therapy: between pro- and antinociception. Pain 2014;155:663–5.
162. Yarnitsky D, Granot M, Nahman-Averbuch H, Khamaisi M, Granovsky Y. Conditioned pain modulation predicts duloxetine efficacy in painful diabetic neuropathy. Pain 2012;153:1193–8.

163. You HJ, Colpaert FC, Arendt-Nielsen L. The novel analgesic and high-efficacy 5-HT1A receptor agonist F 13640 inhibits nociceptive responses, wind-up, and after-discharges in spinal neurons and withdrawal reflexes. Exp Neurol 2005;191:174–83.
164. You HJ, Lei J, Sui MY, Huang L, Tan YX, Tjolsen A, Arendt-Nielsen L. Endogenous descending modulation: spatiotemporal effect of dynamic imbalance between descending facilitation and inhibition of nociception. J Physiol 2010;588:4177–88.
165. You HJ, Morch CD, Chen J, Arendt-Nielsen L. Role of central NMDA versus non-NMDA receptor in spinal withdrawal reflex in spinal anesthetized rats under normal and hyperexcitable conditions. Brain Res 2003;981:12–22.

CHAPTER 9

Electrophysiologic Techniques: Assessment of Spinal Nociceptive Processing Using the Withdrawal Reflex

Ole Kæseler Andersen and José Alberto Biurrun Manresa

Ever since the first descriptions of the spinal flexor reflexes by Sherrington, their relationship to nociception and pain has been in focus. The protective nature of the reflex is linked to actual or potential tissue damage, and hence, the reflex is associated to pain. A polysynaptic reflex arc has been described that integrates almost all sensory input [65], descending control, and spinal motor programs, leading to a multifaceted, functional motor output. In animals, the reflex serves as a key model for assessment of spinal nociception under standardized experimental conditions [45]. With the same arguments, the nociceptive withdrawal reflex (NWR) has also been heavily used for complementing psychophysical assessment of acute, phasic pain or simply for probing *spinal* nociception [1,64,84]. In most studies, electrical stimulation has been used for eliciting the NWR because of efficiency and reproducibility in combination with surface electromyography (EMG) from relevant muscles for assessment of the reflex. For graded suprathreshold stimulation intensities, the pain intensity and NWR size correlate well in healthy volunteers [18,83]. In relation to pain research, the NWR is often termed the RIII reflex [39] to signal that group III or Aδ fibers are mediating the response. The relationship between the NWR threshold and the pain threshold is extremely variable in the literature; to a large extent this can be explained by different reflex threshold definitions. Rhudy and France [60] have presented a thorough work to identify the most reliable definition of the NWR threshold, ending with recommendations for NWR thresholds based on significant EMG deflections from baseline. However, using the NWR threshold as the primary outcome measure in relation to pain in future studies—just like the simple notion of the NWR as an objective measure of a multidimensional pain experience—is too simplistic.

The reflex receptive field (RRF) for a specific muscle is the skin area from which an NWR can be evoked. The reflex exhibits a modular organization, where each muscle or group of synergistic muscles has a well-defined and unique cutaneous RRF [4,69,75]. The RRF adheres to the biomechanical function of the related group of muscles, ensuring adequate withdrawal [19,69,82], and hence, extensor muscles also have an RRF. The net withdrawal is generated by those muscles activated by the current stimulation site. At the spinal cord level, the RRF is most likely organized by a set of deeply located wide dynamic range neurons [70]. In relation to pain research, variation in the sensitivity of such multireceptive neurons in the deep dorsal horn has received substantial attention [29], and therefore, the variation in RRF area as assessed via distributed electrical stimulations [4] is of interest when studying spinal nociceptive mechanisms in humans.

The present chapter will discuss the methodology and primary findings related to the use of the NWR for assessment of spinal nociception in healthy volunteers, in postoperative patients, and in patients with chronic pain.

METHODOLOGY

Stimulation, Recording, and Quantification of the NWR

An NWR can be elicited by natural stimuli, such as heat and mechanical punctuate stimuli, which activate specific pain receptors in the skin [51,69,85]. Although the NWR elicited by these stimuli is easily associated with responses in natural conditions, they present substantial methodological disadvantages in the research context, such as the impossibility of relying on accurate timing from the onset of the stimulus or potential tissue damage after repeated stimulation. Therefore, electrical stimulation is the most widely used "artificial" method for eliciting the NWR because it is easier to control and deliver [79]. The NWR is most commonly recorded from the lower limb after stimulation of the sural, peroneal, tibial, and plantar nerves, either via direct stimulation of the nerve bundle or by stimulation of the skin area innervated by the nerve. This type of stimulus bypasses the skin receptor and generates a synchronous action potential directly in the sensory nerve, depolarizing mainly $A\beta$ and $A\delta$ fibers (usually differentiated by the onset latency of the response) [39]. In relation to the quality of the sensation, the stimulus is often described as a sharp, pricking, and well localized, likely reflecting $A\delta$ afferent inflow [47,48].

Surface EMG is commonly used to record the NWR response from the muscles [1,64]. From these recordings, the NWR can be detected using manual or automatic methods using standardized scoring criteria for NWR detection [40,60]. Once the NWR is detected, a frequently quantified variable is the NWR threshold, i.e., the stimulation intensity required to elicit the NWR with a given probability (commonly 50% of the stimulations). In this regard, reference values for NWR threshold in a normal population are available [52]. Additionally, several methods for further quantification of the NWR in surface EMG recordings are available, such as integrated and mean EMG amplitude [16], area under the curve [30], maximal peak to peak amplitude [42], and root-mean-square amplitude [1]. In all cases, the performance of all detection and quantification methods is negatively affected when the surface EMG signal is contaminated with noise (particularly cross talk between muscles), so newly developed recording and analysis methodologies are suggested for more reliable reflex detection and quantification [40]. The reflex threshold has been used for assessment of anesthetic depth during surgery [80], and the NWR has been used as outcome measure during tests of the anesthetic isoflurane [57].

The Reflex Receptive Field

RRFs are obtained by quantifying the NWR responses elicited after distributed electrical stimulation in humans in which the subject is unaware of the site of the upcoming stimulation. Bidimensional interpolation and extrapolation of NWR amplitudes are then used to generate the RRF [1,53]. This method provides a set of quantitative features (RRF area, RRF volume) that describe the variations in sensitivity of the RRF (Figure 9-1) [53]. As for NWR thresholds, reference values for RRF in a normal population are also available [52]. Another methodology for RRF quantification based on the probability of occurrence has been introduced, which seems to be a robust approach for NWR quantification [49]. A new

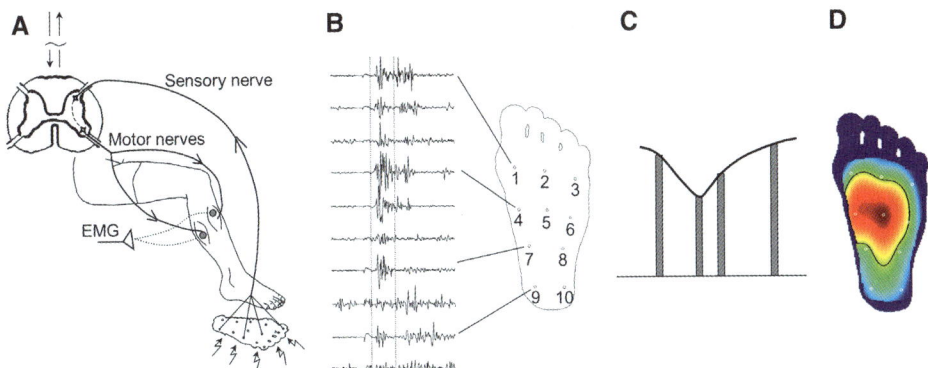

FIGURE 9-1 General methodology for acquisition and recording of nociceptive withdrawal reflex (NWR) and reflex receptive field (RRF). **A:** NWR responses are evoked by electrical stimulation in different locations on the extremities (in the figure, only electrical stimulation at the foot sole is shown). The reflex responses are recorded by surface electromyography (EMG) at any muscle biomechanically involved in the NWR response. **B:** Specifically for RRF recording, stimuli are delivered at several sites in randomized sequence, and the EMG signals are averaged for every stimulation site. The reflex size is typically quantified in the 60 to 180 ms time interval (indicated by the *vertical lines*). **C:** The NWR size detected at each electrode is interpolated and extrapolated. **D:** The two-dimensional interpolation map is then superimposed onto a map of the foot for depicting the NWR sensitivity in a particular muscle. (Modified from Neziri AY, Curatolo M, Bergadano A, Petersen-Felix S, Dickenson A, Arendt-Nielsen L, Andersen OK. New method for quantification and statistical analysis of nociceptive reflex receptive fields in humans. J Neurosci Methods 2009;178:24–30.)

more objective method for assessment of the RRF based on automatic detection of reflex thresholds has been introduced [41] but not yet tested on conditions with changes in spinal nociceptive excitability.

Reliability of the NWR and the RRF

Reliability can be defined as the amount of measurement error that is acceptable for the effective practical use of a measurement tool. Establishing the reliability of a biomarker related to pain is essential if it is to be used for detecting differences within and between healthy individual and patients, to follow up the progression of a given disease, and to investigate the effect of pharmacologic interventions, among others. As such, reliability has to be analyzed before any other experimental hypothesis because its validity could be questioned if such a test is not adequately consistent in whatever value it indicates from repeated (i.e., test–retest) measurements [8].

Previous studies addressed the test–retest reliability of the NWR threshold in populations of healthy volunteers [50]. The absolute reliability (expressed as coefficient of variation) for the NWR threshold was 5% within the same day, 17% after 4 days, and 34% after 16 weeks, whereas the relative reliability (expressed as intraclass correlation coefficient) was 0.98 within the same day and 0.82 after 4 days (no data on relative reliability were reported for the 16 weeks' interval) [27,50]. The test–retest reliability of the NWR threshold was also tested in a population of chronic pain patients, resulting in absolute reliability values of 17% after 7 days and 22% after 14 days, whereas relative reliability values were 0.81 and 0.71 after 7 and 14 days, respectively [13]. In general, the reliability of the NWR in healthy volunteers is comparable with that found in patients with chronic pain, and it is acceptable for experimental and clinical assessment of nociception. However, special caution is necessary when follow-up studies are planned involving long periods of time between sessions (because the reliability decreases with increasing intervals between test and retest).

THE NWR IN THE ASSESSMENT OF SPINAL NOCICEPTION

Relationship to Other Measures of Spinal Nociception

The stimulus–response function to electrical stimulations reveals a linear relationship to stimulus intensity at suprathreshold intensities and a strong correlation to the pain intensity under controlled experimental conditions [18,28,83]. Neurons located in the deep dorsal horn receiving input from both tactile and nociceptive afferents are intercalated in the reflex pathway, and the excitability of these neurons is strongly modulated by robust nociceptive activity [71]. Continued nociceptive input leads to gradual depolarization of spinal neurons and subsequently lower thresholds, leading to stronger neuronal firing for the same afferent input [74]. This kind of temporal summation at spinal level can also be assessed noninvasively using the NWR [5,58]. Stimulation frequencies ranging from 0.5 to 20 Hz and trains lasting up to 5 seconds have been tested [7,9]. A gradual increase in reflex size is observed during the initial phase of repetitive stimulation, which is then followed by a reduction in reflex size [9] most likely reflecting the balance between spinal integration and (delayed) inhibitory mechanisms triggered by the robust input. The reflex buildup most likely resembles the initial phase of the windup phenomenon, which is most pronounced in spinalized animals [31]. Temporal summation has also been tested in relation to RRFs. Summation sensitivity is most pronounced in the center of the RRF, whereas the amount of temporal summation is less in the fringes of the RRF [3].

Modulation of Spinal Nociception in Humans

Under physiologic conditions, descending inhibition and facilitation can adapt the responsiveness of the nociceptive system to protect the body from actual or potential injury. Early research on supraspinal control of reflex excitability mainly focused on descending inhibitory control as a potential target for analgesic mechanisms, although later on it became evident that supraspinal control can be both inhibitory and facilitatory [36,56]. Recent studies involving animals suggest that descending facilitation may have a very rapid onset, whereas descending inhibition shows a late occurrence, probably triggered by sufficient C-fiber afferent activity and temporal summation [89]. The neural basis for bidirectional control from the midline system includes two populations of neurons in the rostroventral medulla (ON-cells and OFF-cells) that are differentially recruited by higher structures to enhance or inhibit pain [36]. Thus, the rostroventral medulla has been suggested as the last relay, but more rostral centers may contribute such as the anterior cingulate cortex, the reticular nuclei, and the periaqueductal gray [63]. These structures can be modulated by cognitive or physiologic factors, and there is increasing evidence that they may contribute to central sensitization in the transition from acute to chronic pain [36,81].

Supraspinal control is strongly modulated via concurrent tonic nociceptive input. Hence, conditioning pain modulation (CPM) has been shown to inhibit the NWR. Immersion of the contralateral hand in ice water results in a clear inhibition of the NWR excitability [78,86], most likely due to activation of descending activity inhibiting dorsal horn neurons [44]. CPM also reduces the reflex temporal summation response [72]. Descending modulation of the NWR due to variation in cognitive activity has also been reported. This includes viewing pictures with strong emotional content [61], anticipatory cues [46], and hypnotic suggestions of analgesia [90]. A recent study has shown enlarged NWR responses following catastrophizing self-statements but interestingly without concurrent modulation of the NWR temporal summation response [62]. Cognitive modulation, by changing the level of attention and distraction, has been shown to lead to reduced and enlarged RRF area, respectively [15], suggesting dynamic modulation of the excitability of deep dorsal horn neurons.

NWR excitability is often used as a biomarker in animal studies. Facilitated reflex responses have been observed following robust activation of nociceptive afferents close to the reflex testing site [35,67,87]. Translation of these models of acute reflex facilitation to humans has been less successful. The few examples available include reflex facilitation following topical application of capsaicin for 30 to 60 minutes [3,34] and a recent study where deep injections of capsaicin resulted in an expansion of RRF area in both spinal intact and complete spinal cord injured (SCI) subjects [11].

The NWR has been used to investigate differences in spinal nociception related to the influence of supraspinal control by testing in SCI individuals [38]. After spinal cord transection, the NWR becomes larger and changes into a stereotyped flexor pattern with flexion of all joints [26,32]. The NWR thresholds also become higher in SCI volunteers compared with those in healthy volunteers [2,37]. In relation to the RRF, it is shaped by excitatory and inhibitory spinal neuronal circuits under supraspinal influence [66]. In volunteers with chronic SCI, the loss of descending control and appropriate peripheral input causes severe changes in the spinal circuitry [24], leading to an abnormal RRF expansion when supraspinal control is impaired and/or when spinal neurons are sensitized [2,25,33,68]. Moreover, a recent study demonstrated that people with complete SCI presented not only larger RRF areas but also a reversed RRF topography compared with RRF of healthy volunteers; e.g., the most sensitive area for the dorsiflexor tibialis anterior in healthy volunteers is the arch of the foot, whereas the arch of the foot became the less sensitive area in people with complete SCI [11]. In any case, the RRF was still able to expand during experimental induction of central sensitization, possibly reflecting that some spinal protective plastic mechanisms may still be partially functional without supraspinal control. A functional model of the NWR has been proposed (Figure 9-2), integrating these new findings with existing knowledge on spinal and supraspinal neural networks involved in the control and modulation of the NWR and the RRF [36,63].

Assessment of Spinal Hyperexcitability in Pain Patients

Experimental and clinical studies in diverse cohorts of patients (e.g., whiplash, fibromyalgia, osteoarthritis, musculoskeletal disorders, headache, and neuropathic, visceral, and postsurgical pain) have shown common traits (dynamic tactile allodynia, secondary punctate or pressure hyperalgesia, aftersensations, enhanced temporal summation and enlargement of referred pain areas), reflecting alterations in central pain processing [21,88]. These traits can be assessed using different experimental tests, such as verbal reports, pain questionnaires, light touch, vibration as well as detection, and first pain and tolerance thresholds to pressure, electrical, heat, and cold stimuli [43,59,73,76,77]. However, these tests are subjective in the sense that they rely on the volunteers' reports after sensory stimulation, and thus, they can be voluntarily and/or involuntarily affected by a number of factors, most notably, the psychological distress associated with chronic pain conditions [17]. In this regard, there is increasing evidence that objective methods, such as those based on the NWR and the RRF, can detect hyperexcitability in the nociceptive pathways without the problems usually associated with subjective assessments. A tendency for lowering of the NWR threshold was also detected in patients undergoing

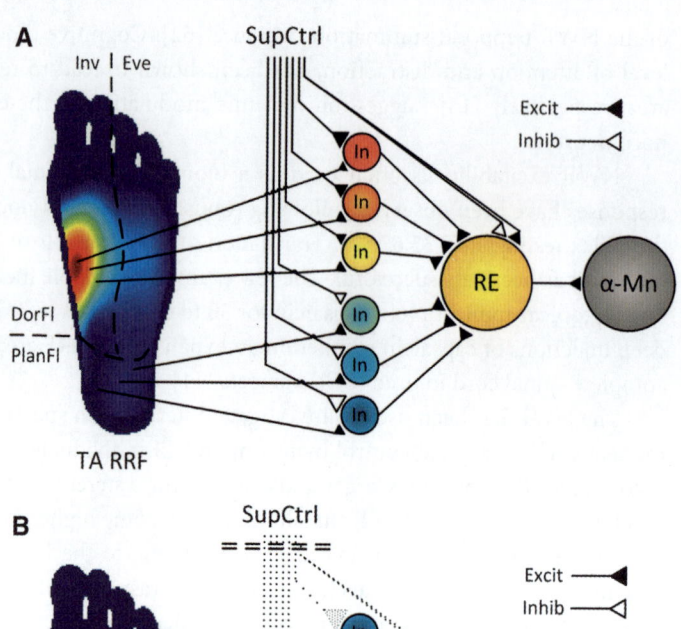

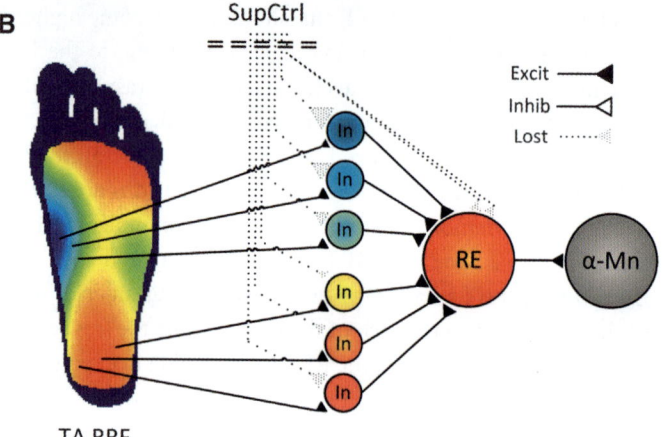

FIGURE 9-2 Functional organization of the nociceptive withdrawal reflex (NWR) pathways. **A:** In healthy volunteers, the reflex receptive field (RRF) of the tibialis anterior (TA) muscle is characterized by a high sensitivity in the medial, distal region, resulting in inversion (Inv) and dorsiflexion (DorFl) of the foot when these sites are activated. Functionally antagonist muscles have RRF that evoke plantarflexion (PlanFl) or eversion (Eve). The RRF is likely shaped by excitatory (Excit) and inhibitory (Inhib) descending control input coming from supraspinal structures (SupCtrl). SupCtrl may act presynaptically (not shown) or postsynaptically on one or more interneurons (In) and/or on reflex encoders (RE) in the NWR pathways modifying their excitability (color-coded similarly to the RRF), adjusting the weight of afferent information from nociceptive input. The net output is translated by α-motoneurons (α-Mn) into efferent signals that evoke a proper contraction in the target muscle(s). **B:** After an injury to the spinal cord, SupCtrl is partially or totally lost, so In that were subjected to tonic inhibitory descending signals increase their excitability as a result of disinhibition and vice versa for excitatory descending pathways. This will result in a reversed topography of RRF maps. (Modified from Biurrun Manresa JA, Finnerup NS, Johannesen IL, Biering-Sorensen F, Jensen TS, Arendt-Nielsen L, Andersen OK. Central sensitization in spinal cord injured humans assessed by reflex receptive fields. Clin Neurophysiol 2014;125:352–62.)

gynecologic laparotomy [22], although further attempts to use the NWR for detecting postoperative spinal hyperexcitability in humans have not been entirely successful. On the other hand, recent studies with patients suffering from different clinical conditions, such as whiplash, fibromyalgia, endometriosis, and acute and chronic musculoskeletal pain, have shown that patients display lower NWR thresholds compared with pain-free volunteers [10,14,23,54]. Temporal summation mechanisms were also altered in patients with significantly lower temporal summation NWR thresholds following repeated

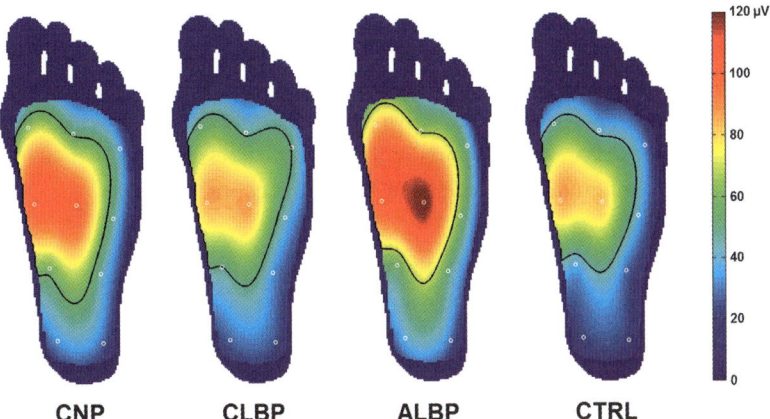

FIGURE 9-3 Grand mean reflex receptive fields (RRF) obtained by averaging the nociceptive withdrawal reflex responses from musculoskeletal pain subjects. CNP, chronic neck pain; CLBP, chronic low-back pain; ALBP, acute low-back pain; CTRL, control. The *white dots* indicate the stimulation sites, the *black line* represents the contour of the RRF area, and the *colors* indicate the reflex amplitude. (Reprinted with permission from Biurrun Manresa JA, Neziri AY, Curatolo M, Arendt-Nielsen L, Andersen OK. Reflex receptive fields are enlarged in patients with musculoskeletal low back and neck pain. Pain 2013;154:1318–24.)

electrical stimulation. Moreover, it was also demonstrated that RRFs are enlarged in acute and chronic musculoskeletal pain patients, as seen in Figure 9-3 [14,54] and in patients with osteoarthritis (preliminary findings, see Figure 9-4).

The fact that the RRF expansion was detected in areas distant from where pain is supposed to originate (i.e., the segment of the putative nociceptive source) indicates a widespread spinal hyperexcitability in these patients [6,76]. This hyperexcitability could be a consequence of increased number of responsive spinal neurons or an expansion of the receptive fields of spinal neurons as a result of increased synaptic sensitivity [20,29].

RRF expansion in patients with musculoskeletal pain as compared with groups of pain-free volunteers [14] holds interesting perspectives for future clinical use. Moreover, the method also allows distinguishing between acute pain patients and chronic pain patients in

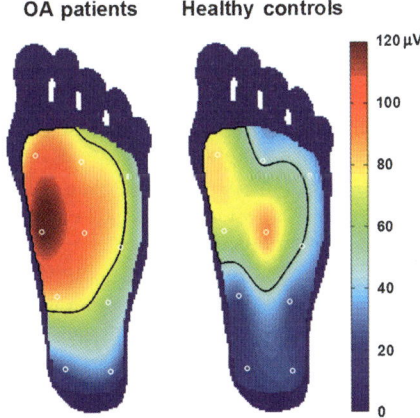

FIGURE 9-4 Grand mean reflex receptive fields (RRF) obtained by averaging the nociceptive withdrawal reflex responses from patients with osteoarthritis (OA) compared with a group of sex- and age-matched healthy volunteers. The *white dots* indicate the stimulation sites, the *black line* represents the contour of the RRF area, and the *colors* indicate the reflex amplitude. Results presented at IASP2016 [12].

some cases, which indicates that it might be possible to perform an early identification of patients at risk of developing chronic pain conditions and follow the effect of proper pain management. More recently, a prediction model based on NWR features was proposed as a new approach for objective assessment of central hyperexcitability in the nociceptive system. This model supports individualized assessment of patients, constituting a first step toward potential applications in daily clinical practice [55].

CONCLUSION AND FUTURE PERSPECTIVES

The NWR is a spinally mediated response that may be used for probing the excitability of the spinal nociceptive system in humans. Outcome measures may include not only reflex threshold and estimates of reflex size to single suprathreshold stimuli but also reflex-based measures of temporal summation involving trains of stimuli. Assessment of RRF areas provides a robust quantification of the excitability of the spinal nociceptive system with minimal subjective bias. Lower threshold and expanded RRFs area have been observed in populations of patients with chronic pain. Future studies should investigate widespread sensitization after surgery and continue to improve the methods for individual assessment that will allow monitoring treatment effects.

REFERENCES

1. Andersen OK. Studies of the organization of the human nociceptive withdrawal reflex. Focus on sensory convergence and stimulation site dependency. Acta Physiol 2007;189(Suppl. 654):1–35.
2. Andersen OK, Finnerup NB, Spaich EG, Jensen TS, Arendt-Nielsen L. Expansion of nociceptive withdrawal reflex receptive fields in spinal cord injured humans. Clin Neurophysiol 2004;115:2798–810.
3. Andersen OK, Gracely RH, Arendt-Nielsen L. Facilitation of the human nociceptive reflex by stimulation of Ab-fibres in a secondary hyperalgesic area sustained by nociceptive input from the primary hyperalgesic area. Acta Physiol Scand 1995;155:87–97.
4. Andersen OK, Sonnenborg FA, Arendt-Nielsen L. Modular organization of human leg withdrawal reflexes elicited by electrical stimulation of the foot sole. Muscle Nerve 1999;22:1520–30.
5. Arendt-Nielsen L, Brennum J, Sindrup S, Bak P. Electrophysiological and psychophysical quantification of temporal summation in the human nociceptive system. Eur J Appl Physiol 1994;68:266–73.
6. Arendt-Nielsen L, Graven-Nielsen T. Muscle pain: sensory implications and interaction with motor control. Clin J Pain 2008;24:291–8.
7. Arendt-Nielsen L, Sonnenborg FA, Andersen OK. Facilitation of the withdrawal reflex by repeated transcutaneous electrical stimulation: an experimental study on central integration in humans. Eur J Appl Physiol 2000;81:165–73.
8. Atkinson G, Nevill AM. Statistical methods for assessing measurement error (reliability) in variables relevant to sports medicine. Sports Med 1998;26:217–38.
9. Bajaj P, Arendt-Nielsen L, Andersen OK. Facilitation and inhibition of withdrawal reflexes following repetitive stimulation: electro- and psychophysiological evidence for activation of noxious inhibitory controls in humans. Eur J Pain 2005;9:25–31.
10. Banic B, Petersen-Felix S, Andersen OK, Radanov BP, Villiger PM, Arendt-Nielsen L, Curatolo M. Evidence for spinal cord hypersensitivity in chronic pain after whiplash injury and in fibromyalgia. Pain 2004;107:7–15.
11. Biurrun Manresa JA, Finnerup NS, Johannesen IL, Biering-Sorensen F, Jensen TS, Arendt-Nielsen L, Andersen OK. Central sensitization in spinal cord injured humans assessed by reflex receptive fields. Clin Neurophysiol 2014;125:352–62.
12. Biurrun Manresa JA, Jensen MB, Petersen KK, Laursen MB, Simonsen O, Arendt-Nielsen L, Andersen OK. Nociceptive reflex receptive fields are enlarged in patients with knee osteoarthritis: preliminary results. In: 16th World Congress on Pain - Yokohama, Japan. 2016. p. PTH025.
13. Biurrun Manresa JA, Neziri AY, Curatolo M, Arendt-Nielsen L, Andersen OK. Test-retest reliability of the nociceptive withdrawal reflex and electrical pain thresholds after single and repeated stimulation in patients with chronic low back pain. Eur J Appl Physiol 2011;111:83–92.

14. Biurrun Manresa JA, Neziri AY, Curatolo M, Arendt-Nielsen L, Andersen OK. Reflex receptive fields are enlarged in patients with musculoskeletal low back and neck pain. Pain 2013;154:1318–24.
15. Bjerre L, Andersen AT, Hagelskjaer MT, Ge N, Morch CD, Andersen OK. Dynamic tuning of human withdrawal reflex receptive fields during cognitive attention and distraction tasks. Eur J Pain 2011;15:816–21.
16. Campbell IG, Carstens E, Watkins LR. Comparisons of human pain sensation and flexion withdrawal evoked by noxious radiant heat. Pain 1991;45:259–68.
17. Carragee EJ, Tanner CM, Khurana S, Hayward C, Welsh J, Date E, Truong T, Rossi M, Hagle C. The rates of false-positive lumbar discography in select patients without low back symptoms. Spine (Phila Pa 1976) 2000;25:1373–80.
18. Chan CWY, Dallaire M. Subjective pain sensation is linearly correlated with the flexion reflex in man. Brain Res 1989;479:145–50.
19. Clarke RW, Harris J. The organization of motor responses to noxious stimuli. Brain Res Brain Res Rev 2004;46:163–72.
20. Cook AJ, Woolf CJ, Wall PD, McMahon SB. Dynamic receptive field plasticity in rat spinal cord dorsal horn following C-primary afferent input. Nature 1987;325:151–53.
21. Curatolo M. Diagnosis of altered central pain processing. Spine (Phila Pa 1976) 2011;36:S200–4.
22. Dahl JB, Erichsen JC, Fuglsang-Frederiksen A, Kehlet H. Pain sensation and nociceptive reflex excitability in surgical patients and human volunteers. Br J Anaesth 1992;69:117–21.
23. Desmeules JA, Cedraschi C, Rapiti E, Baumgartner E, Finckh A, Cohen P, Dayer P, Vischer TL. Neurophysiologic evidence for a central sensitization in patients with fibromyalgia. Arthritis Rheum 2003;48:1420–9.
24. Dietz V. Behavior of spinal neurons deprived of supraspinal input. Nat Rev Neurol 2010;6:167–74.
25. Dietz V, Sinkjaer T. Spastic movement disorder: impaired reflex function and altered muscle mechanics. Lancet Neurol 2007;6:725–33.
26. Dimitrijevic MR, Nathan PW. Studies of spasticity in man. 3. Analysis of reflex activity evoked by noxious cutaneous stimulation. Brain 1968;91:349–68.
27. Dincklage FV, Hackbarth M, Schneider M, Baars JH, Rehberg B. Introduction of a continual RIII reflex threshold tracking algorithm. Brain Res 2009;1260:24–9.
28. Dowman R. Spinal and supraspinal correlates of nociception in man. Pain 1991;45:269–81.
29. Dubner R, Basbaum AI. Spinal dorsal horn plasticity following tissue or nerve injury. In: Melzack R, Wall PD, editors. Textbook of pain. 1994. p. 225–41.
30. Ellrich J, Treede R-D. Convergence of nociceptive and non-nociceptive inputs onto spinal reflex pathways to the tibialis anterior muscle in humans. Acta Physiol Scand 1998;163:391–401.
31. Gozariu M, Bouhassira D, Willer JC, Le Bars D. The influence of temporal summation on a C-fibre reflex in the rat: effects of lesions in the rostral ventromedial medulla (RVM). Brain Res 1998;792:168–72.
32. Grimby L. Normal plantar response: integration of flexor and extensor reflex components. J Neurol Neurosurg Psychiatry 1963;26:39–50.
33. Grimby L. Pathological plantar response: disturbance of the normal integration of flexor and extensor reflex components. J Neurol Neurosurg Psychiatry 1963;26:314–21.
34. Grönross M, Pertovaara A. Capsaicin-induced central facilitation of a nociceptive flexion reflex in humans. Neurosci Lett 1993;159:215–8.
35. Harris J, Clarke RW. Organisation of sensitisation of hind limb withdrawal reflexes from acute noxious stimuli in the rabbit. J Physiol 2003;546:251–65.
36. Heinricher MM, Tavares I, Leith JL, Lumb BM. Descending control of nociception: specificity, recruitment and plasticity. Brain Res Rev 2009;60:214–25.
37. Hiersemenzel LP, Curt A, Dietz V. From spinal shock to spasticity: neuronal adaptations to a spinal cord injury. Neurology 2000;54:1574–82.
38. Hornby TG, Tysseling-Mattiace VM, Benz EN, Schmit BD. Contribution of muscle afferents to prolonged flexion withdrawal reflexes in human spinal cord injury. J Neurophysiol 2004;92(6):3375-84.
39. Hugon M. Exteroceptive reflexes to stimulation of the sural nerve in man. In: Desmedt JE, editor. New developments in electromyography and clinical neurophysiology, vol. 3. Basel: Karger; 1973. p. 713–29.
40. Jensen MB, Manresa JA, Frahm KS, Andersen OK. Analysis of muscle fiber conduction velocity enables reliable detection of surface EMG crosstalk during detection of nociceptive withdrawal reflexes. BMC Neurosci 2013;14:39. doi:10.1186/1471-2202-14-39.
41. Jensen MB, Manresa JB, Andersen OK. A new objective method for acquisition and quantification of reflex receptive fields. Pain 2015;156:555–64.
42. Koceja DM, Bernacki RH, Kamen G. Methodology for the quantitative assessment of human crossed-spinal reflex pathways. Med Biol Eng Comput 1991;29:603–6.

43. Koelbaek JM, Graven-Nielsen T, Schou OA, Arendt-Nielsen L. Generalised muscular hyperalgesia in chronic whiplash syndrome. Pain 1999;83:229–34.
44. Le Bars D, Dickenson AH, Besson JM. Diffuse noxious inhibitory controls (DNIC). I. Effects on dorsal horn convergent neurones in the rat. Pain 1979;6:283–304.
45. Le Bars D, Gozariu M, Cadden SW. Animal models of nociception. Pharmacol Rev 2001;53:597–652.
46. Liebermann DG, Defrin R. Characteristics of the nociceptive withdrawal response elicited under aware and unaware conditions. J Electromyogr Kinesiol 2009;19:e114–22.
47. Mackenzie RA, Burke D, Skuse NF, Lethlean AK. Fibre function and perception during cutaneous nerve block. J Neurol Neurosurg Psychiatry 1975;38:865–73.
48. Magerl W, Ali Z, Ellrich J, Meyer RA, Treede RD. C- and A delta-fiber components of heat-evoked cerebral potentials in healthy human subjects. Pain 1999;82:127–37.
49. Manresa JB, Jensen MB, Andersen OK. Introducing the reflex probability maps in the quantification of nociceptive withdrawal reflex receptive fields in humans. J Electromyogr Kinesiol 2011;21:67–76.
50. Micalos PS, Drinkwater EJ, Cannon J, Arendt-Nielsen L, Marino FE. Reliability of the nociceptive flexor reflex (RIII) threshold and association with pain threshold. Eur J Appl Physiol 2009;105:55–62.
51. Morch CD, Andersen OK, Graven-Nielsen T, Arendt-Nielsen L. Nociceptive withdrawal reflexes evoked by uniform-temperature laser heat stimulation of large skin areas in humans. J Neurosci Methods 2007;160:85–92.
52. Neziri AY, Andersen OK, Petersen-Felix S, Radanov B, Dickenson AH, Scaramozzino P, Arendt-Nielsen L, Curatolo M. The nociceptive withdrawal reflex: normative values of thresholds and reflex receptive fields. Eur J Pain 2010;14:134–41.
53. Neziri AY, Curatolo M, Bergadano A, Petersen-Felix S, Dickenson A, Arendt-Nielsen L, Andersen OK. New method for quantification and statistical analysis of nociceptive reflex receptive fields in humans. J Neurosci Methods 2009;178:24–30.
54. Neziri AY, Haesler S, Petersen-Felix S, Muller M, Arendt-Nielsen L, Manresa JB, Andersen OK, Curatolo M. Generalized expansion of nociceptive reflex receptive fields in chronic pain patients. Pain 2010;151:798–805.
55. Nguyen GP, Biurrun Manresa J, Curatolo M, Moeslund TB, Andersen OK. A prediction model for differentiating chronic pain patients and healthy subjects based on withdrawal reflex EMG signals., Vol. Conference on Neural Engineering (NER). Cancun, Mexico: IEEE Press; 2011. p. 92–5.
56. Ossipov MH, Dussor GO, Porreca F. Central modulation of pain. J Clin Invest 2010;120:3779–87.
57. Petersen-Felix S, Arendt-Nielsen L, Bak P, Fischer M, Bjerring P, Zbinden AM. The effects of isoflurane on repeated nociceptive stimuli (central temporal summation). Pain 1996;64:277–81.
58. Price DD. Characteristics of second pain and flexion reflexes indicative of prolonged central summation. Exp Neurol 1972;37:371–87.
59. Price DD, Staud R, Robinson ME, Mauderli AP, Cannon R, Vierck CJ. Enhanced temporal summation of second pain and its central modulation in fibromyalgia patients. Pain 2002;99:49–59.
60. Rhudy JL, France CR. Defining the nociceptive flexion reflex (NFR) threshold in human participants: a comparison of different scoring criteria. Pain 2007;128:244–53.
61. Rhudy JL, Williams AE, McCabe KM, Nguyen MA, Rambo P. Affective modulation of nociception at spinal and supraspinal levels. Psychophysiology 2005;42:579–87.
62. Ruscheweyh R, Albers C, Kreusch A, Sommer J, Marziniak M. The effect of catastrophizing self-statements on pain perception and the nociceptive flexor reflex (RIII reflex). Clin J Pain 2013;29:725–32.
63. Sandkuhler J. Models and mechanisms of hyperalgesia and allodynia. Physiol Rev 2009;89:707–58.
64. Sandrini G, Serrao M, Rossi P, Romaniello A, Cruccu G, Willer JC. The lower limb flexion reflex in humans. Prog Neurobiol 2005;77:353–95.
65. Schomburg ED. Spinal sensorimotor system and their supraspinal control. Neurosci Res 1990;7:265–340.
66. Schouenborg J. Modular organisation and spinal somatosensory imprinting. Brain Res Rev 2002;40:80–91.
67. Schouenborg J, Dickenson A. Long-lasting activity in rat dorsal horn evoked by impulses in cutaneous C fibres during noxious mechanical stimulation. Brain Res 1988;439:56–63.
68. Schouenborg J, Holmberg H, Weng H-R. Functional organization of the nociceptive withdrawal reflexes. II. Changes of excitability and receptive fields after spinalization in the rat. Exp Brain Res 1992;90:469–78.
69. Schouenborg J, Kalliomäki J. Functional organization of the nociceptive withdrawal reflexes. I. Activation of hindlimb muscles in the rat. Exp Brain Res 1990;83:67–78.
70. Schouenborg J, Kalliomäki J, Weng H-R. Identification of putative reflex interneurones in the nociceptive withdrawal reflex paths. Acta Physiol Scand 1990;140:25A.
71. Schouenborg J, Sjölund BG. Activity evoked by A- and C-afferent fibers in rat dorsal horn neurons and its relation to a flexion reflex. J Neurophysiol 1983;50:1108–21.

72. Serrao M, Rossi P, Sandrini G, Parisi L, Amabile GA, Nappi G, Pierelli F. Effects of diffuse noxious inhibitory controls on temporal summation of the RIII reflex in humans. Pain 2004;112:353–60.
73. Sheather-Reid RB, Cohen ML. Psychophysical evidence for a neuropathic component of chronic neck pain. Pain 1998;75:341–7.
74. Sivilotti LG, Thompson SWN, Woolf CJ. Rate of rise of the cumulative depolarization evoked by repetitive stimulation of small-caliber afferents is a predictor of action potential windup in rat spinal neurons in vitro. J Neurophysiol 1993;69:1621–31.
75. Sonnenborg FA, Andersen OK, Arendt-Nielsen L, Treede R-D. Withdrawal reflex organisation to electrical stimulation of the dorsal foot in humans. Exp Brain Res 2001;136:303–12.
76. Sorensen J, Graven-Nielsen T, Henriksson KG, Bengtsson M, Arendt-Nielsen L. Hyperexcitability in fibromyalgia. J Rheumatol 1998;25:152–5.
77. Staud R, Vierck CJ, Cannon RL, Mauderli AP, Price DD. Abnormal sensitization and temporal summation of second pain (wind-up) in patients with fibromyalgia syndrome. Pain 2001;91:165–75.
78. Terkelsen AJ, Andersen OK, Hansen PO, Jensen TS. Effects of heterotopic- and segmental counter-stimulation on the nociceptive withdrawal reflex in humans. Acta Physiol Scand 2001;172:211–7.
79. Tørring J, Pedersen E, Klemar B. Standardisation of the electrical elicitation of the human flexor reflex. J Neurol Neurosurg Psychiatry 1981;44:129–32.
80. von Dincklage F, Correll C, Schneider MH, Rehberg B, Baars JH. Utility of nociceptive flexion reflex threshold, bispectral index, composite variability index and noxious stimulation response index as measures for nociception during general anaesthesia. Anaesthesia 2012;67:899–905.
81. Wang R, King T, De FM, Guo W, Ossipov MH, Porreca F. Descending facilitation maintains long-term spontaneous neuropathic pain. J Pain 2013;14:845–53.
82. Weng H-R, Schouenborg J. Cutaneous inhibitory receptive fields of withdrawal reflexes in the decerebrate spinal rat. J Physiol 1996;493:253–65.
83. Willer JC. Comparative study of perceived pain and nociceptive flexion reflex in man. Pain 1977;3:69–80.
84. Willer JC. Nociceptive withdrawal reflexes as a tool for pain research in man. In: Desmedt JE, editor. Motor control mechanisms in health and disease. New York: Raven Press; 1983. p. 809–27.
85. Willer JC, Boureau F, Berny J. Nociceptive flexion reflexes elicited by noxious laser radiant heat in man. Pain 1979;7:15–20.
86. Willer JC, Roby A, LeBars D. Psychophysical and electrophysiological approaches to the pain-relieving effects of heterotopic nociceptive stimuli. Brain 1984;107:1095–112.
87. Woolf CJ. Evidence for a central component of post-injury pain hypersensitivity. Nature 1983;306:686–8.
88. Woolf CJ. Central sensitization: implications for the diagnosis and treatment of pain. Pain 2011;152:S2–15.
89. You HJ, Lei J, Sui MY, Huang L, Tan YX, Tjolsen A, Arendt-Nielsen L. Endogenous descending modulation: spatiotemporal effect of dynamic imbalance between descending facilitation and inhibition of nociception. J Physiol 2010;588:4177–88.
90. Zachariae R, Andersen OK, Bjerring P, Jørgensen MM, Arendt-Nielsen L. Effects of an opioid antagonist on pain intensity and withdrawal reflexes during induction of hypnotic analgesia in high- and low-hypnotizable volunteers. Eur J Pain 1998;2:25–34.

CHAPTER 10

Electrophysiologic Techniques to Study the Supraspinal Responses to Nociceptive Input in Humans

André Mouraux

INTRODUCTION

The ongoing electrical activity of the human brain can be sampled noninvasively using an array of electrodes placed against the scalp to measure transient changes in scalp potential (electroencephalography, EEG) or using an array of magnetic sensor coils to measure the transient changes in magnetic fields resulting from that electrical activity (magnetoencephalography, MEG) [90]. This activity can also be sampled invasively using intracerebral electrodes or subdural grids of electrodes implanted for diagnostic and/or therapeutic purpose (local field potentials and electrocorticography).

It is generally accepted that the brain activity recorded using these techniques is mainly the reflection of summated postsynaptic potentials occurring in cortical pyramidal neurons [72]. Sensory, motor, or cognitive events (such as a fast-rising sensory stimulus, a brisk self-paced movement, or a stimulus-triggered cognitive task) can elicit transient changes in this ongoing electrocortical activity [60]. However, only a fraction of these changes actually translates into a measurable signal deflection because the elicited activity must satisfy a number of conditions to be detected [65]. First, it must generate a relatively strong outward electrical field and, therefore, must involve a relatively large population of neurons. Second, the activity elicited within each neuron of the activated population must be synchronous. If unitary activity is dispersed temporally, the resulting electrical or magnetic field will be spread over time, and the related signal deflection will be difficult to measure. Third, the distance between the source of neural activity and the recording sensor must be small.

Whatever the method of sampling this neural activity, the magnitude of the brain potentials or magnetic fields elicited by a given stimulus is often several factors smaller than the magnitude of the background ongoing activity. Therefore, identifying and characterizing event-related brain potentials (ERPs) and magnetic fields relies on signal-processing methods to enhance their signal-to-noise ratio. All of these methods involve repeating the stimulus a given number of times. The recordings are then segmented into epochs, relative to the onset of each stimulus. The simplest and most commonly used procedure consists in averaging all these epochs into a single waveform [65]. The obtained average waveform expresses the average signal as a function of time relative to the onset of the stimulus. The basic assumption underlying this procedure is that the stimulus-evoked activity is *stationary* and, therefore, is unaffected by the averaging procedure because its latency and

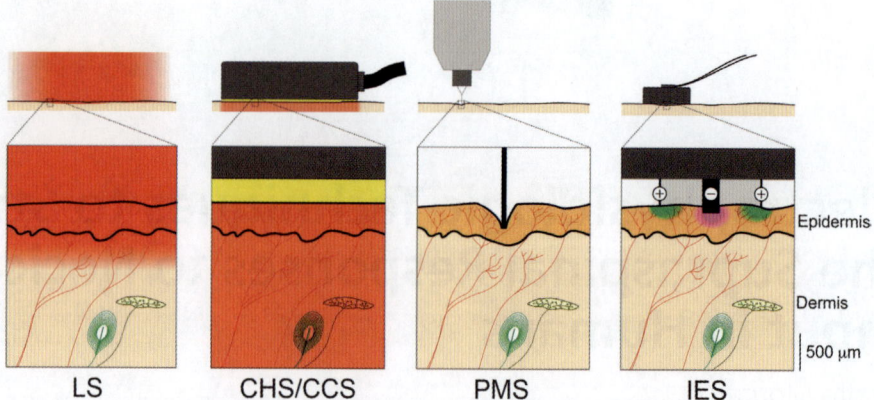

FIGURE 10-1 Infrared laser stimulation (LS) of heat-sensitive nociceptive afferents of the skin is currently the most commonly used method to elicit nociceptive event-related brain potentials (ERPs) in humans. The high energy density of the laser beam allows generating very steep heating ramps, producing a highly synchronous afferent volley well suited to record time-locked responses such as ERPs. Contact heat stimulation (CHS) or contact cold stimulation (CCS) using a thermode applied against the skin has been proposed as a alternative technique to elicit ERPs related to the activation of heat-sensitive (or cold-sensitive) free nerve endings. Punctate mechanical stimulation (PMS) can be used to specifically explore the responses elicited by mechanical nociceptive stimulation. Finally, intraepidermal electrical stimulation (IES) can be used to generate a very focal electric current selectively activating free nerve endings of the epidermis without concurrently activating more deeply located nonnociceptive mechanoreceptors. However, the stimulus will be selective for nociceptive afferents only if low intensities are used.

morphology are invariant across all the repeated epochs. On the contrary, ongoing electrical brain activity, behaving as "noise" unrelated to the event, is largely canceled out by the averaging procedure.

Hence, to record reliably brain potentials or magnetic fields related to the activation of nociceptors requires a method to generate a nociceptive afferent volley that is synchronous, such that it may elicit time-locked and transient brain responses [83,84]. It is for this reason that, in 1976, Carmon et al. [12] introduced the infrared laser as a method to activate skin nociceptors synchronously. The very steep heating ramp produced by the laser is able to activate a population of nociceptors within a few milliseconds, thus generating a highly synchronous and time-locked nociceptive afferent volley (Figure 10-1) [83]. Furthermore, because the method does not require any contact with the skin, it ascertains that the elicited brain responses are triggered by the activation of thermosensitive nociceptive afferents (and not, for example, by the concomitant activation of nonnociceptive low-threshold mechanoreceptors). Although infrared lasers are currently the most widely used technique to elicit thermonociceptive ERPs and magnetic fields, other techniques have been developed, especially in the recent years (Figure 10-2).

For example, thermal stimuli can be delivered using a thermode applied against the skin, and recently, contact thermodes able to achieve temperature rises of up to 70°C/s generate a nociceptive afferent volley that is sufficiently synchronous to elicit measurable ERPs or magnetic fields [1,32]. However, these temperature slopes are still considerably lower than those achieved by laser stimulators (e.g., >1000°C/s) [4,5]. Hence, interpretation of the obtained responses is undermined by the relatively lower signal-to-noise ratio of the elicited brain responses and the need to take into consideration the time required to bring skin temperature above thermal activation threshold when assessing the latency of the elicited responses. An alternative and potentially promising use of these contact stimulators could

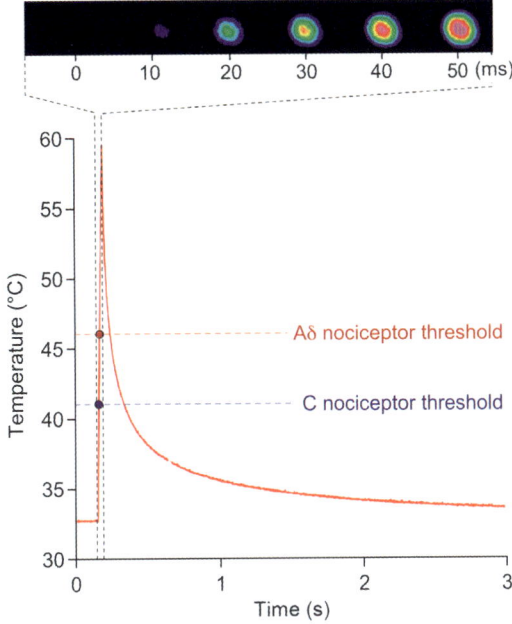

FIGURE 10-2 Skin temperature profile following the delivery of a short-lasting (50 ms) pulse of radiant heat generated by an infrared laser stimulator. The high energy density of the laser beam allows generating a very steep heating ramp, quasisimultaneously activating heat-sensitive C- and Aδ-fiber afferents. The upper inset shows six consecutive images obtained using an infrared camera. The color scale represents skin temperature from black (baseline skin temperature) to purple (maximum target skin temperature).

be the recording of brain responses related to the selective activation of cool-sensitive fibers [5,38]. Indeed, novel stimulators based on micro Peltier elements able to achieve very steep cooling ramps of up to 300°C/s have been developed, making it possible to record reliable cool-evoked potentials with a high signal-to-noise ratio (Figure 10-3), related to the activation of cool-sensitive Aδ fibers.

Another alternative method to elicit ERPs or magnetic fields related to the selective activation of nociceptors is intraepidermal electrical stimulation (IES) [44,50,68]. The technique relies on the fact that a dense network of nociceptive free nerve endings is located in the epidermis, whereas nonnociceptive mechanoreceptors are mainly located more deeply in the dermis. Like cool stimulation, IES could circumvent some limitations of laser stimulation, such as skin overheating and lesion due to stimulus repetition. Furthermore, IES bypasses the transduction of the sensory stimulus into a neural impulse, and this could improve the relative synchronization of the nociceptive afferent volley [64]. However, IES suffers from its own limitations, in particular, the need to use low stimulation intensities to guarantee its selectivity for nociceptors. Indeed, it has been shown that if IES is delivered using a strong intensity (e.g., an intensity corresponding to the pain threshold), the stimulus is not selective for nociceptors because it also activates more deeply located low-threshold mechanoreceptors [78]. The important drawback is that, at such low intensities, a single electrical stimulus elicits a very weak sensation and the signal-to-noise ratio of the elicited ERPs is low, possibly because of the very small number of recruited afferents [54]. To circumvent the lack of spatial summation, some authors have proposed to deliver short trains of stimuli (e.g., three pulses delivered at a 5-ms interstimulus interval) [45,50] or to use multiple electrodes with the aim of increasing the strength of the nociceptive afferent volley

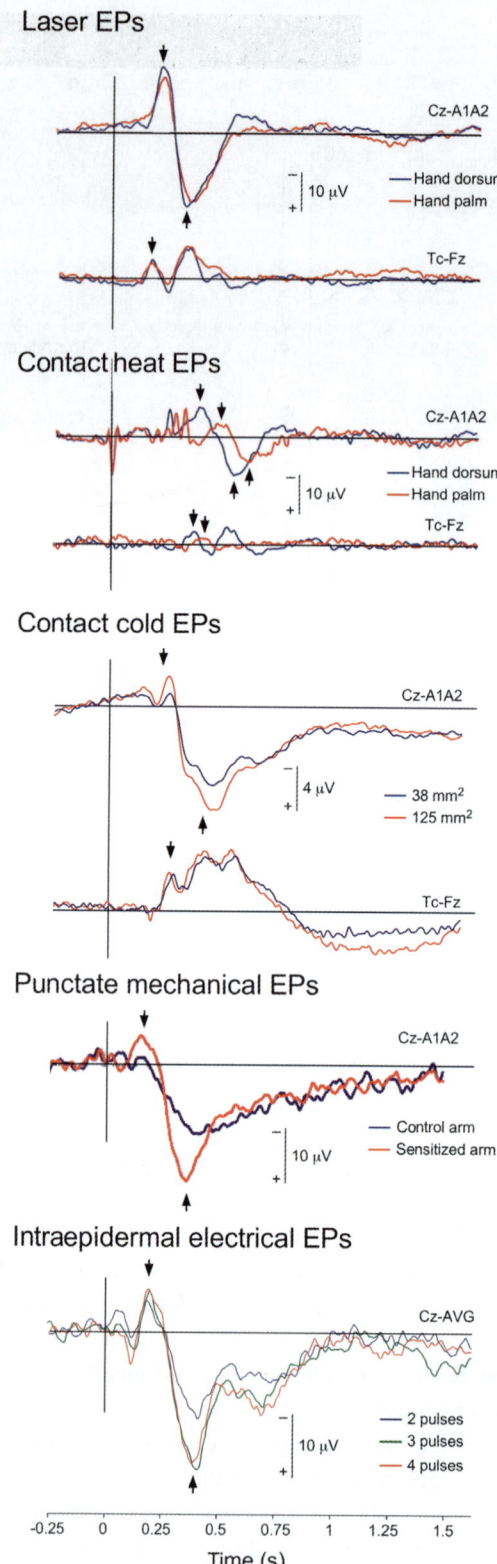

FIGURE 10-3 Nociceptive event-related potentials (EVPs) elicited by laser stimulation (Nd:YAP), contact heat and cold stimulation, punctate mechanical stimulation, and intraepidermal electrical stimulation. Group-level average waveforms of the signals recorded at the scalp vertex (electrode Cz) and/or the contralateral temporal region (electrode Tc reference to electrode Fz) of the hand

through temporal summation. However, repetition of the electrical pulse could activate some additional (nonnociceptive) fibers brought to a subthreshold potential by the preceding pulses.

Finally, it was recently shown that mechanical pinprick stimuli delivered using a thin (e.g., 0.25 mm diameter) flat-tip probe could be used to elicit ERPs related to the activation of mechanosensitive nociceptors [39,107,108]. Interestingly, these studies also showed that, after the experimental induction of secondary mechanical hyperalgesia, the magnitude of pinprick-evoked brain potentials is significantly enhanced, suggesting that these could be used as a clinical tool to assess the presence of central sensitization in patients with chronic pain.

Here, we will focus on the human electrophysiologic brain responses that can be elicited using laser stimulation. In the vast majority of studies, the thermal laser stimuli used to elicit ERPs or magnetic fields activate Aδ and C nociceptors concomitantly, thus eliciting both a sensation of first pain and a sensation of second pain [56,75,84,101]. Only a few studies have focused on the event-related brain responses elicited by stimuli activating C nociceptors selectively [46,82]. Because myelinated Aδ fibers and unmyelinated C fibers have very different conduction velocities [75,82,101], if the thermal stimulus activates both classes of nociceptors quasisimultaneously, it may be expected to generate two distinct nociceptive afferent volleys that will reach their cortical targets at very different latencies, in particular, if the stimulus is applied to the distal part of a body extremity. For example, if a laser stimulus is applied to the dorsum of the hand, the time required to reach the cortex may be expected to be lower than 200 ms for the nociceptive afferent volley conveyed by Aδ fibers and greater than 600 ms for the nociceptive afferent volley conveyed by C fibers. Hence, because electrophysiologic techniques sample brain activity with a temporal resolution lying in the range of milliseconds, it is clearly possible to determine whether the latencies of the elicited responses are compatible with the conduction velocity of Aδ fibers (e.g., latency <650 ms when stimulating the hand dorsum) or with the conduction velocity of C fibers (e.g., latency >650 ms when stimulating the hand dorsum) [14]. However, laser stimuli concomitantly activating Aδ and C fibers elicit ERPs whose latencies are compatible with the conduction velocity of Aδ fibers but do not elicit ERPs whose latencies are compatible with the conduction velocity of C fibers [30]. The responses consists of a large negative–positive complex, maximal at the scalp vertex, whose latency, when stimulating

---

of human volunteers. Note that all waveforms are characterized by a large negative–positive response maximal at the scalp vertex, preceded by a smaller and lateralized negative peak, here visualized at the contralateral temporal electrode (*black arrows*). Also note the important differences in the latency of the responses elicited by the different types of stimuli. These differences can be explained by differences in transduction times. The laser-evoked brain potentials (LEPs) were obtained using an Nd:YAP laser, which penetrates deep in the skin. For this reason, the responses elicited by stimulation of the hand palm and hand dorsum are highly similar [43]. Contact heat ERPs [43] and cold ERPs (unpublished data) can be elicited by a thermode applied against the skin. Note that the contact heat ERPs have a greater latency than LEPs, explained by the longer time required for the relatively slow heating ramps to reach activation threshold. In contrast, the contact cold ERPs have relatively short latency because of the fact that the cold stimulus was delivered using a very steep cooling ramp (200°C/s) and the fact that cool-sensitive afferents respond to very small step decreases of skin temperature. The ERPs elicited by punctate mechanical stimulation were obtained before and after inducing secondary mechanical hyperalgesia using high-frequency electrical stimulation of the skin. Note their clear enhancement after inducing central sensitization [107]. Finally, the ERPs elicited by intraepidermal electrical stimulation [64] have a shorter latency than heat and mechanical ERPs. This can be explained by the fact that direct electrical stimulation bypasses transduction.

the hand dorsum, is approximately 240 (negative wave) and 400 ms (positive wave). In summary, although the stimulus elicits a clear double percept related to the coactivation of Aδ and C nociceptors, the electrophysiologic correlates of the cortical processing of the thermal stimulus, as reflected by laser-evoked brain potentials (LEPs), only include brain responses compatible with the conduction velocity of Aδ fibers.

Furthermore, given the fact that ERPs and magnetic fields reflect only brain responses that are triggered by a very phasic sensory afferent volley, it is generally accepted that LEPs reflect only the activity triggered by nociceptors exhibiting very phasic responses to thermal stimulation. Treede et al. [101] showed that mechanosensitive and heat-sensitive Aδ-fiber (AMH) nociceptors can be subdivided into two relatively distinct populations: type I AMH nociceptors displaying a tonic response to heat consisting in a slow increase of activity peaking only several seconds after stimulus onset and type II AMH nociceptors displaying a very phasic response to heat consisting in a strong but very transient response almost synchronous with stimulus onset. For this reason, it is often considered that LEPs and laser-evoked magnetic fields mainly reflect the activation of type II AMH nociceptors.

LASER-EVOKED BRAIN POTENTIALS (LEPS)

Because EEG is a widely available and noninvasive technique, most studies have relied on this technique to study the electrical brain activity elicited by the thermal activation of nociceptors using lasers.

LEPs Elicited by the Coactivation of Aδ and C Nociceptors

Brief thermal stimuli applied to the skin elicit a large negative–positive potential referred to as the N2 and P2 waves or N2–P2 complex [11] (Figure 10-3). Given their large amplitude, the N2 and P2 waves are often visible in single trials and can be identified and characterized reliably using only a few repeated stimuli (typically, 20-30 stimuli) [18]. The scalp topographies of both the N2 and P2 waves are maximal at the vertex and are largely independent of the location of the stimulus [31]. The N2 and P2 waves are preceded by an earlier negative deflection, often referred to as the N1 wave [37,99,100,102]. At the scalp vertex, the N1 wave often appears embedded in the ascending shoulder of the N2 wave and is thus difficult to isolate. The scalp topography of the N1 wave is clearly lateralized, appearing maximal over central and temporal regions contralateral to the stimulated side. Several studies have suggested that the scalp topography of the N1 wave may be further dependent on the stimulation site [102,114]. They described a contralateral central or temporal topography when stimulating the hand and a more medial scalp topography when stimulating the foot, thus suggesting a somatotopic organization of the neuronal populations contributing to the N1 wave. However, it should be noted that several studies examining LEPs elicited by the stimulation of different body districts have failed to identify such a somatotopic shift of the N1 wave scalp topography [94,96,104].

The latency of the N1, N2, and P2 waves of LEPs is largely dependent on the peripheral conductance distance and is compatible with the conduction velocity of Aδ fibers and incompatible with the conduction velocity of C fibers. Several studies have attempted to estimate the conduction velocity of the spinothalamic tracts conveying the afferent volley leading to LEPs. For example, by comparing the latencies of LEPs elicited by stimuli applied to the skin overlying vertebral spinous processes at various levels (such as to minimize peripheral conduction distance), Cruccu et al. [19] estimated that the conduction velocity of the spinothalamic tracts generating the P2 wave was 11.2 m/s. Using the same method, Valeriani et al. [103] proposed that the conduction velocity of the spinothalamic tracts generating the N1 wave was significantly slower (9 m/s) than the conduction velocity of the spinothalamic tracts generating the later P2 wave (13 m/s), and concluded that both waves reflect nociceptive input conveyed within distinct spinothalamic pathways.

A number of studies have applied source analysis methods to LEPs [31]. Most of these studies have used methods based on the optimization of a fixed spatiotemporal dipole (e.g., [96]). Other studies have used distributed source models, which consist in the reconstruction of the brain electrical activity in each point of a three-dimensional mesh (e.g., [102]). Albeit some exceptions [7,41], most of these studies have suggested that bilateral opercular regions contribute largely to the obtained waveforms. These opercular sources have been hypothesized to reflect neural activity originating from the secondary somatosensory cortex (SII) and, possibly, from the deeper insular cortex [31]. Most studies have identified the contralateral opercular response as the earliest response following laser stimulation, coinciding with the latency of the N1 wave. However, the suggested time courses of opercular activity suggest that they also contribute to the later N2 and P2 waves. In addition to bilateral opercular sources, source analysis studies have repeatedly proposed that LEPs also reflect activity originating from the anterior cingulate cortex, in particular, the midportion corresponding to Brodmann area 24 [31]. In most cases, the latency of this additional source of activity suggests that it contributes mostly to the later N2 and P2 waves. Whether or not the primary somatosensory cortex contributes to the LEP waveform remains a matter of debate. Most source analysis studies have shown that the bulk of the LEPs can be satisfactorily explained without assigning sources in the contralateral primary somatosensory cortex. However, recent studies have provided evidence that the contralateral primary somatosensory cortex does contribute significantly to the early N1 wave [102].

LEPs Elicited by the Selective Activation of C Nociceptors

A number of studies have examined the LEPs elicited by selectively activating C nociceptors, by using various methods to avoid the concomitant activation of Aδ nociceptors, or by blocking the transmission of Aδ-fiber input at peripheral level [82].

The first method takes advantage of the fact that unmyelinated C fibers are more resistant to focal nerve compression than myelinated nerve fibers, including small-diameter Aδ fibers [10]. Using this differential property, several studies have applied pressure to the superficial branch of the radial nerve to induce a selective blockade of myelinated nerve fibers. These studies have shown that after a various delay (usually, 30 to 60 min), brief laser stimuli above the threshold of both Aδ and C nociceptors applied to the skin innervated by the nerve no longer elicit a sensation of first pain but still elicit a sensation of second pain. Furthermore, the Aδ-fiber–related LEPs disappear, and most interestingly, ultralate LEPs appear within a latency range compatible with the conduction of C fibers, i.e., approximately 1 second after stimulus onset [10,71].

The second method takes advantage of the difference in thermal activation threshold between heat-sensitive Aδ-fiber and C-fiber receptors [34,61]. The thermal activation threshold of AMH type II nociceptors, which are thought to underlie LEPs related to the activation of Aδ nociceptors, lies in the range of 46°C. In comparison, heat-sensitive C-fiber mechanoheat nociceptors are thought to have a significantly lower thermal activation threshold, lying in the range of 41°C [101]. Furthermore, C warm receptors can respond to increases in skin temperatures of less than 1°C above baseline skin temperature [51]. Exploiting these differences, Magerl et al. [61] devised an ingenious protocol based on a feedback-controlled CO_2 laser stimulator. At a base temperature of about 33°C, the skin was exposed to two successive heat ramps at 5-second interval. A first heat ramp of 50°C/s lasting 150 ms brought the skin temperature to 40°C, allowing the activation of heat-sensitive C nociceptors. Skin temperature was kept constant at 40°C for an additional 5 seconds, and then, the skin was briefly exposed to a second heat ramp bringing skin temperature to 48°C, allowing this time the activation of Aδ nociceptors. The first heat ramp elicited an ultralate LEP whose latency was compatible with the conduction velocity of C fibers, whereas the second heat ramp elicited a response with a shorter latency, compatible with the conduction velocity of Aδ fibers. Using a similar approach, it was recently shown that the use of temperature-controlled CO_2 laser stimuli can be used to activate C-fiber afferents in a selective fashion and, most importantly, can be used to obtain reliable C-fiber LEPs [46].

The third method takes advantage of the fact that specific pathologies can lead to a selective impairment of myelinated nerve fibers. For example, Lankers et al. [52] observed ultralate LEPs in a patient with hereditary motor and sensory neuropathy type I, indicating the preservation of unmyelinated C-fiber function. Similar anecdotal observations have been made in peripheral neuropathies characterized by a selective loss of Aδ-fiber function (e.g., [13,113]).

Finally, one can exploit the fact that, in the skin, the density of C-fiber free nerve endings is greater than the density of Aδ-fiber free nerve endings. Depending on the species and methods for quantification, the density distribution of C-fiber free nerve endings is about 2 to $8/mm^2$, whereas the density distribution of Aδ-fiber free nerve endings is thought to be $<1/mm^2$ [73,92]. Therefore, if a laser stimulus is applied using a very small stimulus surface area (e.g., $0.15~mm^2$) [9], there is a high probability that the beam will heat C-fiber free nerve endings without concomitantly heating Aδ-fiber free nerve endings. As compared with other methods, the approach has the advantage of not being invasive and not requiring to lower the energy density of the stimulus. Several studies [9,21,22,74–76,88,112] have successfully used this approach to record ultralate LEPs. Very recently, it was suggested that, using laser stimuli of varying beam diameters, the technique could actually be used to assess intraepidermal nerve fiber density noninvasively [69].

Whatever the method used, all of these studies confirmed that when the activation of Aδ-fiber nociceptors is avoided, or when the peripheral Aδ-fiber afferent volley is blocked at peripheral level, the selective activation of C fibers elicits an ultralate negative–positive complex whose latency (750 to 1150 ms after stimulation of the hand) is compatible with the conduction velocity of unmyelinated C fibers. The morphology and scalp topography of these ultralate responses very much resemble the morphology and scalp topography of LEPs elicited by Aδ fibers. The most prominent component of the response also consists of a negative–positive complex, maximal at the vertex, and often referred to as ultralate N2–P2 [82]. Valeriani et al. [105] reported that, in addition to eliciting ultralate N2 and P2 components, the selective activation of C nociceptors could also elicit an earlier negative component, labeled ultralate N1. This ultralate N1 would be similar to the N1 component preceding the Aδ-fiber N2–P2 complex. Indeed, like the Aδ-related N1, the C-fiber–related N1 was described as a peak displaying a lateralized scalp topography, maximal over the temporal region contralateral to the stimulated side.

A small number of studies [20,42,77] have applied source analysis methods to C-fiber LEPs. Like Aδ-fiber LEPs, C-fiber LEPs are best explained by sources originating from bilateral opercular structures, as well as the anterior cingulate cortex [31]. Hence, it would appear that Aδ- and C-fiber afferent volleys elicit brain responses within the same structures.

LASER-EVOKED MAGNETIC FIELDS

The brain responses elicited by thermal stimulation of the skin have also been studied using MEG [111]. Comparing laser-evoked brain responses recorded using EEG with those recorded using MEG could be interesting, as the information recorded by both techniques may be complementary [35]. Deep sources of electrocortical activity are thought to contribute very little to MEG signals, whereas superficial sources could be more accurately and more reliably captured using MEG. In addition, it is often stated that EEG signals mainly reflects sources of electrocortical activity that are radial relative to the scalp surface, whereas MEG signals mainly reflects sources of electrocortical activity that are tangential relative to the scalp surface. Finally, it has also been suggested that MEG recordings are more spatially accurate than EEG recordings because EEG recordings are blurred and distorted by the interposed layers [35]. However, it is important to highlight that these assertions have been questioned by several researchers [3,62,63].

Laser-Evoked Magnetic Fields Elicited by the Coactivation of Aδ and C Nociceptors

Supporting the view that EEG and MEG provide information that is not redundant is the fact that the scalp topography and time course of laser-evoked magnetic fields are not identical to the scalp topography and time course of LEPs. Indeed, laser-evoked magnetic fields mainly consist of an early response peaking at 150 ms when stimulating the hand dorsum and 200 ms when stimulating the foot dorsum [47], whose latency is similar to the laser-evoked N1 wave identified using EEG. In other words, it seems that MEG is very sensitive to the electrocortical activity reflected in the N1 wave of LEPs (and possibly other sources contributing at that latency) but is not very sensitive to the electrocortical activity reflected in the later N2 and P2 waves of LEPs.

A likely explanation as to why MEG does not capture the later cortical activity that is evident in LEPs is that the recording technique is unable to capture activity originating from the cingulate cortex. Supporting this view, unlike source analyses of LEPs, source analyses of laser evoked magnetic fields have mostly failed to reveal responses originating from the cingulate cortex [47,49,111,115]. This could be due to the predominantly radial orientation of this source of activity [31] and/or to its deep location. A notable exception is constituted by the findings of Ploner et al. and Forss et al. [21,86], which did identify laser-evoked cingulate activity using MEG. However, the robustness of this claim is questioned by the fact that Forss et al. identified it in only 3/10 subjects and the fact that the latency of the cingulate response identified by Ploner et al. was unexpected when considering what is usually identified using EEG.

Although MEG studies have failed to consistently identify sources of activity originating from the anterior cingulate cortex, they have shown convincingly that laser stimuli can elicit electrocortical activity originating from the contralateral primary somatosensory cortex [21,49,85,89,97]. Interestingly, in most of these studies, the latency of the activity hypothesized to originate from the contralateral primary somatosensory cortex was concomitant or even slightly delayed as compared with the latency of the activity hypothesized to originate from the SII.

Laser-Evoked Magnetic Fields Elicited by the Selective Activation of C Nociceptors

A small number of studies have examined the MEG response elicited by the selective activation of C nociceptors [21,48,87,98]. The elicited responses were hypothesized to reflect the bilateral activation of opercular regions. Furthermore, with the exception of the study by Forss et al. [21], all these studies included a dipole whose location was compatible with activity originating from the contralateral primary somatosensory cortex. Therefore, the sources contributing to these C-fiber responses appear to be very similar to the sources contributing to the Aδ-fiber responses.

INTRACRANIAL RECORDINGS OF LEPS

Several studies have examined whether noxious thermal stimuli applied to the skin elicit responses within different areas of the brain of awake humans, using surgically implanted intracranial electrodes or subdural electrode grids [79]. In all of these studies, laser stimulators were used to generate very brief stimuli above the thermal activation threshold of both C and Aδ nociceptors.

Intracranial recordings of laser-evoked brain responses have demonstrated that brief thermal stimuli elicit responses that can be recorded in the suprasylvian region. Using a subdural grid, Lenz et al. [55] recorded responses to laser stimuli and described a negative–positive wave that was maximal over the inferior aspect of the central sulcus and appeared to be generated in the vicinity of the suprasylvian opercular region, possibly, the insula or the deep vertical surface of the parietal operculum. The latency of the response coincided with the latency of the N1 and N2 waves of LEPs recorded using scalp EEG. Frot et al. [26,27,29] also identified activity within the suprasylvian opercular region and the insula. Interestingly, they observed an average delay of 50 ms between the responses recorded in the suprasylvian cortex and the responses recorded in the insula, suggesting either sequential activation of the suprasylvian cortex then of the insula or parallel activation of the two structures through distinct pathways with different conduction times. Using subdural grids, Vogel et al. [110] modeled the distribution of the elicited potentials and suggested that the somatotopic organization of the responses elicited by thermal stimulation was different from the somatotopic organization of the responses elicited by innocuous tactile stimulation. This led him to conclude that nociceptive and nonnociceptive somatosensory inputs are processed by distinct populations of operculoinsular neurons. However, Frot et al. [23] did not find any significant difference between the spatial distribution of suprasylvian responses to nociceptive (laser) and nonnociceptive (electrical) stimulation of the upper limb.

Attempts have also been made to identify responses to thermal stimulation in the primary somatosensory cortex contralateral to the stimulated side. Using subdural grids, Kanda et al. [49] found that laser stimuli do elicit activity in the contralateral primary somatosensory cortex. However, contrary to the responses elicited by the electrical stimulation of large-diameter Aβ fibers, the polarity of the identified response did not invert its phase across the central sulcus. This observation suggests that the elicited response was not generated in area 3b (tangential to the sulcus) but, instead, in cortex largely radial to the subdural surface, for example, in areas 3a or 1. Similar observations were recently reported by Baumgartner et al. [6] and Frot et al. [25].

In summary, intracerebral recordings have shown that nociceptive thermal laser stimuli elicit activity in bilateral operculoinsular regions, and, most probably, in the contralateral primary somatosensory cortex. Several studies have attempted to record LEPs in other regions of the awake human brain. Liu et al. [59] showed that laser stimuli could elicit consistent bilateral responses in the amygdala. Valeriani et al. [106] were unable to identify any clear response from deep intracerebral electrodes located around the thalamus. Using subdural grids, Lenz et al. [55] obtained reproducible biphasic responses in the midportion of the anterior cingulate in three epileptic patients when stimulating the face, at a location compatible with Brodmann area 24. However, for an unexplained reason, they failed to elicit similar responses when stimulating the upper limb. Frot et al. [28] reported that laser stimulation of the upper limb elicits consistent responses in the posterior midcingulate cortex.

The latency of all these intracranial responses is only compatible with the conduction velocity of Aδ fibers [2], as they are too early to be possibly conveyed by unmyelinated C fibers. However, most of these studies have restricted the time window of their analysis in such a way that it did not include latencies compatible with the conduction velocity of C fibers. Therefore, whether or not the concomitant activation of C fibers by the laser stimulus also elicits activity that can be captured using these intracranial electrodes or subdural electrode grids remains unknown.

Frot et al. [24] found that increasing stimulus intensity enhances the magnitude of both the SII and the insular responses. They concluded that the dynamics of the changes in response magnitude were different: SII responses encoded gradually the intensity of stimuli and tended to show a ceiling effect for higher intensities. In contrast, the insula did not respond reliably to low-intensity laser pulses but clearly encoded high stimulus intensities, without showing a similar ceiling effect. However, it remains to be determined whether the magnitude of these responses is univocally related to the physical intensity of the stimulus or to the perceptual or contextual appraisal of the stimulus, e.g., its ability to capture attention. Furthermore, it is not known whether various experimental manipulations known to modulate the magnitude of LEPs recorded from the scalp also modulate these responses in a similar fashion, which would constitute an important argument in favor of the claim that these responses contribute significantly to LEPs measured from the scalp.

CLINICAL RELEVANCE

These different methods to sample the electrical brain activity elicited by the selective phasic activation of skin nociceptors offer exciting opportunities for researchers and clinicians: They provide a mean to study where, when, and how nociceptive input is processed in the human brain and how this processing may lead to the perception of pain. However, several important points should be considered when interpreting the functional significance of these responses.

The elicited cortical responses probably reflect only a fraction of the brain activity generated by the nociceptive input.

Because of the variability of the time required for heat conduction and transduction into a neural impulse, the nociceptive afferent volley generated by laser stimulation is probably not as synchronous as, for example, the nonnociceptive afferent volley triggered by the direct electrical activation of Aβ fibers (transcutaneous electrical activation). Furthermore, the target of the laser stimulus must be displaced from trial to trial, and only a relatively small number of stimuli can be applied within a single experimental session to avoid skin overheating, nociceptor habituation, and/or nociceptor sensitization. Therefore, laser-evoked brain responses are usually obtained in conditions that are far from optimal to identify signals that are very transient and/or of very small amplitude.

The magnitude of the elicited brain responses is often correlated with the energy of the eliciting stimulus or with the intensity of the elicited percept. For this reason, investigators often conclude that these responses reflect brain processes related directly to the encoding of pain intensity. However, several studies have shown that this relationship may be disrupted, for example, by stimulus repetition at a short and constant interstimulus interval [66]. In fact, there is a growing amount of evidence indicating that the magnitude of the elicited brain responses may be more related to the saliency of the eliciting stimulus, i.e., its ability to capture attention rather than the intensity of pain perception per se [40,53].

The selectivity of the eliciting stimulus does not preclude the selectivity of the elicited brain responses. There is increasing evidence that LEPs reflect cortical activity that is, in fact, largely unspecific for nociception [40,53]. Indeed, similar brain responses can also be triggered by nonnociceptive visual, auditory, or tactile stimuli provided that they are salient enough to capture attention [57,66], even for intracerebral signals recorded directly from the insula [58]. Importantly, the fact that these responses may reflect cortical processes that are unspecific for nociception does not invalidate its use as a clinical tool to assess the function of nociceptive pathways. Given that the laser stimulus activates nociceptive afferents selectively, the elicited brain responses are still dependent on the state of the nociceptive pathways conveying that input to the brain.

FUTURE PERSPECTIVES

Stimulus-Induced Changes in Ongoing Oscillatory Activity

It is known since the first EEG recordings described by Hans Berger in 1929 [8] that various events, such as closing the eyes, can induce a transient modulation of the magnitude of ongoing EEG rhythms within different frequency bands. These modulations may appear either as a transient increase (event-related synchronization, ERS) or as a transient decrease (event-related desynchronization, ERD) of power, usually confined within a specific frequency band. It is generally considered that the functional significance of ERD and ERS differs according to the affected frequency band. ERS in the alpha frequency band (8 to 12 Hz) is often hypothesized to reflect cortical deactivation, or inhibition [80], whereas ERD in the same frequency band is hypothesized to reflect cortical activation, or disinhibition. These hypotheses rely on experimental results showing, for example, that the power of alpha band rhythms is enhanced over the hand area during visual processing, or during foot movements [81]. In contrast, ERS in the gamma frequency band (25 to 100 Hz) is thought to play an important role for synchronizing cortical processes occurring within and possibly between different brain areas to integrate different features of sensory inputs into a coherent percept [91,93,95]. Assessing ERS and ERD relies on time–frequency decomposition methods to estimate the average amplitude of ongoing oscillations as a function of time and frequency. Because these approaches can disclose an important fraction of the cortical activity to nociceptive stimulation that is lost by conventional time-domain averaging, it may provide a more complete view of how nociceptive input is processed in the human brain.

Recently, using EEG and MEG, it has been reported that nociceptive stimuli elicit such an enhancement of gamma-band oscillations, possibly originating from primary somatosensory cortices [33]. Most interestingly, the magnitude of these responses has been suggested to correlate with the intensity of the elicited pain perception, and for this reason, it has been suggested that they may reflect cortical activity related *directly* to the subjective perception of pain [33,116].

However, one important difficulty in assessing gamma-band oscillations is the possible contamination of the recorded signals by high-frequency muscular and ocular activity, some of which may be stimulus-evoked and, hence, be mistaken for stimulus-evoked gamma activity.

Nociceptive Steady-State Evoked Potentials

In 1966, Regan described the recording of steady-state evoked potentials (SS-EPs) as an alternative approach to characterize stimulus-evoked activity in the ongoing EEG [90]. Unlike conventional transient ERPs, which reflect a phasic cortical response triggered by the occurrence of a brief stimulus (described by Regan as "the response to a kick in the system"), SS-EPs reflect a sustained cortical response induced by the long-lasting periodic repetition of a sensory stimulus (described by Regan as "the response to a gentle shake of the system at a fixed repetition rate"). These steady-state responses remain constant in amplitude and phase over time and are thought to result from an entrainment or resonance of a population of neurons responding to the stimulus at the frequency of stimulation [36,70,109]. Whereas transient ERPs are identified in the time domain as a series of time-locked deflections following the onset of the stimulus, SS-EPs are identified in the frequency domain as peaks appearing at the frequency of the repeated stimulus and/or at harmonics of that frequency.

As compared with methods based on the recording of transient ERPs, but also as compared with other noninvasive methods to sample brain activity in humans such as functional MRI, investigating brain function using SS-EPs offers several advantages. SS-EPs (1) exhibit a particularly high signal-to-noise ratio, (2) reflect neural activity originating mainly from modality-specific sensory cortices, (3) are less contaminated by cortical activity related to stimulus-triggered attentional reorientation, and, most importantly, (4) allow isolating neural activity related specifically to each stream of several, concurrently applied streams of sensory stimuli (reviewed in Ref. [17]).

For these reasons, an increasing number of studies have used this approach successfully to explore the neural activity involved in the cortical processing of sensory modalities, in particular, the visual and auditory. In a series of studies, it was shown that it is possible to record SS-EPs in response to the rapid periodic thermal activation of cutaneous nociceptors in humans by laser stimulation [67] as well as IES [15]. The scalp topography of these nociceptive somatosensory SS-EPs was maximal at the scalp vertex and symmetrically

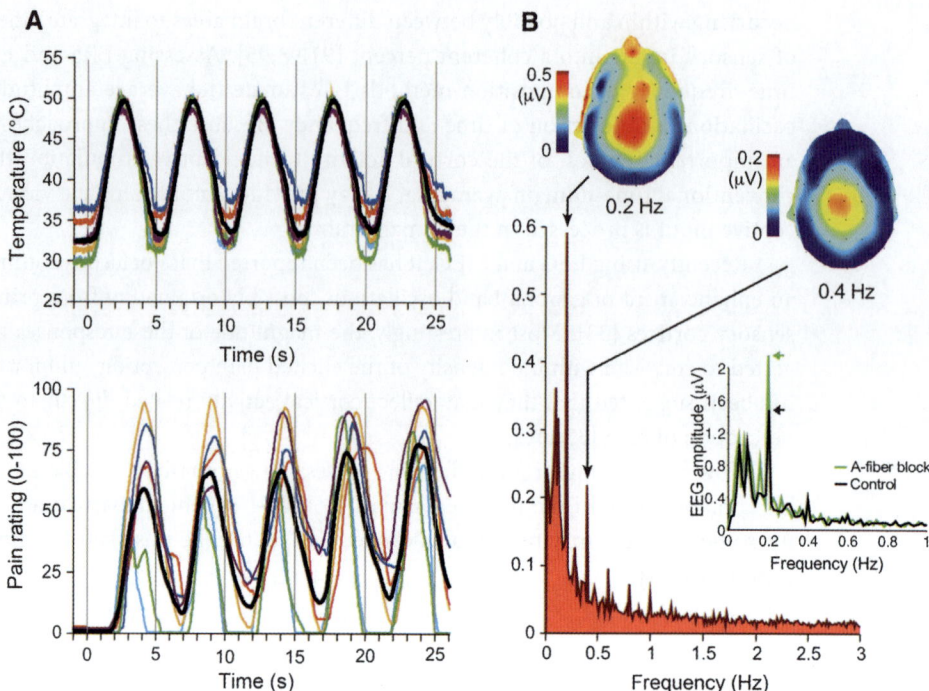

FIGURE 10-4 Nociceptive steady-state evoked potentials (SS-EPs) elicited by periodic sinusoidal heating of the skin at a very low frequency (0.2 Hz). **A:** A temperature-controlled CO_2 laser stimulator was used to slowly oscillate the skin of the hand dorsum between baseline and 50°C, during 75 s. The stimulus generated a sustained oscillating perception of burning pain. The colored waveforms correspond to the across-trial average temperature and pain ratings obtained in each participant. The thick dark waveform corresponds to the group-level average. **B:** The periodic stimulus elicits a clear increase of EEG signal at 0.2 Hz and its harmonics, maximal at the scalp vertex and symmetrically distributed over the two hemispheres. Importantly, this SS-EP was not affected by an A-fiber block, indicating that the elicited brain activity is predominantly related to the activation of C fibers. (Adapted from Colon E, Liberati G, Mouraux A. EEG frequency tagging using ultra-slow periodic heat stimulation of the skin reveals cortical activity specifically related to C fiber thermonociceptors. Neuroimage 2017;146:266–74.)

distributed over both hemispheres. Most interestingly, this midline scalp topography contrasted strongly with the lateralized scalp topography of the SS-EPs obtained by innocuous electrical stimulation of large-diameter Aβ fibers evoking vibrotactile sensations, which displayed a clear maximum over the parietal region contralateral to the stimulated side (primary somatosensory cortex). Because the spatial distribution of nociceptive somatosensory SS-EPs was markedly different from the spatial distribution of nonnociceptive somatosensory SS-EPs, it can be hypothesized that nociceptive SS-EPs reflect the activity of a cortical network spatially distinct from the somatotopically organized cortical network involved in processing innocuous vibrotactile input and, possibly, preferentially involved in processing nociceptive input. Taken together, these results indicate that the recording of nociceptive SS-EPs could contribute to a better understanding of the cortical representation of nociception in humans.

In a recent study, it was shown that periodic sinusoidal heat stimulation of the skin using a very low frequency (0.2 Hz) can be used to elicit robust SS-EPs preferentially related to the activation slowly adapting heat-sensitive C fibers [16] (Figure 10-4). The proposed approach could constitute a mean to study C-fiber function in humans and to explore the cortical processing of tonic heat pain in physiologic and pathologic conditions.

REFERENCES

1. Atherton DD, Facer P, Roberts KM, Misra VP, Chizh BA, Bountra C, Anand P. Use of the novel Contact Heat Evoked Potential Stimulator (CHEPS) for the assessment of small fibre neuropathy: correlations with skin flare responses and intra-epidermal nerve fibre counts. BMC Neurol 2007;7:21.
2. Bastuji H, Frot M, Perchet C, Magnin M, Garcia-Larrea L. Pain networks from the inside: spatiotemporal analysis of brain responses leading from nociception to conscious perception. Hum Brain Mapp 2016;37(12):4301–15.
3. Baumgartner C. Controversies in clinical neurophysiology. MEG is superior to EEG in localization of interictal epileptiform activity: Con. Clin Neurophysiol 2004;115(5):1010–20.
4. Baumgartner U, Cruccu G, Iannetti GD, Treede RD. Laser guns and hot plates. Pain 2005;116(1–2):1–3.
5. Baumgartner U, Greffrath W, Treede RD. Contact heat and cold, mechanical, electrical and chemical stimuli to elicit small fiber-evoked potentials: merits and limitations for basic science and clinical use. Neurophysiol Clin 2012;42(5):267–80.
6. Baumgartner U, Vogel H, Ohara S, Treede RD, Lenz F. Dipole source analyses of laser evoked potentials obtained from subdural grid recordings from primary somatic sensory cortex. J Neurophysiol 2011;106(2):722–30.
7. Bentley DE, Youell PD, Crossman AR, Jones AK. Source localisation of 62-electrode human laser pain evoked potential data using a realistic head model. Int J Psychophysiol 2001;41(2):187–93.
8. Berger H. Über das elektroenkephalogramm des menschen. Arch Psychiatry 1929;87:527–70.
9. Bragard D, Chen ACN, Plaghki L. Direct isolation of ultra-late (C-fibre) evoked brain potentials by CO_2 laser stimulation of tiny cutaneous surface areas in man. Neurosci Lett 1996;209(2):81–4.
10. Bromm B, Neitzel H, Tecklenburg A, Treede RD. Evoked cerebral potential correlates of C-fibre activity in man. Neurosci Lett 1983;43(1):109–14.
11. Bromm B, Treede RD. Nerve fibre discharges, cerebral potentials and sensations induced by CO_2 laser stimulation. Hum Neurobiol 1984;3(1):33–40.
12. Carmon A, Mor J, Goldberg J. Evoked cerebral responses to noxious thermal stimuli in humans. Exp Brain Res 1976;25(1):103–7.
13. Caty G, Hu L, Legrain V, Plaghki L, Mouraux A. Psychophysical and electrophysiological evidence for nociceptive dysfunction in complex regional pain syndrome. Pain 2013;154(11):2521–8.
14. Churyukanov M, Plaghki L, Legrain V, Mouraux A. Thermal detection thresholds of Aδ- and C-fibre afferents activated by brief CO_2 laser pulses applied onto the human hairy skin. PLoS One 2012;7(4):e35817.
15. Colon E, Legrain V, Mouraux A. Steady-state evoked potentials to study the processing of tactile and nociceptive somatosensory input in the human brain. Neurophysiol Clin 2012;42(5):315–23.
16. Colon E, Liberati G, Mouraux A. EEG frequency tagging using ultra-slow periodic heat stimulation of the skin reveals cortical activity specifically related to C fiber thermonociceptors. Neuroimage 2017;146:266–74.
17. Colon E, Nozaradan S, Legrain V, Mouraux A. Steady-state evoked potentials to tag specific components of nociceptive cortical processing. Neuroimage 2012;60(1):571–81.
18. Cruccu G, Aminoff MJ, Curio G, Guerit JM, Kakigi R, Mauguiere F, Rossini PM, Treede RD, Garcia-Larrea L. Recommendations for the clinical use of somatosensory-evoked potentials. Clin Neurophysiol 2008;119(8):1705–19.
19. Cruccu G, Iannetti GD, Agostino R, Romaniello A, Truini A, Manfredi M. Conduction velocity of the human spinothalamic tract as assessed by laser evoked potentials. Neuroreport 2000;11(13):3029–32.
20. Cruccu G, Pennisi E, Truini A, Iannetti GD, Romaniello A, Le Pera D, De Armas L, Leandri M, Manfredi M, Valeriani M. Unmyelinated trigeminal pathways as assessed by laser stimuli in humans. Brain 2003;126(Pt 10):2246–56.
21. Forss N, Raij TT, Seppa M, Hari R. Common cortical network for first and second pain. Neuroimage 2005;24(1):132–42.
22. Franz M, Spohn D, Ritter A, Rolke R, Miltner WH, Weiss T. Laser heat stimulation of tiny skin areas adds valuable information to quantitative sensory testing in postherpetic neuralgia. Pain 2012;153(8):1687–94.
23. Frot M, Garcia-Larrea L, Guenot M, Mauguiere F. Responses of the supra-sylvian (SII) cortex in humans to painful and innocuous stimuli. A study using intra-cerebral recordings. Pain 2001;94(1):65–73.
24. Frot M, Magnin M, Mauguiere F, Garcia-Larrea L. Human SII and posterior insula differently encode thermal laser stimuli. Cereb Cortex 2007;17(3):610–20.
25. Frot M, Magnin M, Mauguiere F, Garcia-Larrea L. Cortical representation of pain in primary sensory-motor areas (S1/M1)–a study using intracortical recordings in humans. Hum Brain Mapp 2013;34(10):2655–68.
26. Frot M, Mauguiere F. Timing and spatial distribution of somatosensory responses recorded in the upper bank of the sylvian fissure (SII area) in humans. Cereb Cortex 1999;9(8):854–63.

27. Frot M, Mauguiere F. Dual representation of pain in the operculo-insular cortex in humans. Brain 2003;126(Pt 2):438–50.
28. Frot M, Mauguiere F, Magnin M, Garcia-Larrea L. Parallel processing of nociceptive A-delta inputs in SII and midcingulate cortex in humans. J Neurosci 2008;28(4):944–52.
29. Frot M, Rambaud L, Guenot M, Mauguiere F. Intracortical recordings of early pain-related CO_2-laser evoked potentials in the human second somatosensory (SII) area. Clin Neurophysiol 1999;110(1):133–45.
30. Garcia-Larrea L. Somatosensory volleys and cortical evoked potentials: 'first come, first served'? Pain 2004;112(1–2):5–7.
31. Garcia-Larrea L, Frot M, Valeriani M. Brain generators of laser-evoked potentials: from dipoles to functional significance. Neurophysiol Clin 2003;33(6):279–92.
32. Gopalakrishnan R, Machado AG, Burgess RC, Mosher JC. The use of contact heat evoked potential stimulator (CHEPS) in magnetoencephalography for pain research. J Neurosci Methods 2013;220(1):55–63.
33. Gross J, Schnitzler A, Timmermann L, Ploner M. Gamma oscillations in human primary somatosensory cortex reflect pain perception. PLoS Biol 2007;5(5):e133.
34. Hallin RG, Torebjork HE, Wiesenfeld Z. Nociceptors and warm receptors innervated by C fibres in human skin. J Neurol Neurosurg Psychiatry 1982;45(4):313–9.
35. Hämäläinen M, Hari R, Ilmoniemi RJ, Knuutila J, Lounasmaa OV. Magnetoencephalography: theory, instrumentation, and applications to noninvasive studies of the working human brain. Rev Mod Phys 1993;65:413–97.
36. Herrmann CS. Human EEG responses to 1-100 Hz flicker: resonance phenomena in visual cortex and their potential correlation to cognitive phenomena. Exp Brain Res 2001;137(3–4):346–53.
37. Hu L, Mouraux A, Hu Y, Iannetti GD. A novel approach for enhancing the signal-to-noise ratio and detecting automatically event-related potentials (ERPs) in single trials. Neuroimage 2010;50(1):99–111.
38. Hullemann P, Nerdal A, Binder A, Helfert S, Reimer M, Baron R. Cold-evoked potentials - ready for clinical use? Eur J Pain 2016;20(10):1730–40.
39. Iannetti GD, Baumgartner U, Tracey I, Treede RD, Magerl W. Pinprick-evoked brain potentials: a novel tool to assess central sensitization of nociceptive pathways in humans. J Neurophysiol 2013;110(5):1107–16.
40. Iannetti GD, Mouraux A. From the neuromatrix to the pain matrix (and back). Exp Brain Res 2010;205(1):1–12.
41. Iannetti GD, Porro CA, Pantano P, Romanelli PL, Galeotti F, Cruccu G. Representation of different trigeminal divisions within the primary and secondary human somatosensory cortex. Neuroimage 2003;19(3):906–12.
42. Iannetti GD, Truini A, Romaniello A, Galeotti F, Rizzo C, Manfredi M, Cruccu G. Evidence of a specific spinal pathway for the sense of warmth in humans. J Neurophysiol 2003;89(1):562–70.
43. Iannetti GD, Zambreanu L, Tracey I. Similar nociceptive afferents mediate psychophysical and electrophysiological responses to heat stimulation of glabrous and hairy skin in humans. J Physiol 2006;577(Pt 1):235–48.
44. Inui K, Tran TD, Hoshiyama M, Kakigi R. Preferential stimulation of Aδ fibers by intra-epidermal needle electrode in humans. Pain 2002;96(3):247–52.
45. Inui K, Tsuji T, Kakigi R. Temporal analysis of cortical mechanisms for pain relief by tactile stimuli in humans. Cereb Cortex 2006;16(3):355–65.
46. Jankovski A, Plaghki L, Mouraux A. Reliable EEG responses to the selective activation of C-fibre afferents using a temperature-controlled infrared laser stimulator in conjunction with an adaptive staircase algorithm. Pain 2013;154(9):1578–87.
47. Kakigi R, Koyama S, Hoshiyama M, Kitamura Y, Shimojo M, Watanabe S. Pain-related magnetic fields following painful CO_2 laser stimulation in man. Neurosci Lett 1995;192(1):45–8.
48. Kakigi R, Tran TD, Qiu Y, Wang X, Nguyen TB, Inui K, Watanabe S, Hoshiyama M. Cerebral responses following stimulation of unmyelinated C-fibers in humans: electro- and magneto-encephalographic study. Neurosci Res 2003;45(3):255–75.
49. Kanda M, Nagamine T, Ikeda A, Ohara S, Kunieda T, Fujiwara N, Yazawa S, Sawamoto N, Matsumoto R, Taki W, Shibasaki H. Primary somatosensory cortex is actively involved in pain processing in human. Brain Res 2000;853(2):282–9.
50. Kaube H, Katsarava Z, Kaufer T, Diener H, Ellrich J. A new method to increase nociception specificity of the human blink reflex. Clin Neurophysiol 2000;111(3):413–6.
51. LaMotte RH, Campbell JN. Comparison of responses of warm and nociceptive C-fiber afferents in monkey with human judgments of thermal pain. J Neurophysiol 1978;41(2):509–28.
52. Lankers J, Frieling A, Kunze K, Bromm B. Ultralate cerebral potentials in a patient with hereditary motor and sensory neuropathy type I indicate preserved C-fibre function. J Neurol Neurosurg Psychiatry 1991;54(7):650–2.
53. Legrain V, Iannetti GD, Plaghki L, Mouraux A. The pain matrix reloaded: a salience detection system for the body. Prog Neurobiol 2011;93(1):111–24.

54. Legrain V, Mouraux A. Activating selectively and reliably nociceptive afferents with concentric electrode stimulation: yes we can! Provided that low stimulus intensities are used! Clin Neurophysiol 2013;124(2):424.
55. Lenz FA, Rios M, Zirh A, Chau D, Krauss G, Lesser RP. Painful stimuli evoke potentials recorded over the human anterior cingulate gyrus. J Neurophysiol 1998;79(4):2231–4.
56. Lewis T, Ponchin EE. The double pain response of the human skin to a single stimulus. Clin Sci 1937;3:67–76.
57. Liang M, Mouraux A, Chan V, Blakemore C, Iannetti GD. Functional characterisation of sensory ERPs using probabilistic ICA: effect of stimulus modality and stimulus location. Clin Neurophysiol 2010;121(4):577–87.
58. Liberati G, Klocker A, Safronova MM, Ferrao Santos S, Ribeiro Vaz JG, Raftopoulos C, Mouraux A. Nociceptive local field potentials recorded from the human insula are not specific for nociception. PLoS Biol 2016;14(1):e1002345.
59. Liu CC, Ohara S, Franaszczuk P, Zagzoog N, Gallagher M, Lenz FA. Painful stimuli evoke potentials recorded from the medial temporal lobe in humans. Neuroscience 2010;165(4):1402–11.
60. Luck SJ. *An introduction to the event-related potential technique*. Cambridge: MIT Press; 2005.
61. Magerl W, Ali Z, Ellrich J, Meyer RA, Treede RD. C- and A delta-fiber components of heat-evoked cerebral potentials in healthy human subjects. Pain 1999;82(2):127–37.
62. Malmivuo J, Suihko V, Eskola H. Sensitivity distributions of EEG and MEG measurements. IEEE Trans Biomed Eng 1997;44(3):196–208.
63. Malmivuo JA, Suihko VE. Effect of skull resistivity on the spatial resolutions of EEG and MEG. IEEE Trans Biomed Eng 2004;51(7):1276–80.
64. Mouraux A, De Paepe AL, Marot E, Plaghki L, Iannetti GD, Legrain V. Unmasking the obligatory components of nociceptive event-related brain potentials. J Neurophysiol 2013;110(10):2312–24.
65. Mouraux A, Iannetti GD. Across-trial averaging of event-related EEG responses and beyond. Magn Reson Imaging 2008;26(7):1041–54.
66. Mouraux A, Iannetti GD. Nociceptive laser-evoked brain potentials do not reflect nociceptive-specific neural activity. J Neurophysiol 2009;101(6):3258–69.
67. Mouraux A, Iannetti GD, Colon E, Nozaradan S, Legrain V, Plaghki L. Nociceptive steady-state evoked potentials elicited by rapid periodic thermal stimulation of cutaneous nociceptors. J Neurosci 2011;31(16):6079–87.
68. Mouraux A, Iannetti GD, Plaghki L. Low intensity intra-epidermal electrical stimulation can activate Aδ-nociceptors selectively. Pain 2010;150(1):199–207.
69. Mouraux A, Rage M, Bragard D, Plaghki L. Estimation of intraepidermal fiber density by the detection rate of nociceptive laser stimuli in normal and pathological conditions. Neurophysiol Clin 2012;42(5):281–91.
70. Muller GR, Neuper C, Pfurtscheller G. "Resonance-like" frequencies of sensorimotor areas evoked by repetitive tactile stimulation. Biomed Tech 2001;46(7–8):186–90.
71. Nahra H, Plaghki L. The effects of A-fiber pressure block on perception and neurophysiological correlates of brief non-painful and painful CO_2 laser stimuli in humans. Eur J Pain 2003;7(2):189–99.
72. Nunez PL, Srinivasan R. *Electric fields of the brain. The neurophysics of EEG*. New York: Oxford University Press; 2006.
73. Ochoa J, Mair WG. The normal sural nerve in man. I. Ultrastructure and numbers of fibres and cells. Acta Neuropathol 1969;13(3):197–216.
74. Opsommer E, Guerit JM, Plaghki L. Exogenous and endogenous components of ultralate (C-fibre) evoked potentials following CO_2 laser stimuli to tiny skin surface areas in healthy subjects. Neurophysiol Clin 2003;33(2):78–85.
75. Opsommer E, Masquelier E, Plaghki L. Determination of nerve conduction velocity of C-fibres in humans from thermal thresholds to contact heat (thermode) and from evoked brain potentials to radiant heat (CO_2 laser). Neurophysiol Clin 1999;29(5):411–22.
76. Opsommer E, Weiss T, Miltner WH, Plaghki L. Scalp topography of ultralate (C-fibres) evoked potentials following thulium YAG laser stimuli to tiny skin surface areas in humans. Clin Neurophysiol 2001;112(10):1868–74.
77. Opsommer E, Weiss T, Plaghki L, Miltner WH. Dipole analysis of ultralate (C-fibres) evoked potentials after laser stimulation of tiny cutaneous surface areas in humans. Neurosci Lett 2001;298(1):41–4.
78. Perchet C, Frot M, Charmarty A, Flores C, Mazza S, Magnin M, Garcia-Larrea L. Do we activate specifically somatosensory thin fibres with the concentric planar electrode? A scalp and intracranial EEG study. Pain 2012;153(6):1244–52.
79. Peyron R, Frot M, Schneider F, Garcia-Larrea L, Mertens P, Barral FG, Sindou M, Laurent B, Mauguiere F. Role of operculoinsular cortices in human pain processing: converging evidence from PET, fMRI, dipole modeling, and intracerebral recordings of evoked potentials. Neuroimage 2002;17(3):1336–46.
80. Pfurtscheller G, Lopes da Silva FH. Event-related EEG/MEG synchronization and desynchronization: basic principles. Clin Neurophysiol 1999;110(11):1842–57.

81. Pfurtscheller G, Neuper C. Event-related synchronization of mu rhythm in the EEG over the cortical hand area in man. Neurosci Lett 1994;174(1):93–6.
82. Plaghki L, Mouraux A. Brain responses to signals ascending through C-fibers. In: Hirata K, editor. *International congress series*, vol. 1232. Amsterdam: Elsevier; 2002. p. 181–92.
83. Plaghki L, Mouraux A. How do we selectively activate skin nociceptors with a high power infrared laser? Physiology and biophysics of laser stimulation. Neurophysiol Clin 2003;33(6):269–77.
84. Plaghki L, Mouraux A. EEG and laser stimulation as tools for pain research. Curr Opin Investig Drugs 2005;6(1):58–64.
85. Ploner M, Gross J, Timmermann L, Schnitzler A. Cortical representation of first and second pain sensation in humans. Proc Natl Acad Sci USA 2002;99(19):12444–8.
86. Ploner M, Schmitz F, Freund HJ, Schnitzler A. Parallel activation of primary and secondary somatosensory cortices in human pain processing. J Neurophysiol 1999;81(6):3100–4.
87. Qiu Y, Inui K, Wang X, Nguyen BT, Tran TD, Kakigi R. Effects of distraction on magnetoencephalographic responses ascending through C-fibers in humans. Clin Neurophysiol 2004;115(3):636–46.
88. Qiu Y, Inui K, Wang X, Tran TD, Kakigi R. Effects of attention, distraction and sleep on CO_2 laser evoked potentials related to C-fibers in humans. Clin Neurophysiol : 2002;113(10):1579–85.
89. Raij TT, Vartiainen NV, Jousmaki V, Hari R. Effects of interstimulus interval on cortical responses to painful laser stimulation. J Clin Neurophysiol 2003;20(1):73–9.
90. Regan D. *Human brain electrophysiology. Evoked potentials and evoked magnetic fields in science and medicine*. New York: Elsevier; 1989.
91. Rodriguez E, George N, Lachaux JP, Martinerie J, Renault B, Varela FJ. Perception's shadow: long-distance synchronization of human brain activity. Nature 1999;397(6718):430–3.
92. Schmidt RF, Schaible HG, Messlinger K, Heppelmann B, Hanesch U, Pawlak M. Silent and active nociceptors: structure, functions, and clinical implications. In: Gebhart GF, Hammond DL, Jensen TA, editors. *Proceedings of the VIIth World Congress on pain*. Seattle: IASP Press; 1994. p. 213–50.
93. Singer W. Synchronization of cortical activity and its putative role in information processing and learning. Annu Rev Physiol 1993;55:349–74.
94. Spiegel J, Hansen C, Treede RD. Laser-evoked potentials after painful hand and foot stimulation in humans: evidence for generation of the middle-latency component in the secondary somatosensory cortex. Neurosci Lett 1996;216(3):179–82.
95. Tallon-Baudry C, Bertrand O. Oscillatory gamma activity in humans and its role in object representation. Trends Cogn Sci 1999;3(4):151–62.
96. Tarkka IM, Treede RD. Equivalent electrical source analysis of pain-related somatosensory evoked potentials elicited by a CO_2 laser. J Clin Neurophysiol 1993;10(4):513–9.
97. Timmermann L, Ploner M, Haucke K, Schmitz F, Baltissen R, Schnitzler A. Differential coding of pain intensity in the human primary and secondary somatosensory cortex. J Neurophysiol 2001;86(3):1499–503.
98. Tran TD, Inui K, Hoshiyama M, Lam K, Qiu Y, Kakigi R. Cerebral activation by the signals ascending through unmyelinated C-fibers in humans: a magnetoencephalographic study. Neuroscience 2002;113(2):375–86.
99. Treede RD, Kief S, Holzer T, Bromm B. Late somatosensory evoked cerebral potentials in response to cutaneous heat stimuli. Electroencephalogr Clin Neurophysiol 1988;70(5):429–41.
100. Treede RD, Meier W, Kunze K, Bromm B. Ultralate cerebral potentials as correlates of delayed pain perception: observation in a case of neurosyphilis. J Neurol Neurosurg Psychiatry 1988;51(10):1330–3.
101. Treede RD, Meyer RA, Raja SN, Campbell JN. Evidence for two different heat transduction mechanisms in nociceptive primary afferents innervating monkey skin. J Physiol 1995;483 (Pt 3):747–58.
102. Valentini E, Hu L, Chakrabarti B, Hu Y, Aglioti SM, Iannetti GD. The primary somatosensory cortex largely contributes to the early part of the cortical response elicited by nociceptive stimuli. Neuroimage 2012;59(2):1571–81.
103. Valeriani M, Le Pera D, Restuccia D, de Armas L, Miliucci R, Betti V, Vigevano F, Tonali P. Parallel spinal pathways generate the middle-latency N1 and the late P2 components of the laser evoked potentials. Clin Neurophysiol 2007;118(5):1097–104.
104. Valeriani M, Rambaud L, Mauguiere F. Scalp topography and dipolar source modelling of potentials evoked by CO_2 laser stimulation of the hand. Electroencephalogr Clin Neurophysiol 1996;100(4):343–53.
105. Valeriani M, Restuccia D, Le Pera D, De Armas L, Maiese T, Tonali P. Attention-related modifications of ultralate CO_2 laser evoked potentials to human trigeminal nerve stimulation. Neurosci Lett 2002;329(3):329–33.
106. Valeriani M, Truini A, Le Pera D, Insola A, Galeotti F, Petrachi C, Mazzone P, Cruccu G. Laser evoked potential recording from intracerebral deep electrodes. Clin Neurophysiol 2009;120(4):790–5.

107. van den Broeke EN, Lambert J, Huang G, Mouraux A. Central sensitization of mechanical nociceptive pathways is associated with a long-lasting increase of pinprick-evoked brain potentials. Front Hum Neurosci 2016;10:531.
108. van den Broeke EN, Mouraux A, Groneberg AH, Pfau DB, Treede RD, Klein T. Characterizing pinprick-evoked brain potentials before and after experimentally induced secondary hyperalgesia. J Neurophysiol 2015;114(5):2672-81.
109. Vialatte FB, Maurice M, Dauwels J, Cichocki A. Steady-state visually evoked potentials: focus on essential paradigms and future perspectives. Prog Neurobiol 2010;90(4):418-38.
110. Vogel H, Port JD, Lenz FA, Solaiyappan M, Krauss G, Treede RD. Dipole source analysis of laser-evoked subdural potentials recorded from parasylvian cortex in humans. J Neurophysiol 2003;89(6):3051-60.
111. Watanabe S, Kakigi R, Koyama S, Hoshiyama M, Kaneoke Y. Pain processing traced by magnetoencephalography in the human brain. Brain Topogr 1998;10(4):255-64.
112. Weiss T, Miltner WH. Double stimulation of tiny skin areas in human subjects increases the number of C- and Aδ-fiber responses. Neurosci Lett 2005;386(3):165-9.
113. Wu Q, Garcia-Larrea L, Mertens P, Beschet A, Sindou M, Mauguiere F. Hyperalgesia with reduced laser evoked potentials in neuropathic pain. Pain 1999;80(1-2):209-14.
114. Xu X, Kanda M, Shindo K, Fujiwara N, Nagamine T, Ikeda A, Honda M, Tachibana N, Barrett G, Kaji R. Pain-related somatosensory evoked potentials following CO_2 laser stimulation of foot in man. Electroencephalogr Clin Neurophysiol 1995;96(1):12-23.
115. Yamasaki H, Kakigi R, Watanabe S, Naka D. Effects of distraction on pain perception: magneto- and electro-encephalographic studies. Brain Res Cogn Brain Res 1999;8(1):73-6.
116. Zhang ZG, Hu L, Hung YS, Mouraux A, Iannetti GD. Gamma-band oscillations in the primary somatosensory cortex–a direct and obligatory correlate of subjective pain intensity. J Neurosci 2012;32(22):7429-38.

CHAPTER 11

Contribution of Positron Emission Tomography (PET) for Understanding Neuronal Activation and Neurotransmission in Pain

Anne Stankewitz, Till Sprenger, Enrico Schulz, and Thomas R. Tölle

The development of positron emission tomography (PET) techniques, about four decades ago, now allows the study of brain activation in humans in vivo with a reasonable anatomical resolution of cortical and subcortical structures. Before this groundbreaking invention, our knowledge about the relationship between structure and function of the brain was based solely on animal studies, postmortem human studies, or electrophysiologic investigations. The development of PET has, in combination with other modern neuroscience methods, strongly improved our understanding of pain-processing networks within the brain during acute pain events in healthy subjects. Additionally, PET has allowed insights into the pathophysiology of chronic pain disorders.

To investigate brain function in humans with PET, a radioactively labeled substance must be administered intravenously or be inhaled by a subject. Through the use of such radioactive compounds, PET allows the study of cerebral hemodynamics and oxygen consumption ($H_2^{15}O$-PET) [1], glucose metabolism (^{18}F-fluoro-2-deoxy-D-glucose-PET; FDG-PET) [2], and specific neurotransmitter receptor systems (ligand-PET) [3].

In neuroscience, the most frequently applied PET technique uses O-15 labeled water for the noninvasive measurement of the regional cerebral blood flow ($H_2^{15}O$-PET). By assuming a tight connection between neuronal and vascular changes, inferences can be drawn about neuronal activity patterns in the brain. The second method relies on injection of radioactively labeled glucose (FDG), which accumulates in brain regions with high metabolism (FDG-PET) because of the high demand for energy. The third method allows us to characterize and map receptor availability in different neurotransmitter systems in vivo (ligand-PET).

Although there are limitations, specifically of a spatial and temporal nature, PET allows the absolute level of blood flow, metabolism, and receptor availability to be quantified without the need for any baseline corrections. PET is thus perfectly suited to assess pathologic states in chronic pain disorders without additional stimulation or baseline assessment. Additionally, PET allows for the detection of changes in response to various treatments. In the healthy brain, PET can be used to assess increases or decreases in cortical glucose consumption in response to a variety of experimental conditions (such as heat pain) as well as to variations of cognitive factors.

PET STUDIES ON PAIN PROCESSING IN THE HEALTHY BRAIN

Before being applied as a means of studying pain processing in *pathologic* conditions (such as chronic pain) in vivo, a number of studies focused primarily on how pain is processed in the healthy human brain. Some of the earliest studies determined changes of cortical blood flow in response to experimentally administered pain stimuli with means of $H_2^{15}O$-PET. These early studies showed consistently that pain activates an extended network of brain regions, such as the thalamus, the primary and secondary somatosensory cortex (SI and SII), the insular cortex, the middle and anterior cingulate cortex (ACC), the prefrontal cortex, the amygdala, and the cerebellum [32]. Later, PET studies revealed that specific brain regions contribute to specific aspects of pain sensation: The affective–emotional component of pain perception is processed in the medial thalamic nuclei, the anterior insula [34] as well as in the ACC [40], whereas the sensory–discriminative component is encoded in the lateral thalamic nuclei, the posterior insular cortex as well as in SI and SII.

Subsequent PET studies aimed at characterizing, in vivo, the opioid receptor density of pain-processing structures. The first tracer studies demonstrated a higher receptor binding in the more medial structures of the cerebral pain processing network, such as in medial thalamic nuclei and the cingulate cortex, than in more lateral regions, which include the lateral thalamic nuclei and the somatosensory cortex [16]. However, a further ligand-PET study revealed that there is also a relevant density of opioid receptors in the lateral regions, particularly in the operculoinsular cortex [1]. Owing to these findings, the authors argued that in fact both systems—the sensory–discriminative and the affective–motivational pain components—are influenced by opioid receptor agonists and antagonists.

It was through the means of ligand-PET that specific characteristics of binding patterns were explored for the opioid agonist ^{11}C-carfentanil and the opioid antagonist ^{11}C-diprenorphine [8]. The results of these experiments showed a stronger binding of diprenorphine in the striatum, cingulate cortex, and frontal cortex, which suggested a relatively high concentration of the κ- and δ-opioidergic receptors in these brain regions.

A further study investigated the μ-opioidergic receptor system in response to nociceptive stimulation of the masseter muscles in healthy subjects. The dorsal ACC, insula, thalamus, hypothalamus, amygdala, and the lateral prefrontal regions all displayed reduced binding of the exogenous opioidergic ligand in response to the stimulus, probably reflecting release of endogenous opioids. A further investigation showed that receptor availability correlated with sensory and affective pain ratings, thus indicating an important role of these receptors in the regulation of individual pain experiences [48]. On a similar note, alterations of the binding potential were observed in various pain-processing regions of the brain in response to heat pain [38] as well as during the cold pressor test [29].

Other ligand-PET studies explored the interactions between the different receptor systems that are involved in pain processing in a healthy brain. These studies were able to show that opioids modulate the neurotransmission in the nigrostriatal dopaminergic pathway. Additionally, the administration of the μ-antagonist alfentanil increased the receptor binding potential of the dopamine D2 radioligand raclopride in the putamen and in the caudate nucleus [11].

PET FOR ASSESSING THE ENDOGENOUS PAIN CONTROL SYSTEM

There are a few PET studies that have focused in particular on the descending pain system that controls and modulates the transmission of pain signals from the periphery to the cerebral cortex. In these studies, increased brain activity was observed in the ACC, the midbrain, and prefrontal regions after administrations of intravenous opioidergic medications (fentanyl or remifentanil) [30,43]. Interestingly, a similar activation pattern was observed with placebo analgesia [41].

There is strong evidence that the perigenual ACC (pACC) contributes to pain modulatory circuits via efferent connections to the periaqueductal gray (PAG). During pain stimulation and the concomitant application of an analgesic opioid, a strong coupling of the pACC and the PAG was observed through the use of PET. This coupling, however, was not observed during unmedicated painful stimulation [41]. A further study found a higher activity in ACC and PAG in response to painful heat stimulation than in response to nonpainful heat stimulation under remifentanil [42].

The pACC has therefore been proposed as a major modulator of pain signals in the brain that regulates brainstem structures (including the PAG), which in turn project to the medullary and spinal dorsal horn to enhance or diminish nociception.

PET STUDIES IN CLINICAL PAIN CONDITIONS

Neuropathic Pain

For central poststroke pain (CPSP), tracer studies have revealed reduced opioid receptor binding in a variety of cortical and subcortical brain regions including the ACC, the dorsolateral cingulate cortex, the insula, the inferior parietal cortex, and the thalamus. These receptor binding changes were not restricted to the localization of stroke-related lesions but were rather widespread [17,21,46]. A further study demonstrated that the alteration of receptor binding was not symmetrically distributed in the patients' brains; abnormalities occurred predominantly contralateral to the pain side [46].

In peripheral neuropathic pain patients (peripheral NP), similar reductions of opioidergic binding were observed [21]. Although peripheral NP and CPSP patients did not differ in any clinical characteristic (such as pain intensity scores), changes of the receptor binding were found in both hemispheres in peripheral NP patients, and thus, peripheral NP patients may be characterized by a globally altered opioidergic tone. The bilateral changes in these patients may relate to the permanent nociceptive input.

Similar alterations of the opioidergic receptor function were found in trigeminal neuralgia [15] and rheumatoid arthritis [14]. A recently published tracer PET study observed that in a small group of trigeminal neuropathic pain patients, there was reduced μ-opioid receptor availability in the left nucleus accumbens that was negatively correlated with the subjective pain ratings. Interestingly, the nucleus accumbens is thought to be involved in pain modulation as well as in reward and aversive learning behavior [7].

Opioidergic changes were also observed in brain regions contributing to the affective–motivational component of pain in patients suffering from complex regional pain syndrome (CRPS). Using PET and the opioidergic radioligand ^{18}F-fluoroethyl-diprenorphine, a decreased opioid receptor binding was found in the amygdalohippocampal region contralateral to the painful limb. Additionally, the scores of anxiety and depression were significantly related to the opioid receptor binding potential in various brain regions [20]. Given that the intensity of perceived endogenous pain in CRPS is often associated with psychological stress, anxiety or depression, this finding is in line with the clinical picture in this disorder.

Fibromyalgia

Because pain is usually permanently present in fibromyalgia patients, $H_2^{15}O$-PET measurements are perfectly suited to study the potentially abnormal, disease-related brain activity in these patients. One $H_2^{15}O$-PET study found reduced blood flow in a variety of cortical regions, including the temporal, parietal, occipital, and frontal cortices. By contrast, increased activation was observed in the retrosplenial cortex. This region has dense, reciprocal connections to both the thalamus and the hippocampus and has been shown to be involved in encoding and integrating sensory information and memories. The authors of the study hypothesized that increased neuronal activity in this region may pathologically amplify incoming noxious pain signals from the periphery (muscles and tendons) in patients suffering from fibromyalgia [45]. Clinical experiences and neuropsychological tests demonstrating a decreased cognitive performance as well as a prevalent history of psychological traumas in these patients are in line with these findings. With the means of ligand-PET, studies have also demonstrated that both the dopaminergic and the opioidergic systems are involved in the pathogenesis of the disease. Reduced binding potential in the dopaminergic system has been observed in various brain areas including the brainstem, thalamus, and the limbic system [46]. Reductions of μ-opioidergic binding potential were found in brain areas associated with the affective modulation of pain, e.g., the ventral striatum, the amygdala, and the cingulate cortex. Additionally, the opioid receptor binding potential in the nucleus accumbens, cingulate cortex, and striatum was negatively correlated with affective pain ratings [12] (see Figure 11-1). These findings may explain the supposedly limited efficacy of opioids in patients with fibromyalgia.

Cluster Headache

The application of PET has contributed profoundly to our knowledge on the pathogenesis of trigeminal autonomic cephalalgias such as cluster headache. An increase of cerebral blood flow in the midbrain at the border of the hypothalamus to the ventral tegmental area ipsilaterally to the headache side was observed during but not outside of acute cluster headache attacks [10,35]. Hyperactivity of this region was also observed in other trigeminal autonomic headache syndromes, namely in hemicrania continua [27] and paroxysmal hemicrania [26]. Because the hypothalamus regulates autonomic functions and acts as an internal biologic clock controlling the sleep–wake rhythm, this region has been discussed as a potential structure initiating and maintaining trigeminoautonomic headaches. However, its activation may indeed also relate to the termination of attacks, as the posterior hypothalamus is integrated in antinociceptive networks. Finally, hypothalamic hyperactivity may explain autonomic symptoms that accompany cluster headache attacks such as ptosis, meiosis, conjunctival injection, and lacrimation.

Compared with healthy control subjects, another PET study found reduced glucose uptake in cluster headache patients in the pACC, prefrontal cortex, and orbitofrontal cortex (OFC). Interestingly, this reduction of metabolism was detectable not only during the acute cluster period ("in bout") but also during the remission period ("out of the bout"). This study also revealed that the glucose uptake was significantly higher in patients in bout compared with out-of-the-bout period in brain areas involved in top–down pain-modulating circuits such as the pACC and the frontal brain structures. These findings emphasize notions about an altered endogenous pain control system in cluster headache patients [37].

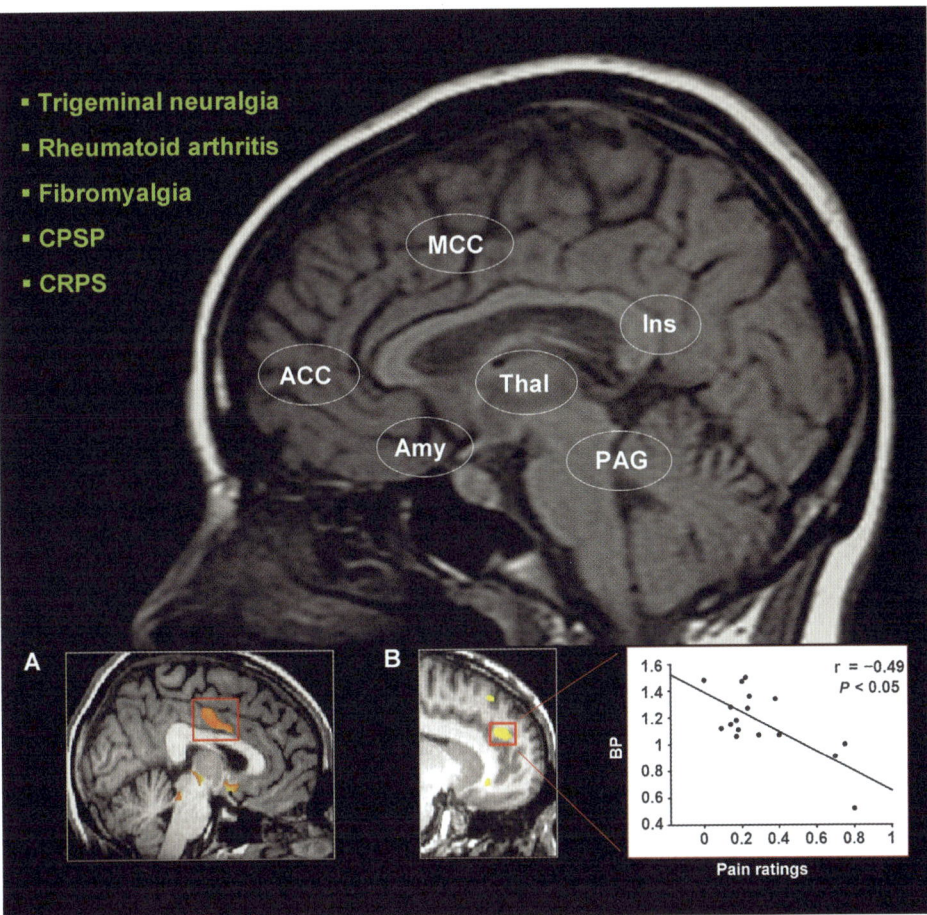

FIGURE 11-1 This figure visualizes findings of ligand-PET studies in chronic pain states: Alterations of the opioidergic binding potential (BP) were observed in various pain-processing and pain-modulating brain regions including the anterior (ACC) and middle cingulate cortex (MCC), thalamus (Thal), insula (Ins), and amygdala (Amy). Patients suffering from trigeminal neuralgia, rheumatoid arthritis, fibromyalgia, central poststroke pain (CPSP), and complex regional pain syndrome (CRPS) show a reduced opioidergic receptor availability in brain areas encoding the sensory-discriminative and/or the emotional–affective component of pain. As an example, the lower left part of the figure **(A)** depicts the results of ligand-PET demonstrating decreased BP in MCC, periaqueductal gray (PAG), and amygdala in fibromyalgia. The lower right picture **(B)** shows a strong correlation between the BP in the MCC and individual rating scores of the sensory and affective quality of pain [12]. As opioids have a strong analgesic effect, these findings may explain some aspects of the pathogenesis of chronic pain.

Furthermore, a tracer study explored the opioidergic system in cluster headache patients and found an opioidergic dysfunction in the pineal gland [39]. This part of the brain produces the hormone melatonin that modulates circadian rhythms. At the molecular level, melatonin affects the β-endorphin level, which has a strong analgesic effect, and as opioids can stimulate the secretion of melatonin, an opioidergic dysfunction in cluster headache may cause an impaired melatonin homeostasis in the pineal gland, which could explain some rhythmic characteristics of the disorder. With longer disease duration, the authors of this study further observed that the receptor availability decreased in the ACC and in the hypothalamus [39].

Migraine

Although the pathophysiology of migraine is not yet completely understood, several PET studies have substantially improved our knowledge about underlying mechanisms of the disorder. Through the means of $H_2^{15}O$-PET, hyperactivity in the rostral part of the pons was consistently shown in migraineurs, both during headache attacks and even after the injection of sumatriptan (and resulting pain relief), but not during the interictal interval. This finding suggests that the activity of the brainstem is not the result of pain perception but might be in fact related to the migraine attack itself. It would appear as though this hyperactivity persists for the entire length of the migraine attack and does not decrease before the attack is remitting. This part of the brainstem has thus been suggested to be a "migraine generator", although clearly more evidence is necessary to substantiate this concept [3,4,44]. A seminal ligand-PET study demonstrated alterations of the 5-HT (5-hydroxytryptamine) synthesis in migraine patients in several cortical regions as well as in the dorsal part of the brainstem [5], where a large amount of the neurotransmitter serotonin is localized (in the dorsal raphe nucleus and the nucleus raphe magnus). The highest ligand binding values were detected during acute migraine attacks, the lowest binding values were detected after the administration of sumatriptan, and intermediate values were observed during the pain-free period. As serotonin levels in migraineurs were similar during attacks to those of healthy controls (but decreased interictally), these findings point to the contribution of reduced serotonin levels in the pathogenesis of migraine [33].

Increased blood flow was further observed in the hypothalamus not only during the headache phase of migraine attacks [6] but already at the earliest clinical stage of an attack, the so-called premonitory phase, when patients experience symptoms such as yawning, tiredness, reduced concentration, or cravings [25,36]. Hypothalamic dysfunction would be in line with the clinical picture of the disease, as nonheadache symptoms often occur before (e.g., fatigue), during (e.g., nausea, vomiting), and after headache attacks (e.g., hyperuricemia). Moreover, many trigger factors of migraine attacks are related to hypothalamic (dys) functions, namely hormonal fluctuations, alterations of the sleep–wake cycle, delaying a meal, or stress.

Using FDG-PET, a further study was able to examine glucose metabolism in migraine patients during the pain-free interval and reported reduced glucose uptake in numerous pain-processing brain areas such as the ACC, the insula, and the posterior cortex, prefrontal cortex, and SI. Interestingly, the abnormal hypometabolism corresponds to an increasing disease duration and attack frequency. The authors thus speculated that an altered metabolism in the pain-processing network may be the result of recurrent head pain and might, therefore, be reversible [18]. In line with this finding, a further FDG-PET study showed that the process in which medication overuse transforms episodic migraine into chronic daily headache is generally reversible. Before withdrawal of analgesics, hypometabolism was present in the thalamus, OFC, ACC, inferior parietal cortex, insula, and striatum, whereas hypermetabolism was observed in the cerebellar vermis. Except for the OFC, metabolism normalized in each of these regions after withdrawal (some months later). The authors hypothesized that the persistent hypometabolism in the OFC is related to an abuse trait that most likely persists even after 3 months of withdrawal and increases the risk for recurrent overuse of analgesic medications [9].

LONGITUDINAL PET STUDIES FOR ASSESSING TREATMENT OUTCOMES

The efficacy of pain treatments is usually assessed using subjective verbal reports of the patients. The next paragraph describes examples of how imaging methods such as PET can be used to objectively characterize dynamic changes in the neurotransmission following various interventions.

Motor Cortex Stimulation

In two seminal studies, motor cortex and spinal cord stimulation–induced changes of brain activation were studied in patients suffering from neuropathic pain with $H_2^{15}O$-PET [19,31]. The authors were able to show decreased pain intensity ratings in response to both stimulation techniques. In the brain, this was reflected by increases of cerebral blood flow in specific regions involved in the descending pain modulatory system (e.g., the ACC).

A further PET study explored the effect of motor cortex stimulation in neuropathic pain on the opioidergic receptor occupancy using the tracer ^{11}C-diprenorphine. After several months of invasive motor cortex stimulation, a decrease of the ligand binding potential was observed in brain areas belonging to the endogenous pain control system, i.e., in the prefrontal and the cingulate cortex as well as in the PAG. These findings were accompanied by reduced pain intensity ratings. Thus, motor cortex stimulation likely induces an enhanced release of endogenous opioids. The data provide further evidence for the relevance of an impaired endogenous opioidergic system in chronic pain [22]. Using the ligand ^{11}C-diprenorphine, another recent PET study further explored longitudinal effects of motor cortex stimulation induced by implanted electrodes in refractory neuropathic pain patients. PET scans were assessed in both preoperative and postoperative sessions, and it was shown that the level of preoperative opioid binding in some key regions (i.e., the insula, thalamus, PAG, ACC, and OFC) was positively correlated with postoperative pain relief after 7 months; i.e., patients with the lowest preoperative opioid receptor density benefited the least from the procedure. The authors of the study argued that these findings may aid clinicians in selecting appropriate candidates for surgery who likely benefit from the invasive procedure [23].

Deep Brain Stimulation

In chronic cluster headache patients, neuromodulatory effects were studied in response to hypothalamic deep brain stimulation [28]. The authors reported reduced attack frequency with hypothalamic stimulation and demonstrated stimulator-related brain activity changes in the ipsilateral hypothalamus at the site of stimulation and in various other brain regions, which are known to process trigeminal nociceptive input [28].

Occipital Nerve Stimulation

Cluster headache patients who underwent occipital nerve stimulation demonstrated a reduction of attack frequency after several months of treatment. Simultaneously FDG-PET was used to study brain metabolism, which was shown to normalize in all but one brain region, the hypothalamus. Cluster headache attacks recurred after turning off the stimulator; these findings enhance further evidence for the principle role of the hypothalamus for initiating and maintaining the disease [24] (Figure 11-2).

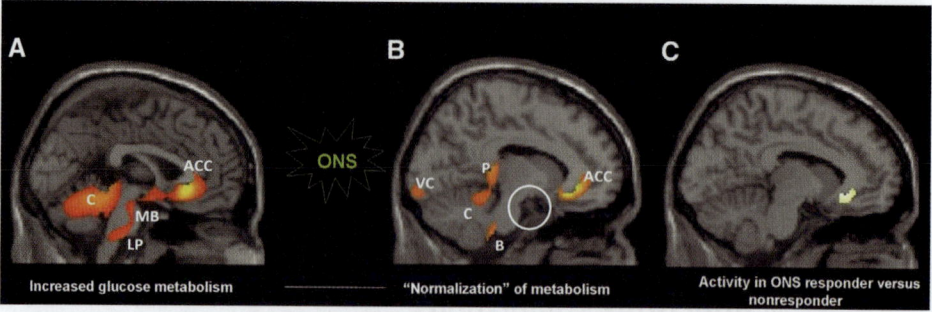

FIGURE 11-2 As an example for numerous PET studies investigating supraspinal mechanisms of various treatments, the figure depicts the effect of occipital nerve stimulation (ONS) on the brain's glucose metabolism (measured by means of FDG-PET) in chronic cluster headache patients. Before treatment, cluster headache patients showed an increased glucose metabolism in the anterior cingulate cortex (ACC), the hypothalamus, the cerebellum (C), the midbrain (MB), and the lower pons (LP) **(A)**. From 1 to 30 mo after ONS, a "normalization" of the same brain areas was progressively observed in the ACC and brainstem but not in the hypothalamus (marked with a *white circle* in the middle picture) **(B)**. This finding provides further evidence for a dysfunction of this region in cluster headache. A cortical hyperactivity in the ACC is present in treatment responders (pain-free or >90% attack frequency reduction) but not in nonresponders [24] **(C)**. P, pulvinar; VC, visual cortex; and B, brainstem.

Endurance Training

A longitudinal study, using ligand-PET, demonstrated how physical activity may contribute to reduced pain perception by release of endogenous opioids in healthy subjects: After 2 hours of running, the release of endogenous opioids was shown in a distributed network of brain regions, particularly in the pACC and the ventromedial and dorsolateral prefrontal cortex [2]. As stated earlier, these regions are thought to play an important role for the endogenous opioid-mediated modulation of pain.

Acupuncture

In recent years, traditional Chinese acupuncture has been receiving increasing attention in the treatment of different kinds of diseases. With means of PET, the cerebral effect of acupuncture was explored in migraine and fibromyalgia.

An FDG-PET study investigated the effect of acupuncture on the glucose metabolism in migraine patients during acute headache attacks. The treatment group received traditional acupuncture, and a control group received an unspecific stimulation. The main result was that the treatment group reported significantly lower pain ratings after the acupuncture treatment compared with the control group. At the same time, the treatment group showed higher glucose uptake in several cortical regions including the frontal, temporal, insular, and cingulate cortices and the precuneus but decreased metabolism in the hippocampus, the fusiform and postcentral gyri, and the cerebellum compared with the control group [47].

A longitudinal PET study using the ligand ^{11}C-carfentanil further explored metabolic changes induced by traditional Chinese acupuncture compared with sham acupuncture in fibromyalgia patients [13]. An increased μ-opioid receptor binding potential was found in key regions of the pain-processing network (including the pACC, the amygdala, and the insular cortex) in response to both short-term (during the first session) and long-term stimulation (over 4 weeks). At a behavioral level, patients reported lower pain scores, suggesting an analgesic effect. Given that a decrease of μ-opioid receptor binding has been previously found (as described earlier) in fibromyalgia patients [12], the authors hypothesized that acupuncture may lead to a "normalization" of μ-opioid receptor binding.

CONCLUSION

The introduction of PET for the study of acute and chronic pain has allowed us to examine hemodynamics ($H_2^{15}O$-PET), glucose metabolism (FDG-PET), and specific neurotransmitter systems (ligand-PET) in vivo. The resulting PET studies have had a truly profound impact on the increase of knowledge and the discussions within the scientific community. Although further advancement in PET technology must still be achieved to provide more sensitive and more specific data, PET has, nonetheless, been crucial to the understanding of pain processing and pain modulation in the brain. It has successfully been used to assess the outcomes and mechanisms of various treatment approaches. PET has also provided important insights into abnormal brain activation patterns in clinical pain conditions. Lastly, the study of receptor availability is particularly unique in neuroscience and has largely improved our understanding of the various releases of neurotransmitters across the entire brain. In the future, the combination of PET and MRI techniques will allow even more comprehensive insights into brain dysfunction in pain conditions, as noninvasive functional MRI techniques can then be combined with, e.g., receptor studies in just one examination.

REFERENCES

1. Baumgartner U, Buchholz HG, Bellosevich A, et al. High opiate receptor binding potential in the human lateral pain system. Neuroimage 2006;30(3):692–9.
2. Boecker H, Sprenger T, Spilker ME, et al. The runner's high: opioidergic mechanisms in the human brain. Cereb Cortex 2008;18(11):2523–31.
3. Borsook D, Burstein R. The enigma of the dorsolateral pons as a migraine generator. Cephalalgia 2012;32(11):803–12.
4. Dahlem MA, Rode S, May A, et al. Towards dynamical network biomarkers in neuromodulation of episodic migraine. Transl Neurosci 2013;4(3).
5. Demarquay G, Lothe A, Royet JP, et al. Brainstem changes in 5-HT1A receptor availability during migraine attack. Cephalalgia 2011;31(1):84–94.
6. Denuelle M, Fabre N, Payoux P, et al. Hypothalamic activation in spontaneous migraine attacks. Headache 2007;47(10):1418–26.
7. DosSantos MF, Martikainen IK, Nascimento TD, et al. Reduced basal ganglia mu-opioid receptor availability in trigeminal neuropathic pain: a pilot study. Mol Pain 2012;8:74.
8. Frost JJ, Mayberg HS, Sadzot B, et al. Comparison of [^{11}C] diprenorphine and [^{11}C] carfentanil binding to opiate receptors in humans by positron emission tomography. J Cereb Blood Flow Metab 1990;10(4):484–92.
9. Fumal A, Laureys S, Di Clemente L, et al. Orbitofrontal cortex involvement in chronic analgesic-overuse headache evolving from episodic migraine. Brain 2006;129(Pt 2):543–50.
10. Goadsby PJ, May A. PET demonstration of hypothalamic activation in cluster headache. Neurology 1999;52(7):1522.
11. Hagelberg N, Kajander JK, Nagren K, et al. Mu-receptor agonism with alfentanil increases striatal dopamine D2 receptor binding in man. Synapse 2002;45(1):25–30.
12. Harris RE, Clauw DJ, Scott DJ, et al. Decreased central mu-opioid receptor availability in fibromyalgia. J Neurosci 2007;27(37):10000–6.
13. Harris RE, Zubieta JK, Scott DJ, et al. Traditional Chinese acupuncture and placebo (sham) acupuncture are differentiated by their effects on mu-opioid receptors (MORs). Neuroimage 2009;47(3):1077–85.
14. Jones AK, Cunningham VJ, Ha-Kawa S, et al. Changes in central opioid receptor binding in relation to inflammation and pain in patients with rheumatoid arthritis. Br J Rheumatol 1994;33(10):909–16.

15. Jones AK, Kitchen ND, Watabe H, et al. Measurement of changes in opioid receptor binding in vivo during trigeminal neuralgic pain using [^{11}C] diprenorphine and positron emission tomography. J Cereb Blood Flow Metab 1999;19(7):803–8.
16. Jones AK, Qi LY, Fujirawa T, et al. In vivo distribution of opioid receptors in man in relation to the cortical projections of the medial and lateral pain systems measured with positron emission tomography. Neurosci Lett 1991;126(1):25–8.
17. Jones AK, Watabe H, Cunningham VJ, Jones T. Cerebral decreases in opioid receptor binding in patients with central neuropathic pain measured by [^{11}C] diprenorphine binding and PET. Eur J Pain 2004;8(5):479–85.
18. Kim JH, Kim S, Suh SI, et al. Interictal metabolic changes in episodic migraine: a voxel-based FDG-PET study. Cephalalgia 2010;30(1):53–61.
19. Kishima H, Saitoh Y, Oshino S, et al. Modulation of neuronal activity after spinal cord stimulation for neuropathic pain; $H_2^{15}O$ PET study. Neuroimage 2010;49(3):2564–9.
20. Klega A, Eberle T, Buchholz HG, et al. Central opioidergic neurotransmission in complex regional pain syndrome. Neurology 2010;75(2):129–36.
21. Maarrawi J, Peyron R, Mertens P, et al. Differential brain opioid receptor availability in central and peripheral neuropathic pain. Pain 2007;127(1–2):183–94.
22. Maarrawi J, Peyron R, Mertens P, et al. Motor cortex stimulation for pain control induces changes in the endogenous opioid system. Neurology 2007;69(9):827–34.
23. Maarrawi J, Peyron R, Mertens P, et al. Brain opioid receptor density predicts motor cortex stimulation efficacy for chronic pain. Pain 2013;154(11):2563–8.
24. Magis D, Bruno MA, Fumal A, et al. Central modulation in cluster headache patients treated with occipital nerve stimulation: an FDG-PET study. BMC Neurol 2011;11:25.
25. Maniyar FH, Sprenger T, Monteith T, Schankin C, Goadsby PJ. Brain activations in the premonitory phase of nitroglycerin-induced migraine attacks. Brain 2014; 137(1):232–41.
26. Matharu MS, Cohen AS, Frackowiak RS, Goadsby PJ. Posterior hypothalamic activation in paroxysmal hemicrania. Ann Neurol 2006;59(3):535–45.
27. Matharu MS, Cohen AS, McGonigle DJ, et al. Posterior hypothalamic and brainstem activation in hemicrania continua. Headache 2004;44(8):747–61.
28. May A, Leone M, Boecker H, et al. Hypothalamic deep brain stimulation in positron emission tomography. J Neurosci 2006;26(13):3589–93.
29. Mueller C, Klega A, Buchholz HG, et al. Basal opioid receptor binding is associated with differences in sensory perception in healthy human subjects: a [^{18}F] diprenorphine PET study. Neuroimage 2010;49(1):731–7.
30. Petrovic P, Kalso E, Petersson KM, Ingvar M. Placebo and opioid analgesia– imaging a shared neuronal network. Science 2002;295(5560):1737–40.
31. Peyron R, Faillenot I, Mertens P, et al. Motor cortex stimulation in neuropathic pain. Correlations between analgesic effect and hemodynamic changes in the brain. A PET study. Neuroimage 2007;34(1):310–21.
32. Peyron R, Laurent B, Garcia-Larrea L. Functional imaging of brain responses to pain. A review and meta-analysis (2000). Neurophysiol Clin 2000;30(5):263–88.
33. Sakai Y, Dobson C, Diksic M, et al. Sumatriptan normalizes the migraine attack-related increase in brain serotonin synthesis. Neurology 2008;70(6):431–9.
34. Schreckenberger M, Siessmeier T, Viertmann A, et al. The unpleasantness of tonic pain is encoded by the insular cortex. Neurology 2005;64(7):1175–83.
35. Sprenger T, Boecker H, Tolle TR, et al. Specific hypothalamic activation during a spontaneous cluster headache attack. Neurology 2004;62(3):516–7.
36. Sprenger T, Maniyar FH, Monteith TS, et al. Midbrain activation in the premonitory phase of migraine: a $H_2^{15}O$-positron emission tomography study. Headache 2012;52(863).
37. Sprenger T, Ruether KV, Boecker H, et al. Altered metabolism in frontal brain circuits in cluster headache. Cephalalgia 2007;27(9):1033–42.
38. Sprenger T, Valet M, Boecker H, et al. Opioidergic activation in the medial pain system after heat pain. Pain 2006;122(1–2):63–7.
39. Sprenger T, Willoch F, Miederer M, et al. Opioidergic changes in the pineal gland and hypothalamus in cluster headache: a ligand PET study. Neurology 2006;66(7):1108–10.
40. Tolle TR, Kaufmann T, Siessmeier T, et al. Region-specific encoding of sensory and affective components of pain in the human brain: a positron emission tomography correlation analysis. Ann Neurol 1999;45(1):40–7.
41. Wager TD, Scott DJ, Zubieta JK. Placebo effects on human mu-opioid activity during pain. Proc Natl Acad Sci USA 2007;104(26):11056–61.

42. Wagner KJ, Sprenger T, Kochs EF, et al. Imaging human cerebral pain modulation by dose-dependent opioid analgesia: a positron emission tomography activation study using remifentanil. Anesthesiology 2007;106(3):548–56.
43. Wagner KJ, Willoch F, Kochs EF, et al. Dose-dependent regional cerebral blood flow changes during remifentanil infusion in humans: a positron emission tomography study. Anesthesiology 2001;94(5):732–9.
44. Weiller C, May A, Limmroth V, et al. Brain stem activation in spontaneous human migraine attacks. Nat Med 1995;1(7):658–60.
45. Wik G, Fischer H, Bragee B, et al. Retrosplenial cortical activation in the fibromyalgia syndrome. Neuroreport 2003;14(4):619–21.
46. Willoch F, Schindler F, Wester HJ, et al. Central poststroke pain and reduced opioid receptor binding within pain processing circuitries: a [^{11}C] diprenorphine PET study. Pain 2004;108(3):213–20.
47. Yang J, Zeng F, Feng Y, et al. A PET-CT study on the specificity of acupoints through acupuncture treatment in migraine patients. BMC Complement Altern Med 2012;12:123.
48. Zubieta JK, Smith YR, Bueller JA, et al. Regional mu opioid receptor regulation of sensory and affective dimensions of pain. Science 2001;293(5528):311–5.

SECTION 4

Researching Mechanisms of Chronification of Acute Pain

CHAPTER 12

Predicting Chronic Pain After Joint Surgery

Kristian Kjær Petersen and Lars Arendt-Nielsen

Osteoarthritis (OA) is an increasing problem because of an increasingly aging population and lifestyle changes, and OA generally affects more women than men. Pain is the most common symptom leading individuals to seek medical attention and approx. 20% of the European population is estimated to suffer from pain caused by OA [40]. Patients can obtain pain relief by nonsurgical methods such as exercise, pain education, or pharmaceutical interventions in the early stages of OA [53]. The most severe OA patients will obtain pain relief from total joint arthroplasty (TJA), but some patients report severe pain after TJA and revision surgery based on the indications of pain does not seem to improve the pain state [46]. A US survey has estimated a sixfold increase in TJA, which will cause various problems including the increased number of patients developing chronic postoperative pain [34]. A better understanding of the factors important for developing chronic postoperative pain after this procedure is highly warranted, and the present chapter focuses on some of the pain mechanisms that may identify the patients most vulnerable to develop continued postoperative pain.

CHRONIC POSTOPERATIVE PAIN AFTER TOTAL JOINT ARTHROPLASTY

OA is defined by loss of cartilage with associated pain and function impairment. Severe obesity has been associated with acceleration of the osteoarthritic process [16], and because obesity is a growing problem [41], the number of patients with OA is expected to increase. Social factors have been found to play a significant role in the progression of arthritis [60].

Several pharmacologic and nonpharmacologic treatment guidelines are available for the early stages of OA [53]. End-stage OA is the main reason for TJA, and the incidence of TJA is increasing dramatically in these years [34] with total knee arthroplasty (TKA) and total hip arthroplasty (THA) expected to increase by 200% and 700%, respectively, before 2030 [34]. Chronic postoperative pain is defined by the International Association for the Study of Pain (IASP) as persistent pain 6 months after surgery. Increasing evidence suggests that nonpharmacologic approaches including exercise and BMI reduction will decrease pain in patients with joint pain [53]. However, a recent study showed that joint replacement surgery is still superior compared with exercise in patients with severe knee osteoarthritis (KOA) [59] although the exercise may postpone surgery. So far no randomized control studies have defined the most optimal exercise modality.

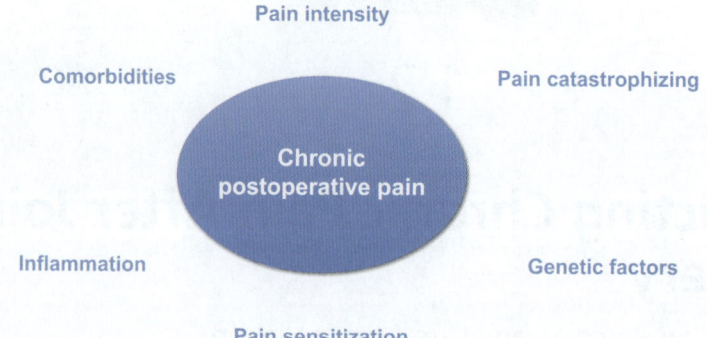

FIGURE 12-1 Preoperative risk factors for chronic postoperative pain following total joint arthroplasty.

TKA and THA have a low rate of technical errors. However, 20% of TKA patients and 10% of THA patients will suffer from chronic postoperative pain [7]. Around 80% to 90% of TKA and THA revision surgeries are performed because of pain, aseptic loosing, infection, instability, and stiffness. Following TKA revision surgery, up to 50% of the patients will continue to suffer from chronic postoperative pain [45]. Furthermore, TKA revision surgery is associated with a high risk of multiple revision surgeries [25]. In addition, revision TKA patients have been found to be less satisfied with the surgery compared with primary TKA patients [45].

Few attempts have been made to phenotype OA patients. However, the phenotyping studies have demonstrated different degeneration of the joint, different sensory pain profiles [2,19], and different outcomes after total joint replacement surgery [28,44,48,64] (Figure 12-1).

Clinical Assessment of Osteoarthritis

OA is recognized as a disease involving all joint tissues. However, the specific pain mechanisms and the actual origin of pain in OA are largely unknown. KOA is traditionally diagnosed based on a combination of symptomatic pain and stiffness indications and radiographic cartilage assessments such as the Kellgren and Lawrence (KL) score. Interestingly, the pain intensity reported by the patient and the radiologic score seem to be weakly correlated [1,17], suggesting that other extra-articular factors than cartilage might be important for OA pain. Biopsies of different joint tissues have found that, e.g., the synovium membrane, the Hoffa fat pad, and the subchondral bone are highly innervated, whereas the cartilage is minimally innervated under normal conditions although this may change in the progress of OA [17,26].

The preoperative pain intensity has been shown to be a clinical predictor of the development of chronic pain, and acute postoperative pain is correlated with the development of chronic postoperative pain [32]. In addition, higher analgesia consumption in the acute postoperative phase has been shown to be a risk factor [32,42].

Recent studies have investigated specific groups of patients with OA characterized by high pain intensities but low radiologic severity, and these patients seem to be highly pain-sensitive [3,19]. Furthermore, low radiologic severity before TKA has been linked to a low functional level after surgery [52], and recently low radiologic scores in combination with pain sensitivity profiles were found to be associated with less pain relief following TKA [47,65].

Comorbidities

Several preoperative comorbidities have been found to be associated directly or indirectly with chronic postoperative pain, and the following section will cover some of the more common comorbidities and the association with pain after TJA.

High preoperative fibromyalgia scores (defined by the American College of Rheumatology survey criteria) have been associated with less satisfaction, high opioid consumption, high risk of complications, and high postoperative pain levels [10]. Furthermore, an increased number of joints affected by OA have been associated with a high risk of chronic postoperative pain following TJA [43]. Interestingly, postoperative outcomes after TJA in patients with rheumatoid arthritis (RA) are still debated, and a large study by Goodman et al. [21] found that patients with RA had similar postoperative outcomes compared with patients with OA.

Increasing evidence suggests that obesity is associated with the progression of OA in both weight-bearing and non-weight-bearing joints [18]. Obese patients are known to present with higher preoperative pain intensities compared with nonobese patients [55]. However, the association between preoperative obesity and chronic postoperative pain is still debated. A recent study found that preoperative BMI was not associated with increasing postoperative complications [14]. Furthermore, obesity has been associated with increased inflammatory levels and development of diabetes, which is associated with a risk of neuropathy, which again is associated with pronociceptive sensory profiles [29].

Inflammation

Cytokines are known not only to contribute to the degradation of the joint but also to play an important role in pain generation [54]. In disease-free conditions the balance between proinflammatory and anti-inflammatory cytokines enables, e.g., a stable level of cartilage and does not interfere with pain. In recent years, the role of the synovium and synovitis in OA has attracted increased attention, and a systematic review from 2011 [67] concluded that synovitis is associated with knee OA pain. Serologic levels of interleukin (IL)-2, IL-4, and IL-10 have been detected in OA patients in the early and advanced stages [6]. One study found that the synovial fluid levels of IL-6 and tumor necrosis factor alpha (TNF-α) were associated with chronic postoperative pain after TKA [20]. Furthermore, proinflammatory cytokines, such as IL-1β, IL-6, IL-17, and TNF-α, are known to sensitize the peripheral nociceptors [54], which may potentially lead to facilitation of central pain pathways and an increased risk of chronic postoperative pain. Figure 12-2 illustrates this hypothesis; however, more research is required within this field.

Anti-inflammatory treatment is known to reduce the inflammatory response and potentially lower the risk of chronic postoperative pain. Based on this hypothesis, several small studies have investigated the effect of perioperative administration of cortisol and found this to reduce IL-6 and pain 24 to 48 hours postoperatively in both THA [56] and TKA [30] patients compared with placebo. However, further large studies with a long follow-up period are required to confirm the association with chronic postoperative pain following TJA.

Sensitization of the Nervous System

Sensitization of nociceptive fibers has been widely studied in the last decade with special focus on comparison between healthy and OA-affected subjects and recently also on the prognostic information in preoperative screening using quantitative sensory testing (QST).

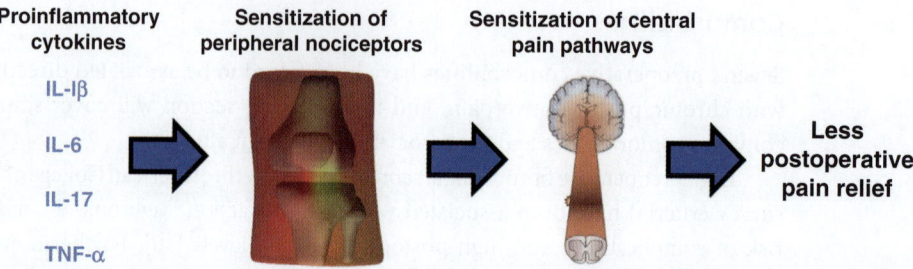

FIGURE 12-2 Proinflammatory cytokines have been associated with sensitization of peripheral nerve fibers. Ongoing nociceptive input can lead to sensitization of central pain pathways, which have been associated with chronic postoperative pain following total joint arthroplasty. This figure illustrates a working hypothesis. IL, interleukin; TNF-α, tumor necrosis factor alpha.

QST has been widely used to study peripheral and central sensitization in patients with musculoskeletal pain [4]. The concept of QST is to apply standardized stimuli under standardized conditions while the subject rates the pain perceived during the stimulus. The use of multiple stimulus modalities with different intensities or one prolonged stimulus with increasing intensity enables determination of stimulus–response relationships to characterize the pain sensitivity of the subjects. Hyperalgesia in an OA patient can objectively be quantified by a leftward shift in the stimulus–response curve compared with a healthy control subject.

QST aims at giving an insight into the pain mechanisms compared with, e.g., the simple visual analogue scale (VAS). However, QST is time-consuming and requires training of the subject to perform a reliable and accurate rating of the pain stimuli. Combining different stimulation techniques allows for a more "complete" quantification of the state of the nervous system [4]. A simple bedside testing test platform to assess sensitization is highly warranted, but currently no simplistic device has been developed despite various attempts [13].

Three main measurements are generally applied when assessing the pain sensitivity in OA, i.e., pressure pain thresholds, temporal summation of pain (TSP), and conditioned pain modulation (CPM) [4]. In general, patients with OA present with widespread hyperalgesia, facilitated TSP, and impaired CPM compared with healthy controls [4], indicating that the central pain pathways have been changed in these patients. A few studies have investigated changes in central pain pathways when comparing OA patients with other patients. However, the results indicate that these different sensory profiles may hold information on pain after TJA, and the following section will cover different sensory profiles in OA patients.

A recent study investigated the range of early to severe OA, defined by pain and radiologic OA, and found that the pressure pain sensitivity increased with increasing pain and structural damage [2]. Furthermore, the study found a specific phenotype based on low structural OA but high pain intensity. This group was characterized by facilitated TSP and impaired CPM [2], indicating a pronociceptive profile in this specific group.

Several studies have attempted to apply phenotyping of patients before or after TJA. First, Petersen et al. [48] investigated knee OA patients based on clinical pain intensities 12 months following TKA and found that patients with chronic postoperative pain had preoperatively facilitated TSP compared with patients with a normal recovery after TKA. Furthermore, Petersen et al. [44] phenotyped patients based on preoperative TSP and CPM and found that patients with preoperatively facilitated TSP and impaired CPM had less pain relief 12 months following TKA compared with patients with other preoperative sensory profiles. Wylde et al. [65] found that preoperative widespread hyperalgesia in combination with low structural damage (low radiologic OA) was associated with less pain relief following TJA. Similarly, Petersen et al. [47] found that preoperative low radiologic OA and facilitated TSP were associated with chronic postoperative pain following TKA. Recently, Izumi et al. [28] found that preoperatively facilitated TSP was associated with less pain relief 6 weeks after THA. Furthermore, preoperative TSP [47,48] and widespread hyperalgesia [44] have been found independently of preoperative VAS in association with chronic postoperative pain, suggesting that the addition of preoperative measures of central sensitization provides information on patient risk compared with the VAS measure alone.

Collectively, these studies indicate that the state of the central nervous system before TJA may hold information on postoperative pain outcomes following TJA. However, future studies are required to validate this.

Sensitization seems to be normalized in patients with a pain-free recovery when comparing pre- and postoperative QST measurements following TKA [23] and THA [33]. However, patients with ongoing pain after primary TKA can be offered revision TKA surgery (re-TKA). In general, re-TKA involves a high risk of a poor outcome [45], and after re-TKA, patients with pain show widespread hyperalgesia, facilitated TSP, and impaired CPM compared with patients with no pain after re-TKA [58]. Facilitated temporal summation is more predominant in KOA patients with widespread hyperalgesia after re-TKA compared with KOA patients before primary TKA [57]. Despite the removal of the OA-affected joint, this could indicate a continued nociceptive drive, further indicating that sensitization could play a key role in the chronification of postoperative pain. This suggests that sensitization should also be considered before re-TKA.

Different pharmaceutical treatments have been applied to improve pronociceptive profiles. Duloxetine has been found to increase CPM in patients with painful neuropathy [66], ketamine has been shown to reduce TSP and widespread hyperalgesia in patients with fibromyalgia [24], and pregabalin has been found to decrease widespread hyperalgesia in patients with chronic pancreatitis [9], indicating that these drugs could improve preoperative sensory profiles. Buvanendran et al. [12] found perioperative administration of pregabalin to reduce neuropathic pain 6 months after TKA, but a recent systematic review [37] found that perioperative pregabalin had no effect on chronic postoperative pain. Similarly, Lunn et al. [36] found no effect of perioperative gabapentin on postoperative pain following TKA. However, more research is required to describe the association between pharmaceutical interventions and pronociceptive profiles and the potential to reduce chronic postoperative pain.

Genetics and Joint Pain

Genetic epidemiology is the study of genetic factors influencing the dynamics of disease in populations. Studies have shown that genetics can influence the risk of developing OA and the progression in the different stages of OA. Obesity, gender, age, skeletal shape, and bone mass are examples of genetic factors that can influence the progression of OA. Low age is linked with a more vigorous neoplastic response, and gender differences have been shown in relation to pain modulation. Therefore, low age and gender differences are classified as risk factors for postoperative pain after joint replacement. More women than men are diagnosed with OA [61], and in general women report higher postoperative pain than men [32].

If possible, untreated comorbidities and other pain problems than the primary reason for surgery should be identified and treated to minimize the risk of postoperative chronic pain [32].

Less known examples of genetic factors are genetically increased pain sensitivity or genes encoding for, e.g., ILs. The catechol-O-methyltransferase (COMT gene) has been shown to be associated with hip pain in patients with hip OA, and the gene coding for IL-6 has been positively correlated with osteolysis in patients after THA [22]. Other genetic factors include the single nucleotide polymorphism (SNP) in the SCN9A gene (encoding for specific sodium channels), which is associated with increased pain levels if present in OA patients leading to changed pain thresholds [49]. In recent years, epigenetic modifications have been found to be a new and important factor in pain [39] and may show to be important for developing chronic postoperative pain.

Psychological Factors

During the last decade, depression and anxiety have been studied as potential underlying mechanisms for pain in patients with OA. For specific causes of pain, self-efficacy (the belief that one has the ability to control pain) [35], pain catastrophizing (the belief that pain will get worse and that one cannot deal with it) [31], and fear of movement (the belief that movement will generate pain and additional injury) [27] have been studied. Pain catastrophizing and chronic postoperative pain have been widely studied, and it has been demonstrated that overall high levels of preoperative pain catastrophizing is associated with a high level of chronic postoperative pain [11]. A recent review concluded that the preoperative presence of catastrophic thinking and poor coping strategies predicts high postoperative pain, that there is no association between preoperative fear of movement and postoperative pain, and that there is conflicting evidence whether preoperative depressive symptoms and anxiety predict postoperative pain after TKA [5].

Cognitive behavioral therapy (CBT) aims to identify maladaptive thoughts and change these into more realistic and constructive thoughts consequently reducing the pain experience. Riddle et al. [50] investigated preoperative administration of CBT in 18 KOA patients and found this to reduce the pain severity and pain catastrophizing 2 months after TKA compared with usual care. Other psychological interventions such as acceptance and commitment therapy [62] and mindfulness-based stress reduction [63] have been found as effective as the traditional CBT [15,68].

Currently, no studies have investigated the effect of treatment targeting preoperative pain catastrophizing and the potential reduction of chronic postoperative pain after TJA; however, several randomized control trial protocols are currently being conducted [8,38,51].

CONCLUSION

Pain following TJA is an increasing clinical problem with 20% of TKA patients and 10% of THA patients developing chronic postoperative pain.

Preoperative pain sensitization has been shown to predict the development of chronic postoperative pain in patients undergoing TKA and THA. Furthermore, patients with a preoperatively low degree of radiologic OA but with a high pain level seem to be highly sensitized, and these patients seem to have high risk of chronic postoperative pain.

Pharmaceutical intervention aiming at improving central sensitization is still debated, and currently no pharmaceutical intervention can be recommended to lower the risk of chronic postoperative pain.

The preoperative pain intensity has been shown to be a clinical predictor of the development of chronic pain, and acute postoperative pain is correlated with the development of chronic postoperative pain. In addition, high analgesia consumption in the acute postoperative phase has been shown to be a risk factor. Women seem to have a higher risk of chronic postoperative pain than men, and an association between low age and the development of chronic postoperative pain has been shown.

Inflammation can lead to sensitization of the nervous fibers, and a preoperative imbalance of specific cytokines has been linked to chronic postoperative pain after TKA; however, further research is required within this field.

Pain catastrophizing has been shown to be a preoperative risk factor for chronic postoperative pain following TJA, and several studies are currently being conducted to investigate if preoperative pain catastrophizing can be lowered, thereby reducing the risk of chronic postoperative pain.

Currently, several preoperative risk factors have been identified, but evidence on preoperative treatment of these risk factors and the associated lowering of the incidence of chronic postoperative is still missing.

REFERENCES

1. Arendt-Nielsen L. Joint pain: more to it than just structural damage? Pain 2017;158:66–73.
2. Arendt-Nielsen L, Egsgaard LL, Petersen KK, Eskehave TN, Graven-Nielsen T, Hoeck HC, Simonsen O. A mechanism-based pain sensitivity index to characterize knee osteoarthritis patients with different disease stages and pain levels. Eur J Pain 2015;19:1406–17.
3. Arendt-Nielsen L, Eskehave TN, Egsgaard LL, Petersen KK, Graven-Nielsen T, Hoeck HC, Simonsen O, Siebuhr AS, Karsdal M, Bay-Jensen AC. Association between experimental pain biomarkers and serologic markers in patients with different degrees of painful knee osteoarthritis. Arthritis Rheumatol 2014;66:3317–26.
4. Arendt-Nielsen L, Skou ST, Nielsen TA, Petersen KK. Altered central sensitization and pain modulation in the CNS in chronic joint pain. Curr Osteoporos Rep 2015;13:225–34.
5. Baert IAC, Lluch E, Mulder T, Nijs J, Noten S, Meeus M. Does pre-surgical central modulation of pain influence outcome after total knee replacement? A systematic review. Osteoarthritis Cartilage 2016;24:213–23.
6. Barker T, Rogers VE, Henriksen VT, Aguirre D, Trawick RH, Rasmussen GL, Momberger NG. Serum cytokines are increased and circulating micronutrients are not altered in subjects with early compared to advanced knee osteoarthritis. Cytokine 2014;68:133–6.
7. Beswick AD, Wylde V, Gooberman-Hill R, Blom A, Dieppe P. What proportion of patients report long-term pain after total hip or knee replacement for osteoarthritis? A systematic review of prospective studies in unselected patients. BMJ Open 2012;2:e000435.
8. Birch S, Stilling M, Mechlenburg I, Hansen TB. Effectiveness of a physiotherapist delivered cognitive-behavioral patient education for patients who undergoes operation for total knee arthroplasty: a protocol of a randomized controlled trial. BMC Musculoskelet Disord 2017;18:116.
9. Bouwense SA, Olesen SS, Drewes AM, Poley J-W, van Goor H, Wilder-Smith OHG. Effects of pregabalin on central sensitization in patients with chronic pancreatitis in a randomized, controlled trial. PLoS One 2012;7:e42096.
10. Brummett CM, Janda AM, Schueller CM, Tsodikov A, Morris M, Williams DA, Clauw DJ. Survey criteria for fibromyalgia independently predict increased postoperative opioid consumption after lower-extremity joint arthroplasty: a prospective, observational cohort study. Anesthesiology 2013;119:1434–43.
11. Burns LC, Ritvo SE, Ferguson MK, Clarke H, Seltzer Z, Katz J. Pain catastrophizing as a risk factor for chronic pain after total knee arthroplasty: a systematic review. J Pain Res 2015;8:21–32.
12. Buvanendran A, Kroin JS, Della Valle CJ, Kari M, Moric M, Tuman KJ. Perioperative oral pregabalin reduces chronic pain after total knee arthroplasty: a prospective, randomized, controlled trial. Anesth Analg 2010;110:199–207.

13. Eaton T, Osgood E, Trudeau J, Jensen M, Gammaitoni A, Simon L, Katz N. Development of a bedside sensory testing kit for the neurologic classification of patients with osteoarthritis. J Pain 2012;13:S10.
14. Edelstein AI, Suleiman LI, Alvarez A, Sacotte R, Qin CD, Beal M, Manning DW. The interaction of obesity and metabolic syndrome in determining risk of complication following total joint arthroplasty. J Arthroplasty 2016;31(9 Suppl.):192-6.
15. Ehde DM, Dillworth TM, Turner JA. Cognitive-behavioral therapy for individuals with chronic pain: efficacy, innovations, and directions for research. Am Psychol 2014;69:153–66.
16. Eymard F, Parsons C, Edwards MH, Petit-Dop F, Reginster JY, Bruyère O, Richette P, Cooper C, Chevalier X. Diabetes is a risk factor for knee osteoarthritis progression. Osteoarthritis Cartilage 2015;23:851–9.
17. Felson DT. The sources of pain in knee osteoarthritis. Curr Opin Rheumatol 2005;17:624–8.
18. Felson DT. Weight and osteoarthritis. Am J Clin Nutr 1996;63:430S–2S.
19. Finan PH, Buenaver LF, Bounds SC, Hussain S, Park RJ, Haque UJ, Campbell CM, Haythornthwaite JA, Edwards RR, Smith MT. Discordance between pain and radiographic severity in knee osteoarthritis: findings from quantitative sensory testing of central sensitization. Arthritis Rheum 2013;65:363–72.
20. Gandhi R, Santone D, Takahashi M, Dessouki O, Mahomed NN. Inflammatory predictors of ongoing pain 2 years following knee replacement surgery. Knee 2013;20:316–8.
21. Goodman SM, Johnson B, Zhang M, Huang W-T, Zhu R, Figgie M, Alexiades M, Mandl LA. Patients with rheumatoid arthritis have similar excellent outcomes after total knee replacement compared with patients with osteoarthritis. J Rheumatol 2015;43:46–53.
22. Gordon A, Kiss-Toth E, Stockley I, Eastell R, Wilkinson JM. Polymorphisms in the interleukin-1 receptor antagonist and interleukin-6 genes affect risk of osteolysis in patients with total hip arthroplasty. Arthritis Rheum 2008;58:3157–65.
23. Graven-Nielsen T, Wodehouse T, Langford RM, Arendt-Nielsen L, Kidd BL. Normalization of widespread hyperesthesia and facilitated spatial summation of deep-tissue pain in knee osteoarthritis patients after knee replacement. Arthritis Rheum 2012;64:2907–16.
24. Graven-Nielsen T, Aspegren Kendall S, Henriksson KG, Bengtsson M, Sörensen J, Johnson A, Gerdle B, Arendt-Nielsen L, Sörensen J, Johnson A, Gerdle B, Arendt-Nielsen L. Ketamine reduces muscle pain, temporal summation, and referred pain in fibromyalgia patients. Pain 2000;85:483–91.
25. Graves S. Australian Orthopaedic Association National Joint Replacement Registry. 2001.
26. Grässel S. The role of peripheral nerve fibers and their neurotransmitters in cartilage and bone physiology and pathophysiology. Arthritis Res Ther 2014;16:485.
27. Heuts PHTG, Vlaeyen JWS, Roelofs J, De Bie RA, Aretz K, Van Weel C, Van Schayck OCP. Pain-related fear and daily functioning in patients with osteoarthritis. Pain 2004;110:228–35.
28. Izumi M, Petersen KK, Laursen MB, Arendt-Nielsen L, Graven-Nielsen T. Facilitated temporal summation of pain correlates with clinical pain intensity after hip arthroplasty. Pain 2017;158:323–32.
29. Jensen TS, Finnerup NB. Allodynia and hyperalgesia in neuropathic pain: clinical manifestations and mechanisms. Lancet Neurol 2014;13:924–35.
30. Jules-Elysee KM, Wilfred SE, Memtsoudis SG, Kim DH, YaDeau JT, Urban MK, Lichardi ML, McLawhorn AS, Sculco TP. Steroid modulation of cytokine release and desmosine levels in bilateral total knee replacement. J Bone Joint Surg Am 2012;94:2120–7.
31. Keefe F, Smith S, Buffington A. Recent advances and future directions in the biopsychosocial assessment and treatment of arthritis. J Consult Clin Psychol 2002;70:640.
32. Kehlet H, Jensen TS, Woolf CJ, Centre M. Persistent postsurgical pain: risk factors and prevention. Lancet 2006;367:1618–25.
33. Kosek E, Ordeberg G. Lack of pressure pain modulation by heterotopic noxious conditioning stimulation in patients with painful osteoarthritis before, but not following, surgical pain relief. Pain 2000;88:69–78.
34. Kurtz S, Ong K, Lau E, Mowat F, Halpern M. Projections of primary and revision hip and knee arthroplasty in the United States from 2005 to 2030. J Bone Joint Surg Am 2007;89:780–5.
35. Lorig K, González VM, Laurent DD, Morgan L, Laris BA. Arthritis self-management program variations: three studies. Arthritis Care Res 1998;11:448–54.
36. Lunn TH, Husted H, Laursen MB, Hansen LT, Kehlet H. Analgesic and sedative effects of perioperative gabapentin in total knee arthroplasty: a randomized, double-blind, placebo-controlled, dose-finding study. Pain 2015;156:1.
37. Martinez V, Pichard X, Fletcher D. Perioperative pregabalin administration does not prevent chronic postoperative pain. Systematic review with a meta-analysis of randomized trials. Pain 2017;158(5):775–83.
38. das Nair R, Anderson P, Clarke S, Leighton P, Lincoln NB, Mhizha-Murira JR, Scammell BE, Walsh DA. Home-administered pre-surgical psychological intervention for knee osteoarthritis (HAPPiKNEES): study protocol for a randomised controlled trial. Trials 2016;17:54.

39. Niederberger E, Resch E, Parnham MJ, Geisslinger G. Drugging the pain epigenome. Nat Rev Neurol 2017;13(7):434–47.
40. O'Brien T, Breivik H. The impact of chronic pain-European patients' perspective over 12 months. Scand J Pain 2012;3:23–9.
41. Ogden CL, Carroll MD, Fryar CD, Flegal KM. Prevalence of obesity among adults and youth: United States, 2011-2014. NCHS Data Brief 2015:1–8.
42. Perkins FM, Kehlet H. Chronic pain as an outcome of surgery. A review of predictive factors. J Am Soc Anesthesiol 2000;93:1123–33.
43. Perruccio AV., Power JD, Evans HMK, Mahomed SR, Gandhi R, Mahomed NN, Davis AM. Multiple joint involvement in total knee replacement for osteoarthritis: effects on patient-reported outcomes. Arthritis Care Res 2012;64:838–46.
44. Petersen KK, Graven-Nielsen T, Simonsen O, Laursen MB, Arendt-Nielsen L. Preoperative pain mechanisms assessed by cuff algometry are associated with chronic postoperative pain relief after total knee replacement. Pain 2016;157:1400–6.
45. Petersen KK, Simonsen O, Laursen MB, Nielsen TA, Rasmussen S, Arendt-Nielsen L. Chronic postoperative pain after primary and revision total knee arthroplasty. Clin J Pain 2015;31:1–6.
46. Petersen KK, Simonsen O, Laursen MB, Rasmussen S, Arendt-Nielsen L. Persisting postoperative pain following primary and revision total knee arthroplasty. [n.d.].
47. Petersen KK, Simonsen O, Laursen MB, Arendt-Nielsen L. The role of preoperative radiologic severity, sensory testing, and temporal summation on chronic postoperative pain following total knee arthroplasty. Clin J Pain 2018;34(3):193–7.
48. Petersen KK, Arendt-Nielsen L, Simonsen O, Wilder-Smith O, Laursen MB. Presurgical assessment of temporal summation of pain predicts the development of chronic postoperative pain 12 months after total knee replacement. Pain 2015;156:55–61.
49. Reimann F, Cox JJ, Belfer I, Diatchenko L, Zaykin DV, McHale DP, Drenth JPH, Dai F, Wheeler J, Sanders F, Wood L, Wu T-X, Karppinen J, Nikolajsen L, Männikkö M, Max MB, Kiselycznyk C, Poddar M, Te Morsche RHM, Smith S, Gibson D, Kelempisioti A, Maixner W, Gribble FM, Woods CG. Pain perception is altered by a nucleotide polymorphism in SCN9A. Proc Natl Acad Sci USA 2010;107:5148–53.
50. Riddle D, Keefe F, Nay W, McKee D, Attarian D, Jensen M. Pain coping skills training for patients with elevated pain catastrophizing who are scheduled for knee artroplasty: a quasi-experimental study. Arch Phys Med Rehabil 2011;92:859–65.
51. Riddle DL, Keefe FJ, Ang D, Khaled J, Dumenci L, Jensen MP, Bair MJ, Reed SD, Kroenke K. A phase III randomized three-arm trial of physical therapist delivered pain coping skills training for patients with total knee arthroplasty: the KASTPain protocol. BMC Musculoskelet Disord 2012;13:149.
52. Riis A, Rathleff MS, Jensen MB, Simonsen O. Low grading of the severity of knee osteoarthritis pre-operatively is associated with a lower functional level after total knee replacement: a prospective cohort study with 12 months' follow-up. Bone Joint J 2014;96–B:1498–502.
53. Roos EM, Juhl CB. Osteoarthritis 2012 year in review: rehabilitation and outcomes. Osteoarthritis Cartilage 2012;20:1477–83.
54. Schaible HG. Nociceptive neurons detect cytokines in arthritis. Arthritis Res Ther 2014:470.
55. Schett G, Kleyer A, D'Agostino MA, Perricone C, Iagnocco A, Sahinbegovic E, Berenbaum F, Zwerina J, Willeit J, Kiechl S. Diabetes mellitus as an independent predictor for severe osteoarthritis. Ann Rheum Dis 2013;71:403–9.
56. Sculco PK, McLawhorn AS, Desai N, Su EP, Padgett DE, Jules-Elysee K. The effect of perioperative corticosteroids in total hip arthroplasty: a prospective double-blind placebo controlled pilot study. J Arthroplasty 2016;31:1208–12.
57. Skou ST, Graven-Nielsen T, Rasmussen S, Simonsen OH, Laursen MB, Arendt-Nielsen L. Facilitation of pain and sensitization in knee osteoarthritis – a cross-sectional study on symptomatic osteoarthritis and revision total knee arthroplasty pain patients. Eur J Pain 2014;18(7):1024–31.
58. Skou ST, Graven-Nielsen T, Rasmussen S, Simonsen OH, Laursen MB, Arendt-Nielsen L. Widespread sensitization in patients with chronic pain after revision total knee arthroplasty. Pain 2013;154:1588–94.
59. Skou ST, Roos EM, Laursen MB, Rathleff MS, Arendt-Nielsen L, Simonsen O. A randomized, controlled trial of total knee replacement. N Engl J Med 2015;373:1597–606.
60. Sokka T, Abelson B, Pincus T. Mortality in rheumatoid arthritis: 2008 update. Clin Exp Rheumatol 2008;26.
61. Suokas A, Walsh D, McWilliams D, Condon L, Moreton B, Wylde V, Arendt-Nielsen L, Zhang W. Quantitative sensory testing in painful osteoarthritis: a systematic review and meta-analysis (structured abstract). Osteoarthritis Cartilage 2012;20:1075–85.

62. Trompetter HR, Bohlmeijer ET, Fox JP, Schreurs KMG. Psychological flexibility and catastrophizing as associated change mechanisms during online Acceptance & Commitment Therapy for chronic pain. Behav Res Ther 2015;74:50–9.
63. Turner JA, Anderson ML, Balderson BH, Cook AJ, Sherman KJ, Cherkin DC. Mindfulness-based stress reduction and cognitive-behavioral therapy for chronic low back pain: similar effects on mindfulness, catastrophizing, self-efficacy, and acceptance in a randomized controlled trial. Pain 2016;157:2434–44.
64. Wylde V, Sayers A, Lenguerrand E, Gooberman-Hill R, Pyke M, Beswick AD, Dieppe P, Blom AW. Preoperative widespread pain sensitization and chronic pain after hip and knee replacement. Pain 2015;156:47–54.
65. Wylde V, Sayers A, Odutola A, Gooberman-Hill R, Dieppe P, Blom AW. Central sensitization as a determinant of patients' benefit from total hip and knee replacement. Eur J Pain 2017;21:357–65.
66. Yarnitsky D, Granot M, Nahman-Averbuch H, Khamaisi M, Granovsky Y. Conditioned pain modulation predicts duloxetine efficacy in painful diabetic neuropathy. Pain 2012;153:1193–8.
67. Yusuf E, Kortekaas MC, Watt I, Huizinga TWJ, Kloppenburg M. Do knee abnormalities visualised on MRI explain knee pain in knee osteoarthritis? A systematic review. Ann Rheum Dis 2011;70:60–7.
68. Öst LG. Efficacy of the third wave of behavioral therapies: a systematic review and meta-analysis. Behav Res Ther 2008;46:296–321.

CHAPTER 13

Altered Perioperative Pain Processing and Persistent Pain After Surgery

Oliver H.G. Wilder-Smith

It is generally accepted that patients with chronic pain exhibit altered pain processing [3,11,41,59]. Typically, these changes affect pain processing by the central nervous system (CNS), in the sense of the CNS becoming more sensitive to painful sensory inputs [42,43]. Hyperalgesia due to such "central sensitization" is frequently segmental in earlier disease stages, tending to spread away from the initial source of nociception with disease progression [47]. In advanced or severe chronic pain disorders, spreading hyperalgesia can be generalized all over the body [16], classically also affecting heterotopic deep tissues such as muscle [5,10,19,32]. Many patients with chronic pain further suffer from the disorder of their endogenous pain modulation systems, which can additionally contribute to increased pain sensitivity [12,24,25,27,33,36,51]. Key in this context is the function of the pathways descending from the brainstem to the posterior spinal horn, where disorder can range from inadequate inhibitory control to overt descending facilitation [22,50,60].

The clinical factors most frequently associated with increased risk of chronic pain development after surgery include the presence of pre- and postoperative pain, type and extent of surgery, and nerve damage [1,23,34]. All of these factors have in common that they can be expressions of increased pain sensitivity or hyperalgesia (more pre- or postoperative pain, more postoperative analgesia consumption) or a cause thereof (nerve damage, more extensive surgery) [1,23,29,31,34,54]. Furthermore, nerve damage is not only directly associated with hyperalgesia, it is also linked to more central sensitization and reorganization as well as loss of descending inhibitory controls and even conversion to descending facilitation [4,7,13,17,18,35,37,46,48,49,59].

Taking these two aspects together (Figure 13-1), it would seem that a crucial step in understanding why certain patients develop chronic pain after surgery would be to document the *changes in CNS pain processing*, which take place after surgery. Appreciating how these changes develop in time, and how they are affected by a variety of pre-, intra-, and postoperative factors internal and external to the patient, could then provide the foundation for effective prediction/monitoring and prevention/treatment of chronic pain development in clinical practice. The present chapter seeks to summarize what is known to date regarding these issues.

MEASURING ALTERED PAIN PROCESSING IN PATIENTS

With the advent of validated quantitative sensory testing (QST) methods suitable for use in patients, it has become feasible to research the alterations in pain processing following

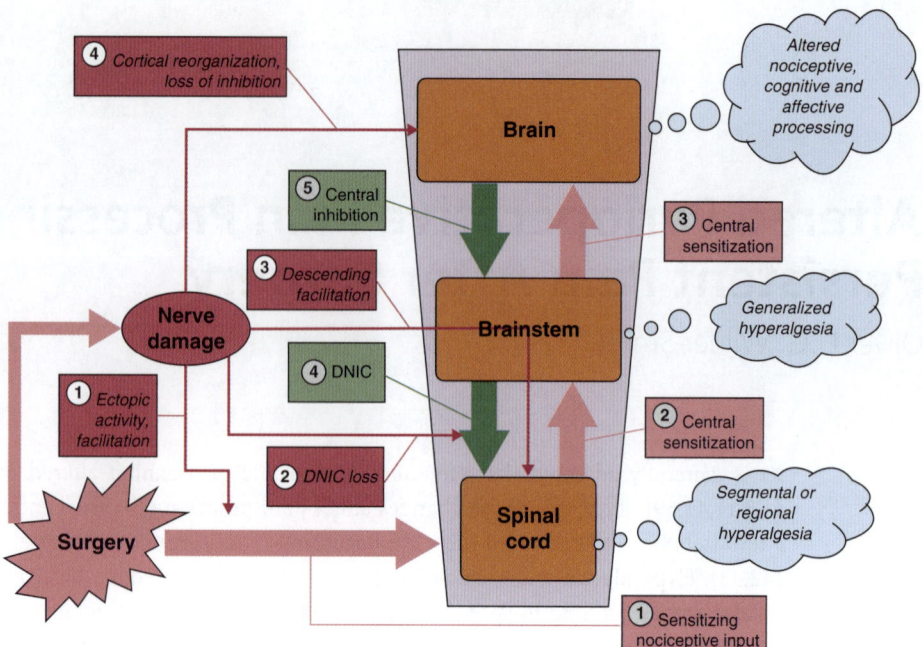

FIGURE 13-1 Effects of ongoing nociception (e.g., due to surgery) on central pain processing. There is progressive rostral neuraxial spread of central sensitization, *filled circles* 1 to 3. Nerve damage results in altered CNS function, *unfilled circles* 1 to 4. Manifestations of CNS sensitization are listed in the *gray clouds*. Rostral spread of central sensitization is subject to descending modulation, *filled circles* 4 to 5. DNIC, diffuse noxious inhibitory controls.

surgery in clinical patient cohorts [14,15,26,28,55–58]. Reliable QST techniques are now available to assess the time course of both aspects of altered central pain processing named earlier, namely spreading central sensitization and dysfunction of inhibitory descending pain modulation. Databases documenting pain sensitivities in healthy volunteers are now available, permitting assessment of individual degree of deviation from normal values [39,40]. We have developed and implemented a clinical screening QST paradigm suitable for this purpose [52]. The Nijmegen–Aalborg Screening QST (NASQ) paradigm detects spreading central sensitization by bilaterally mapping pain sensitivity at several standardized body sites [52]. Heterotopic spread of sensitization is assessed by measuring skin as well as deep tissue pain sensitivity using electric and pressure algometry devices. The NASQ investigates dysfunction of descending endogenous pain modulation using a conditioned pain modulation (CPM) paradigm [21,38,61]. The NASQ CPM paradigm uses the cold pressor task as conditioning stimulation and electric and pressure pain tolerance thresholds as test stimuli before and after conditioning stimulation. As an alternative QST approach, other groups have implemented mapping techniques, e.g., using pinprick stimulation, to detect areas of hyperalgesia surrounding sites of surgery [14,15,26,28,44].

Using such QST paradigms, we are now in a position to explore the alterations in central pain processing resulting from the ongoing nociception of surgery, their relationship to chronic pain development after surgery, and the factors influencing postsurgical altered pain processing and chronic pain.

EARLY POSTOPERATIVE PERIOD: PAIN PROCESSING IN THE FIRST WEEK AFTER SURGERY

A number of studies have followed alterations in central pain processing using pain thresholds in the first week after surgery [55,57,58]. Figure 13-2 shows a typical example from this first type of studies [58].

Taken together, such studies show a biphasic response in the first week after surgery regarding pain sensitivity. In the first 24 hours postoperatively there is a generalized, predominantly hypoalgesic response, more marked caudally. This is followed by hyperalgesia both close to—and distant from—surgery 5 days after the operation. Postoperative alterations in pain processing do not correlate well with clinical pain measures such as visual analogue scale (VAS) or morphine patient-controlled analgesia use. Pre- and intraoperative analgesic supplementation (e.g., opioids, ketamine, magnesium) increases hypoalgesia in the first 24 hours after surgery, particularly distant from surgery. It also markedly decreases hyperalgesia distant from surgery 5 days postoperatively, with smaller effects on peri-incisional hyperalgesia. This positive effect is not seen with ketorolac supplementation. The marked day 5 hyperalgesia seen after back surgery is not seen after abdominal hysterectomy, probably because of the absence of the extensive nerve damage seen in back pain and surgery. Of interest is the fact that the presence of pain preoperatively in back surgery patients is linked to much more—and increasing—hyperalgesia after surgery, particularly at 5 days (Figure 13-3).

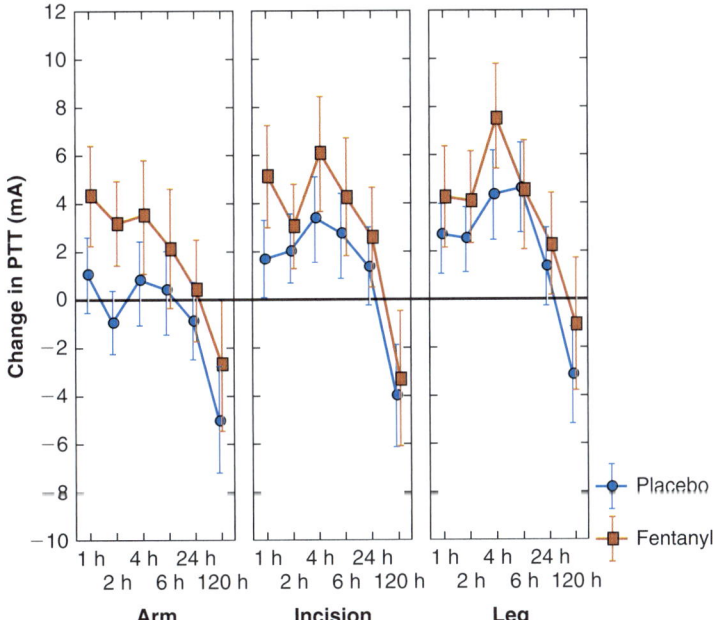

FIGURE 13-2 Alterations in electric pain tolerance thresholds in patients after back surgery. They show a predominantly hypoalgesic response, greater in the presence of analgesic opioid (fentanyl) supplementation, for the first 24 h postoperatively. Five days postoperatively, significant segmental and spreading hyperalgesia appears, predominantly in the placebo group. The vertical axis shows change in electric pain tolerance thresholds (PTT) preoperatively (in mA). The upper horizontal axis shows time postoperatively in hours; the lower horizontal axis shows site of threshold measurement (arm, peri-incisionally in the back, leg). Values are means and 95% confidence intervals. (Modified from Wilder-Smith OH, Tassonyi E, Senly C, et al. Surgical pain is followed not only by spinal sensitization but also by supraspinal antinociception. Br J Anaesth 1996;76(6):816–21.)

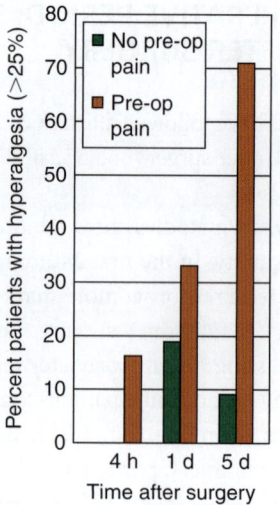

FIGURE 13-3 Effects of presence or absence of preoperative pain on incidence (in percent) of postoperative hyperalgesia greater than 25% (vertical axis) in back surgery patients. Horizontal axis gives hours (H) or days (D) postoperatively. (Modified after Wilder-Smith OH. Chronic pain and surgery: a review of new insights from sensory testing. J Pain Palliat Care Pharmacother 2011;25(2):146–59.)

A second type of study uses pinprick stimulation to map early peri-incisional changes in pain processing [14,15,26,28,44]. An example of such a study is summarized in Figure 13-4 [26]. The findings are congruent with those of the first type of studies. Again there is no strong link between postoperative hyperalgesia and clinical measures of pain. The area of peri-incisional hyperalgesia increases with time the first few days after surgery, and perioperative analgesic supplementation or locoregional analgesia use is associated with smaller areas of postoperative peri-incisional hyperalgesia. Of particular importance is the demonstration of a strong link between greater areas of early (week 1) postoperative peri-incisional hyperalgesia and more chronic pain up to 1 year after surgery [15,26,28]. Moreover, nerve damage is not only associated with larger areas of hyperalgesia but also with more chronic pain [28].

In summary, pain processing during the first postoperative week initially shifts in the direction of acute, generalized inhibition (the first day or so). This is followed by the development and rapid spread of hyperalgesia not only over the skin but also to deeper tissues. Worse perioperative analgesia and nerve damage are associated with more week-1 spreading hyperalgesia; this in turn is associated with more persisting pain up to 1 year postoperatively. Subjective pain experience (e.g., pain scores) does not reliably reflect these alterations in central pain processing.

LATE POSTOPERATIVE PERIOD: PAIN PROCESSING UP TO 6 MONTHS AFTER SURGERY

We are aware of only one study prospectively, systematically, and longitudinally documenting the long-term time course of alterations in central pain processing after surgery [56]. The main results of this study recruiting patients undergoing major abdominal surgery in standardized general anesthesia are summarized in Figure 13-5. Compared with patients not reporting chronic pain, patients with chronic pain show significantly more skin and deep tissue hyperalgesia distant from the surgical site 1 day to 6 months

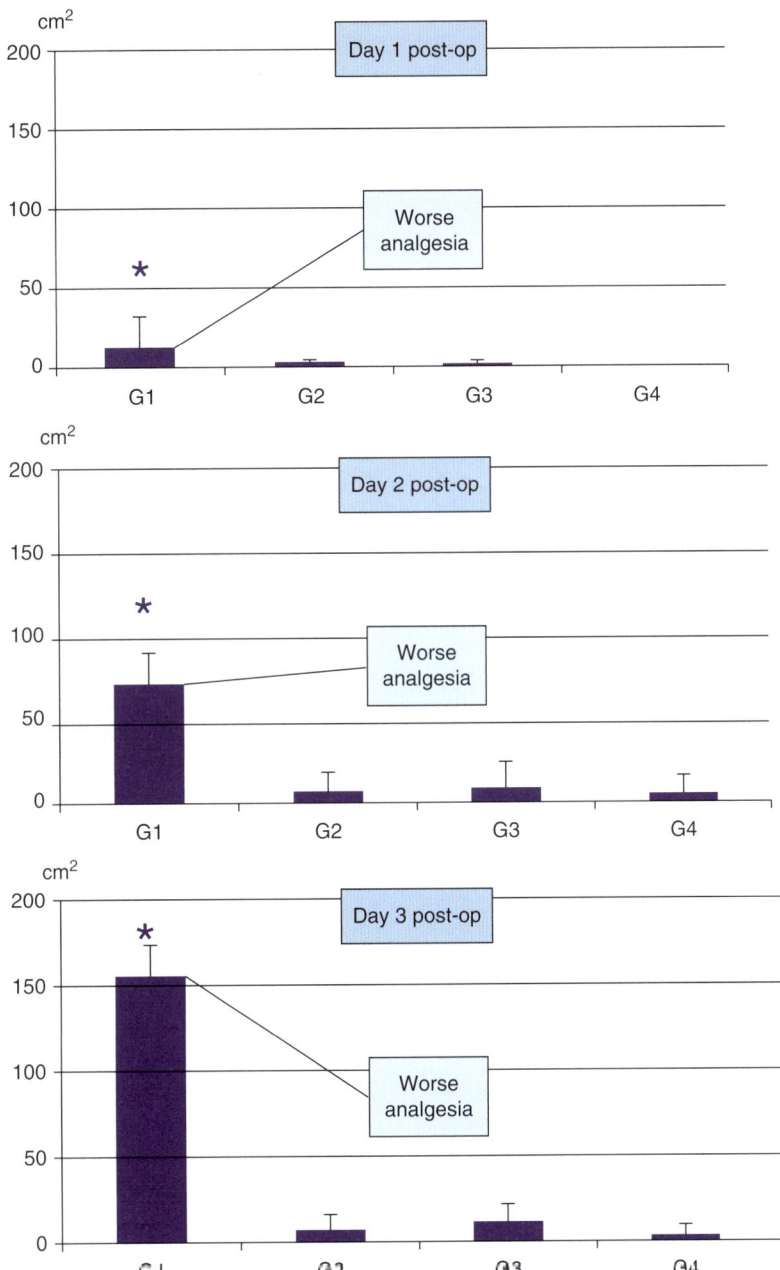

FIGURE 13-4 Area (vertical axis) of secondary mechanical hyperalgesia surrounding abdominal incision for colectomy measured using von Frey filaments at 24, 48, and 72 h post-op. At all times hyperalgesic area was larger in group 1 than in groups 2 to 4 ($*P < 0.05$). Grouping was according to intra/postoperative analgesia. Group 1 (G1): IV–IV (systemic analgesia); G2: IV–epidural; G3: epidural–epidural; and G4: epidural–IV. (Modified after Lavand'homme P, De Kock M, Waterloos H. Intraoperative epidural analgesia combined with ketamine provides effective preventive analgesia in patients undergoing major digestive surgery. Anesthesiology 2005;103(4):813–20.)

after surgery. Patients with chronic pain also exhibit more peri-incisional skin hyperalgesia in the 6-month postoperative time course. As with the studies covering the early postoperative period, the differences in central pain processing up to 3 months postoperatively are also not well reflected in clinical pain measures. The prominent

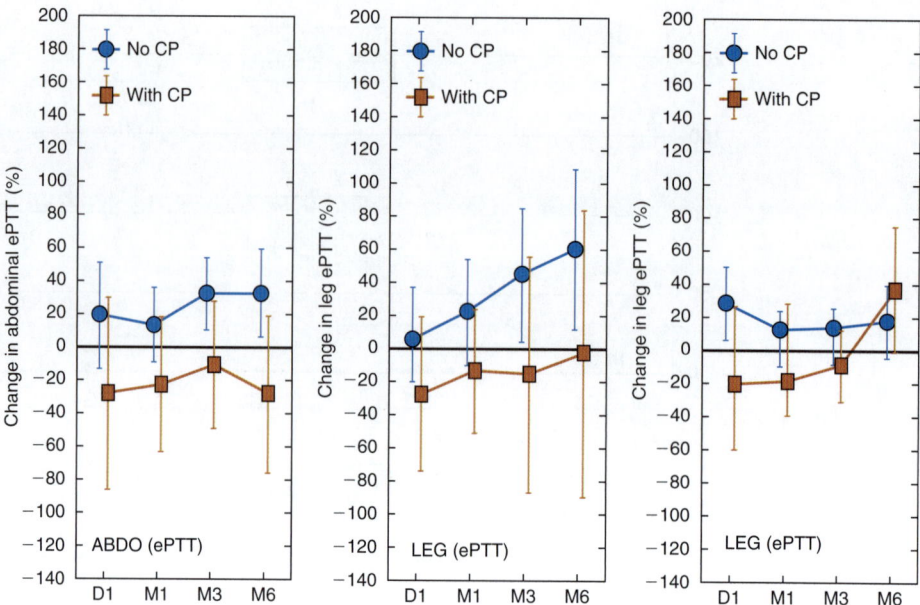

FIGURE 13-5 Postoperative time course of change in percent versus preoperative values of electric pain tolerance thresholds (ePTT) and pressure pain tolerance thresholds (pPTT) peri-incisionally (ABDO) and distant from surgery (LEG) after major abdominal surgery in standard general anesthesia. Values are means and 95% confidence intervals. D1, post-op day 1; M1, M3, M6, 1, 3, 6 mo after surgery; No CP, no chronic pain reported at 6 mo post-op; With CP, with chronic pain reported at 6 mo post-op [53]. (Modified after Wilder-Smith OH, Schreyer T, Scheffer GJ, Arendt-Nielsen L. Patients with chronic pain after abdominal surgery show less preoperative endogenous pain inhibition and more postoperative hyperalgesia: a pilot study. J Pain Palliat Care Pharmacother 2010;24(2):119–28.)

presence and role of hyperalgesia in the development of chronic pain after surgery are supported by a number of cross-sectional studies documenting excitatory alterations of pain processing in patients reporting chronic pain after surgery [6,20,29,30], thus also confirming that chronic pain after surgery shares mechanisms with other types of chronic pain regarding altered central pain processing. A recent study tried to find association between postoperative pain and changes in sensory state after surgery. The authors reported that pain after breast surgery was associated with presence of sensory loss, the more widespread the loss, the more the pain. This suggests that at least for the neuropathic component of the pain, higher extent of nerve damage corroborates with higher pain reports [2].

Use of COX2 inhibitors started before breast surgery and, given for 5 days thereafter, did not reduce postoperative hyperalgesia compared with placebo but did reduce certain aspects of the clinical pain [45].

In summary, early evidence suggests that patients who manifest persistent or chronic pain up to 6 months after surgery show increased and marked spread of sensitization (expressed as spreading hyperalgesia) in their CNS. This spread is both rostral (toward supraspinal structures) and heterotopic (to other, deeper tissues). Furthermore, nerve damage inflicted by surgery is associated with higher clinical pain. Effects of therapeutic interventions on this process have been minimally explored. In one study nonsteroidal anti-inflammatory drugs did not change postoperative hyperalgesia yet reduced pain. It seems that subjective pain experience poorly reflects the alterations in central pain processing.

PREOPERATIVE PAIN MODULATION: EFFECTS ON POSTOPERATIVE CHRONIC PAIN AND PAIN PROCESSING

In the recently reported study [56], preoperative descending pain modulating ability showed significant effects on postoperative chronic pain and pain processing. Thus greater intensity of pain at rest and on movement 6 months after surgery significantly correlated with decreased preoperative ability to inhibit skin pain sensitivity (CPM paradigm with electric test stimuli and cold pressor task for conditioning stimulation). Moreover, decreased ability to inhibit deep tissue pain sensitivity (CPM paradigm with pressure test stimuli) highly significantly correlated with deep tissue hyperalgesia distant from surgery (leg) 1, 3, and 6 months after surgery. These results are in concordance with those of an earlier study in thoracotomy patients, where increased risk of chronic pain after surgery correlated with less inhibitory descending modulation preoperatively using a CPM paradigm based on heat test and conditioning stimulation [62]. This issue is discussed in more detail in another chapter in this book (Chapter 15).

To summarize, poor descending inhibitory pain modulation before surgery appears to be associated with (1) more spread and persistence of central sensitization (expressed as hyperalgesia) 6 months postoperatively and (2) more pain 6 months postoperatively. No effects of therapeutic intervention have been published to date in this context.

OUTLOOK

Pain and hyperalgesia after surgery are increased in the presence of pain before surgery, poor intraoperative analgesia, and perioperative nerve damage. Combining these facts with the results reported earlier regarding perioperative pain processing, we would suggest that better long-term pain outcomes after surgery may be facilitated by implementation of the following measures for perioperative pain management:

1. *Preoperative*
   a. Systematic identification of patients at risk for poor pain outcomes, particularly those with chronic pain and nerve damage
   b. Testing for presence of central sensitization and effectiveness of descending inhibitory pain modulation
   c. Treating identified pronociceptive alterations in central pain processing, e.g., by specific treatment of central sensitization via antihyperalgesic agents (e.g., pregabalin or S-ketamine [8,9]), or using agents improving descending inhibitory controls (c.g., duloxctinc [63])
2. *Intraoperative*
   a. Pay particular attention to patients preoperatively identified as being at risk for poor pain outcomes (e.g., via a special management track)
   b. Anesthesiologists: optimize analgesia, antinociception, and antihyperalgesia
   c. Surgeons: avoid nerve damage or extensive tissue damage
3. *Postoperative*
   a. Specifically and systematically monitor for and treat progression to chronic pain
   b. Monitoring: serial mapping of pain sensitivity to detect persistence and spread of deep tissue hyperalgesia
   c. Early and effective treatment: manage central sensitization using specific antihyperalgesic agents (pregabalin, S-ketamine [8,9]) or improve descending inhibitory controls using agents such as duloxetine [63]

SYNOPSIS

First studies are now available documenting alterations in pain processing after surgery, how these relate to chronic pain development, and the influence of some factors internal and external to the patient on altered pain processing and chronic pain after surgery. It would appear that the development of chronic pain is related to the heterotopic spread of central sensitization along the neuraxis, expressed as spread and generalization of deep tissue hyperalgesia. Moreover, there is first evidence that development and persistence of chronic pain and hyperalgesia are facilitated by poor or absent descending inhibitory controls before surgery. Few data are available to date regarding therapeutic interventions in this area, but promising approaches would appear to include optimization of antinociceptive measures intraoperatively and targeted management of pronociceptive shifts in central pain processing throughout the perioperative period.

Clearly further research is needed to confirm and expand the early results described and discussed earlier. There is a particularly urgent need for large prospective observational and interventional longitudinal studies documenting central pain processing and its alterations together with clinical pain measures before and after surgery. Of great importance is that such future studies use a common standard paradigm such as the NASQ to document altered pain sensitivity and modulation over a sufficiently long time, i.e., at least 6 months after surgery. Only on the basis of such concerted and multicenter studies accompanying clinical practice will we be able to acquire the reliable mechanistic knowledge about chronic pain development after surgery necessary to predict and diagnose—and then to prevent or treat—this challenging condition effectively on the group and individual level.

REFERENCES

1. Aasvang E, Kehlet H. Chronic postoperative pain: the case of inguinal herniorrhaphy. Br J Anaesth 2005;95(1):69–76.
2. Andersen KG, Duriaud HM, Kehlet H, Aasvang EK. The relationship between sensory loss and persistent pain 1 year after breast cancer surgery. J Pain 2017;18(9):1129–38. doi:10.1016/j.jpain.2017.05.002 [PMID:28502878].
3. Apkarian AV, Baliki MN, Geha PY. Towards a theory of chronic pain. Prog Neurobiol 2009;87(2):81–97.
4. Apkarian AV, Sosa Y, Sonty S, et al. Chronic back pain is associated with decreased prefrontal and thalamic gray matter density. J Neurosci 2004;24(46):10410–5.
5. Arendt-Nielsen L, Graven-Nielsen T. Central sensitization in fibromyalgia and other musculoskeletal disorders. Curr Pain Headache Rep 2003;7(5):355–61.
6. Baad-Hansen L, Arima T, Arendt-Nielsen L, et al. Quantitative sensory tests before and 1(1/2) years after orthognathic surgery: a cross-sectional study. J Oral Rehabil 2010;37(5):313–21.
7. Birklein F, Riedl B, Sieweke N, et al. Neurological findings in complex regional pain syndromes—analysis of 145 cases. Acta Neurol Scand 2000;101(4):262–9.
8. Bouwense SA, Buscher HC, van Goor H, Wilder-Smith OH. S-ketamine modulates hyperalgesia in patients with chronic pancreatitis pain. Reg Anesth Pain Med 2011;36(3):303–7.
9. Bouwense SA, Olesen SS, Drewes AM, et al. Effects of pregabalin on central sensitization in patients with chronic pancreatitis in a randomized, controlled trial. PLoS One 2012;7(8):e42096.
10. Buscher HC, Wilder-Smith OH, van Goor H. Chronic pancreatitis patients show hyperalgesia of central origin: a pilot study. Eur J Pain 2006;10(4):363–70.
11. Cervero F. Visceral pain-central sensitisation. Gut 2000;47(Suppl. 4):iv56–7 [discussion iv58].
12. Chua NH, Vissers KC, Arendt-Nielsen L, Wilder-Smith OH. Do diagnostic blocks have beneficial effects on pain processing? Reg Anesth Pain Med 2011;36(4):317–21.
13. Costigan M, Scholz J, Woolf CJ. Neuropathic pain: a maladaptive response of the nervous system to damage. Annu Rev Neurosci 2009;32:1–32.
14. De Kock M, Lavand'homme P, Waterloos H. 'Balanced analgesia' in the perioperative period: is there a place for ketamine? Pain 2001;92(3):373–80.

15. De Kock M, Lavand'homme P, Waterloos H. The short-lasting analgesia and long-term antihyperalgesic effect of intrathecal clonidine in patients undergoing colonic surgery. Anesth Analg 2005;101(2):566–72 [table of contents].
16. Diatchenko L, Nackley AG, Slade GD, et al. Idiopathic pain disorders – pathways of vulnerability. Pain 2006;123(3):226–30.
17. Freynhagen R, Baron R, Tolle T, et al. Screening of neuropathic pain components in patients with chronic back pain associated with nerve root compression: a prospective observational pilot study (MIPORT). Curr Med Res Opin 2006;22(3):529–37.
18. Freynhagen R, Rolke R, Baron R, et al. Pseudoradicular and radicular low-back pain – a disease continuum rather than different entities? Answers from quantitative sensory testing. Pain 2008;135(1–2):65–74.
19. Giamberardino MA, Affaitati G, Lerza R, et al. Relationship between pain symptoms and referred sensory and trophic changes in patients with gallbladder pathology. Pain 2005;114(1–2):239–49.
20. Gottrup H, Andersen J, Arendt-Nielsen L, Jensen TS. Psychophysical examination in patients with post-mastectomy pain. Pain 2000;87(3):275–84.
21. Granot M, Weissman-Fogel I, Crispel Y, et al. Determinants of endogenous analgesia magnitude in a diffuse noxious inhibitory control (DNIC) paradigm: do conditioning stimulus painfulness, gender and personality variables matter? Pain 2008;136(1–2):142–9.
22. Heinricher MM, Tavares I, Leith JL, Lumb BM. Descending control of nociception: specificity, recruitment and plasticity. Brain Res Rev 2009;60(1):214–225.
23. Kehlet H, Jensen TS, Woolf CJ. Persistent postsurgical pain: risk factors and prevention. Lancet 2006;367(9522):1618–25.
24. Kosek E, Ordeberg G. Lack of pressure pain modulation by heterotopic noxious conditioning stimulation in patients with painful osteoarthritis before, but not following, surgical pain relief. Pain 2000;88(1):69–78.
25. Lautenbacher S, Rollman GB. Possible deficiencies of pain modulation in fibromyalgia. Clin J Pain 1997;13(3):189–96.
26. Lavand'homme P, De Kock M, Waterloos H. Intraoperative epidural analgesia combined with ketamine provides effective preventive analgesia in patients undergoing major digestive surgery. Anesthesiology 2005;103(4):813–20.
27. Leffler AS, Kosek E, Lerndal T, et al. Somatosensory perception and function of diffuse noxious inhibitory controls (DNIC) in patients suffering from rheumatoid arthritis. Eur J Pain 2002;6(2):161–76.
28. Martinez V, Ben Ammar S, Judet T, et al. Risk factors predictive of chronic postsurgical neuropathic pain: the value of the iliac crest bone harvest model. Pain 2012;153(7):1478–83.
29. Mikkelsen T, Werner MU, Lassen B, Kehlet H. Pain and sensory dysfunction 6 to 12 months after inguinal herniotomy. Anesth Analg 2004;99(1):146–51.
30. Moiniche S, Dahl JB, Erichsen CJ, et al. Time course of subjective pain ratings, and wound and leg tenderness after hysterectomy. Acta Anaesthesiol Scand 1997;41(6):785–9.
31. Nikolajsen L, Kristensen AD, Thillemann TM, et al. Pain and somatosensory findings in patients 3 years after total hip arthroplasty. Eur J Pain 2009;13(6):576–81.
32. O'Neill S, Manniche C, Graven-Nielsen T, Arendt-Nielsen L. Generalized deep-tissue hyperalgesia in patients with chronic low-back pain. Eur J Pain 2007;11(4):415–20.
33. Olesen SS, Brock C, Krarup AL, et al. Descending inhibitory pain modulation is impaired in patients with chronic pancreatitis. Clin Gastroenterol Hepatol 2010;8(8):724–30.
34. Perkins FM, Kehlet H. Chronic pain as an outcome of surgery. A review of predictive factors. Anesthesiology 2000;93(4):1123–33.
35. Peyron R, Schneider F, Faillenot I, et al. An fMRI study of cortical representation of mechanical allodynia in patients with neuropathic pain. Neurology 2004;63(10):1838–46.
36. Pielsticker A, Haag G, Zaudig M, Lautenbacher S. Impairment of pain inhibition in chronic tension-type headache. Pain 2005;118(1–2):215–23.
37. Porreca F, Ossipov MH, Gebhart GF. Chronic pain and medullary descending facilitation. Trends Neurosci 2002;25(6):319–25.
38. Pud D, Granovsky Y, Yarnitsky D. The methodology of experimentally induced diffuse noxious inhibitory control (DNIC)-like effect in humans. Pain 2009;144(1–2):16–9.
39. Rolke R, Baron R, Maier C, et al. Quantitative sensory testing in the German Research Network on Neuropathic Pain (DFNS): standardized protocol and reference values. Pain 2006;123(3):231–43.
40. Rolke R, Magerl W, Campbell KA, et al. Quantitative sensory testing: a comprehensive protocol for clinical trials. Eur J Pain 2006;10(1):77–88.
41. Ruscheweyh R, Wilder-Smith O, Drdla R, et al. Long-term potentiation in spinal nociceptive pathways as a novel target for pain therapy. Mol Pain 2011;7:20.

42. Sandkuhler J. Models and mechanisms of hyperalgesia and allodynia. Physiol Rev 2009;89(2):707–58.
43. Sandkuhler J. Central sensitization versus synaptic long-term potentiation (LTP): a critical comment. J Pain 2010;11(8):798–800.
44. Stubhaug A, Breivik H, Eide PK, et al. Mapping of punctuate hyperalgesia around a surgical incision demonstrates that ketamine is a powerful suppressor of central sensitization to pain following surgery. Acta Anaesthesiol Scand 1997;41(9):1124–32.
45. van Helmond N, Steegers MA, Filippini-de Moor GP, Vissers KC, Wilder-Smith OH. Hyperalgesia and persistent pain after breast cancer surgery: a prospective randomized controlled trial with perioperative COX-2 inhibition. PLoS One 2016;11(12):e0166601. doi:10.1371/journal.pone.0166601 [PMID:27935990; PMCID:PMC5147830].
46. Vanegas H, Schaible HG. Descending control of persistent pain: inhibitory or facilitatory? Brain Res Brain Res Rev 2004;46(3):295–309.
47. Vaneker M, Wilder-Smith OH, Schrombges P, et al. Patients initially diagnosed as 'warm' or 'cold' CRPS 1 show differences in central sensory processing some eight years after diagnosis: a quantitative sensory testing study. Pain 2005;115(1–2):204–11.
48. Vera-Portocarrero LP, Xie JY, Kowal J, et al. Descending facilitation from the rostral ventromedial medulla maintains visceral pain in rats with experimental pancreatitis. Gastroenterology 2006;130(7):2155–64.
49. Vera-Portocarrero LP, Zhang ET, Ossipov MH, et al. Descending facilitation from the rostral ventromedial medulla maintains nerve injury-induced central sensitization. Neuroscience 2006;140(4):1311–20.
50. Villanueva L. Diffuse Noxious Inhibitory Control (DNIC) as a tool for exploring dysfunction of endogenous pain modulatory systems. Pain 2009;143(3):161–2.
51. Wilder-Smith CH, Schindler D, Lovblad K, et al. Brain functional magnetic resonance imaging of rectal pain and activation of endogenous inhibitory mechanisms in irritable bowel syndrome patient subgroups and healthy controls. Gut 2004;53(11):1595–601.
52. Wilder-Smith O. A paradigm shift in pain medicine: implementing a systematic approach to altered pain processing in everyday clinical practice based on quantitative sensory testing. Aalborg: River Publishers; 2014. p. 120.
53. Wilder-Smith OH. Chronic pain and surgery: a review of new insights from sensory testing. J Pain Palliat Care Pharmacother 2011;25(2):146–59.
54. Wilder-Smith OH, Arendt-Nielsen L. Postoperative hyperalgesia: its clinical importance and relevance. Anesthesiology 2006;104(3):601–7.
55. Wilder-Smith OH, Arendt-Nielsen L, Gaumann D, et al. Sensory changes and pain after abdominal hysterectomy: a comparison of anesthetic supplementation with fentanyl versus magnesium or ketamine. Anesth Analg 1998;86(1):95–101.
56. Wilder-Smith OH, Schreyer T, Scheffer GJ, Arendt-Nielsen L. Patients with chronic pain after abdominal surgery show less preoperative endogenous pain inhibition and more postoperative hyperalgesia: a pilot study. J Pain Palliat Care Pharmacother 2010;24(2):119–28.
57. Wilder-Smith OH, Tassonyi E, Crul BJ, Arendt-Nielsen L. Quantitative sensory testing and human surgery: effects of analgesic management on postoperative neuroplasticity. Anesthesiology 2003;98(5):1214–22.
58. Wilder-Smith OH, Tassonyi E, Senly C, et al. Surgical pain is followed not only by spinal sensitization but also by supraspinal antinociception. Br J Anaesth 1996;76(6):816–21.
59. Woolf CJ, Salter MW. Neuronal plasticity: increasing the gain in pain. Science 2000;288(5472):1765–9.
60. Yarnitsky D. Conditioned pain modulation (the diffuse noxious inhibitory control-like effect): its relevance for acute and chronic pain states. Curr Opin Anaesthesiol 2010;23(5):611–5.
61. Yarnitsky D, Arendt-Nielsen L, Bouhassira D, et al. Recommendations on terminology and practice of psychophysical DNIC testing. Eur J Pain 2010;14(4):339.
62. Yarnitsky D, Crispel Y, Eisenberg E, et al. Prediction of chronic post-operative pain: pre-operative DNIC testing identifies patients at risk. Pain 2008;138(1):22–8.
63. Yarnitsky D, Granot M, Nahman-Averbuch H, et al. Conditioned pain modulation predicts duloxetine efficacy in painful diabetic neuropathy. Pain 2012;153(6):1193–8.

CHAPTER 14

Electroencephalography: A Potentially Valuable Tool for Measuring Central Neuroplasticity in the Context of Acute Postoperative Pain

Emanuel N. van den Broeke

Assessing changes in nociceptive processing in humans in the context of acute and persistent postoperative pain mostly relies on psychophysical assessments. However, the recording of laser-evoked brain potentials (LEPs) is considered as the best available tool to assess the functional status of heat-sensitive nociceptive pathways [4]. LEPs are voltage polarity changes recorded in the electroencephalogram (EEG) in response to a laser stimulus (see Chapter 10). Laser stimuli selectively activate cutaneous heat-sensitive nociceptors without concomitant activation of low-threshold mechanoreceptors. However, besides the availability to assess thermonociceptive pathways, it would also be valuable to be able to assess mechanical nociceptive pathways, in particular, because mechanical hyperalgesia (increased pain sensitivity) is a major clinical symptom in acute postoperative pain [14]. The aim of this chapter is (1) to discuss the relevance of assessing mechanical nociceptive pathways in the context of acute and persistent postoperative pain and (2) to show new developments regarding the recording of pinprick-evoked brain responses (PEPs) as a novel tool to assess the functional status of mechanical nociceptive pathways.

HUMAN SURROGATE MODEL OF ACUTE POSTOPERATIVE PAIN

Hyperalgesia is a predominant clinical symptom of acute postoperative pain. This increased pain sensitivity is present in and surrounding the region subjected to surgical damage. One aspect contributing to this postsurgical hyperalgesia is the tissue damage due to the surgical incision. To achieve a better understanding of the development of this incision-induced pain and hyperalgesia, an experimental incision model has been developed [5,8,9]. In this model, a 4 mm length incision is made through the skin, fascia, and muscle. When performed, this incision induces a moderate to strong ongoing pain, which then progressively declines. Directly after the incision, the skin develops a flare reaction in the skin surrounding the injured area, suggesting inflammation and the activation of peptidergic nociceptive afferents. Moreover, two types of cutaneous hyperalgesia are observed: (1) hyperalgesia at the site of incision, referred to as "primary" hyperalgesia and characterized by reduced thresholds to heat and mechanical pinprick stimuli, and (2) hyperalgesia in the skin surrounding the incision, referred to as "secondary" hyperalgesia and characterized by reduced thresholds and increased perceived intensity to mechanical pinprick stimuli [5].

SECONDARY PINPRICK HYPERALGESIA IS MEDIATED BY HEAT-INSENSITIVE NOCICEPTORS

Secondary hyperalgesia can be induced experimentally, for example, after intradermal capsaicin injection (which selectively activates the transient receptor potential vanilloid 1(TRPV1) receptor [3]) [1,12,15,31] or via high-frequency electrical stimulation (HFS) of the skin (Figure 14-1; [10,11,26,27,29,30]). HFS consists of five trains of 100 Hz delivered during 1 second at a 10-second intertrain interval and is delivered to the skin via a specific electrode consisting of multiple pins to strongly activate nociceptive free nerve endings located in the superficial layer of the skin. The stimulus is typically delivered at an intensity corresponding to 10 or 20 times the absolute detection threshold to a single electrical pulse.

By using these methods, in combination with selectively blocking subpopulations of primary nociceptive afferents, researchers have attempted to investigate which population of nociceptors induce and mediate secondary hyperalgesia. Henrich et al. [6] showed that the induction of secondary hyperalgesia mainly depends on the activation of unmyelinated nociceptors expressing the TRPV1 receptor. Other studies showed that secondary hyperalgesia (1) is characterized by increased pain to mechanical but not short-lasting heat stimuli [1], (2) is abolished during an A-fiber nerve conduction block [31], and (3) is still present in skin pretreated with capsaicin to denervate the skin of nociceptive afferents expressing

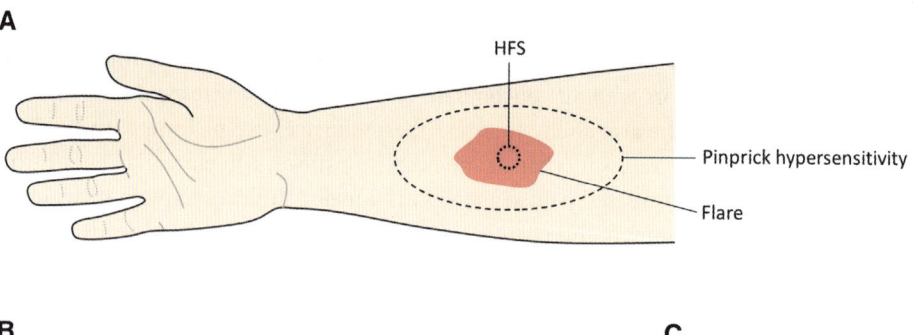

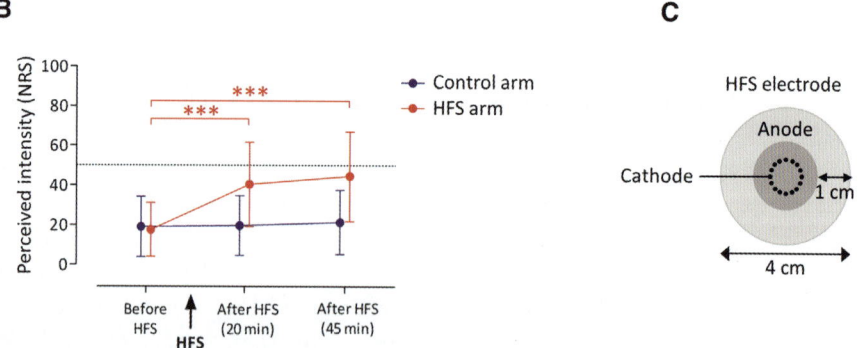

FIGURE 14-1   A: High-frequency electrical stimulation (HFS) delivered to the ventral forearm typically induces (1) a flare response that gradually disappears within approximately 30 to 40 min after applying HFS and (2) a large area of increased pinprick sensitivity (secondary hyperalgesia) that remains for several hours. B: Pinprick stimuli (64 mN) applied in the area of increased pinprick sensitivity induced by HFS elicits an increase in pinprick perception at least up to 45 min after applying HFS. The ratings were obtained using an Numeric Rating Scale (NRS) that ranged from 0 (no detection) to 100 (maximal imaginable pain) with 50 being the transition between the nonpainful and painful domain. *** denotes $P < 0.001$ (paired t tests). C: Characteristics of the HFS electrode. The cathode consists of 16 blunt stainless steel pins with a diameter of 0.2 mm protruding 1 mm from the base. The 16 pins are placed in a circle with a diameter of 10 mm. The anode consists of a surrounding stainless steel ring having an inner diameter of 22 mm and an outer diameter of 40 mm.

the TRPV1 receptor [15]. These results suggest that secondary hyperalgesia is mediated by mechanosensitive A fibers that do not express the TRPV1 receptor (capsaicin-insensitive) and are heat-insensitive (or have high heat thresholds) [17]. Two populations of nociceptors fulfill these criteria: type I mechano- and heat-sensitive Aδ fibers (type I AMH) and high-threshold mechanoreceptors (HTMs; [15,18]).

We recently investigated the contribution of type I AMH nociceptors to secondary hyperalgesia [27]. Single fiber recordings in monkeys have shown that type I AMH nociceptors do not respond to short-lasting 1-second heat stimuli, even at 53°C; however, when they are exposed to sustained heat (30 seconds, 53°C), they start responding after a few seconds, with an average peak latency around 16 or 21 seconds, depending on the study [24,25]. Using a temperature-controlled CO_2 laser, we delivered sustained heat stimuli (30 seconds) at an intensity above the type II AMH heat threshold, before and after the experimental induction of secondary hyperalgesia. We observed that the perceived intensity elicited by sustained heat stimulation of the skin was not increased in the area of secondary hyperalgesia (Figure 14-2), suggesting that secondary hyperalgesia is predominantly mediated by HTMs [27].

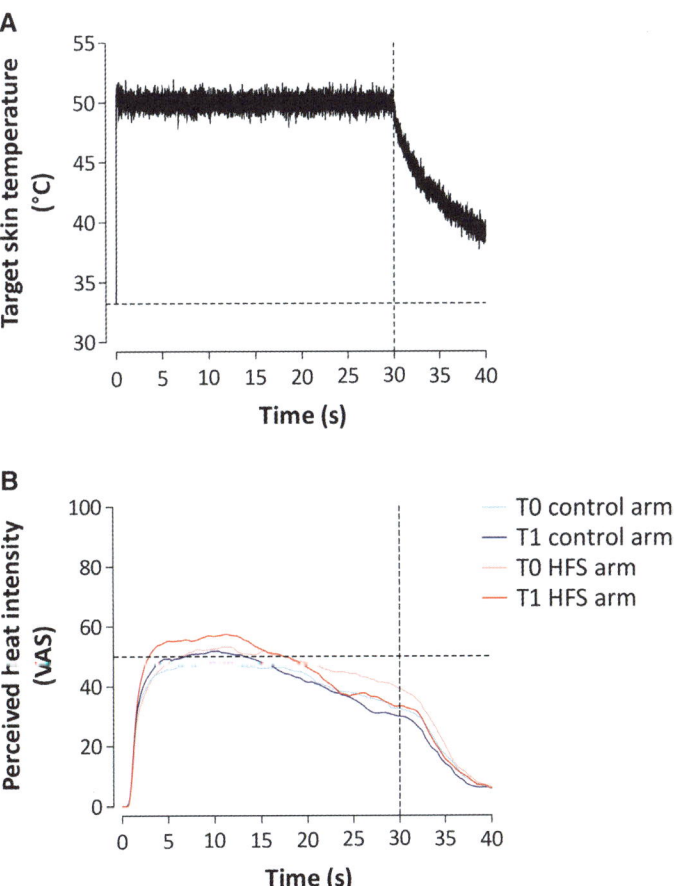

FIGURE 14-2 **A:** Example of the time course of the target skin temperature during a long-duration heat stimulus (30 s) delivered by a temperature-controlled CO_2 laser. **B:** Long-duration heat stimuli delivered before (T0) and 20 min after (T1) inducing increased pinprick sensitivity using high-frequency electrical stimulation (HFS) of the skin. No significant increase in heat pain is observed when the long-duration heat stimuli were are delivered inside the area of increased pinprick sensitivity. (Adapted from Van den Broeke EN, Lenoir C, Mouraux A. Secondary hyperalgesia is mediated by heat-insensitive A-fibre nociceptors. J Physiol 2016;594:6767–76.)

SECONDARY HYPERALGESIA IS THOUGHT TO BE THE RESULT OF CENTRAL SENSITIZATION

Secondary hyperalgesia is thought to be the result of central sensitization [2,12,20], which is defined by the International Association for the Study of Pain (IASP) as *"increased responsiveness of nociceptive neurons within the central nervous system to their normal or subthreshold afferent input"* [13]. This notion is supported by studies showing that once secondary hyperalgesia has developed, it appears to be less dependent or even independent of peripheral neural activity [8,9]. Moreover, Baumann et al [2], using single fiber recordings in monkeys, found no evidence for a peripheral sensitization of mechano- and heat-sensitive C-fiber (CMH) nociceptors and type I AMH in the area of secondary hyperalgesia. Also, Serra et al. [21] did not observe signs of peripheral sensitization of CMH nociceptors using microneurography recordings performed in humans. However, they did find that mechanoinsensitive C fibers became responsive to mechanical stimulation after remote intradermal injection of capsaicin. However, this result is in contradiction with that of Schmelz et al. [22], who did not observe a sensitization of mechanoinsensitive C fibers in the area adjacent to the site of intradermal capsaicin injection. Specifically, injection of capsaicin in one part of the receptive field of a mechanoinsensitive C fiber did not change the activity of the same C fiber when stimulating another part of the receptive field.

Further support for a central origin of secondary hyperalgesia comes from a study conducted by Simone et al. [20], who made electrophysiologic recordings of spinothalamic tract neurons before and after injecting capsaicin into the arm of monkeys. They showed an increased responsiveness of both high-threshold (HT) and wide-dynamic-range (WDR) neurons after capsaicin injection to punctate stimuli delivered 1 to 3 cm away from the capsaicin injection site.

At present the exact spinal mechanism underlying secondary hyperalgesia has not yet been elucidated [19]; however, Torsney [23], using complete Freund adjuvant (CFA) to induce inflammation in rats, showed with whole-cell patch-clamp recordings that inflammation recruits silent monosynaptic Aδ-fiber input to dorsal horn lamina I (neurokinin-1-positive) neurons. This novel Aδ-fiber input may strengthen the input to the lamina I neurons and could potentially be a possible mechanism underlying secondary hyperalgesia.

SECONDARY PINPRICK HYPERALGESIA IS ASSOCIATED WITH INCREASED EEG RESPONSES

To explore changes in brain activity related to secondary hyperalgesia, we recently recorded pinprick-evoked brain potentials (PEPs) before and after experimentally induced secondary hyperalgesia [29]. For this purpose, we used a custom-built calibrated handheld pinprick stimulator consisting of a cylindrical stainless steel flat tip probe on top of which rests a calibrated cylindrical weight (Figure 14-3; [26]). The probe and weight are mounted inside an aluminum tube. When applied perpendicular to the skin, the probe and weight slide freely inside the tube. Once the probe is maintained against the skin, it generates a constant normal force entirely determined by the mass of the probe and weight [26]. To generate a trigger in the EEG that marked the actual time at which the probe touched the skin, we used a high-resistance switch triggered by the change in impedance occurring between the probe and a ground electrode placed against the skin at the wrist [26]. A thin layer of conductive gel was used to lower the impedance between the probe and the skin. The delay between the contact of the skin and the generation of the trigger was almost zero (0.046 ± 0.015 ms; [26]).

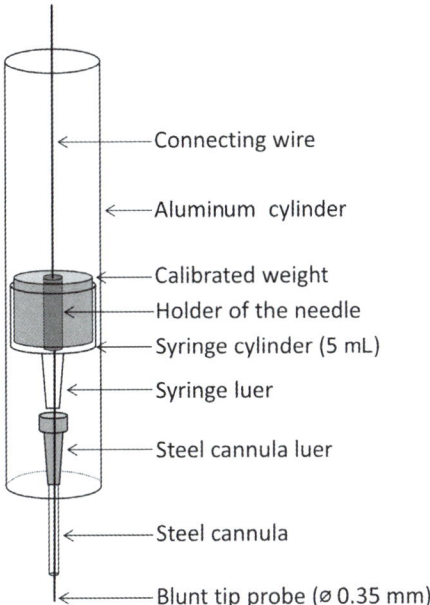

FIGURE 14-3 Characteristics of the pinprick stimulator used to record pinprick-evoked brain potentials. (Adapted from Van den Broeke EN, Lambert J, Huang G, Mouraux A. Central sensitization of mechanical nociceptive pathways is associated with a long-lasting increase of pinprick-evoked brain potentials. Front Hum Neurosci 2016;10:531.)

Pinprick stimuli (64 mN) delivered to normal skin of the volar forearm elicited a clear positive wave peaking approximately 350 ms after stimulus onset (Figure 14-4). When the same pinprick stimuli were applied inside the area of pinprick hypersensitivity, the magnitude of this positivity was significantly increased compared with the PEPs elicited by stimulation of normal skin (Figure 14-4). The latency at which the increase in PEP was observed was 290 to 470 ms, compatible with the conduction velocity of Aδ-fiber nociceptors. The increase in PEP magnitude was maximal at central–posterior brain regions. We also showed that the increase in PEP followed the same time course as the increase in pinprick perception [26].

In addition, we found that the increase in PEP magnitude is dependent on stimulation intensity [28]. Specifically, we observed a nonlinear inverted U-shape relationship between the increase in PEP and stimulation intensity. The maximal (and significant) increase in PEP was observed at the intermediate pinprick intensity (64 mN). It remains unclear why at higher stimulation intensities (>64 mN) pinprick perception is significantly enhanced but the PEP not [29]. Possible explanations for this dissociation should be explored in future studies.

PERSISTENT POSTOPERATIVE PAIN

At present there are no studies that have investigated the clinical usefulness of PEPs in patients with persistent postoperative pain. In some cases persistent pain after surgery might be neuropathic pain. Mechanical hyperalgesia is a frequently observed symptom in neuropathic pain [7,16]. The recording of PEPs could constitute a way to assess the functional status of mechanical nociceptive pathways and to provide a less subjective measure for central sensitization.

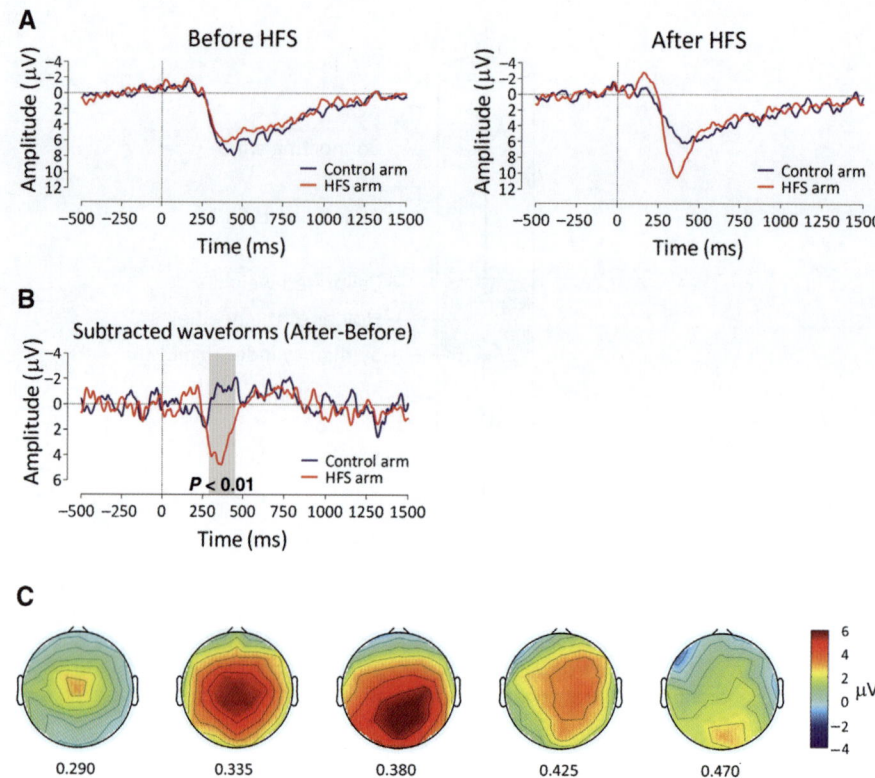

FIGURE 14-4 **A:** Pinprick-evoked brain potentials (PEPs) elicited by a 64 mN stimulation intensity before and 20 min after inducing increased pinprick sensitivity using high-frequency electrical stimulation (HFS) of the skin. The PEPs are recorded at Cz versus A1A2. **B:** Difference waveforms (after minus before HFS) of the PEPs obtained by stimulation of the HFS-treated arm and the contralateral control arm. The *gray rectangle* shows the time window in which the two waveforms were significantly different. **C:** Scalp topography of the difference waveform, showing that the change in PEPs induced by HFS is maximal at central–posterior scalp locations. (Adapted from Van den Broeke EN, de Vries B, Lambert J, Torta DM, Mouraux A. Phase-locked and non-phase-locked EEG responses to pinprick stimulation before and after experimentally-induced secondary hyperalgesia. Clin Neurophysiol 2017;128(8):1445–56.)

Acknowledgment

E.N.vdB. is supported by the ERC "Starting Grant" (PROBING PAIN 336130).

REFERENCES

1. Ali Z, Meyer RA, Campbell JN. Secondary hyperalgesia to mechanical but not heat stimuli following a capsaicin injection in hairy skin. Pain 1996;68(2–3):401–11.
2. Baumann TK, Simone DA, Shain CN, LaMotte RH. Neurogenic hyperalgesia: the search for the primary cutaneous afferent fibers that contribute to capsaicin-induced pain and hyperalgesia. J Neurophysiol 1991;66:212–27.
3. Caterina MJ, Schumacher MA, Tominaga M, Rosen TA, Levine JD, Julius D. The capsaicin receptor: a heat-activated ion channel in the pain pathway. Nature 1997;389(6653):816–24.
4. Cruccu G, Sommer C, Anand P, Attal N, Baron R, Garcia-Larrea L, Haanpaa M, Jensen TS, Serra J, Treede R-D. EFNS guidelines on neuropathic pain assessment: revised 2009. Eur J Neurol 2010;17:1010–8.
5. Fißmer I, Klein T, Magerl W, et al. Modality-specific somatosensory changes in a human surrogate model of postoperative pain. Anesthesiology 2011;115:387–97.
6. Henrich F, Magerl W, Klein T, Greffrath W, Treede RD. Capsaicin-sensitive C- and A-fibre nociceptors control long-term potentiation-like pain amplification in humans. Brain 2015;138(9):2505–20.

7. Jensen TS, Finnerup NB. Allodynia and hyperalgesia in neuropathic pain: clinical manifestations and mechanisms. Lancet Neurol 2014;13(9):924–35.
8. Kawamata M, Watanabe H, Nishikawa K, et al. Different mechanisms of development and maintenance of experimental incision-induced hyperalgesia in human skin. Anesthesiology 2002;97:550–9.
9. Kawamata M, Takahashi T, Watanabe H, et al. Experimental incision-induced pain in human skin: effects of systemic lidocaine on flare formation and hyperalgesia. Pain 2002;100:77–89.
10. Klein T, Magerl W, Hopf H-C, Sandkühler J, Treede R-D. Perceptual correlates of nociceptive long-term potentiation and long-term depression in humans. J Neurosci 2004;24(4):964–71.
11. Klein T, Stahn S, Magerl W, Treede R-D. The role of heterosynaptic facilitation in long-term potentiation (LTP) of human pain perception. Pain 2008;139:507–19.
12. LaMotte RH, Shain CN, Simone DA, Tsai E-F. Neurogenic hyperalgesia: psychophysical studies of underlying mechanisms. J Neurophysiol 1991;66:190–211.
13. Loeser JD, Treede RD. The Kyoto protocol of IASP Basic Pain Terminology. Pain 2008;137(3):473–7.
14. Lavand'homme P, De Kock M, Waterloos H. Intraoperative epidural analgesia combined with ketamine provides effective preventive analgesia in patients undergoing major digestive surgery. Anesthesiology 2005;103:813–20.
15. Magerl W, Fuchs PN, Meyer RA, Treede RD. Roles of capsaicin-insensitive nociceptors in cutaneous pain and secondary hyperalgesia. Brain 2001;124:1754–64.
16. Maier C, Baron R, Tölle TR, Binder A, Birbaumer N, Birklein F, Gierthmühlen J, Flor H, Geber C, Huge V, Krumova EK, Landwehrmeyer GB, Magerl W, Maihöfner C, Richter H, Rolke R, Scherens A, Schwarz A, Sommer C, Tronnier V, Uçeyler N, Valet M, Wasner G, Treede RD. Quantitative sensory testing in the German Research Network on Neuropathic Pain (DFNS): somatosensory abnormalities in 1236 patients with different neuropathic pain syndromes. Pain 2010;150(3):439–50.
17. Meyer RA, Treede R-D. Mechanisms of secondary hyperalgesia: a role for myelinated nociceptors in punctate hyperalgesia. In: Brune K, Handwerker HO, editors. Hyperalgesia: molecular mechanisms and clinical implications. Progress in pain research and management. Seattle: IASP-Press; 2004. p. 143–55.
18. Ringkamp M, Peng YB, Wu G, Hartke TV, Campbell JN, Meyer RA. Capsaicin responses in heat-sensitive and heat-insensitive A-fiber nociceptors. J Neurosci 2001;21(12):4460–8.
19. Sandkühler J, Gruber-Schoffnegger D. Hyperalgesia by synaptic long-term potentiation (LTP): an update. Curr Opin Pharmacol 2012;12(1):18–27.
20. Simone DA, Sorkin LS, Oh U, Chung JM, Owens C, LaMotte RH, Willis WD. Neurogenic hyperalgesia: central neural correlates in responses to spinothalamic tract neurons. J Neurophysiol 1991;66:228–46.
21. Serra J, Campero M, Bostock H, Ochoa J. Two types of C nociceptors in human skin and their behavior in areas of capsaicin-induced secondary hyperalgesia. J Neurophysiol 2004;91(6):2770–81.
22. Schmelz M, Schmid R, Handwerker HO, Torebjörk HE. Encoding of burning pain from capsaicin-treated human skin in two categories of unmyelinated nerve fibres. Brain 2000;123(3):560–71.
23. Torsney C. Inflammatory pain unmasks heterosynaptic facilitation in lamina I neurokinin 1 receptor-expressing neurons in rat spinal cord. J Neurosci 2011;31(13):5158–68.
24. Treede RD, Meyer RA, Campbell JN. Myelinated mechanically insensitive afferents from monkey hairy skin: heat-response properties. J Neurophysiol 1998;80:1082–93.
25. Treede RD, Meyer RA, Raja SN, Campbell JN. Evidence for two different heat transduction mechanisms in nociceptive primary afferents innervating monkey skin. J Physiol 1995;483:747–58.
26. Van den Broeke EN, Lambert J, Huang G, Mouraux A. Central sensitization of mechanical nociceptive pathways is associated with a long-lasting increase of pinprick-evoked brain potentials. Front Hum Neurosci 2016;10:531.
27. Van den Broeke EN, Lenoir C, Mouraux A. Secondary hyperalgesia is mediated by heat-insensitive A-fibre nociceptors. J Physiol 2016;594:6767–76.
28. Van den Broeke EN, Mouraux A, Groneberg AH, Pfau DB, Treede RD, Klein T. Characterizing pinprick-evoked brain potentials before and after experimentally induced secondary hyperalgesia. J Neurophysiol 2015;114(5):2672–81.
29. Van den Broeke EN, de Vries B, Lambert J, Torta DM, Mouraux A. Phase-locked and non-phase-locked EEG responses to pinprick stimulation before and after experimentally-induced secondary hyperalgesia. Clin Neurophysiol 2017;128(8):1445–56.
30. Vo L, Drummond PD. High frequency electrical stimulation concurrently induces central sensitization and ipsilateral inhibitory pain modulation. Eur J Pain 2013;17:357–68.
31. Ziegler EA, Magerl W, Meyer RA, Treede R-D. Secondary hyperalgesia to punctate mechanical stimuli: central sensitization to A-fibre nociceptor input. Brain 1999;122:2245–57.

CHAPTER 15

Drug Effects and Altered Perioperative Pain Processing

David Yarnitsky and Lee-Bareket Kisler

Assessment of the way pain is processed in the CNS of humans can be done in several ways—psychophysical, using various arrays of stimuli and asking subjects to describe the evoked sensations; neurophysiologic, using brain waves as the venue of response; and by imaging, using various MRI protocols or PET in gathering the responses. This chapter will focus on the psychophysical response, which is the most ready and intuitive way of obtaining data from patients yet is not free of drawbacks, such as the reports' subjectivity and often low reliability of responses, with a large interindividual variability. It is now customary to divide the psychophysical pain measurement tools into static and dynamic ones. The first group depicts the psychophysical response to a single point in a spectrum of possible intensities, usually at one time epoch, such as measuring threshold of pain, its tolerance, or magnitude of suprathreshold stimuli (briefly called "suprathreshold"), where a stimulus of a certain intensity is administered and subjects are asked to evaluate the magnitude of their perceived pain on a pain scale of any kind.

Pain thresholds have been used extensively and found their application mainly in documenting neurologic deficit in neuropathic pain cases, although they were shown to describe sensitization as well [9]. The parameter of suprathreshold was examined, in several articles published during the recent decade, as a potential predictor of acute postoperative pain and found so by several, mainly when heat energy is used to deliver the stimulus [6,7,16,31,39,41,62]; for review see Ref. [1]. Overall, suprathreshold stimuli seem to carry the potential of reflecting on the state of pain modulation in the studied patients; those reporting higher pain perception at a pain-free time before surgery seem to have a more pronociceptive pain-perceiving system, expressed in higher response to the noxious stimuli evoked by the operation. This is one of the first cases where consistent data have been collected to show that the laboratory-based psychophysical assessment of pain is correlated with the clinical pain phenotype. This suggests that the laboratory-based pain modulation profile (PMP) is of value in prediction of clinical pain levels in response to substantially noxious events such as surgery.

The advent of dynamic psychophysical protocols upgraded our ability to describe pain modulation of individuals. This line includes tests that try to evoke an experimental process of pain modulation in the examined subject, thus, bringing us closer to the "real" pain experience patients undergo. There are two commonly used protocols under this category—temporal summation (TS) and conditioned pain modulation (CPM). They depict the state of ascending facilitation and descending inhibition, respectively. In the TS protocol, subjects receive a series of identical painful stimuli and report the perceived intensity along

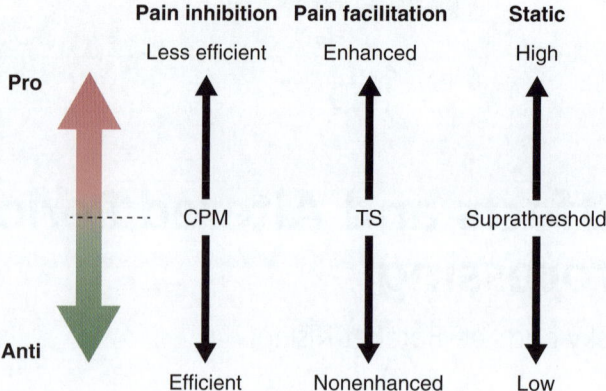

FIGURE 15-1 The three pain laboratory tests on which the suggested construct of pain modulation profile is based. CPM, conditioned pain modulation; TS, temporal summation.

the series, or at least at its start and end. Typically, given that the first stimulus is painful, subjects will report an increase in pain intensity along the series. In the CPM protocol, two remote painful stimuli are given, a test-stimulus and a conditioning-stimulus. The pain intensity rating given for the test-stimulus when applied alone usually decreases when it is reapplied concomitantly or immediately after administration of the conditioning-stimulus, which should be painful as well (see Refs. [11,38,50], for methodology) (Figure 15-1). Not all healthy individuals express this inhibition, under the various specific test protocols used to elicit CPM, up to one-third of individuals express an increase of the pain rating to the test-stimulus due to conditioning stimulation.

Using the two tests, TS and CPM, one can characterize the PMP of any patient as being either pro- or antinociceptive. Because in most studies there has not been a correlation between TS and CPM, it is likely that they represent mostly independent lines of physiologic pain processing, and hence, the characterization of each patient's PMP should take into consideration the function of the two lines. Thus, along the ascending facilitatory line, patients can be either facilitatory pronociceptive, if they express enhanced TS, or facilitatory antinociceptive, if the TS is lower than normal. For easier communication, we suggest the use of the terms ascending pronociceptive and ascending antinociceptive, respectively. In line, along the descending inhibitory line, one can be inhibitory pronociceptive if CPM is less efficient and inhibitory antinociceptive if CPM is highly efficient. The equivalent suggested terms will be descending pronociceptive and descending antinociceptive, respectively. Consequently, patients can be classified as dual pronociceptive (high TS and less efficient CPM), descending pronociceptive (normal TS and less efficient CPM), ascending pronociceptive (high TS and efficient CPM), and antinociceptive (i.e., nonpronociceptive) on both lines (normal TS and efficient CPM).

Clinical implications of pronociceptivity are under current research, and understanding is cumulating. One part of the puzzle, which is already well described, is that groups of patients with chronic pain express pronociceptive profile when compared with groups of controls. This has been shown repeatedly for both the descending and the ascending lines, via inhibitory and the facilitatory tests, in many pain syndromes; for CPM, less efficient inhibitory pain modulation was reported for fibromyalgia [21,26], irritable bowel syndrome [12,25,56], migraine [53], tension headache [8,46], temporomandibular disorder [32,40], osteoarthritis (OA) and muscle pain [3,5,27], and whiplash [13]. For TS, enhanced pain facilitation was documented for fibromyalgia [29,49,57–59], OA [3,5], migraine [63], temporomandibular disorder [17,33,54,55], and whiplash [30,61]. In recent papers, there has been an attempt to identify subgroups of patients according to their PMP, and it is generally found that patients with the dual pronociceptive profile express higher pain intensity and lower extent of pain relief after treatment, compared with those with less pronociceptive profile [44,45], (Figure 15-2).

In the context of pain in the perioperative period, data are available on three important aspects: (1) prediction of pain acquisition after surgery, both acute and chronic; (2) prediction of the effect of pain-reducing medications in prevention and treatment of postoperative pain; and (3) prediction of success of surgery performed for pain reduction, as expressed by reduction in preexisting pain.

For the first, there are a good number of papers exploring the predictive value of suprathreshold magnitude estimation of pain on the acute postoperative pain, as briefly

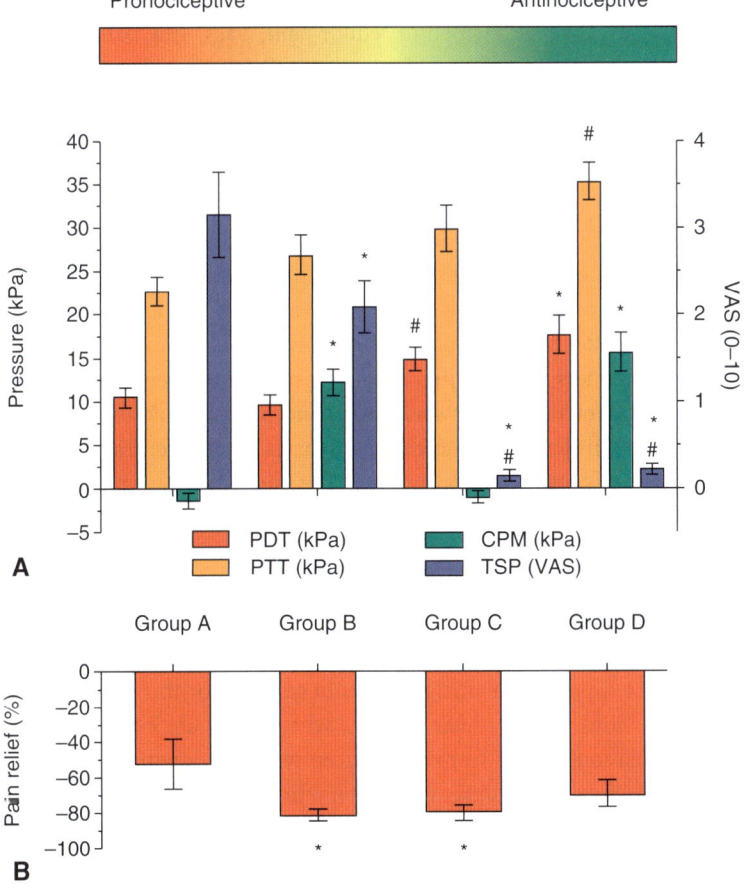

FIGURE 15-2 **A:** Mean (±SEM) preoperative pressure pain detection thresholds (PDTs) (*red bars*, [kPa]), pressure pain tolerance thresholds (PTTs) (*yellow bars*, [kPa]), conditioned pain modulation (CPM) (*green bars*, [kPa]), and temporal summation of pain (TSP) (*blue bars*, [VAS]) were measured using cuff algometry at the lower leg. Groups are defined by facilitated TSP and impaired CPM (Group A, N = 16), facilitated TSP and normal CPM (Group B, N = 15), normal TSP and impaired CPM (Group C, N = 44), and normal TSP and normal CPM (Group D, N = 28). **B:** Mean (±SEM) pain relief from the four groups after total knee replacement. *Significant difference ($P < 0.05$) compared with group A. #Significant difference ($P < 0.05$) compared with group B. (Taken from Petersen KK, Graven-Nielsen T, Simonsen O, et al. Preoperative pain mechanisms assessed by cuff algometry are associated with chronic postoperative pain relief after total knee replacement. Pain 2016;157:1400–6 [Figure 1].)

mentioned previously. Data were reviewed by Abrishami [1], showing that from all the static parameters, suprathreshold heat pain magnitude estimation is most likely to correlate with postoperative pain in the acute phase. A few studies examined the predictive value of dynamic psychophysical parameters on postoperative pain. Our group had shown that CPM predicts chronic postoperative pain. In a cohort of patients scheduled for thoracotomy, an efficient CPM was found to predict lower rates of chronic postthoracotomy pain [66]. Similar data were also obtained by Wilder-Smith et al. for abdominal surgery [64]. In these two studies the preoperative assessment did not predict the levels of acute postoperative pain. Landau et al. reported prediction of acute post–cesarean section pain by preoperative CPM [28]. An interesting recent finding is that CPM did predict pain levels after mastectomy but only if there was no preoperative pain [52], insinuating that the presence of previous pain might have changed, or "consumed" the CPM resources of the patients, to the point of losing the ability to predict future pain behavior. Grosen et al. [18] have found that preoperative CPM predicted acute morphine consumption following funnel chest surgery. For operations performed to reduce pain, classifying painful knee OA patients by a combination of CPM and TS before surgery, Petersen et al. [45] found that dual pronociceptive patients (high TS and less efficient CPM) were those to gain the least pain reduction by total knee replacement (TKR), compared with patients who were pronociceptive in either the ascending or descending line only, although not compared with antinociceptive on both lines.

For TS, Weissman-Fogel et al. [62] found higher acute postthoracotomy pain for subjects with enhanced summation. For pain reduction after surgery, a similar direction was found in hip OA, where high preoperative TS was associated with less clinical pain relief 6 weeks after hip arthroplasty [20]. As for chronic pain, high TS preceding TKR in knee OA predicted less relief in clinical pain 1 year after surgery [44].

The interaction between drugs and pain modulation depends on the drug's mode of action. This text will concentrate on drugs that act centrally and can be considered as modulators of central pain processing. The interaction is expected to be bidirectional: Effect of the drug should be determined by the modulation state, and the modulation state should be altered by the effect of the drug (this text will refer to human studies only; for animal based studies see Refs. [34,43], and for a review see Ref. [47]). Drugs can be used (1) before surgery, to potentially render the system more antinociceptive and therefore more resistant to the nociceptive neuronal barrages, resulting in lower clinical pain. The term preemptive, or better, preventive analgesia has been used for this concept (see Ref. [23] for elaborate discussion), and (2) after surgery, when drugs are expected to lower the pronociceptive modulation derived from the nociceptive exposure during surgery.

As far as the nature of the interaction, we would like to introduce the leading concept of "fix the dysfunction." This concept suggests that for analgesic drugs that have a CNS-modulating effect, coupling of drug's mode of action with the patient's dysfunction of pain modulation would lead to efficacious use of the drug. This way, if a specific patient shows a certain dysfunctional mechanism, for example, descending pronociceptive expressed by less efficient CPM, a drug that augments pain inhibition, and therefore improves CPM, would be the likely drug to cause pain amelioration for this individual. For another individual, whose CPM is efficient, one would expect a little, if any, effect of such a drug. For the latter patient, drugs that exert their analgesic effect via other modes of action should be used. Our group has recently shown that painful diabetic neuropathy patients responded to duloxetine along this line of reasoning [67]. Duloxetine is a serotonin–norepinephrine reuptake inhibitor (SNRI), whose main action is to inhibit reuptake of noradrenalin and serotonin, the two neurotransmitters that exert the descending pain inhibition effect at the spinal dorsal horn level. We found that patients with less efficient CPM were the ones to respond to the drug, whereas those with efficient CPM to begin with did not respond to the drug. Furthermore, for the former, CPM improved in parallel to the decrease in pain, whereas for the latter, it did not change. Our results have been supported by Niesters et al. [36], who found a similar effect for tapentadol, a combined SNRI–μ opioid drug.

A parallel line can be drawn for the facilitatory tests. Ascending pronociceptive patients with enhanced TS would most likely best respond to drugs of the gabapentinoid family, which are Ca^{++} channel ligands, whose main mode of action is reduction of neuronal sensitization. Reduction of TS by pregabalin (PGB) has been demonstrated in healthy volunteers [4]. Patients whose summation is nonenhanced are less likely to respond to this line of drug and should use other medications. In a study on prediction of PGB efficacy in chronic pancreatitis patients [39], those reporting lower pain tolerance thresholds, measured by tetanic electrical skin stimulation in the pancreatic dermatome (as compared with a distant dermatome), were the ones to best respond to PGB. As could be expected, CPM did not predict PGB efficacy (Figure 15-3), although PGB was recently shown to have some effect on the descending system, improving CPM in healthy subjects [60].

The preemptive analgesia concept has been extensively studied, and several reviews and meta-analyses had been published along the years [14,22,35,37,48]. Typically, an analgesic of any kind is given before surgery, and the patient is followed up for acute postoperative pain and analgesic consumption after surgery. Some studies also look at the long-term effects. Generally, the concept is considered as interesting and seems as a "more useful approach" [47]. Nonetheless, the use of preemptive, or as often termed, preventive analgesia for surgery has not been implemented as a standard practice. Over the past decade, data have been accumulated on this topic, and it is now possible to draw some conclusions regarding the combined effect of some preoperative drugs such as ketamine and pain-reducing surgeries [47]. Recently published meta-analysis concluded that NSAIDs, more specifically COX2 inhibitors and gabapentin seem to be effective at reducing analgesic consumption 24 hours after surgery [37]. Even though much progress has been made, there are still many unanswered questions and the large heterogeneity between the different studies makes it difficult to draw clear conclusions. PMP had not been so far a consideration in the use of preemptive analgesia, and we will try to reason why it should be. Taking into

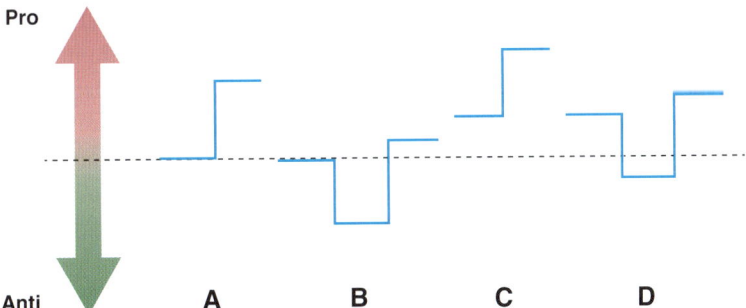

FIGURE 15-3 Changes in pain modulation due to surgery: An individual with normal modulation profile becomes pronociceptive due to surgery **(A)**. If preemptive analgesia is successfully given **(B)**, the individual becomes antinociceptive at surgery, and the same shift caused by surgery will lead to a better modulation profile than without treatment. An individual with an a priori pronociceptive profile will become much more pronociceptive due to surgery **(C)**. If preemptive analgesia is successfully given, a better final modulation profile will be achieved **(D)**.

consideration the concept of coupling a drug by its mode of action with the individual's dysfunction in pain modulation, as shown for chronic pain, one can design a treatment to improve postoperative pain outcomes by use of individually tailored preemptive analgesia: (1) We expect pain-free individuals who are pronociceptive to be more susceptible to acquire pain, having a higher pain phenotype expression, i.e., more frequent and more intense pain, in the context of surgery. Thus, pronociceptive individuals would be the prime target population for preemptive treatment. It is currently unclear whether antinociceptive persons would gain some benefit from preemptive treatment. (2) Individuals who are descending pronociceptive, based on less efficient CPM, should be given a drug that can reverse this dysfunction, to better prepare them for the nociceptive challenge of surgery. In this case, SNRIs, and maybe tricyclics, should be appropriate drugs. (3) Individuals who are ascending pronociceptive, based on enhanced TS, should be given a drug that can reverse this dysfunction, such as a gabapentinoid, or maybe, another antiepileptic medication. (4) Dual pronociceptive individuals who express both reduced inhibition and enhanced facilitation should probably receive a combination of two drugs.

Some of the placebo-controlled studies exploring preemptive analgesia for surgery used drugs that can be considered as pain modulating, such as duloxetine and PGB. In most of these studies that explored the acute postoperative phase, the drug was given for a very short period, usually 1 or 2 hours before surgery [2,15,19,24,42,51,65], and its effects were evaluated against placebo. In studies that looked on chronic postoperative pain, drugs were usually administered for a longer period [35] after surgery but started only 1 to 2 hours before the procedure [10]. Many studies, though not all, showed acute postoperative pain reduction in the treated group. In a recent meta-analysis, PGB was shown to reduce pain and analgesic consumption in the acute phase after surgery [14]. In regard to prevention of chronic postoperative pain, a recent review and meta-analysis on the use of PGB in preemptive analgesia concluded that its effect is not superior to placebo [35]. Nevertheless, pain modulation had not been assessed in these patients, and data on this line of thinking are awaited. There are many open questions, such as how long should the drug be used. On the one hand, studies in diabetic painful neuropathy and postherpetic neuralgia have shown a curve of gradual pain reduction along the first 2 to 4 weeks of administration of the agent, suggesting that longer periods of time are required; on the other hand, the few articles that used PGB perioperatively found an effect on acute postoperative pain even after 1 hour of use just before surgery. It is likely that for pain-free individuals there should be a shorter time period than several weeks preoperatively to attain an effect, but, likely, it will be optimal to use drugs for longer than 1 hour preoperatively. Another question is for how long the drug should be used after surgery. Mechanistic thinking will indicate that as long as the nociceptive activity from the site of surgery is still active, there should be a drug in the system to protect the CNS from its effects. On the other hand, these drugs do have side effects, and one would like to shorten their use to the minimum necessary.

The "fix the dysfunction" concept can be straightforwardly extended to the postoperative period. Even if preemptive analgesia is not used, the concept of individual tailoring of analgesia is relevant here as well. It is unclear whether the individual tailoring concept is relevant to opioids use in the postoperative period; the relatively high rate of response makes the search for individual tailoring less relevant. Nevertheless, current developments regarding the prevalence of opioid-induced hyperalgesia and its undesirable effects might generate a need for individual tailoring for opioids as well.

In summary, this manuscript proposes a pain modulation mechanism–based approach to the prevention and treatment of acute and chronic pain in the perioperative period. We believe that assessing patient's pain modulation using quantitative sensory testing and tailoring treatment in a way that reverses dysfunctions of modulation can improve our ability to manage postoperative pain, both acute and chronic.

REFERENCES

1. Abrishami A, Chan J, Chung F, Wong J. Preoperative pain sensitivity and its correlation with postoperative pain and analgesic consumption: a qualitative systematic review. Anesthesiology 2011;114:445–57.
2. Agarwal A, Gautam S, Gupta D, et al. Evaluation of a single preoperative dose of pregabalin for attenuation of postoperative pain after laparoscopic cholecystectomy. Br J Anaesth 2008;101:700–4.
3. Arendt-Nielsen L, Egsgaard LL, Petersen KK, et al. A mechanism-based pain sensitivity index to characterize knee osteoarthritis patients with different disease stages and pain levels. Eur J Pain 2015;19:1406–17.
4. Arendt-Nielsen L, Frøkjaer JB, Staahl C, et al. Effects of gabapentin on experimental somatic pain and temporal summation. Reg Anesth Pain Med 2007;32:382–8.
5. Arendt-Nielsen L, Nie H, Laursen MB, et al. Sensitization in patients with painful knee osteoarthritis. Pain 2010;149:573–81.
6. Bisgaard T, Klarskov B, Rosenberg J, Kehlet H. Characteristics and prediction of early pain after laparoscopic cholecystectomy. Pain 2001;90:261–9.
7. Brandsborg B, Dueholm M, Kehlet H, et al. Mechanosensitivity before and after hysterectomy: a prospective study on the prediction of acute and chronic postoperative pain. Br J Anaesth 2011;107:940–7.
8. Buchgreitz L, Egsgaard LL, Jensen R, et al. Abnormal pain processing in chronic tension-type headache: a high-density EEG brain mapping study. Brain 2008;131:3232–8.
9. Burstein R, Yarnitsky D, Goor-Aryeh I, et al. An association between migraine and cutaneous allodynia. Ann Neurol 2000;47:614–24.
10. Buvanendran A, Kroin JS, Della Valle CJ, et al. Perioperative oral pregabalin reduces chronic pain after total knee arthroplasty: a prospective, randomized, controlled trial. Anesth Analg 2010;110:199–207.
11. Cathcart S, Winefield AH, Rolan P, Lushington K. Reliability of temporal summation and diffuse noxious inhibitory control. Pain Res Manag 2009;14:433–8.
12. Chang L. Brain responses to visceral and somatic stimuli in irritable bowel syndrome: a central nervous system disorder? Gastroenterol Clin North Am 2005;34:271–9.
13. Daenen L, Nijs J, Roussel N, et al. Dysfunctional pain inhibition in patients with chronic whiplash-associated disorders: an experimental study. Clin Rheumatol 2013;32:23–31.
14. Dong J, Li W, Wang Y. The effect of pregabalin on acute postoperative pain in patients undergoing total knee arthroplasty: a meta-analysis. Int J Surg 2016;34:148–60.
15. Gianesello L, Pavoni V, Barboni E, et al. Perioperative pregabalin for postoperative pain control and quality of life after major spinal surgery. J Neurosurg Anesthesiol 2012;24:121–6.
16. Granot M, Lowenstein L, Yarnitsky D, et al. Post-cesarean section pain prediction by preoperative experimental pain assessment. Anesthesiology 2003;98:1422–6.
17. Greenspan JD, Slade GD, Bair E, et al. Pain sensitivity risk factors for chronic TMD: descriptive data and empirically identified domains from the OPPERA case control study. J Pain 2011;12(Suppl.):T61–74.
18. Grosen K, Vase L, Pilegaard HK, et al. Conditioned pain modulation and situational pain catastrophizing as preoperative predictors of pain following chest wall surgery: a prospective observational cohort study. PLoS One 2014;9:e90185.
19. Ho KY, Tay W, Yeo MC, et al. Duloxetine reduces morphine requirements after knee replacement surgery. Br J Anaesth 2010;105:371–6.
20. Izumi M, Petersen KK, Laursen MB, et al. Facilitated temporal summation of pain correlates with clinical pain intensity after hip arthroplasty. Pain 2017;158:323–32.
21. Julien N, Goffaux P, Arsenault P, Marchand S. Widespread pain in fibromyalgia is related to a deficit of endogenous pain inhibition. Pain 2005;114:295–302.
22. Katz J, McCartney CJ. Current status of preemptive analgesia. Curr Opin Anesthesiol 2002;15:435–41.
23. Katz J, Clarke H, Seltzer Z. Preventive analgesia: quo vadimus? Anesth Analg 2011;113:1242–53.
24. Kim JC, Choi YS, Kim KN, et al. Effective dose of peri-operative oral pregabalin as an adjunct to multimodal analgesic regimen in lumbar spinal fusion surgery. Spine 2011;36:428–33.
25. King C, Wong F, Currie T, et al. Deficiency in endogenous modulation of prolonged heat pain in patients with Irritable Bowel Syndrome and Temporomandibular Disorder. Pain 2009;143:172–8.

26. Kosek E, Hansson P. Modulatory influence on somatosensory perception from vibration and heterotopic noxious conditioning stimulation (HNCS) in fibromyalgia and healthy subjects. Pain 1997;70:41–51.
27. Kosek E, Ordeberg G. Lack of pressure pain modulation by heterotopic noxious conditioning stimulation in patients with painful osteoarthritis before, but not following, surgical pain relief. Pain 2000;88:69–78.
28. Landau R, Kraft JC, Flint LY, et al. An experimental paradigm for the prediction of Post-Operative Pain (PPOP). J Vis Exp 2010;27:35.
29. Lautenbacher S, Rollman GB. Possible deficiencies of pain modulation in fibromyalgia. Clin J Pain 1997;13:189–96.
30. Lemming D, Graven-Nielsen T, Sörensen J, et al. Widespread pain hypersensitivity and facilitated temporal summation of deep tissue pain in whiplash associated disorder: an explorative study of women. J Rehabil Med 2012;44:648–57.
31. Lunn TH, Gaarn-Larsen L, Kehlet H. Prediction of postoperative pain by preoperative pain response to heat stimulation in total knee arthroplasty. Pain 2013;154:1878–85.
32. Maixner W, Fillingim R, Booker D, Sigurdsson A. Sensitivity of patients with painful temporomandibular disorders to experimentally evoked pain. Pain 1995;63:341–51.
33. Maixner W, Fillingim R, Sigurdsson A, et al. Sensitivity of patients with painful temporomandibular disorders to experimentally evoked pain: evidence for altered temporal summation of pain. Pain 1998;76:71.
34. Matsuoka H, Suto T, Saito S, Obata H. Amitriptyline, but not pregabalin, reverses the attenuation of noxious stimulus–induced analgesia after nerve injury in rats. Anesth Analg 2016;123:504–10.
35. Martinez V, Pichard X, Fletcher D. Perioperative pregabalin administration does not prevent chronic postoperative pain: systematic review with a meta-analysis of randomized trials. Pain 2017;158:775–83.
36. Niesters M, Proto P, Aarts L, et al. Tapentadol potentiates descending pain inhibition in chronic pain patients with diabetic polyneuropathy. Br J Anaesth 2014;113:148–56.
37. Nir RR, Nahman-Averbuch H, Moont R, et al. Preoperative preemptive drug administration for acute postoperative pain: a systematic review and meta-analysis. Eur J Pain 2016;20:1025–43.
38. Nir R-R, Yarnitsky D. Conditioned pain modulation. Curr Opin Support Palliat Care 2015;9:131–7.
39. Olesen SS, Graversen C, Bouwense SA, et al. Quantitative sensory testing predicts pregabalin efficacy in painful chronic pancreatitis. PLoS One 2013;8:e55460.
40. Oono Y, Wang K, Baad-Hansen L, et al. Conditioned pain modulation in temporomandibular disorders (TMD) pain patients. Exp Brain Res 2014;232:3111–9.
41. Pan PH, Coghill R, Houle TT, et al. Multifactorial preoperative predictors for postcesarean section pain and analgesic requirement. Anesthesiology 2006;104:417–25.
42. Peng PW, Li C, Farcas E, et al. Use of low-dose pregabalin in patients undergoing laparoscopic cholecystectomy. Br J Anaesth 2010;105:155–61.
43. Peters CM, Hayashida K-i, Suto T, et al. Individual differences in acute pain-induced endogenous analgesia predict time to resolution of postoperative pain in the rat. Anesthesiology 2015;122:895–907.
44. Petersen KK, Arendt-Nielsen L, Simonsen O, et al. Presurgical assessment of temporal summation of pain predicts the development of chronic postoperative pain 12 months after total knee replacement. Pain 2015;156:55–61.
45. Petersen KK, Graven-Nielsen T, Simonsen O, et al. Preoperative pain mechanisms assessed by cuff algometry are associated with chronic postoperative pain relief after total knee replacement. Pain 2016;157:1400–6.
46. Pielsticker A, Haag G, Zaudig M, Lautenbacher S. Impairment of pain inhibition in chronic tension-type headache. Pain 2005;118:215–23.
47. Pogatzki-Zahn EM, Segelcke D, Schug SA. Postoperative pain—from mechanisms to treatment. Pain Rep 2017;2:e588.
48. Pogagtzki-Zahn EM, Zahn PK. From pre-emptive to preventive analgesia. Curr Opin Anesthesiol 2006;19:551–5.
49. Price DD, Staud R. Neurobiology of fibromyalgia syndrome. J Rheumatol 2005;75(Suppl.):22–8.
50. Pud D, Granovsky Y, Yarnitsky D. The methodology of experimentally induced diffuse noxious inhibitory control (DNIC)-like effect in humans. Pain 2009;144:16–9.
51. Reuben SS, Buvanendran A, Kroin JS, Raghunathan K. The analgesic efficacy of celecoxib, pregabalin, and their combination for spinal fusion surgery. Anesth Analg 2006;103:1271–7.
52. Ruscheweyh R, Viehoff A, Tio J, Pogatzki-Zahn EM. Psychophysical and psychological predictors of acute pain after breast surgery differ in patients with and without pre-existing chronic pain. Pain 2017;158:1030–8.
53. Sandrini G, Rossi P, Milanov I, et al. Abnormal modulatory influence of diffuse noxious inhibitory controls in migraine and chronic tension-type headache patients. Cephalalgia 2006;26:782–9.

54. Sarlani E, Garrett PH, Grace EG, Greenspan JD. Temporal summation of pain characterizes women but not men with temporomandibular disorders. J Orofac Pain 2007;21:309–17.
55. Sarlani E, Grace EG, Reynolds MA, Greenspan JD. Evidence for up-regulated central nociceptive processing in patients with masticatory myofascial pain. J Orofac Pain 2004;18:41–55.
56. Song GH, Venkatraman V, Ho KY, et al. Cortical effects of anticipation and endogenous modulation of visceral pain assessed by functional brain MRI in irritable bowel syndrome patients and healthy controls. Pain 2006;126:79–90.
57. Staud R, Robinson ME, Price DD. Temporal summation of second pain and its maintenance are useful for characterizing widespread central sensitization of fibromyalgia patients. J Pain. 2007;8:893–901.
58. Staud R. Abnormal endogenous pain modulation is a shared characteristic of many chronic pain conditions. Expert Rev Neurother 2012;12:577–85.
59. Staud R, Weyl EE, Riley III JL, Fillingim RB. Slow temporal summation of pain for assessment of central pain sensitivity and clinical pain of fibromyalgia patients. PLoS One 2014;9:e89086.
60. Sugimine S, Saito S, Araki T, Yamamoto K, Obata H. Endogenous analgesic effect of pregabalin: a double-blind and randomized controlled trial. Eur J Pain 2017. doi:10.1002/ejp.1007.
61. Van Oosterwijck J, Nijs J, Meeus M, Paul L. Evidence for central sensitization in chronic whiplash: a systematic literature review. Eur J Pain 2013;17:299–312.
62. Weissman-Fogel I, Granovsky Y, Crispel Y, et al. Enhanced presurgical pain temporal summation response predicts post-thoracotomy pain intensity during the acute postoperative phase. J Pain 2009;10:628–36.
63. Weissman-Fogel I, Sprecher E, Granovsky Y, Yarnitsky D. Repeated noxious stimulation of the skin enhances cutaneous pain perception of migraine patients in-between attacks: clinical evidence for continuous sub-threshold increase in membrane excitability of central trigeminovascular neurons. Pain 2003;104:693–700.
64. Wilder-Smith OH, Schreyer T, Scheffer GJ, Arendt-Nielsen L. Patients with chronic pain after abdominal surgery show less preoperative endogenous pain inhibition and more postoperative hyperalgesia: a pilot study. J Pain Palliat Care Pharmacother 2010;24:119–28.
65. YaDeau JT, Lin Y, Mayman DJ, et al. Pregabalin and pain after total knee arthroplasty: a double-blind, randomized, placebo-controlled, multidose trial. Br J Anaesth 2015;115:285–93.
66. Yarnitsky D, Crispel Y, Eisenberg E, et al. Prediction of chronic post-operative pain: pre-operative DNIC testing identifies patients at risk. Pain 2008;138:22–8.
67. Yarnitsky D, Granot M, Nahman-Averbuch H, et al. Conditioned pain modulation predicts duloxetine efficacy in painful diabetic neuropathy. Pain 2012; 153:1193–8.

SECTION 5

Researching Interventions to Inhibit or Prevent Chronification of Acute Pain

CHAPTER 16

Pain Sensitization: A Critical Process in the Transition from Acute to Chronic Postsurgical Pain (CPSP)

Guy Simonnet

Pain after surgery is the theme of the IASP's 2017 global year against pain. Twenty years ago, Crombie et al. [16] noted that 22.5% of patients attending pain clinics attributed their pain to a previous surgery. Therefore, the prevention of chronic postsurgical pain (CPSP) is an actual challenge in clinical practice [25]. In spite of numerous clinical studies to identify risk factors, the nature of CPSP is still poorly characterized. Today, clinical research has mainly focused on preoperative risk factors and the type of surgery [34,57]. Recently, a multicenter, prospective, observational study within the European registry PAIN OUT (http:www.pain-out.eu/) generates new hypothesis suggesting the percentage of time in severe pain during the first 24 hours after surgery (acute postsurgical pain) is also an important risk factor for CPSP: A 10% in time spent in severe pain on day 1 after surgery is associated with a 30% increase of CPSP incidence at 12 months [19]. This European clinical trial confirms the prevalence of neuropathic signs because an incidence of 11.8% for moderate to severe CPSP 12 months after surgery is revealed with neuropathic signs in 39.2%. In contrast, studies investigating the associated CPSP with 90 genetic markers found no evidence for genetic predisposition [57]. Therefore, the time of the acute postsurgical pain appears as a critical episode for CPSP.

To better understand this new hypothesis, a modern concept suggests that exaggerated acute pain after surgery is not only the result of surgical nociceptive inputs but also the reflection of an increased pain sensitivity associated with central sensitization induced by pre- and perioperative factors [8,20,32,35,46,47,53,55,60,61]. From a theoretical viewpoint, the existence of a postsurgical central sensitization suggests that nociceptive and nonnociceptive postsurgical events may reactivate pain in sensitized patients, leading to abnormal pain and probably to CPSP. Of noteworthy is that neuronal sensitization processes are different from nociceptive processes. In other words, an effective prevention of CPSP cannot to be limited to a pure analgesic strategy, as it has been previously suggested with the preemptive analgesia concept. A careful antisensitization strategy has also to be developed before and after surgery for specifically preventing an enhancement in pain sensitivity leading to exaggerated acute postsurgical pain and CPSP.

Because it is difficult to examine central sensitization associated with surgical situation in clinical trials, the aim of this chapter is to provide a comprehensive review of the neurobiologic processes underlying pain hypersensitivity development in experimental animal models of surgery. To identify risk factors inducing central sensitization, we and others initiated a "reverse translational research" by developing experimental animal models mimicking situations with persistent pain after surgery in humans. Obviously, the validation of these preclinical results requires a rigorous comparison with human clinical trial data. Therefore, we examined, in animal models, the ability of factors to trigger or reactivate pain hypersensitivity. Based on data obtained in these experimental CPSP models, pharmacologic and nutritional therapies able to prevent pain hypersensitivity induced by pre-, peri-, and postsurgical events will be briefly discussed.

PAIN ASSOCIATED WITH TISSUE INJURY INDUCES LATENT PAIN HYPERSENSITIVITY

It is generally recognized that tissue damage associated with surgical lesions or inflammation often produces peripheral and central sensitization that may outlast the stimuli leading to sustained hyperalgesia, allodynia, and persistent pain [18,31,49]. The abnormal persistence of nervous system sensitization subsequent to acute nociception is now considered a major candidate mechanism for the development of chronic pain [37]. A rarely appreciated fact is that all chronic pain was once acute. Despite difficulties in obtaining evidence in clinical practice, the phenomenon of pain hypersensitivity is strongly suspected to exist in humans after a surgical insult. A *princeps* observation was reported in young children: Those who had been circumcised 6 months earlier showed an increase in their pain response to a vaccination procedure [56].

This phenomenon has been clearly observed in animals. In rats [29], the existence of an initial painful lesion, even if it is healed (e.g., a surgical incision in a paw), causes pain hypersensitivity that is revealed if a second tissue damage (inflammation) is incurred several days later in another area of the body (Figure 16-1A and B). This observation is particularly interesting because it is indicative of a sensitization process of central origin or at least of bilateral communication at the spinal cord level. In humans, the presence of contralateral pain has been occasionally observed in some types of chronic pain [50]. In other words, although the postsurgical pain had disappeared, its imprint in the central nervous system remained because pain hypersensitivity was observed at both the ipsilateral and contralateral levels. This phenomenon has been referred to as latent pain hypersensitivity [29,46]. Although these animal experiments were limited to a time span of several weeks, the results suggest that a prior pain experience can facilitate the development of CPSP. This central sensitization process could explain some "spontaneous pain" or exaggerated pain in individuals with pain history.

From a mechanistic standpoint, there is a compelling body of evidence that neural N-methyl-D-aspartate receptor (NMDA-R) activation plays a critical role in the development and maintenance of pain hypersensitivity. In a *princeps* paper, Stubhaug et al. [55] reported that the intravenous infusion of ketamine in humans during and after surgery reduced mechanical punctate hyperalgesia surrounding a surgical lesion for several days after surgery. Although a single preadministration of ketamine had only moderate effects on early postsurgical pain (1 to 5 postsurgical days), injection of this NMDA-R antagonist completely prevented the latent pain hypersensitivity in rats that experienced pain, as revealed by the disappearance of abnormal hyperalgesia associated with an additional tissue injury (inflammation) 2 weeks after the initial surgical pain [47]. Nevertheless, although NMDA-Rs appear to play a critical role, other mechanisms closely related with long-term potentiation (LTP) [23,49] may participate in chronic postoperative pain [18,60].

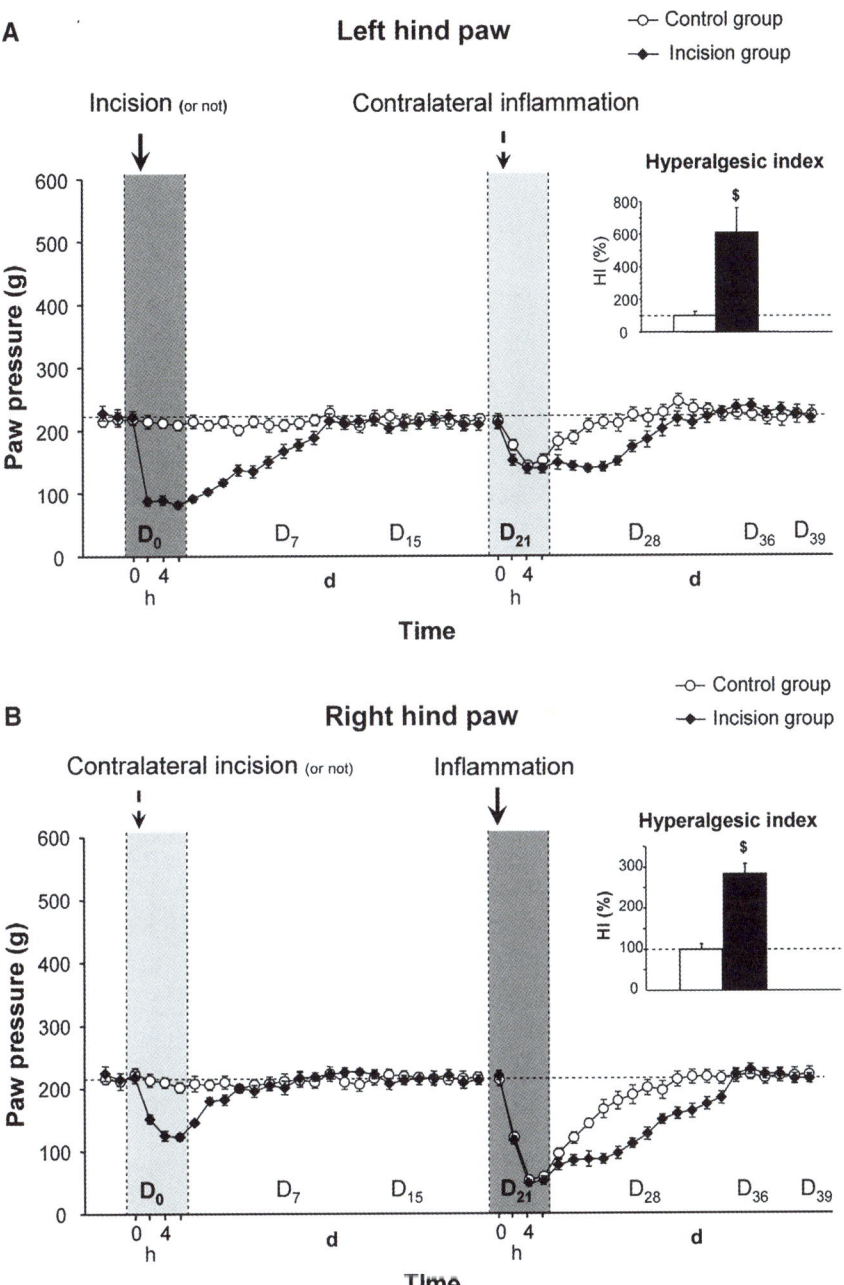

FIGURE 16-1 Latent pain hypersensitivity induced by a surgical lesion and its amplification by the administration of opioid analgesics. The mechanical nociceptive threshold (vocalization elicited in response to pressure) in rats was assessed using a Randall–Selitto test on the posterior paws. On D_0, the rats received four injections of saline or fentanyl (100 µg/kg) at intervals of 15 min, and an incision was made in the plantar muscle of the left paw 5 min after the first injection of fentanyl or saline. Incision was not performed on control animals. Three weeks later (D_{21}), an injection of carrageenan, which causes inflammation, was administered to the posterior right paw. The new inflammatory lesion created on D_{21} induced an exaggerated pain response (hyperalgesia) in the inflamed paw (**B and D**—right hind paw) but was capable of reactivating the pain hypersensitivity in the healed paw, in which there was a surgical lesion, regardless of whether the animals received fentanyl treatment 3 weeks prior (**A and C**—left hind paw). (Adapted from Laboureyras E, Chateauraynaud J, Richebe P, Simonnet G. Long-term pain vulnerability after surgery in rats: prevention by nefopam, an analgesic with antihyperalgesic properties. Anesth Analg 2009;109:623–31.)

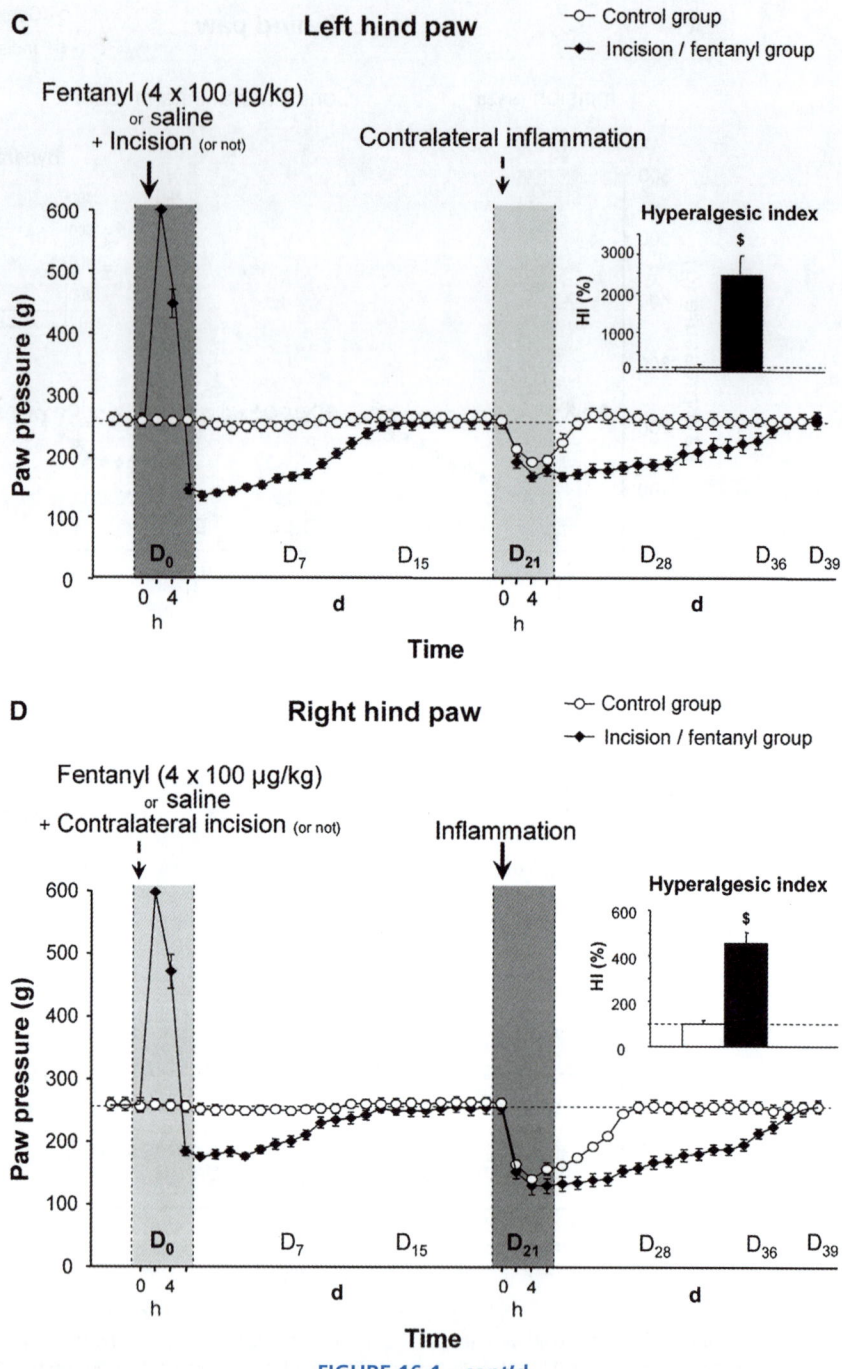

FIGURE 16-1 cont'd

OPIOID-INDUCED HYPERALGESIA (OIH)

Although it is comprehensible that previous experiences of pain can leave a biologic mark and may play a critical role in the development of the pain sensitization processes, it may seem paradoxical to highlight the role of opioids (either exogenous or endogenous) in the development of certain types of chronic pain. Nevertheless, although opioids are recognized as unsurpassed analgesics for moderate to severe pain (i.e., most surgical pain), for more than a century, clinical studies have reported that hyperalgesia is the most common symptom of withdrawal after prolonged opioid administration [15]. Indeed, this problem has been marginalized in surgical practice, as it is logical that a patient who undergoes an operation would have postoperative pain and would require opioid administration.

Mao documented the first occurrence of opioid-induced hyperalgesia (OIH) in laboratory animals, indicating that thermal hyperalgesia was associated with the development of tolerance in rats induced by prolonged morphine administration [38,39]. To mimic the clinical use of opioids for surgery, we performed a long-term animal study to examine both acute and long-lasting effects induced by a single administration of an opioid, such as fentanyl. By measuring changes in the nociceptive threshold, we [8] showed that in addition to the immediate analgesic effect observed in rats receiving four subcutaneous fentanyl boluses within 1 hour, a degree of pain hypersensitivity was always observed (Figure 16-2A) and continued for several days after opioid administration was discontinued. The amplitude of hyperalgesia was higher if the dose of opioid was higher. It is apparent that the time course of this biphasic effect, i.e., analgesia followed by hyperalgesia, is very different compared with that of a monophasic effect. The first effect only lasts as long as the opioid receptors are being stimulated (hours), and the second effect is far longer in duration (days), which suggests that a system of memorization or imprinting is being activated. Similar OIHs were observed following the administration of alfentanil and remifentanil [1,6]. This phenomenon of pain hypersensitivity induced by opioids has also been observed in healthy volunteers given remifentanil [28] and in heroin addicts [15].

From a mechanistic standpoint, we and others have demonstrated the critical role of NMDA-Rs in OIH by showing that a single administration of an NMDA-R antagonist, such as ketamine, MK-801, or BN2572 completely prevented OIH in animals [7,8,30,32]. Electrophysiologic studies have demonstrated that µ-opioid receptor (MOR) stimulation activates intracellular protein kinase C (PKC), which reduces Mg^{2+} blocking, thereby activating NMDA-Rs [10]. The subsequent increase in the intracellular Ca^{2+} concentration has been suggested to further stimulate PKC activity, leading to a lasting enhancement of glutamatergic synaptic efficiency in a positive feedback loop (Figure 16-3), a process resembling LTP. Recently, it has been proposed that opioid-induced LTP in the spinal cord results from increased presynaptic glutamate release from the transient receptor potential vanilloid 1 (TRPV1)–expressing primary afferents [62]. Activation of TRPV1 has been reported to contribute to OIH via glutamate release [59], and TRPV1 blockers reduce OIH [11]. Interestingly, blocking of the NMDA-NO cascade using the nitric oxide synthase (NOS) inhibitor N^G-nitro-L-arginine methyl ester (L-NAME) has been reported to produce effects similar to those of NMDA-R antagonists. This result suggests a critical role for this intracellular secondary messenger system in OIH because NO release facilitates the glutamate release at the spinal cord level; this is also consistent with the observation that OIH is significantly attenuated in mutant mice lacking inducible nitric oxide synthase (iNOS) [6]. Taken together, these results indicate that the spinal NMDA-Rs/iNOS system plays a critical role at the dorsal horn level in OIH. Other mechanisms underlying OIH could not be excluded at either the spinal or supraspinal level, such as the involvement of the β-adrenergic receptor [13], α2-adrenoreceptors [43], Ca^{2+}/calmodulin-dependent protein kinase IIα (CAMKIIα) [12], and local cytokine production [36]. CAMKIIα has been described to interact with the NMDA-R system [27]. Therefore, CAMKIIα and the NMDA receptor systems may interact in a feed-forward manner in OIH. Antiopioid

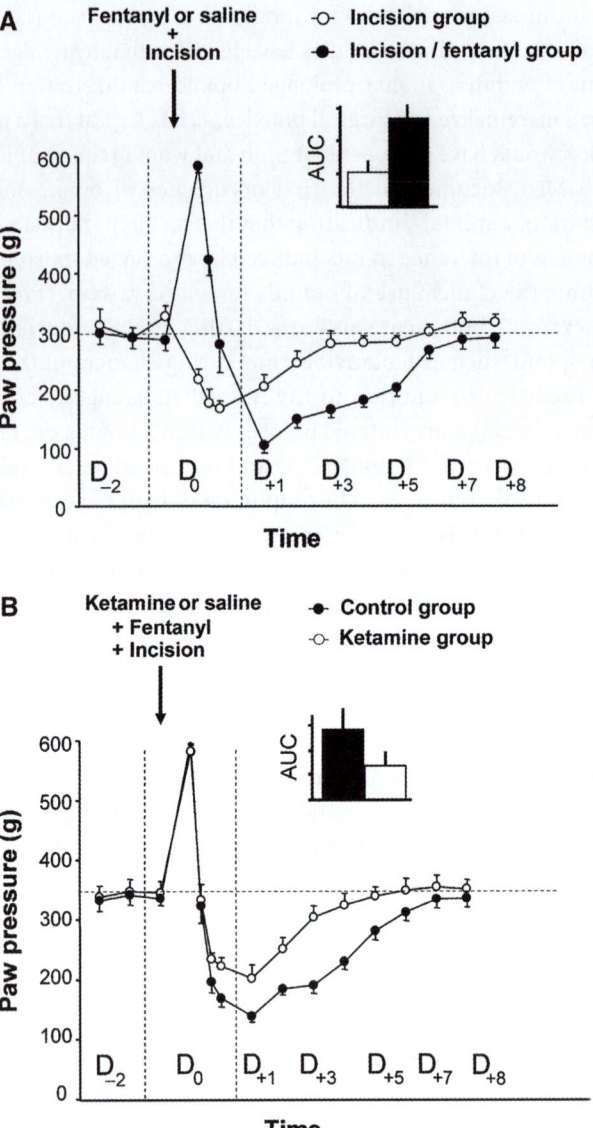

FIGURE 16-2 Amplification of surgical injury–induced hyperalgesia via the administration of an opioid analgesic and the reduction of this amplification by the administration of ketamine, an NMDA receptor antagonist. **A:** On D_0, the rats received four injections of saline or fentanyl (100 µg/kg) at intervals of 15 min and an incision was made in the plantar muscle of the left paw 15 min after the first injection of fentanyl or saline. The administration of fentanyl resulted in an immediate analgesic effect but also potentiated the pain hypersensitivity induced by a surgical lesion, which is expressed as an amplification of the postsurgical hyperalgesia for several days. **B:** Using the same experimental design, three injections of ketamine (3 × 10 mg/kg) or saline were administered subcutaneously. The first injection was administered 30 min before surgery, and the subsequent injections were administered every 5 h. The administration of ketamine results in a reduction of hyperalgesia induced by a surgical lesion associated with fentanyl administration. (From Richebe P, Rivat C, Laulin JP, et al. Ketamine improves the management of exaggerated postoperative pain observed in perioperative fentanyl-treated rats. Anesthesiology 2005;102:421–8.)

peptides (AOPs), such as cholecystokinin (CCK), neuropeptide FF (NPFF), dynorphin, and orphanin FQ/nociceptin, are endogenous peptides released following opioid receptor stimulation. AOPs have been proposed to be involved in OIH because specific AOP receptor antagonists prevent OIH [51]. AOPs promote the release of glutamate, and AOP release

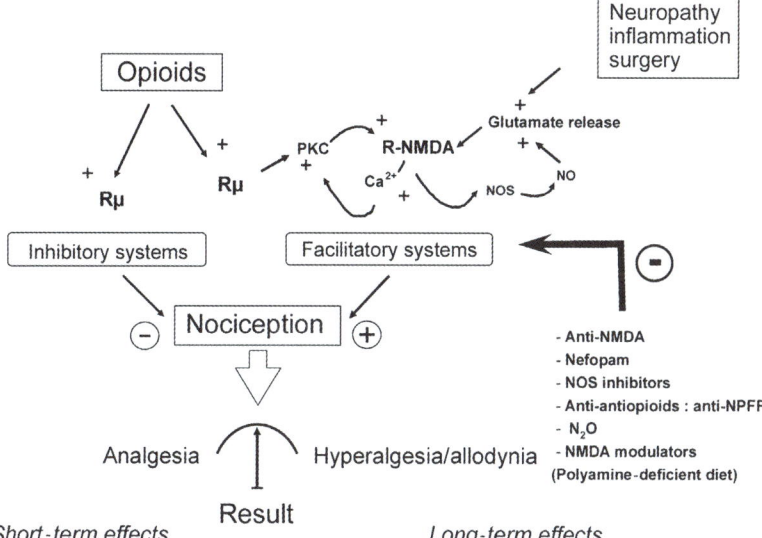

FIGURE 16-3 Model of the dual effects of opioids. Opioids simultaneously activate pain inhibitory systems (analgesia) and *N*-methyl-D-aspartate (NMDA)–dependent pain facilitatory systems, inducing pain hypersensitivity that outlasts opioid analgesia. The analgesic effect of opioid administration results from these two opposing processes, suggesting that the effect is partially masked as early as the first opioid exposure and that it is followed by hyperalgesia/allodynia. Repeated opioid administration induces lasting enhancement of glutamate synaptic efficiency in a positive feedback loop, increasing the activation level of NMDA-dependent pain facilitatory systems (sensitization); however, opioid analgesia remains unchanged. This effect leads to an apparent decrease in opioid analgesic potency (apparent tolerance). PKC, protein kinase C; NOS, nitric oxide synthase; NPFF, neuropeptide FF.

is facilitated by NMDA-R stimulation [26,52]. Finally, numerous studies have indicated that the rostral ventromedial medulla (RVM) and the surrounding tissue are a prominent source of descending pain modulation.

From an adaptive viewpoint, OIH, which involves experiencing paradoxical or abnormal pain, may be considered a physiologic or normal response if opioid-induced analgesia is considered a disturbance of homeostatic equilibrium [53]. In this context, pain hypersensitivity appears to be an effective response through which a new homeostatic equilibrium can be achieved (i.e., allostasis). The concept of a perturbed equilibrium, described by Canon, exists alongside the concept of physiologic balance: The imbalance that has been induced (analgesia) must be compensated for a return to a new equilibrium via the activation of an opponent process [54], such as pronociceptive system recruitment. Similar pain hypersensitivity has been observed following administration of triptans and α2-adrenoreceptor agonists [17,43].

THE ADMINISTRATION OF EXOGENOUS OPIOIDS AMPLIFIES THE LONG-LASTING HYPERALGESIA INDUCED BY A SURGICAL LESION

Considering these new physiologic concepts, we must evaluate whether the treatment with an opioid during the perioperative period is likely to amplify postsurgical pain and to promote the development of chronic postsurgical pain. This question is difficult to address in clinical practice because it is difficult to differentiate between normal and abnormal postsurgical pain. To mimic such a surgical situation, we used the preclinical incisional pain model (unilateral incision of a hind paw) developed by Brennan and colleagues [4], in association with the administration of fentanyl administration, an opioid drug that is extensively used by anesthesiologists.

In the first series of experiments, we evaluated the putative enhancement of postsurgical pain in rats receiving a series of four subcutaneous fentanyl boluses within 1 hour. Pain scoring was performed by measuring changes in the nociceptive threshold (heat and mechanical tests) or by evaluating changes in postural disequilibrium (weight bearing test) before, during, and several days after surgery. These preclinical studies showed that the administration of fentanyl not only produces an immediate analgesia, as expected, but also acts in a dose-dependent manner to strongly potentiate the pain hypersensitivity induced by the surgical lesion [29,45] (Figure 16-1C and D). These results have been reproduced in the mouse model by other groups after injections of fentanyl, remifentanil, alfentanil, or sufentanil [5,9,41].

As in OIH, this process of sensitization to pain is NMDA-dependent and can be prevented by a single injection of an NMDA-R antagonist, such as ketamine or other medications that are classified as antihyperalgesics (NO inhibitors [3], nefopam,[29] or gabapentin [58]). The amplification of postsurgical pain was considerably reduced in mice lacking the iNOS gene, confirming the critical role of the NMDA-R/iNOS system. Interestingly, this pain hypersensitivity is not only localized to the injured hind paw but also present on the contralateral uninjured hind paw, which confirms the central origin of this process [29,47].

It is questionable whether opioids enhance postsurgical pain in humans. Among various clinical studies, one quantitative sensory test (QST) has clinically demonstrating postsurgical pain enhancement via perioperative opioid use [24]. This study revealed that a relatively large dose of intraoperative remifentanil (0.40 μg/kg per minute) increases pain sensitivity, as evidenced by a reduction of the postsurgical pain threshold proximal to the surgical wound and an extension of peri-incisional hyperalgesia. This phenomenon lasted throughout the postoperative period and was associated with an increase in the postoperative self-administration of morphine (patient-controlled analgesia or PCA). In agreement with preclinical observations, a small dose of ketamine during and after surgery prevented the increase in postsurgical pain sensitivity and punctate hyperalgesia and reduced the morphine requirement by PCA. However, human studies have led to conflicting results, most likely because the potential existence of such a phenomenon is framed within the current understanding of opioids as analgesic drugs, rather than hyperalgesic drugs. Moreover, physicians are reticent to undertreat pain, and the idea that potent analgesic such as opioids may actually worsen pain symptoms appears paradoxical and needs to be better incorporated into our philosophy of pain management. The suggestion that perioperative opioids may actually worsen pain presents new challenges. As it has been suggested [60], the demonstration of such a phenomenon requires rigorous research protocols for serial determination of stimulus dose–response curves under standardized conditions, such as QST, as it has been performed for OIH in human volunteers.

In a second series of experiments, we evaluated the level of long-term pain vulnerability induced by surgery associated with fentanyl by testing the pain response induced by an experimental inflammation performed 3 weeks after surgery. Indeed, it is unclear how long the change of state, in terms of sensitivity to pain, persists beyond the early postoperative period of hyperalgesia induced by tissue injury, even in a latent form when nociceptive inputs have stopped. This question is clinically important because some patients must undergo treatments during the postsurgical period that are potentially painful, while others must undergo further surgical procedures in the short- or medium-term that are sometimes performed on the contralateral side, such as surgery for hallux valgus, hip prosthesis, or cataracts.

In our experimental model, we observed [29] that the amplitude and duration of the hyperalgesia induced by an experimental inflammation in a hind paw (e.g., the right hind paw) were dramatically enhanced when it was performed in rats that had experienced a prior tissue injury, such as a surgical lesion on the contralateral side (e.g., on the left hind paw) (Figure 16-1B). This phenomenon, which is referred to as latent pain sensitization [35,46], was strongly amplified in the animals that received fentanyl boluses after a surgical incision was performed 3 weeks earlier (Figure 16-1D). Similar results were obtained in the same mouse model after perioperative remifentanil administration [5]. These preclinical studies indicate that the administration of an opioid analgesic amplified the development of a latent pain sensitization: Despite tissue healing, the individual did not return to the initial physiologic state (homeostatic state) but rather developed long-lasting pain vulnerability (allostatic state). This latent pain vulnerability has not yet been explored in surgical patients and must be examined. These data suggest that the evaluation of individual pain and opioid histories in humans may help identify patients at risk for exaggerated postsurgical pain, which may result in chronic postsurgical pain.

ENDOGENOUS OPIOIDS RELEASED DURING PRE- OR POSTSURGICAL ENVIRONMENTAL STRESS INDUCE PAIN VULNERABILITY

On the basis of the aforementioned data, questions arise concerning the ability of endogenous opioids to induce pain facilitatory effects. It is well known that stressful situations produce analgesia (stress-induced analgesia or SIA) through the release of endogenous opioid peptides in the CNS [21,44]. However, consistent with the biopsychosocial conceptual framework, there is a compelling body of evidence in humans that unmanaged negative emotion associated with stressful events is a psychological predictor of exaggerated pain, manifesting as postsurgical pain [22]. Pain hypersensitivity induced by stress is a lesser-known phenomenon compared with SIA, despite being more relevant from clinical and therapeutic standpoints because pain hypersensitivity leads to exaggerated pain and the enhancement of medical care.

To gain a better understanding of the underlying mechanisms and the pathophysiologic relevance of changes in pain sensitivity induced by prior endogenous opioid release, we developed an experimental animal model. In this model, animals underwent a series (one to three) of nonnociceptive stress episodes for 1 hour, which induced an opioid-dependent SIA (reversible by naltrexone) and were performed several days before a tissue injury (inflammation in a hind paw). We observed that prestressed rats showed a dramatic enhancement (three to four times the normal level if there were three stress episodes) of hyperalgesia induced by inflammation (Figure 16-4A). Rats experienced greater and more prolonged inflammatory hyperalgesia with an increased number of stress sessions. Notably, the blockade of opioid receptors by naltrexone before each stress event completely prevented SIA and suppressed the exaggerated inflammatory hyperalgesia (Figure 16-4B). These results demonstrate that, similar to exogenous opioids (see above), endogenous opioid systems play a critical role in the development of pain vulnerability. Consistent with data obtained using with exogenous opioids, the blockade of NMDA-Rs with an antagonist

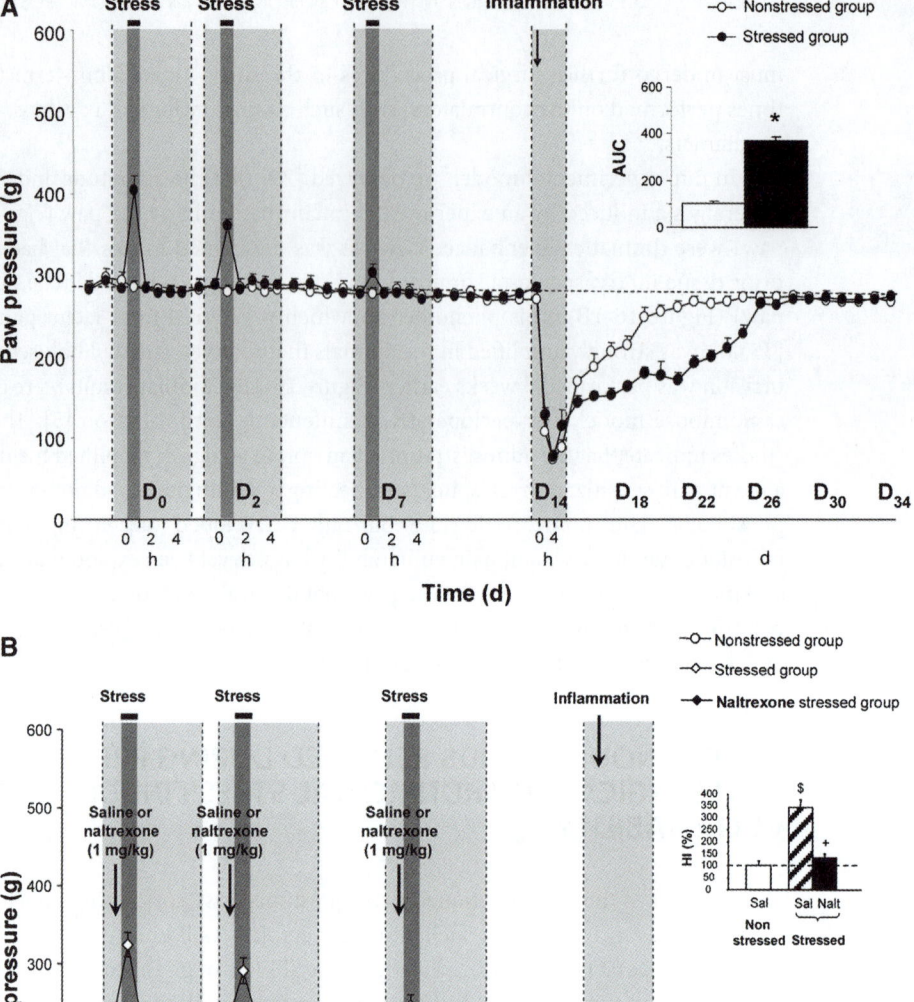

FIGURE 16-4 Endogenous opioids released during nonnociceptive stress induced latent pain sensitization via an NMDA-dependent process. The mechanical nociceptive threshold (vocalization in response to pressure) in rats was assessed using the Randall–Selitto test on a posterior paw. **A:** Rats were exposed to nonnociceptive environmental stress (changes in the cage, litter, and lighting intensity) for 1 h on D_0, D_2, and D_7 (stressed group). Control rats were not exposed to stress (nonstressed group). On D_{14}, inflammation was induced in the left paw (injection of carrageenan). In stressed rats, postinflammatory hyperalgesia was strongly enhanced compared with nonstressed rats. **B:** In stressed rats, naltrexone (1 mg/kg) or saline was injected 30 min before exposure to each stress (D_0, D_2, and D_7). On D_{14}, inflammation was induced in the left paw (injection of carrageenan). The administration of naltrexone before each stress blocked the enhancement of postinflammatory hyperalgesia observed 14 d later. **C:** Rats were exposed to nonnociceptive environmental stress (changes in the cage, litter, and lighting intensity) for 1 h on D_0, D_2, and D_7. Saline or the NMDA-R antagonist BN2572 (0.3 mg/kg) was injected 30 min before inflammation (injection of carrageenan) on D_{14}. Rats in the ketamine group received three injections of ketamine (3 × 10 mg/kg). The first injection was performed 30 min before inflammation, and the subsequent injections were performed every 5 h. The administration of ketamine or BN2572 resulted in a reduction of postinflammatory hyperalgesia in stressed rats. (From Le Roy C, Laboureyras E, Gavello-Baudy S, et al. Endogenous opioids released during non-nociceptive environmental stress induce latent pain sensitization via a NMDA-dependent process. J Pain 2011;12:1069–79.)

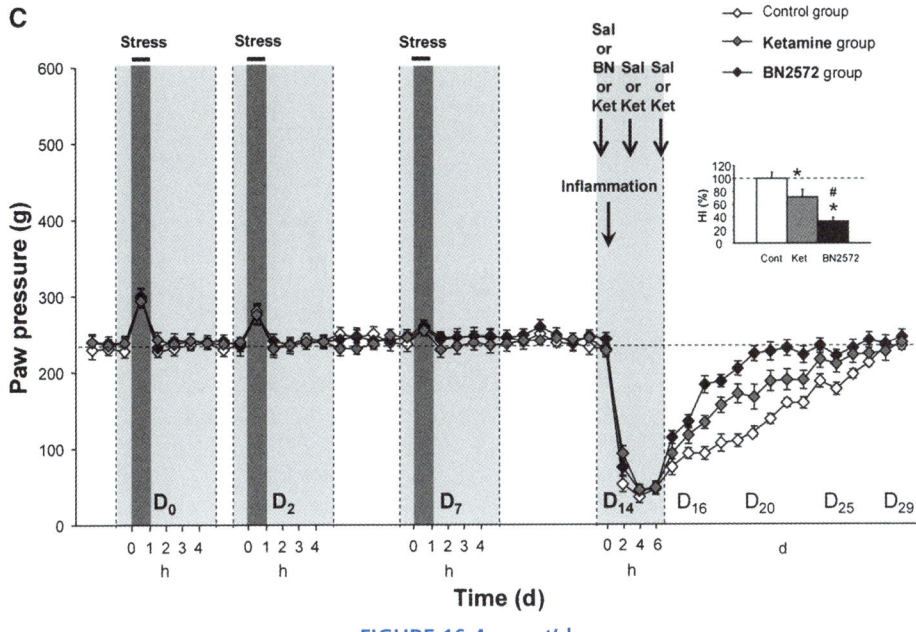

FIGURE 16-4 cont'd

immediately before inflammation also prevented the exaggerated inflammatory hyperalgesia (Figure 16-4C), suggesting common mechanisms. These results indicate that the individual's postsurgical perception of pain (intensity and duration) reflects not only the severity of the injury, as expected, but also the individual's history, particularly in terms of preoperative stress, and the conscious or unconscious feelings that may influence the individual's fear of surgery. These preclinical data may, at least in part, explain the clinical observations of unexpected hyperalgesia and unsatisfactory opioid analgesia in stressed patients [33,40]. Interestingly, we also demonstrated in animals that postoperative nonnociceptive environmental stress induced hyperalgesia, not analgesia, in pain- and opioid-experienced rats (Figure 16-5A). These results suggest that endogenous opioids released before or after surgery may facilitate the development of CPSP [46]. They also indicate that some social postsurgical events, not only preoperative events, may trigger or unmask latent pain sensitization leading to pain vulnerability and CPSP.

FROM PAIN TO PAIN VULNERABILITY: A NEW CONCEPT FOR THE IMPROVED UNDERSTANDING AND ENHANCED ALLEVIATION OF BOTH EXAGGERATED ACUTE POSTSURGICAL PAIN AND CPSP

Although speculative at present, the process of pain sensitization, which is described as abnormal in the literature, may not be paradoxical and should be interpreted as an adaptive response by an organism that is suddenly subjected to the activation of endogenous systems in response to an insult (stress or tissue injury). The administration of exogenous opioids in modern medicine could mimic this response. From an adaptive viewpoint, it is not abnormal for such a process to be remembered and therefore sensitize the individual to further nociceptive inputs, similar to how the immune system responds after an initial encounter with a pathogenic agent.

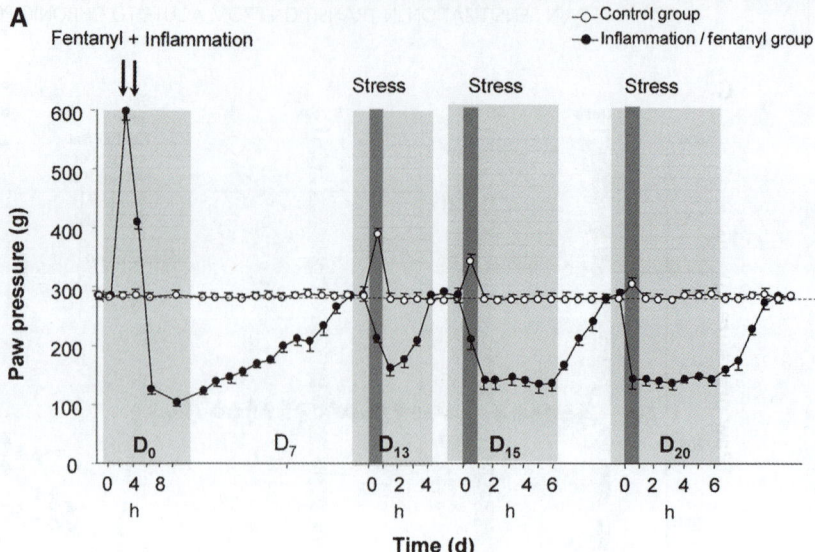

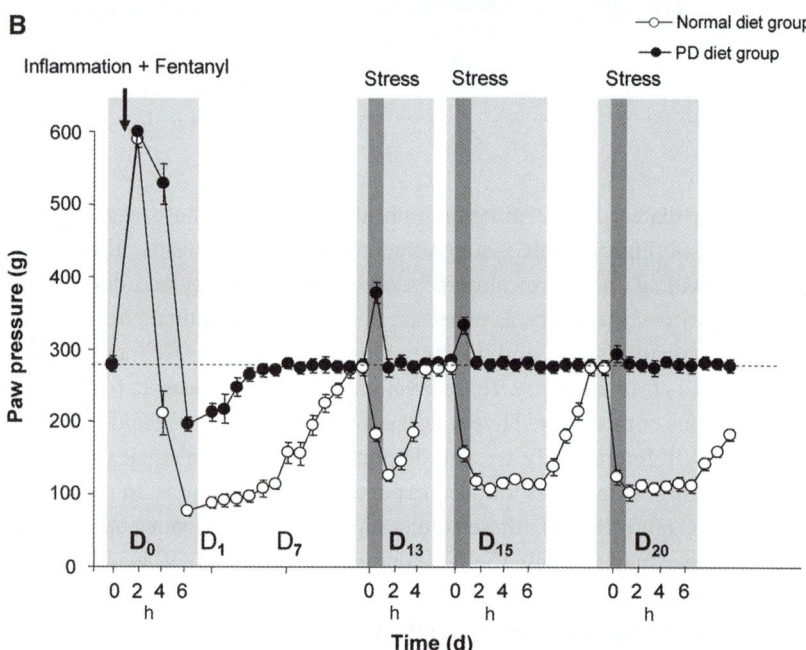

FIGURE 16-5 Release of endogenous opioids due to nonnociceptive stress induces hyperalgesia rather than analgesia in pain- and opioid-experienced rats. The mechanical nociceptive threshold (vocalization in response to pressure) in rats was assessed using the Randall–Selitto test on a posterior paw. **A:** On D_0, the rats received four injections of fentanyl (100 µg/kg), at intervals of 15 min, and inflammation was induced in the left paw (injection of carrageenan) 5 min after the first fentanyl injection. Inflammation was not induced, and fentanyl was not administered in the control group. Two weeks later (D_{13}), the rats were exposed to the first nonnociceptive environmental stress for 1 h (changes in the cage, litter, and lighting intensity). This stress was repeated on D_{15} and D_{20}. Unlike the control animals, which developed an analgesic response that was limited to the duration of the stress, the animals that had experienced inflammatory pain treated with fentanyl developed hyperalgesia that lasted several hours (first episode of stress). This hyperalgesia was amplified (over several days) when the animals were subjected to a second and third stress. **B:** Using the same experimental design, the rats were fed a normal diet or a polyamine-deficient diet (PD diet) for 7 d before injury and during the entire experiment. The PD diet prevented long-lasting hyperalgesia induced by inflammatory pain in fentanyl-treated rats and completely abolished hyperalgesia induced by the three stress exposures. ((A) From Rivat C, Laboureyras E, Laulin JP, et al. Non-nociceptive environmental stress induces hyperalgesia, not analgesia, in pain and opioid-experienced rats. Neuropsychopharmacology 2007;32:2217–28. (B) From Rivat C, Laulin JP, Corcuff JB, et al. Fentanyl enhancement of carrageenan-induced long-lasting hyperalgesia in rats: prevention by the N-methyl-D-aspartate receptor antagonist ketamine. Anesthesiology 2002;96:381–91.)

The fact that opioid administration would induce hyperalgesia following analgesia is in agreement with the opponent-process theory [54], which postulates that drug effects are automatically opposed by centrally mediated mechanisms. Briefly, this theory postulates that positive reinforcers, such as drugs, engage positive hedonic processes (*a-processes*) that are opposed by negative hedonic processes (*b-processes*). The positive hedonic processes are assumed to be simple and stable, and they immediately follow the administration of the drug. In contrast, negative hedonic processes have a long latency, slowly build up strength, and are slow to decay. Considering that the analgesic effect of opioids reflects a positive hedonic process (*a-process*), it is possible that the associated negative hedonic process will involve a hyperalgesic effect (*b-process*). This suggests that the net analgesic effect is then the sum of the two opposing process, which mask one another from the very first exposure to an opioid. Consequently, delayed hyperalgesia appears as an allostatic outcome of analgesia induced by an opioid, and not as an abnormal or paradoxical phenomenon because *b-processes* have a longer latency period than *a-processes*. The opposing process underlying delayed hyperalgesia (i.e., pain hypersensitivity, which may appear harmful, because of the undefined role of exaggerated or chronic pain) may, in reality, represent a fundamental strategy for adaptation that was selected for during evolution. Pain hypersensitivity likely favored an individual's survival in the threatening, nonmedicalized world of prehistory, by priming recovery strategies. Although unpleasant from an individual viewpoint, pain hypersensitivity encouraged individuals to seek care and facilitated the avoidance of dangerous situations for endurance. It can be argued that a modern, medicalized society no longer forces humans to use such strategies, which have lost physiologic function and are considered prehistoric. This viewpoint, however, fails to take into account the mismatch between the timing of the biologic evolution of complex multicultural organisms on one hand and the changes in our environment, particularly with respect to social and technical aspects. As Nesse suggests [42], we were not designed by natural selection for our present environments and lifestyles. Some paradoxical responses are likely to occur because natural selection has not had the time to transform us to adapt to life in the modern environment. Although our medical technology, including analgesic procedures, has improved in recent decades, the biologic evolution of our brain proceeds much more slowly. These ideas open new perspectives that can improve our understanding of the transition from acute to chronic pain.

Therefore, it would be advantageous to revisit the WHO classification to introduce the concept of the risk of pain hypersensitivity. From this point of view, four types of analgesic strategies could be proposed: (1) pure antinociceptive analgesics, such as paracetamol; (2) antinociceptive agents that are also able to induce delayed and sustained pain hypersensitivity, such as opioids, α2 adrenoreceptor agonists [43], and triptans [17]; (3) true antihyperalgesic agents, such as NMDA-R antagonists and gabapentinoids [58]; and (4) antinociceptive agents with antihyperalgesic properties such as NO [3] and nefopam [29].

Interestingly, it has been demonstrated that the level of our individual pain sensitivity is also dependent on our diet [2,48]. Therefore, the reduction or prevention of pain sensitization offers new possibilities for innovative therapeutic strategies, such as nutritional therapies. Because pain sensitization is an NMDA-dependent process and NMDA-R antagonists have unacceptable side effects, an alternative strategy is the negative modulation of NMDA-R function without blocking NMDA-R basal activity by targeting allosteric receptor sites rather than binding receptor sites. Because polyamines, which mainly originate from daily dietary intake, are positive modulators of NMDA-Rs, we developed a nutritional strategy based on a polyamine-deficient diet (PD diet). The rationale is that a PD diet can prevent the development of pain sensitization. Preclinical studies in rats have shown that the administration of a PD diet for 7 days before surgery had no effect on basal pain sensitivity, which is indicative of the absence of antinociceptive properties; however, postsurgical hyperalgesia was strongly reduced, especially in fentanyl-treated rats. A PD diet also decreased the hyperalgesia induced by pre- or postsurgical nonnociceptive environmental stress (Figure 16-5B) and reduced hyperalgesia in some models of chronic pain [46]. From a mechanistic standpoint, this diet prevented the enhanced tyrosine phosphorylation of the spinal NR2B subunit–containing NMDA-R, which is associated with tissue injury in fentanyl-treated rats. The PD diet did not induce any noticeable side effects in animals [48] or humans [14], and it restored the analgesic effect of morphine in some preclinical models of chronic pain that are poorly sensitive to opioids, such as neuropathic pain models [48]. Therefore, this nutritional approach could be part of an effective and safe strategy for preemptive analgesia and for reducing the transition from acute to CPSP.

Acknowledgments

G.S. was supported by the Université de Bordeaux, the Ministère de l'Education Nationale, de l'Enseignement Supérieur et de la Recherche, and the Centre National de la Recherche Scientifique (CNRS). G.S. also wishes to thank Jean-Paul Laulin, Emilie Laboureyras, Evelyne Célérier, Cyril Rivat, Baptiste Bessière, Chloé Le Roy, and Méric Ben Boujema, who participated in most of the experimental studies developed by our research team that were described in this review.

Conflict of Interest

The University of Bordeaux and the University of Rennes 1 have a patent (G. Simonnet and J.P. Moulinoux are coinventors) on a polyamine-deficient diet for humans that was adapted and modified from rat chow. A patent licensing arrangement for this nutritional therapy has been established between the University of Bordeaux, the University of Rennes 1, and Nutrialys Medical Nutrition SA and Effinov, France (G. Simonnet and J.P. Moulinoux were founder members in Nutrialys Medical Nutrition SA). Nutrialys and Effinov have not provided financial supports for these experimental studies.

REFERENCES

1. Angst MS, Clark JD. Opioid-induced hyperalgesia: a qualitative systematic review. Anesthesiology 2006;104:570–87.
2. Bell RF, Borzan J, Kalso E, Simonnet G. Food, pain, and drugs: does it matter what pain patients eat? Pain 2012;153:1993–6.
3. Bessiere B, Richebe P, Laboureyras E, et al. Nitrous oxide (N_2O) prevents latent pain sensitization and long-term anxiety-like behavior in pain and opioid-experienced rats. Neuropharmacology 2007;53:733–40.
4. Brennan TJ, Vandermeulen EP, Gebhart GF. Characterization of a rat model of incisional pain. Pain 1996;64:493–501.
5. Cabanero D, Campillo A, Celerier E, et al. Pronociceptive effects of remifentanil in a mouse model of postsurgical pain: effect of a second surgery. Anesthesiology 2009;111:1334–45.
6. Célèrier E, Gonzalez JR, Maldonado R, et al. Opioid-induced hyperalgesia in a murine model of postoperative pain: role of nitric oxide generated from the inducible nitric oxide synthase. Anesthesiology 2006;104:546–55.
7. Célèrier E, Laulin J, Larcher A, et al. Evidence for opiate-activated NMDA processes masking opiate analgesia in rats. Brain Res 1999;847:18–25.
8. Célèrier E, Rivat C, Jun Y, et al. Long-lasting hyperalgesia induced by fentanyl in rats: preventive effect of ketamine. Anesthesiology 2000;92:465–72.

9. Célèrier E, Simonnet G, Maldonado R. Prevention of fentanyl-induced delayed pronociceptive effects in mice lacking the protein kinase C gamma gene. Neuropharmacology 2004;46:264–72.
10. Chen L, Huang LY. Sustained potentiation of NMDA receptor-mediated glutamate responses through activation of protein kinase C by a mu opioid. Neuron 1991;7:319–26.
11. Chen Y, Geis C, Sommer C. Activation of TRPV1 contributes to morphine tolerance: involvement of the mitogen-activated protein kinase signaling pathway. J Neurosci 2008;28:5836–45.
12. Chen Y, Yang C, Wang ZJ. Ca^{2+}/calmodulin-dependent protein kinase II alpha is required for the initiation and maintenance of opioid-induced hyperalgesia. J Neurosci 2010;30:38–46.
13. Chu LF, Cun T, Ngai LK, et al. Modulation of remifentanil-induced postinfusion hyperalgesia by the beta-blocker propranolol in humans. Pain 2012;153:974–81.
14. Cipolla BG, Havouis R, Moulinoux JP. Polyamine contents in current foods: a basis for polyamine reduced diet and a study of its long term observance and tolerance in prostate carcinoma patients. Amino Acids 2007;33:203–12.
15. Compton P, Charuvastra VC, Ling W. Pain intolerance in opioid-maintained former opiate addicts: effect of long-acting maintenance agent. Drug Alcohol Depend 2001;63:139–46.
16. Crombie IK, Davies HT, Macrae WA. Cut and thrust: antecedent surgery and trauma among patients attending a chronic pain clinic. Pain 1998;76(1–2):167–71.
17. De Felice M, Ossipov MH, Wang R, et al. Triptan-induced latent sensitization: a possible basis for medication overuse headache. Ann Neurol 2010;67:325–37.
18. Deumens R, Steyaert A, Forget P, et al. Prevention of chronic postoperative pain: cellular, molecular, and clinical insights for mechanism-based treatment approaches. Prog Neurobiol 2013;104:1–37.
19. Fletcher D, Stamer UM, Pogatzki-Zahn E, Zaslansky R, Tanase NV, Perruchoud C, Kranke P, Komann M, Lehman T, Meissner W, euCPSP group for the Clinical Trial Network group of the European Society of Anaesthesiology. Chronic postsurgical pain in Europe: an observational study. Eur J Anaesthesiol 2015;32(10):725–34.
20. Grosu I, de Kock M. New concepts in acute pain management: strategies to prevent chronic postsurgical pain, opioid-induced hyperalgesia, and outcome measures. Anesthesiol Clin June 2011;29(2):311–27.
21. Imbe H, Iwai-Liao Y, Senba E. Stress-induced hyperalgesia: animal models and putative mechanisms. Front Biosci 2006;11:2179–92.
22. Ip HY, Abrishami A, Peng PW, et al. Predictors of postoperative pain and analgesic consumption: a qualitative systematic review. Anesthesiology 2009;111:657–77.
23. Ji RR, Kohno T, Moore KA, Woolf CJ. Central sensitization and LTP: do pain and memory share similar mechanisms? Trends Neurosci 2003;26:696–705.
24. Joly V, Richebe P, Guignard B, et al. Remifentanil-induced postoperative hyperalgesia and its prevention with small-dose ketamine. Anesthesiology 2005;103:147–55.
25. Kehlet H, Jensen TS, Woolf CJ. Persistent postsurgical pain: risk factors and prevention. Lancet 2006;367:1618–25.
26. King T, Ossipov MH, Vanderah TW, et al. Is paradoxical pain induced by sustained opioid exposure an underlying mechanism of opioid antinociceptive tolerance? Neurosignals 2005;14:194–205.
27. Kitamura Y, Miyazaki A, Yamanaka Y, Nomura Y. Stimulatory effects of protein kinase C and calmodulin kinase II on N-methyl-D-aspartate receptor/channels in the postsynaptic density of rat brain. J Neurochem 1993;61:100–9.
28. Koppert W, Sittl R, Scheuber K, et al. Differential modulation of remifentanil-induced analgesia and postinfusion hyperalgesia by S-ketamine and clonidine in humans. Anesthesiology 2003;99:152–9.
29. Laboureyras E, Chateauraynaud J, Richebe P, Simonnet G. Long-term pain vulnerability after surgery in rats: prevention by nefopam, an analgesic with antihyperalgesic properties. Anesth Analg 2009;109:623–31.
30. Larcher A, Laulin JP, Célèrier E, et al. Acute tolerance associated with a single opiate administration: involvement of N-methyl-D-aspartate-dependent pain facilitatory systems. Neuroscience 1998;84:583–9.
31. Latremoliere A, Woolf CJ. Central sensitization: a generator of pain hypersensitivity by central neural plasticity. J Pain 2009;10:895–926.
32. Laulin JP, Célèrier E, Larcher A, et al. Opiate tolerance to daily heroin administration: an apparent phenomenon associated with enhanced pain sensitivity. Neuroscience 1999;89:631–6.
33. Lautenbacher S, Huber C, Schofer D, et al. Attentional and emotional mechanisms related to pain as predictors of chronic postoperative pain: a comparison with other psychological and physiological predictors. Pain 2010;151:722–31.
34. Lavand'homme P. Transition from acute to chronic pain after surgery. Pain 2017;158(Suppl. 1):S50–4.

35. Le Roy C, Laboureyras E, Gavello-Baudy S, et al. Endogenous opioids released during non-nociceptive environmental stress induce latent pain sensitization via a NMDA-dependent process. J Pain 2011;12:1069–79.
36. Liang D, Shi X, Qiao Y, et al. Chronic morphine administration enhances nociceptive sensitivity and local cytokine production after incision. Mol Pain 2008;4:7.
37. Macrae WA. Chronic post-surgical pain: 10 years on. Br J Anaesth 2008;101:77–86.
38. Mao J. Opioid-induced abnormal pain sensitivity: implications in clinical opioid therapy. Pain 2002;100:213–7.
39. Mao J, Price DD, Mayer DJ. Thermal hyperalgesia in association with the development of morphine tolerance in rats: roles of excitatory amino acid receptors and protein kinase C. J Neurosci 1994;14:2301–12.
40. Masselin-Dubois A, Attal N, Fletcher D, et al. Are psychological predictors of chronic postsurgical pain dependent on the surgical model? A comparison of total knee arthroplasty and breast surgery for cancer. J Pain 2013;14:854–64.
41. Minville V, Fourcade O, Girolami JP, Tack I. Opioid-induced hyperalgesia in a mice model of orthopaedic pain: preventive effect of ketamine. Br J Anaesth 2009;104:231–8.
42. Nesse RM, Williams GC. On Darwinian medicine. Life Sci Res 1999;3:1–17.
43. Quartilho A, Mata HP, Ibrahim MM, et al. Production of paradoxical sensory hypersensitivity by alpha 2-adrenoreceptor agonists. Anesthesiology 2004;100:1538–44.
44. Quintero L, Moreno M, Avila C, et al. Long-lasting delayed hyperalgesia after subchronic swim stress. Pharmacol Biochem Behav 2000;67:449–58.
45. Richebe P, Rivat C, Laulin JP, et al. Ketamine improves the management of exaggerated postoperative pain observed in perioperative fentanyl-treated rats. Anesthesiology 2005;102:421–8.
46. Rivat C, Laboureyras E, Laulin JP, et al. Non-nociceptive environmental stress induces hyperalgesia, not analgesia, in pain and opioid-experienced rats. Neuropsychopharmacology 2007;32:2217–28.
47. Rivat C, Laulin JP, Corcuff JB, et al. Fentanyl enhancement of carrageenan-induced long-lasting hyperalgesia in rats: prevention by the N-methyl-D-aspartate receptor antagonist ketamine. Anesthesiology 2002;96:381–91.
48. Rivat C, Richebe P, Laboureyras E, et al. Polyamine deficient diet to relieve pain hypersensitivity. Pain 2008;137:125–37.
49. Sandkuhler J. Understanding LTP in pain pathways. Mol Pain 2007;3:9.
50. Shenker N, Haigh R, Roberts E, et al. A review of contralateral responses to a unilateral inflammatory lesion. Rheumatology (Oxford) 2003;42:1279–86.
51. Simonin F, Schmitt M, Laulin JP, et al. RF9, a potent and selective neuropeptide FF receptor antagonist, prevents opioid-induced tolerance associated with hyperalgesia. Proc Natl Acad Sci USA 2006;103:466–71.
52. Simonnet G, Le Moal M. Vulnerability to opioid tolerance, dependence, and addiction – an individual-centered versus drug-centered paradigm analysis. Seattle: IASP Press; 2010:405–30.
53. Simonnet G, Rivat C. Opioid-induced hyperalgesia: abnormal or normal pain? Neuroreport 2003;14:1–7.
54. Solomon RL, Corbit JD. An opponent-process theory of motivation. I. Temporal dynamics of affect. Psychol Rev 1974;81:119–45.
55. Stubhaug A, Breivik H, Eide PK, et al. Mapping of punctuate hyperalgesia around a surgical incision demonstrates that ketamine is a powerful suppressor of central sensitization to pain following surgery. Acta Anaesthesiol Scand 1997;41:1124–32.
56. Taddio A, Katz J, Ilersich AL, Koren G. Effect of neonatal circumcision on pain response during subsequent routine vaccination. Lancet 1997;349:599–603.
57. VanDenKerkhof EG, Hopman WM, Goldstein DH, Wilson RA, Towheed TE, Lam M, Harrison MB, Reitsma ML, Johnston SL, Medd JD, Gilron I. Impact of perioperative pain intensity, pain qualities, and opioid use on chronic pain after surgery: a prospective cohort study. Reg Anesth Pain Med 2012;37(1):19–27.
58. Van Elstraete AC, Sitbon P, Mazoit JX, Benhamou D. Gabapentin prevents delayed and long-lasting hyperalgesia induced by fentanyl in rats. Anesthesiology 2008;108:484–94.
59. Vardanyan A, Wang R, Vanderah TW, et al. TRPV1 receptor in expression of opioid-induced hyperalgesia. J Pain 2009;10:243–52.
60. Wilder-Smith OH, Arendt-Nielsen L. Postoperative hyperalgesia: its clinical importance and relevance. Anesthesiology 2006;104:601–7.
61. Woolf CJ, Salter MW. Neuronal plasticity: increasing the gain in pain. Science 2000;288(5472):1765–9.
62. Zhou HY, Chen SR, Chen H, Pan HL. Opioid-induced long-term potentiation in the spinal cord is a presynaptic event. J Neurosci 2010;30:4460–6.

CHAPTER 17

The Role of Intraoperative Nerve Injury in Persistent Postoperative Pain

Eske Kvanner Aasvang

Surgical procedures invariably result in tissue trauma including damage to cutaneous and deep tissue sensory nerve fibers and nociceptors, suggesting that intraoperative nerve injury is a key factor when investigating the potential pathogenetic factors in persistent postoperative pain [22]. Thus, large epidemiologic data reveal neuropathy as a frequent finding after surgery, although procedure related [18,26]. Surgical pain models, such as inguinal herniotomy, thoracotomy, and mastectomy, allow for detailed studies of the relative role of nerve injury in the development of persistent postsurgical pain together with other potential predisposing factors, including gender, age, genetics, and psychosocial variables [28,34,39], *before* injury, as opposed to other chronic pain conditions such as low-back pain and headache. Understanding the role of nerve injury and separating it from other causes of PPSP are essential in future advances in treatment and preventive strategies, and the findings may be expanded into the understanding of other nonsurgical pain syndromes. This chapter will focus on the current knowledge mainly from three intensely studied surgical procedures (mastectomy, herniotomy, and thoracotomy) and discuss the need for future research areas regarding nerve injury, including the role of cutaneous versus deep nerve injury and hyperalgesia in the development and maintenance of persistent postoperative pain.

THE CASE OF INGUINAL HERNIOTOMY

Inguinal herniotomy has been one of the most studied surgical procedures as a model for persistent postoperative pain, especially for the role of intraoperative nerve injury, as three to four nerves transverse the surgical field in groin hernia surgery, depending on the surgical approach. Thus, in open repair the ilioinguinal, iliohypogastric, and genitofemoral nerves, and in laparoscopic repair, also the lateral femoral cutaneous nerve are at risk for intraoperative nerve damage [40,51]. Furthermore, herniotomy is performed in large numbers of patients by standardized procedures, has low occurrence of psychopathology, and has no exposure to radiotherapy or chemotherapy, which is a well-documented risk factor for sensory disturbances and pain, making it a potential ideal model for the study of nerve damage as a risk factor for persistent postoperative pain [3,28].

Preoperative Sensory Function

Before postoperative neuropathy is assumed to have a causal relationship to intraoperative nerve injury, it is critical to assess the preoperative sensory function. In groin herniotomy, preoperative hernia pain has been shown to be related to development of persistent pain [3,35], which may suggest that preoperative hernia pain induces nociceptive neuroplastic changes that facilitates nociceptive signaling to the central nervous system (CNS) and ultimately leads to continuation of pain after surgery. Preoperative neuroplastic changes are reported in other visceral pain syndromes (such as gallstone and appendicitis) [19,47,48] or osteoarthritis [12], where sensory changes such as hyperalgesia in the painful or referred area are related to pain intensity. Thus, the preoperative peripheral sensory function in groin hernia patients could potentially be affected by the hernia, either owing to the physical protrusion causing stretching of the tissue or more likely from nociceptive-induced neuroplasticity.

However, in a large prospective study (n = 442) on predictive factors for persistent postherniotomy pain, warmth and heat pain detection thresholds (WDT and HPDT) and response to a tonic 47°C heat stimulation on the arm and groin *preo*perative pain were not associated with alterations in local preoperative nociceptive function in the groin. The finding that the sensory function in the groin and arm was closely related also supports that the preoperative groin hernia pain does not cause general hyperalgesia [3]. These findings are similar to previous smaller but more detailed investigations where sensory function was assessed by a standardized QST protocol, where no correlation between any test and pain on the hernia side was found, and sensory function was not significantly different between the two groins [4].

Thus, assessment of preoperative sensory function has not revealed signs of pain-induced neuroplasticity in groin hernia patients or other changes when compared with the naïve side. In this sense, hernia patients do not exhibit the hyperalgesia seen in other pain syndromes (such as gallstone, migraine, appendicitis, and osteoarthritis) [12,30,47,48,54]. These findings have advocated for similar assessment of preoperative sensory in other procedures before postoperative sensory findings are contributed to intraoperative nerve damage.

Acute Sensory Dysfunction and Development of Persistent Postoperative Pain

Acute postoperative pain is correlated to and predicts persistent postoperative pain [28,34,39]. But it remains unsettled whether acute pain causes persistent pain directly or in contrast, whether acute and persistent pain share the same preoperative and intraoperative factors without a direct causal relationship. Information on acute postoperative sensory function would benefit our understanding of *why* acute pain predicts persistent pain and if it could be due to nociceptive plasticity. In a 20-patient pilot study of the role of diffuse noxious inhibitory control (DNIC) on acute and postoperative pain and hyperalgesia after abdominal surgery, acute postsurgical pressure hyperalgesia was seen more often in patients who later reported pain at 6 months and at that time also had pressure hyperalgesia [55]. However, the data are not clear because hyperalgesia was seen more often in the pain-free group at 3 months, and the surgical group consisted of various upper and lower abdominal and urogenital surgical procedures, making the findings intriguing but inconclusive. Another study investigating areas of acute poststernotomy hyperalgesia by pinprick did not find any correlation to persistent pain 4 to 6 months later, but the single modality assessment and exclusion of thermal stimuli may have resulted in low detection of hyperalgesia [44]. Only a small study has assessed sensory function between the operated and contralateral sides by QST before groin herniotomy, 1 week and 2½ years postoperatively, where acute thermal and mechanical hypoesthesia and pressure hyperalgesia were found on the operated side, but no relationship between acute pressure hyperalgesia and persistent pain were seen after 2½ years. However, the limited number of studies hinders firm conclusions [5].

Thus, inguinal herniotomy results in acute cutaneous hypoesthesia and deep hyperalgesia, but the data on the effect on persistent pain are sparse and supported by other surgical models.

Late Sensory Function and Pain—Pain-Free Patients

One of the main advantages of investigating postoperative pain is the availability of an optimal control group of pain-free patients treated for the same illness with the same procedure as those who develop pain. As opposed to comparing pain patients with healthy volunteers, the pain-*free control* group allows for understanding the specific role of nerve injury (i.e., sensory dysfunction) while controlling for other potential factors [28].

Several studies using questionnaires and bedside sensory testing to describe the relationship between pain and sensory dysfunction after groin herniotomy show a clear trend of sensory disturbances (such as numbness, paraesthesia, and foreign body sensations) occurring not only in 40% to 50% of pain patients but also in 10% to 40% of pain-free patients [11,17,32,41]. More details on the characteristics of sensory function in pain-free patients come from a study of 40 patients with unilateral herniotomy 2 years before [7]. Sensory mapping on the operated side showed that 52% of patients had areas of cold hypoesthesia, 40% brush hypoesthesia, 35% pinprick hypoesthesia, and 5% pinprick hyperalgesia. When the two sides were compared, QST revealed that hypoesthesia and hypoalgesia to cold, warmth, heat, and tactile stimulations were found on the operated side. Pressure and pressure tolerance thresholds were significantly lower (hyperalgesia) on the operated side than those on the contralateral side.

Pain thresholds on both sides were significantly correlated suggesting that the clinically irrelevant cutaneous hypoalgesia and deep hyperalgesia found in pain-free operated patients may sensitize contralateral neurons on a central nervous level (a so-called mirror effect), similar to what is seen other nerve injuries [11,36,38]. However, there is little or no indication of central/peripheral nociceptive hyperexcitability in pain-free operated hernia patients as evidenced by the finding that although repetitive stimulation with a von Frey fiber elicited pain in 15% of patients, pain ceased when stimulation stopped in all patients and without aftersensations.

These findings show that hernia surgery leads to cutaneous hypoesthesia and hypoalgesia and deep tissue hyperalgesia in pain-free patients similar to other surgical models, including thoracotomy [56], mastectomy [11], and traumatic peripheral nerve injury after various surgical procedures [31].

The reason why these patients do not experience pain despite having reduced pain thresholds is not clarified but may be that a relevant pain stimulus like the pressure algometry does not occur in everyday life or that these patients have a better inhibitory pain modulation than pain patients [49]. However, the findings from the operated side clearly show that a pain-free *operated* control group is essential when sensory findings in persistent postoperative pain are interpreted to evaluate the role of intraoperative nerve injury. Thus assessment of sensory function should not only compare side-to-side differences, adjusting for mirror effects or generalized sensitization, but also perform individual characterization based on normative data from the pain-free operated patients, and that reference data from an unoperated side should be used with caution.

Late Sensory Function and Pain—Pain Patients

When postherniotomy pain patients are compared with a pain-free operated control group, they do not only have a higher incidence of sensory disturbances [1,33], assessed by sensory mapping, but also have more severe disturbances and include positive phenomena such as hyperalgesia and temporal summation wind-up-like pain [27,33]. The first QST study involved a combination of 20 persistent pain patients and 52 pain-free operated patients [33] with a 6- to 12-month follow-up. Hypoesthesia and allodynia were seen significantly more often in pain patients, but pressure pain thresholds and cutaneous thresholds were not significantly different between the two groups, which may be explained by the fact that pain patients only had mild pain (median visual analogue scale [VAS] 22, range 12 to 30), thereby not including those patients that may have more severe nerve damage and/or nociceptive sensitization.

Later—and larger—detailed QST studies comparing patients with moderate/severe persistent postherniotomy pain have revealed significant lower mechanical and pressure pain thresholds (hyperalgesia) and significantly increased thermal thresholds (hypoesthesia/hypoalgesia) in pain patients compared with values from pain-free patients [1-3]. Thus the relative role of 23 potentially relevant patient- and surgery-related risk factors were assessed in a large prospective study and showed that postoperative impairment of warmth detection—compared with preoperative values—was one of only four independent factors significantly related to severe pain-related activity impairment 6 months postoperatively [3]. For each degree Celsius of sensory loss in warmth detection, the risk for severe postoperative pain increased by 7%. When patients were divided into those with a good outcome and those who favored less well, there was a significant increase in warmth detection (4.8°C vs. 2.7°C) and heat pain detection (2.5°C vs. 1.5°C) thresholds in patients with a poor versus good outcome. Further analysis showed that changes in sensory function before and after surgery was local around the operated area, as the sensory function on the arm remained intact, supporting that change must have occurred as a result of localized surgical trauma and not as part of a generalized hypersensitivity. These findings are supported by a large and detailed mastectomy QST study where mechanical and thermal hypoesthesia and the area size of hypoesthesia were significantly related to the occurrence of persistent pain [11].

Individual Characterization of Pain Patients

Several pain states shows signs of heterogeneous pain processing despite a common etiology. This has been shown in persistent postherniotomy pain [2], postmastectomy pain syndrome [11,20], postthoracotomy pain [21,56], and postherpetic neuralgia [37]. Thus, from the detailed sensory studies of persistent postherniotomy pain patients [1,33], there is an evident large interindividual variation in sensory function on the operated side in pain patients [1] in contrast to the smaller variation in pain-free operated patients [1,7], especially when compared with hernia patients before surgery [2], suggesting that the patient group may be heterogeneous. To investigate this, a normalized data from 40 pain-free operated patients [7] were used to construct individual sensory profiles in a cohort of 70 persistent postherniotomy patients with moderate to severe pain. Of those studied, 80% had hyperalgesia (50% to two or more modalities and 30% had unimodal hyperalgesia), but 20% were not different from pain-free patients with regards to sensory function. The study showed that nociceptive heterogeneity exists not only for parameters where a group-to-group difference is not detected (heat pain detection) but also where a difference was shown (mechanical pain detection). Thus, postherniotomy patients can be divided into those who only have cutaneous hyperalgesia (cold, heat, and mechanical) (6%), only pinch (6%), only pressure (17%), or combined cutaneous, pinch, and pressure hyperalgesia (48%). One in four (25%) of patients had a combination of significant sensory loss *and* hypersensitivity. Again, similar results are found in other procedures including mastectomy, showing that the degree of sensory hyperexcitability is highly variable, with some only having a slightly reduced pain detection threshold, whereas others had a severe sensory disturbance [2,11]. However, the finding that the degree of sensory dysfunction was not related to pain intensity suggests that QST does not cover all the factors for pain processing, in particular it may not sufficiently assess central modulating mechanisms [49] and pain from deeper tissues [45].

Nerve Identification and Handling

If one is to avoid nerve injury, it would seem obvious to identify nerves before potentially putting them at harm by placing sutures, tacks, or dissecting tissues. However, this is challenging because of the variation in anatomical distribution, where the ilioinguinal or iliohypogastric nerves has an aberrant course 40% of 110 explorations [8], but sparse data support the identification of nerves. A study of 525 patients found that nonidentification of nerves was significantly associated with postoperative pain at 3 months [46], and in 895 patients (973 hernioplasties), there were no cases of moderate or severe pain in the 380 patients if all three nerves were identified, but in the 40 patients where all three nerves were transected, there was a 10% incidence of moderate/severe pain at 6 months [9]. In a prospective cohort study, 241 patients were treated by open hernia repair and neurectomy if technically necessary to perform the hernia repair. At the 5-year follow-up, 16% with an ilioinguinal neurolysis reported pain in contrast to only 1.4% of those without neurolysis [41]. One of the major problems when interpreting these studies and most studies on nerve identification and subsequent pain is the lack of data on sensory disturbances from *all* the pain-free patients. A detailed study with a full preoperative and 6 months postoperative QST protocol in *all* 244 patients undergoing hernia repair found a high identification rate of the ilioinguinal and iliohypogastric nerves (95% and 98%, respectively), whereas the genitofemoral nerve was only identified in 21% of cases [15]. This study failed to show a difference in pain-related functional impairment and sensory dysfunction between those with or without nerve identification, supporting that other factors than nerve injury are important in the development of persistent postoperative pain.

Another reason for the failure of the latter study to show a relation between nerve identification and pain and sensory disturbances may be the fact that even when the nerves are macroscopically intact, they may suffer from severe axonal damage from stretching or crushing injury. This has been shown by intraoperative neurography in bilateral sagittal split osteotomy (BSSO). In this procedure the lower jaw is elongated with possible bilateral damage to the inferior alveolar nerve (IAN), and the neurography allows on-line accurate detection, classification, and grading of nerve injury of the IAN [23,24]. In 95% of BSSO, an IAN injury of various degrees occurred [50]. Importantly, this was the case even when no macroscopic injury was seen, and severe axonal injury was observed in apparently intact nerves [24,50]. The most frequent occurring intraoperative injury was demyelinating damage (−50%), assumed to have occurred from compression with retractors, and partial axonal damage (−40%) from stretching, cuts, and/or ischemia. A combination of both was seen in 15% of cases. The recovery was highly dependent on the type of injury as almost all demyelinating injuries recovered back to baseline values, but 80% axonal lesions had incomplete subjective and neurophysiologic recovery at 4 months postoperatively [25]. Persistent pain (5% overall) only occurred after axonal lesions where it was seen in 13% of cases [25]. At 4 months there was a normal bedside examination in pain patients, but QST revealed impaired sensory function to warmth and cold detection in patients with axonal damage. In mesh-based herniotomy, a microscopically detected increased nerve regrowth ("sprouting") has been demonstrated in persistent pain patients compared with pain-free patients, despite macroscopically intact nerves [13]. Thus, the inflammation caused by the mesh, together with overlooked and microscopic nerve injuries, may stimulate nerve regrowth and increased/spontaneous nociceptive input.

However, despite these caveats when assuming that a macroscopically intact nerve is uninjured, the role of nerve identification as a protective factor for persistent postoperative pain in herniotomy remains in favor of nerve identification and is supported by studies in mastectomy regarding identification of the intercostobrachial nerve (ICBN) although the handling differs. As in herniotomy, identification and preservation of the ICBN is difficult during axillary surgery and may result in complete or partial transection of the nerve. Although preservation of the ICBN has been shown to result in less hypoesthesia postoperatively, detailed data from breast cancer surgery show that in case of axillary dissection, preservation of the ICBN increases the risk for persistent pain, suggesting that a macroscopically intact nerve may be injured by tension or crushing, causing spontaneous activity [10].

In thoracotomy, intraoperative neurography has shown that rib retractors can result in loss of conduction in up to 100% of segments [42], which has been shown to subsequently correlate to long-term (1 month) pain [14]. Furthermore, various nerve sparring techniques (such as intercostal sutures, muscle flap, and nerve identification) has shown a reduced risk for acute and persistent postthoracotomy pain [29,52].

In conclusion, nerve identification should be attempted to avoid injury, and preservation may reduce the risk for persistent postherniotomy pain, whereas transection in mastectomy seems to reduce the risk for persistent pain after breast cancer surgery.

Deep Versus Superficial Pain

Deep tissue pain is the predominate clinical pain syndrome when compared with solely cutaneous pain syndromes (such as postherpetic neuralgia and diabetic neuropathy) [45], and nonmalignant musculoskeletal pain (such as osteoarthritis, back pain, muscle damage/overuse, fibromyalgia, and other disorders) is the most common clinical symptom that causes patients to seek medical attention and a prevalent cause of disability worldwide [45]. In persistent postoperative pain, the previous sections have shown that in the case of postherniotomy pain, the majority of patients report deep, rather than cutaneous-related, pains—supported by QST where pressure algometry reveals deep tissue hyperalgesia in about 70% of patients [1,2] similar to patients with persistent postmastectomy pain [11]. Patients scheduled for hysterectomy have significantly lower pain pressure thresholds if they have concomitant pelvic pain compared with those without [16]. In patients with severe persistent postherniotomy pain, reoperation with removal of mesh and entrapped nerves has been shown to reverse deep tissue hyperalgesia with simultaneous cutaneous hypoesthesia [6], although these findings need further confirmation and a long-term follow-up. Taken together, the available literature shows that cutaneous *hypoalgesia* to various modalities of stimulation (heat, cold, mechanical) is consistent in persistent pain across surgical procedures, with concomitant deep tissue *hyperalgesia* documented in specific procedures [45].

These prevailing syndromes characterized by deep pains necessitate an integrated approach to viewing the deeper somatic tissues, including muscle and viscera and not only the skin, as nociceptive organs. Deep tissues are three dimensional and although many pains from cutaneous tissues are localized and relate to nerve distributions or areas of tissue damage, deep pains can present as more diffuse and are distributed over large areas. Part of these differences may relate to peripheral innervation mechanisms, but other contributions from central processes may be important. Furthermore, the majority of investigations target the skin to assess the role of nerve injury/neuropathy in pain, despite the fact that activation of nociceptors from deep tissue results in a longer lasting and more intense activation of dorsal horn neurons than activation of cutaneous nociceptors [53], and that deep experimental stimulation alters cutaneous nociception, calling for further investigations into the intricate interaction between deep and cutaneous sensory function. Thus, the current standard for assessing pain from deeper structures is pressure algometry, which has several shortcomings when it comes to interpretation of the results. Pressure algometry is an *unspecific* indirect stimulation of all tissues beneath the stimulation probe, without tissue discrimination (e.g., skin, subcutis, fascia, muscle, periost, bone) and in contrast to the majority of tests in a standard QST protocol [2,43].

In conclusion, nerve injury, either direct or from surrounding inflammation, is a necessary but insufficient factor for persistent postoperative pain. Future research should look toward nerve handling and deep tissue hyperalgesia to expand our understanding of nerve injury in persistent postoperative pain to improve prevention and treatment options.

REFERENCES

1. Aasvang EK, Brandsborg B, Christensen B, Jensen TS, Kehlet H. Neurophysiological characterization of postherniotomy pain. Pain 2008;137:173–81.
2. Aasvang EK, Brandsborg B, Jensen TS, Kehlet H. Heterogeneous sensory processing in persistent postherniotomy pain. Pain 2010;150:237–42.
3. Aasvang EK, Gmaehle E, Hansen JB, Gmaehle B, Forman JL, Schwarz J, Bittner R, Kehlet H. Predictive risk factors for persistent postherniotomy pain. Anesthesiology 2010;112:957–69.
4. Aasvang EK, Hansen JB, Kehlet H. Pre-operative pain and sensory function in groin hernia. Eur J Pain 2009;13:1018–22.
5. Aasvang EK, Hansen JB, Kehlet H. Late sensory function after intraoperative capsaicin wound instillation. Acta Anaesthesiol Scand 2010;54:224–31.
6. Aasvang EK, Kehlet H. The effect of mesh removal and selective neurectomy on persistent postherniotomy pain. Ann Surg 2009;249:327–34.
7. Aasvang EK, Kehlet H. Persistent sensory dysfunction in pain free herniotomy. Acta Anaesthesiol Scand 2010;54:291–8.
8. Al-dabbagh AK. Anatomical variations of the inguinal nerves and risks of injury in 110 hernia repairs. Surg Radiol Anat 2002;24:102–7.
9. Alfieri S, Rotondi F, Di GA, Fumagalli U, Salzano A, Di MD, Ridolfini MP, Sgagari A, Doglietto G. Influence of preservation versus division of ilioinguinal, iliohypogastric, and genital nerves during open mesh herniorrhaphy: prospective multicentric study of chronic pain. Ann Surg 2006;243:553–8.
10. Andersen KG, Duriaud HM, Jensen HE, Kroman N, Kehlet H. Predictive factors for the development of persistent pain after breast cancer surgery. Pain 2015;156:2413–22.
11. Andersen KG, Duriaud HM, Kehlet H, Aasvang EK. The relationship between sensory loss and persistent pain 1 year after breast cancer surgery. J Pain 2017;18(9):1129–38.
12. Arendt-Nielsen L, Eskehave TN, Egsgaard LL, Petersen KK, Graven-Nielsen T, Hoeck HC, Simonsen O, Siebuhr AS, Karsdal M, Bay-Jensen AC. Association between experimental pain biomarkers and serological markers in patients with different degree of painful knee osteoarthritis. Arthritis Rheumatol 2014;66(12):3317–26.

13. Bendavid R, Lou W, Grischkan D, Koch A, Petersen K, Morrison J, Iakovlev V. A mechanism of mesh-related post-herniorrhaphy neuralgia. Hernia 2016;20:357–65.
14. Benedetti F, Vighetti S, Ricco C, Amanzio M, Bergamasco L, Casadio C, Cianci R, Giobbe R, Oliaro A, Bergamasco B, Maggi G. Neurophysiologic assessment of nerve impairment in posterolateral and muscle-sparing thoracotomy. J Thorac Cardiovasc Surg 1998;115:841–7.
15. Bischoff JM, Aasvang EK, Kehlet H, Werner MU. Does nerve identification during open inguinal herniorrhaphy reduce the risk of nerve damage and persistent pain? Hernia 2012;16:573–7.
16. Brandsborg B, Dueholm M, Kehlet H, Jensen TS, Nikolajsen L. Mechanosensitivity before and after hysterectomy: a prospective study on the prediction of acute and chronic postoperative pain. Br J Anaesth 2011;107:940–7.
17. Cunningham J, Temple WJ, Mitchell P, Nixon JA, Preshaw RM, Hagen NA. Cooperative hernia study. Pain in the postrepair patient. Ann Surg 1996;224:598–602.
18. Duale C, Ouchchane L, Schoeffler P, Dubray C. Neuropathic aspects of persistent postsurgical pain: a French multicenter survey with a 6-month prospective follow-up. J Pain 2014;15:24.
19. Giamberardino MA, Affaitati G, Lerza R, Lapenna D, Costantini R, Vecchiet L. Relationship between pain symptoms and referred sensory and trophic changes in patients with gallbladder pathology. Pain 2005;114:239–49.
20. Gottrup H, Andersen J, Arendt-Nielsen L, Jensen TS. Psychophysical examination in patients with post-mastectomy pain. Pain 2000;87:275–84.
21. Guastella V, Mick G, Soriano C, Vallet L, Escande G, Dubray C, Eschalier A. A prospective study of neuropathic pain induced by thoracotomy: incidence, clinical description, and diagnosis. Pain 2011;152:74–81.
22. Haroutiunian S, Nikolajsen L, Finnerup NB, Jensen TS. The neuropathic component in persistent postsurgical pain: a systematic literature review. Pain 2013;154:95–102.
23. Jaaskelainen SK, Peltola JK, Forssell K, Vahatalo K. Evaluating function of the inferior alveolar nerve with repeated nerve conduction tests during mandibular sagittal split osteotomy. J Oral Maxillofac Surg 1995;53:269–79.
24. Jaaskelainen SK, Teerijoki-Oksa T, Forssell K, Vahatalo K, Peltola JK, Forssell H. Intraoperative monitoring of the inferior alveolar nerve during mandibular sagittal-split osteotomy. Muscle Nerve 2000;23:368–75.
25. Jaaskelainen SK, Teerijoki-Oksa T, Virtanen A, Tenovuo O, Forssell H. Sensory regeneration following intraoperatively verified trigeminal nerve injury. Neurology 2004;62:1951–7.
26. Johansen A, Schirmer H, Nielsen CS, Stubhaug A. Persistent post-surgical pain and signs of nerve injury: the Tromsø Study. Acta Anaesthesiol Scand 2016;60:380–92.
27. Kalliomaki ML, Meyerson J, Gunnarsson U, Gordh T, Sandblom G. Long-term pain after inguinal hernia repair in a population-based cohort; risk factors and interference with daily activities. Eur J Pain 2008;12:214–25.
28. Kehlet H, Jensen TS, Woolf CJ. Persistent postsurgical pain: risk factors and prevention. Lancet 2006;367:1618–25.
29. Koop O, Gries A, Eckert S, Ellermeier S, Hoksch B, Branscheid D, Beshay M. The role of intercostal nerve preservation in pain control after thoracotomy. Eur J Cardio Thorac Surg 2013;43:808–12.
30. Ladda J, Straube A, Forderreuther S, Krause P, Eggert T. Quantitative sensory testing in cluster headache: increased sensory thresholds. Cephalalgia 2006;26:1043–50.
31. Landerholm SH, Ekblom AG, Hansson PT. Somatosensory function in patients with and without pain after traumatic peripheral nerve injury. Eur J Pain 2010;14:847–53.
32. Loos MJ, Roumen RM, Scheltinga MR. Chronic sequelae of common elective groin hernia repair. Hernia 2007;11:169–73.
33. Mikkelsen T, Werner MU, Lassen B, Kehlet H. Pain and sensory dysfunction 6 to 12 months after inguinal herniotomy. Anesth Analg 2004;99:146–51.
34. Niraj G, Rowbotham DJ. Persistent postoperative pain: where are we now? Br J Anaesth 2011;107:25–9.
35. O'Dwyer PJ, Alani A, McConnachie A. Groin hernia repair: postherniorrhaphy pain. World J Surg 2005;29:1062–5.
36. Oaklander AL, Brown JM. Unilateral nerve injury produces bilateral loss of distal innervation. Ann Neurol 2004;55:639–44.
37. Pappagallo M, Oaklander AL, Quatrano-Piacentini AL, Clark MR, Raja SN. Heterogenous patterns of sensory dysfunction in postherpetic neuralgia suggest multiple pathophysiologic mechanisms. Anesthesiology 2000;92:691–8.
38. Pedersen JL, Kehlet H. Hyperalgesia in a human model of acute inflammatory pain: a methodological study. Pain 1998;74:139–51.

39. Reddi D, Curran N. Chronic pain after surgery: pathophysiology, risk factors and prevention. Postgrad Med J 2014;90:222–7.
40. Reinpold W, Schroeder AD, Schroeder M, Berger C, Rohr M, Wehrenberg U. Retroperitoneal anatomy of the iliohypogastric, ilioinguinal, genitofemoral, and lateral femoral cutaneous nerve: consequences for prevention and treatment of chronic inguinodynia. Hernia 2015;19:539–48.
41. Reinpold WM, Nehls J, Eggert A. Nerve management and chronic pain after open inguinal hernia repair: a prospective two phase study. Ann Surg 2011;254:163–8.
42. Rogers ML, Henderson L, Mahajan RP, Duffy JP. Preliminary findings in the neurophysiological assessment of intercostal nerve injury during thoracotomy. Eur J Cardio Thorac Surg 2002;21:298–301.
43. Rolke R, Baron R, Maier C, Tolle TR, Treede RD, Beyer A, Binder A, Birbaumer N, Birklein F, Botefur IC, Braune S, Flor H, Huge V, Klug R, Landwehrmeyer GB, Magerl W, Maihofner C, Rolko C, Schaub C, Scherens A, Sprenger T, Valet M, Wasserka B. Quantitative sensory testing in the German Research Network on Neuropathic Pain (DFNS): standardized protocol and reference values. Pain 2006;123:231–43.
44. Setala P, Kalliomaki ML, Jarvela K, Huhtala H, Sisto T, Puolakka P. Postoperative hyperalgesia does not predict persistent post-sternotomy pain; observational study based on clinical examination. Acta Anaesthesiol Scand 2016;60:520–8.
45. Sikandar S, Aasvang EK, Dickenson AH. Scratching the surface: the processing of pain from deep tissues. Pain Manag 2016;6:95–102.
46. Smeds S, Lofstrom L, Eriksson O. Influence of nerve identification and the resection of nerves 'at risk' on postoperative pain in open inguinal hernia repair. Hernia 2010;14:265–70.
47. Stawowy M, Funch-Jensen P, Arendt-Nielsen L, Drewes AM. Somatosensory changes in the referred pain area in patients with cholecystolithiasis. Eur J Gastroenterol Hepatol 2005;17:865–70.
48. Stawowy M, Rossel P, Bluhme C, Funch-Jensen P, Arendt-Nielsen L, Drewes AM. Somatosensory changes in the referred pain area following acute inflammation of the appendix. Eur J Gastroenterol Hepatol 2002;14:1079–84.
49. Suzuki R, Rygh LJ, Dickenson AH. Bad news from the brain: descending 5-HT pathways that control spinal pain processing. Trends Pharmacol Sci 2004;25:613–7.
50. Teerijoki-Oksa T, Jaaskelainen SK, Forssell K, Forssell H, Vahatalo K, Tammisalo T, Virtanen A. Risk factors of nerve injury during mandibular sagittal split osteotomy. Int J Oral Maxillofac Surg 2002;31:33–9.
51. Tomaszewski KA, Popieluszko P, Henry BM, Roy J, Sanna B, Kijek MR, Walocha JA. The surgical anatomy of the lateral femoral cutaneous nerve in the inguinal region: a meta-analysis. Hernia 2016;20:649–57.
52. Visagan R, McCormack DJ, Shipolini AR, Jarral OA. Are intracostal sutures better than pericostal sutures for closing a thoracotomy? Interact Cardiovasc Thorac Surg 2012;14:807–15.
53. Wall PD, Woolf CJ. Muscle but not cutaneous C-afferent input produces prolonged increases in the excitability of the flexion reflex in the rat. J Physiol 1984;356:443–58.
54. Weissman-Fogel I, Sprecher E, Granovsky Y, Yarnitsky D. Repeated noxious stimulation of the skin enhances cutaneous pain perception of migraine patients in-between attacks: clinical evidence for continuous sub-threshold increase in membrane excitability of central trigeminovascular neurons. Pain 2003;104:693–700.
55. Wilder-Smith OH, Schreyer T, Scheffer GJ, Arendt-Nielsen L. Patients with chronic pain after abdominal surgery show less preoperative endogenous pain inhibition and more postoperative hyperalgesia: a pilot study. J Pain Palliat Care Pharmacother 2010;24:119–28.
56. Wildgaard K, Ringsted TK, Aasvang EK, Ravn J, Werner MU, Kehlet H. Neurophysiological characterization of persistent postthoracotomy pain. Clin J Pain 2012;28(2):136–42.

CHAPTER 18

Prevention of Pain Persistence: Anesthesiologic Aspects

Patricia Lavand'homme

For years, anesthesiologists have explored in increasing depth the long term effects of patients' perioperative pain management including potential benefits for preventing persistent pain. Any tissue trauma can lead to "chronic pain," pain which by definition persists past normal healing time [63]. Actually, the persistence of pain after a surgical procedure, trauma, or ICU stay has become a major focus of interest, and its prevention now represents a challenge as an index of the quality of health care. Long-term pain after surgery is the cause of disability and suffering, associated with reduced quality of life and increase of health care use. For that reason, persistent postsurgical pain (PPSP) has become a health priority, and the entity will be included in the new version of the *International Classification of Diseases (ICD-11)*, which results from the joint efforts of WHO and IASP [63]. Any chronic pain condition, including PPSP, is a complex problem, multifaceted, with a multifactorial etiology. It is worth noting that patients who attribute their pain to a specific cause such as surgery or trauma are more prone to suffer higher emotional distress and pain than others whose pain has an insidious or spontaneous onset [18]. Several studies have analyzed the risk factors involved in the development of PPSP after various surgical procedures [25,35]; among them, severe poorly relieved acute postoperative pain is one of the most frequently reported. For a long time, anesthesiologists have focused on intraoperative pharmacologic treatments able to control postoperative pain, unfortunately with inconsistent clinical results. Moreover, some patients presenting with severe acute pain will never develop persistent pain, supporting the fact that individuals are not equal facing pain. Other risk factors then have been raised such as dysfunction of endogenous pain modulation and psychosocial factors that may place people at lower or higher risk for severe acute and chronic pain. Thereby, the anesthesiologic aspects of PPSP prevention have been extended to the global perioperative period from preoperative selection until late postoperative follow-up with the aim to better target patients at high risk and to provide them tailored treatment [38].

FROM PRECLINICAL MODELS TO PATIENTS: EVOLUTION OF THE CONCEPT OF PPSP PREVENTION

Postsurgical pain is driven by nociceptive inputs from the wound that are amplified by sensitized peripheral and central neurons [10,52]. Central nervous system sensitization accompanies the acute pain experienced by the patient although its exact role in the magnitude and duration of postoperative pain is not yet fully understood. Central sensitization represents an abnormal state of responsiveness, an increased gain of the nociceptive system [37,71] that translates clinically into higher pain, i.e., hyperalgesia (specifically for mechanical stimuli), which is a major feature of central sensitization. This activity-dependent sensitization may be an early adaptive or protective mechanism serving to reduce mobilization and to promote healing [37,71]. In the acute postoperative period, incisional pain is associated with secondary mechanical (punctate) hyperalgesia in uninjured tissues surrounding the wound. This area of secondary punctate hyperalgesia is ketamine-sensitive and reflects the magnitude of central sensitization [27,50]. Later, ongoing pain caused by persistent tissue damage (e.g., nonresolving inflammation at the surgical site, nerve injury) may lead to a second-phase central sensitization and sometimes to a persistent state of central sensitization. Ultimately, central sensitization may even become independent of peripheral nociceptive inputs, resulting in both spontaneous pain and evoked pain [37,71].

Because central sensitization is one of the mechanisms underlying the maintenance of pain [37], its control has been and still remains a major target in the prevention of PPSP. *Preemptive analgesia*, which should prevent nociceptive inputs from injured tissues from reaching and sensitizing the central nervous system, has only brought controversial results in the perioperative setting. Experimental models of incisional pain clearly show that any analgesic treatment administered before incision is not superior to the same treatment provided after incision because, when the effects of the analgesic treatment abate, the wound is able to reinitiate the central sensitization [10]. These experimental findings, supported by many clinical observations, have led to two major implications for perioperative management. First, preemptive analgesia has evolved into the concept of *preventive analgesia*, a broader definition that involves any perioperative treatments aiming to control central nervous system sensitization and to reduce the development of PPSP. In preventive analgesia, both the duration and the efficacy of the treatment are more important than the timing of administration of the drugs [53]. Second, the wound has a major role in postoperative pain (peripheral sensitization) and drives central sensitization. Thus, actual *protective analgesia* involves any combination of potent analgesic techniques and antihyperalgesic drugs (e.g., epidural analgesia and systemic ketamine) to maximally reduce both primary and secondary hyperalgesias and to put the central nervous system in a limited reactive state [20].

PERIOPERATIVE DRUGS AND TECHNIQUES TO PREVENT PPSP: THE CLINICAL EVIDENCE

Actual perioperative management is procedure-specific and relies on the use of multimodal or balanced analgesia. Besides improving postoperative pain control, an important goal of balanced analgesia is also to minimize the intraoperative administration of opioids. Indeed, opioids provoke side effects that delay rehabilitation and are involved in the phenomenon called "opioid-induced hyperalgesia (OIH)," which enhances nociceptive central sensitization i.e., sensitization caused by noxious inputs from the surgical wound [68]. Beyond afferent barrage from damaged tissues, humoral factors released locally and systemically also contribute to central sensitization. Pain perception is strongly linked to the immune system, particularly in the context of tissue injury, and the inflammatory reaction is a key player in both acute postoperative pain and PPSP. Nociceptive pain is enhanced by inflammatory pain caused by mediators released in the wound, which reduce the threshold of local nerve endings (peripheral sensitization). In the central nervous system, the traditional view that persistent pain is a neuronal-based phenomenon has broadened to a concept including the microglia and the astrocytes as key players [66]. Experimental studies have underlined the important inflammatory reaction that occurs in the central nervous system and takes part in the central sensitization process. Glial activation participates in the amplification of neural signaling, which elicits pain hypersensitivity [66]. Consequently, preventive strategies should take into account those two components (by definition "protective analgesia").

Locoregional Analgesia

Locoregional analgesia provides better postoperative pain control than opioids at least during the first 24 hours after major surgery. Intraoperative and postoperative use of regional anesthesia rather than only postoperative treatment is mandatory to block nociceptive inputs from the wound [10,52]. Epidural analgesia or even better spinal analgesia decreases the area of secondary mechanical hyperalgesia surrounding the wound, e.g., the extent of central sensitization after open abdominal surgery, and reduces the risk of developing PPSP (15% PPSP at 6 months by comparison with 37% in patients without neuraxial block) [39]. Perioperative use of thoracic epidural anesthesia may prevent PPSP in one out every four patients at 6 months after thoracotomy with an odds ratio (OR) of 0.33 (95% confidence interval [CI], 0.20 to 0.56) [4]. Noxious inputs associated with both abdominal and thoracic surgery are conveyed by segmental (i.e., spinal nerves) and heterosegmental (i.e., vagus and phrenic nerves) innervation. Thereby, an effective block of these components may require the combination of both analgesic and antihyperalgesic drugs, in other words, the use of protective analgesia [39]. Subanesthetic doses of ketamine strongly potentiate epidural analgesia either by a supraspinal effect blocking brainstem sensitization or by an anti-inflammatory effect [22]. Clonidine, an α2-adrenergic agonist which mimics noradrenergic descending inhibitory system, displays antihyperalgesic properties after neuraxial (intrathecal and epidural) but not systemic administration. Clinical modulation of secondary punctate hyperalgesia by intrathecal clonidine has been demonstrated in abdominal procedures, colonic resection, and cesarean section and has been associated with a significant reduction of PPSP in patients undergoing major digestive surgery [21]. Peripheral nerve blocks allow a better control of postoperative pain than opioids, particularly during mobilization, and mainly during the first 12 to 24 hours [2]. Although paravertebral block seems to prevent PPSP 6 months after breast cancer surgery in one woman out of every five women [4], peripheral nerve blocks, in contrast, have brought controversial results in orthopedic procedures despite improved acute postoperative pain control. After total knee arthroplasty, extended-duration continuous femoral nerve block up to 4 days was no more effective than 24 hours' block in preventing PPSP and improving health-related quality of life between 7 days and 12 months. Moreover, the addition of a sciatic nerve block to the continuous femoral block did not improve the expected long term benefits [67].

The effect of local anesthetic wound infiltration on the risk of PPSP remains unclear. After cesarean section, continuous infiltration of the wound with either a local anesthetic or an anti-inflammatory drug decreases the incidence (25% vs. 43% in saline infiltration) but not the extent of secondary punctate hyperalgesia at 48 hours [41]. Both treatment groups demonstrated a trend to a lower incidence of PPSP at 6 months, but the study was not powered to evaluate that effect. In a recent study, continuous surgical site infiltration with local anesthetic reduced the area of secondary hyperalgesia as much as does epidural analgesia after open nephrectomy [11]. Moreover, local wound infiltration also decreases the severity of residual pain at 1 month and optimizes quality-of-life parameters at 3 months. A previous study has demonstrated a reduction of PPSP at 4 years, both in intensity and incidence of neuropathic characteristics, e.g., dysesthesia, after a 48 hours' local infiltration of the site of iliac bone graft harvest [60]. A large trial in the context of hip and knee replacement (638 patients undergoing either procedure) assessed the impact of intraoperative local infiltration analgesia (LIA) of the joint [72]. Although very effective to reduce acute postoperative pain, LIA impact on the development of PPSP was very modest and only worked in some patients undergoing hip replacement. In these ones, LIA was more likely to result in no pain or moderate pain than severe pain at 12 months compared with standard care. LIA also decreased the neuropathic component of PPSP. No benefit of LIA was observed after knee replacement.

Ketamine

Ketamine, an old anesthetic drug, increases the quality of postoperative pain control in addition to demonstrating an interesting opioid-sparing effect. Ketamine is best known as an antagonist of the excitatory neurotransmission (*N*-methyl-D-aspartate [NMDA] receptor antagonist), but the drug also interacts with several other receptors and possesses anti-inflammatory properties [22]. Both its anti-NMDA effect and its anti-inflammatory properties may account for the reduction of secondary punctate hyperalgesia, thereby the reduction of central sensitization observed in postoperative patients. In a meta-analysis focusing on systemic drugs for the prevention of PPSP, among 40 RCTs identified, 14 included intravenous ketamine. The results of the meta-analysis suggest a modest (small study size) but significant reduction of PPSP at 3 months and later following ketamine treatment [14]. Another meta-analysis focusing on ketamine (17 studies included) supported a significant reduction in risk of developing PPSP at 3 and 6 months with perioperative intravenous but not epidural ketamine use [46]. The preventive effect was particularly evident in orthopedic procedures. As usually observed in meta-analysis, timing and dosing regimens varied greatly between trials, precluding any recommendation for effective regimen.

Gabapentin and Pregabalin

Perioperative use of **gabapentin and pregabalin**, two oral anticonvulsants which bind to the δ2 subunit of calcium channels, has become widespread. Several meta-analyses of RCTs have brought conflicting results [43]. The conclusions of a very recent large systematic review with meta-analysis (18 studies, 2485 patients) concluded that perioperative pregabalin administration does not prevent PPSP at 3 months after surgery [43]. For the first time, results from unpublished trials, i.e., 79% of the patients, were included in the meta-analysis. Furthermore, a subanalysis seemed to show a decreased incidence of PPSP of neuropathic origin with pregabalin use (0.7% vs. 11% in placebo groups) but with no difference in neuropathic PPSP intensity at 3 months. These observations need to be confirmed (low-quality evidence). To date, clinical studies that have objectively assessed the antihyperalgesic effect of gabapentin and pregabalin are scarce. One randomized placebo-controlled study involving a small number of patients has demonstrated a reduction of 48 hours' secondary mechanical hyperalgesia after elective transperitoneal nephrectomy in patients who received 300 mg pregabalin before surgery but did not inquire about pain persistence [9].

Antidepressant Drugs

Antidepressant drugs are often prescribed for the treatment of chronic pain, specifically when a neuropathic component is present. To date, there is insufficient evidence to support the clinical use of antidepressants both for treatment of acute postoperative pain and for prevention of PPSP according to a systematic review of 15 studies including 1000 patients [70]. Three RCTs included in this meta-analysis used repeated doses of duloxetine (knee replacement), venlafaxine (breast cancer surgery), and escitalopram (coronary artery bypass grafting, treatment beginning up to 2 weeks preoperatively and lasting for up to 6 months after surgery) for prevention of PPSP. Clinical heterogeneity of trials with respect to drug, dosing regimen, and outcome measures once again precluded any meta-analysis and definitive conclusion.

Choice of Anesthetics

The **choice of anesthetics** also might not be innocent [61]. In a retrospective study, intravenous propofol anesthesia seemed to be associated with a decreased incidence of PPSP after breast cancer surgery than sevoflurane inhaled anesthesia (44.2% vs. 67.4%; OR 1.51, 95% CI, 1.15 to 1.81) [17]. However, propofol did not have a significant effect on severity and duration of persistent pain. It is worth noting that propofol might display antihyperalgesic properties counterbalancing hyperalgesia caused by intraoperative use of high doses of opioids [24].

Nitrous oxide has antihyperalgesic properties that rely on direct inhibition of spinal NMDA receptors and activation of descending inhibitory pathways leading to spinal release of norepinephrine. More, nitrous oxide modulates postoperative OIH in humans. A first outcome analysis in patients who received nitrous oxide 70% in oxygen during their surgical procedure (ENIGMA trial) seemed to show both a lower incidence (7% vs. 14% in the air-oxygen group) and reduced severity of PPSP at 3 months after surgery [13]. The aforementioned observations were not confirmed in subsequent analysis of data [12]. Nitrous oxide does not affect PPSP rate or intensity, except in a subgroup of Asian patients with genotype variant.

Nonsteroidal anti-inflammatory drugs have a major role in multimodal analgesia, but their preventive effect on PPSP is still inconclusive [14]. **Cyclooxygenase 2 (COX2) inhibitors** have attracted attention because peripheral and central COX2 induction after tissue injury may be a key player in central sensitization [37,71]. Prolonged administration of celecoxib for 6 weeks after knee arthroplasty provides less painful and more rapid recovery with functional benefits still present at 1 year postsurgery [58]. In contrast, addition of celecoxib (preoperative and 5 days postoperative treatment) to paravertebral block of nociceptive sensitization in the context of breast cancer surgery reduced acute pain during mobilization but did not affect PPSP at 12 months [64]. The authors also assessed generalized pressure hyperalgesia, which was not modified by celecoxib, but remained present during all the follow-ups in patients who developed PPSP.

Corticosteroids are currently used to reduce postoperative nausea and vomiting improve postoperative analgesia. They exert a different modulation of the inflammatory reaction, as they act upstream the regular nonsteroidal anti-inflammatory drugs and also block the production of proinflammatory cytokines. Despite that, their role in the prevention of PPSP remains largely unexplored [14]. In patients undergoing augmentation mammoplasty, single preoperative dose of methylprednisolone resulted in less hyperesthesia by comparison with parecoxib or placebo but did not significantly reduce the prevalence of spontaneous or evoked PPSP at 1 year [56]. It is interesting to point out that the incidence of PPSP after lateral thoracotomy is lower in patients who undergo lung transplantation and receive long-lasting immunosuppressive treatment including corticosteroids (18% vs. 30% to 60%) [69]. Finally, it is worth noting that local anesthetics, ketamine, and even gabapentinoids possess anti-inflammatory properties and may act as immune modulators affecting central sensitization.

Intravenous lidocaine infusion (up to 36 hours after the procedure) reduces postoperative pain and improves bowel function after digestive surgery. To date, a single study has found a preventive effect at 3 months after breast cancer surgery in terms of PPSP incidence (11.8% vs. 47.4% in the placebo group) and intensity [27]. In the retrospective study from Joris et al. [32], ketamine combined with intravenous lidocaine, but not lidocaine alone, was associated to a reduced risk of PPSP after laparoscopic colorectal surgery. As glial activation plays a major role in the development and the maintenance of central sensitization, a selective block of microglial activation may represent an interesting target to modulate PPSP development. Such approach (e.g., propentophylline) has been successful in animal models but rather disappointing in humans. In a recent study, 8 days' postoperative administration of **minocycline**, a broad-spectrum antibiotic with antiapoptotic, anti-inflammatory properties and inhibitory effect on microglial activation, did not reduce acute pain, failed to decrease the incidence and intensity of neuropathic pain, and did not improve functional scores at 3 months after lumbar discectomy [44]. Several explanations including too low a dose and an insufficient duration of treatment may account for the lack of effect of minocycline treatment. Furthermore, it is interesting to point out that microglial activation has a greater role in the initiation than in the maintenance of central sensitization, whereas astroglial activation, which is not affected by minocycline treatment, plays a major role in the maintenance of central sensitization [44]. Nevertheless, a subanalysis of the results seems to suggest that minocycline might be effective in a subgroup of patients with predominantly deep spontaneous pain at baseline. Such finding highlights the interest of assessing the efficacy of phenotype-based treatment according to neuropathic characteristics.

Perioperative Opioid Use

Prevention of PPSP also involves the problem of **perioperative opioid use**. Opioids have been used for decades as the cornerstone of perioperative analgesia, a very comfortable choice, but are now considered as a significant cause of problems at the individual level (delayed recovery and poorer outcome) and social level (prolonged use after surgery, even after minor procedure, and gateway to addiction) [36]. Although opioids remain the most potent drugs to control severe pain, neuroadaptation impairs opioids' ability to provide long-term analgesia and produces opposite effects, i.e., enhancement of existent pain and facilitation of chronic pain development [55]. Neuroadaptation to opioids use yields to the development of tolerance and to a phenomenon called "opioid-induced hyperalgesia." Opioids recruit endogenous pronociceptive systems mainly through central NMDA receptor activation [55]. They are also able to enhance the glial inflammatory reaction secondary to tissue injury, a state which contributes to central nervous system sensitization [55]. OIH is dependent on the dose of opioid administered and exacerbates postoperative pain through acute hyperalgesia and tolerance, two interrelated phenomena. With *intraoperative administration of opioids*, and particularly the ultrashort-acting opioid remifentanil, a dose-related increase of the area of secondary mechanical hyperalgesia was found [31]. A potential connection between OIH and PPSP has been recently suggested as there is a dose-dependent relationship between intraoperative remifentanil use and PPSP after thoracic surgery [57,63]. Indirectly, in comparison with general anesthesia, the use of intraoperative neuraxial anesthesia reduces the risk of severe PPSP at 1 year after total hip and knee replacement (OR 2.5; 95% CI, 1.3 to 4.8), a benefit partly attributed to the opioid-sparing effect of the analgesic technique [30]. Therefore, the concept of **opioid-sparing anesthesia** (and ultimately "opioid-free anesthesia") may be a major step in the prevention of PPSP. Several strategies currently used as preventive analgesia, besides their effectiveness to modulate central sensitization process, also reduce the perioperative need for opioids (e.g., locoregional analgesic techniques, antihyperalgesic drugs such as ketamine) [54]. Preoperative pain, at the site of surgery and elsewhere, is very common and stands as an important risk factor for PPSP [3,35,38]. When preoperative pain is associated with *preoperative use of opioids,* it not only worsens acute postoperative pain but also increases the risk of PPSP with an RR of 2.0 (95% CI, 1.2 to 3.3) [65] and poorer outcome after orthopedic [48] and major abdominal [19] procedures. A recent study in the context of joint arthroplasty highlighted the fact that patients who successfully decrease their use of opioids before surgery (50% weaning of opioid dose) demonstrate substantially improved clinical outcomes, comparable to those of patients who did not use opioids preoperatively, and superior to those of patients who did not wean opioids preoperatively [49].

THE FAILURE OF ACTUAL PERIOPERATIVE STRATEGIES: A CLUE FOR THE DEVELOPMENT OF FUTURE IMPROVED STRATEGIES

Inconsistent clinical results of preventive analgesia warrant analysis and explanation. Undoubtedly, **the extent and the duration of central sensitization**, i.e., its involvement in pain chronification process, may highly differ among individuals even after similar injury. Preliminary results show that, after limb amputation, prolonged and individualized (from 4 to 83 days) perineural infusion of local anesthetic allows a significantly reduction in the incidence of phantom pain (16% instead of 67% as usually reported with shorter-lasting therapeutic interventions) [8]. Preoperative chronic pain is not unusual (50% to 62% of the patients) and may favor a state of preoperative central sensitization precluding the expected benefits of preemptive and preventive analgesia. Moreover, in some of these patients, long-term opioid intake also might have further sensitized the central nervous system. This is particularly evident for orthopedic procedures [48]. Patients with poorly controlled preoperative pain will have less favorable outcome after surgery and might be more prone to develop PPSP. A clinical trial regarding limb amputation has highlighted the impact of effective preoperative pain control (whatever the technique used) on PPSP development [33]. Preoperative opioid weaning before joint arthroplasty, thereby improved control of preoperative pain, and had better surgical outcomes including less PPSP 6 to 12 months postoperatively [49].

Perioperative management includes **preoperative identification of patients at risk** for PPSP. Validated tools already exist to predict the risk of severe acute postoperative pain (Table 18-1)

Among many other studies in the field, the observational study from Fletcher [25] also identified risk factors for the development of PPSP. Preoperative pain and the percentage of time in severe acute pain currently stand as major risk factors. These factors are also part of a prospective risk-factor index [3], which identified five key predictors: emotional overload/overstrain, preoperative pain at the operative site, other chronic preoperative pain (e.g., headache, fibromyalgia, and backache), acute postoperative pain, and comorbid stress symptoms such as anxiety or disturbed sleep (including the intake of medications to treat those symptoms). It is worth noting that, despite the hopes and promises of genetics that unveiled several links between gene polymorphisms and sensitivity to pain, clinical risk factors remain the best available predictors of PPSP, including neuropathic PPSP [45,47]. Other developments should involve preoperative psychophysical measures of individuals'

> **TABLE 18-1 Perioperative Risk Factors for the Development of Persistent Postsurgical Pain (PPSP)**
>
> 1. Preoperative pain at surgical site (odds ratio: 3.2)
> 2. Preoperative pain elsewhere (odds ratio: 2.4)
> 3. One or more comorbid stress symptoms (odds ratio: 2.4)
> 4. Capacity overload in the past 6 mo (odds ratio: 3.6)
> 5. Postoperative acute pain (with a pain score > 3 on a scale from 0, no pain, to 10, the worst pain) (odds ratio: 3.1).
>
> According to the preliminary risk index developed by Althaus et al. [3]. Regarding the risk index, the authors suggest the following classifications: zero to one risk factor present, low risk of developing PPSP; two risk factors present, moderate risk of developing PPSP; three to five risk factors present, high risk of developing PPSP.

endogenous pain processing i.e., quantitative sensory testing (QST). One day, it may become mandatory to determine whether some patients have an inherited propensity for developing central sensitization. Central sensitization process reflects the balance between endogenous inhibitory and excitatory systems, which modulate pain processing. Endogenous differences among patients place them at lower or higher risk to present with severe acute and chronic pain [23]. Several chronic pain conditions are linked to altered pain transmission and pathologic QST (e.g., fibromyalgia, osteoarthritis, etc.) where patients present with enhanced excitatory processes (i.e., positive temporal summation) and poor inhibitory systems [73]. Some QST techniques are easier than others to apply in clinical setting, including during the preoperative evaluation of the patient. In example, presurgical assessment of mechanical temporal summation of pain predicts the development of PPSP 12 months after knee replacement [51]. Chronic use of opioid analgesics also modulates the balance of pain processing toward an enhanced proexcitatory state as found in 30% of the patients scheduled for an orthopedic procedure [29]. A better knowledge of patient's endogenous pain processing may allow the individualization of perioperative management [26,73]. Facilitated temporal summation may be modulated by administration of NMDA inhibitors or COX2 inhibitors as recently found in patients suffering painful osteoarthritis [5]. Finally, besides inquiring about memories of previous long-lasting pain after surgical procedure or trauma, the physical examination of previous scars in patients might demonstrate the existence of preoperative hyperalgesia as demonstrated in 41% of women scheduled for repeat cesarean delivery [50]. The phenomenon correlated with enhanced postoperative pain and as a sign of persistent sensitization might predict PPSP (unfortunately not reported in the study).

Acute and Subacute Postoperative Pain Control: A Better View of Pain Resolution

Although pain is a dynamic process, the current postoperative pain management is not. The development of pain trajectories as proposed by Chapman [15] from day 1 to day 6, and even longer, should allow to identify abnormal pain resolution. Looking at the pain trajectory pattern, specifically at the slope (e.g., the rate of pain resolution), 25% of patients have a flat slope and 12% show a positive slope (e.g., increase of pain), indicating that 37% of patients are living with unresolved postoperative pain at day 6 after surgery [15] and perhaps later. After total knee replacement, the laters were still in severe pain at 3 months after surgery with their CPSP including a neuropathic component [40]. The control of severe acute pain after surgery requires a correct **assessment of the type of postoperative pain** with the aim to provide an accurate treatment. Recent observations support this assertion. First, early acute postsurgical neuropathic pain, for which diagnosis is often neglected, significantly increases the risk of neuropathic PPSP [6]. Second, after abdominal surgery, the visceral component of the pain might be the one to target. Indeed, the risk of chronic pain after laparoscopic cholecystectomy seems significantly related to the visceral pain response during the first week after surgery [7]. Subacute pain that can last for several weeks after surgery represents a neglected area of clinical investigation [16,38], although some prospective studies have demonstrated the predictive value of 30-day or 6-week postoperative pain intensity as a risk factor for PPSP after inguinal hernia repair [1] and cosmetic breast surgery [55]. The nature of PPSP remains unclear because inflammatory mechanisms play an important role even in the development of neuropathic pain. However, recent arguments are in favor of a predominant **neuropathic origin**, as there is a strong association between sensory disturbances (hypoesthesia and hyperesthesia) and the presence and the intensity of PPSP [25,30], some procedures carrying higher risk. Pain intensity and incidence may increase during the subacute pain period as shown postherniotomy (14% at day 30 vs. 7% at day 7) [1] and postthoracotomy (from 8% at day 7 to 22% at 3 months) [59], perhaps revealing a neuropathic pain process. Although data are still scarce, neuropathic pain characteristics may appear very early after surgery [6] and if underrecognized may lead to long-lasting severe pain, in other words to neuropathic PPSP. Among patients diagnosed with acute neuropathic pain, 78% still reported PPSP at 6 months and 56% at 12 months [28]. A recent study, using the iliac crest bone harvest model, demonstrates that both nerve lesion and central sensitization are involved in persistent neuropathic pain [42]. Patients who developed PPSP of neuropathic origin displayed higher acute pain intensity at 48 hours postsurgery, cutaneous mechanical hyperalgesia, and neuropathic pain characteristics on the Douleur Neuropathic 4 questionnaire. Consequently, the anesthesiologists should pay particular attention to the patients' clinical course early during recovery. Prompt administration of analgesic and antihyperalgesic treatments should be possible from the immediate postoperative period (during hospital stay) until weeks later (follow-up in "transitional pain units") [20,34].

CONCLUSIONS

Because inconsistent clinical results have underlined the failure of purely intraoperative treatments (e.g., mainly those aiming to prevent central neuroplastic changes) to stop the development of persistent pain after surgery, a different approach has been developed, which involves the entire perioperative period from preoperative patient selection until late follow-up pain management (Table 18-2).

A key goal is to target high-risk patients and to provide them the most personally adapted treatment. Severe preoperative pain at surgical site and elsewhere as well as unrelieved postoperative pain remains a strong predictor of PPSP that leads to the supposition that some patients might be genetically predisposed to pain, both acute and persistent. Future developments in genetic factors might help to further select patients at risk for severe pain as well as those susceptible to develop OIH. Finally, it is important to point out that, beside pharmacologic treatments, the future perioperative prevention of PPSP should also include psychological treatments aiming to reduce patients' anxiety, catastrophizing, and posttraumatic stress, all negative mental factors which certainly play an important role in the maintenance of pain after surgery.

TABLE 18-2 Anesthesiologic Aspects of the Prevention of Persistent Postsurgical Pain (PPSP)

	Preoperative	Intraoperative	Postoperative
Traditional view	Inconsistent, not addressed	Preemptive analgesia	Acute pain control (24–48 h)
Actual view optimized	Use of index of risk factors for • severe acute pain • PPSP	Providing preventive/protective analgesia to all patients	Acute pain control (24–48 h) with antihyperalgesic medications as needed
Future developments	Individualization of high-risk patients (selected by risk index) • evaluation of endogenous pain process (QST) • genetic background • psychological and social risk factors • opioid intake weaning	Protective analgesia tailored on • preoperative QST evaluation (and perhaps genetic evaluation) • multimodal opioid-sparing anesthesia and analgesia	Objective evaluation of severe pain • neuropathic, visceral component • hypersensitivity (mechanical hyperalgesia) Adequate treatments and long-term follow-up (subacute pain) Use of pain trajectories as a tool to assess pain resolution

REFERENCES

1. Aasvang EK, Gmaehle E, Hansen JB, Gmaehle B, Forman JL, Schwarz J, Bittner R, Kehlet H. Predictive risk factors for persistent postherniotomy pain. Anesthesiology 2010;112(4):957–69.
2. Abdallah FW, Halpern SH, Aoyama K, Brull R. Will the real benefits of single-shot interscalene block please stand up? A systematic review and meta-analysis. Anesth Analg 2015;120(5):1114–29.
3. Althaus A, Hinrichs-Rocker A, Chapman R, Arranz Becker O, Lefering R, Simanski C, Weber F, Moser KH, Joppich R, Trojan S, Gutzeit N, Neugebauer E. Development of a risk index for the prediction of chronic post-surgical pain. Eur J Pain 2012;16(6):901–10.
4. Andreae MH, Andreae DA. Local anaesthetics and regional anaesthesia for preventing chronic pain after surgery. Cochrane Database Syst Rev 2012;10:CD007105.
5. Arendt-Nielsen L, Egsgaard LL, Petersen KK. Evidence for a central mode of action for etoricoxib (COX-2 inhibitor) in patients with painful knee osteoarthritis. Pain 2016;157(8):1634–44.
6. Beloeil H, Sion B, Rousseau C, Albaladejo P, Raux M, Aubrun F, Martinez V, SFAR research network. Early postoperative neuropathic pain assessed by the DN4 score predicts an increased risk of persistent postsurgical neuropathic pain. Eur J Anaesthesiol 2017;34(10):652–7.
7. Blichfeldt-Eckhardt MR, Ording H, Andersen C, Licht PB, Toft P. Early visceral pain predicts chronic pain after laparoscopic cholecystectomy. Pain 2014;155(11):2400–7.
8. Borghi B, D'Addabbo M, White PF, Gallerani P, Toccaceli L, Raffaeli W, Tognu A, Fabbri N, Mercuri M. The use of prolonged peripheral neural blockade after lower extremity amputation: the effect on symptoms associated with phantom limb syndrome. Anesth Analg 2010;111(5):1308–15.
9. Bornemann-Cimenti H, Lederer AJ, Wejbora M, Michaeli K, Kern-Pirsch C, Archan S, Rumpold-Seitlinger G, Zigeuner R, Sandner-Kiesling A. Preoperative pregabalin administration significantly reduces postoperative opioid consumption and mechanical hyperalgesia after transperitoneal nephrectomy. Br J Anaesth 2013;108(5):845–9.
10. Brennan TJ. Pathophysiology of postoperative pain. Pain 2011;152(3 Suppl.):S33–40.
11. Capdevila X, Moulard S, Plasse C, Peshaud JL, Molinari N, Dadure C, Bringuier S. Effectiveness of epidural analgesia, continuous surgical site analgesia, and patient-controlled analgesic morphine for postoperative pain management and hyperalgesia, rehabilitation, and health-related quality of life after open nephrectomy: a prospective, randomized, controlled study. Anesth Analg 2017;124(1):336–45.

12. Chan MT, Peyton PJ, Myles PS, Leslie K, Buckley N, Kasza J, Paech MJ, Beattie WS, Sessler DI, Forbes A, Wallace S, Chen Y, Tian Y, Wu WK, and the Australian and New Zealand College of Anaesthetists Clinical Trials Network for the ENIGMA-II investigators. Chronic postsurgical pain in the evaluation of nitrous oxide in the gas mixture for anaesthesia (ENIGMA)-II trial. Br J Anaesth 2016;117(6):801–11.
13. Chan MT, Wan AC, Gin T, Leslie K, Myles PS. Chronic postsurgical pain after nitrous oxide anesthesia. Pain 2011;152(11):2514–20.
14. Chaparro LE, Smith SA, Moore RA, Wiffen PJ, Gilron I. Pharmacotherapy for the prevention of chronic pain after surgery in adults. Cochrane Database Syst Rev 2013;7:CD008307.
15. Chapman CR, Donaldson GW, Davis JJ, Bradshaw DH. Improving individual measurement of postoperative pain: the pain trajectory. J Pain 2011;12(2):257–62.
16. Chapman CR, Vierck CJ. The transition of acute postoperative pain to chronic pain: an integrative overview of research on mechanisms. J Pain 2017;18(4):359.e351-38.
17. Cho AR, Kwon JY, Kim KH, Lee HJ, Kim HK, Kim ES, Hong JM, Kim C. The effects of anesthetics on chronic pain after breast cancer surgery. Anesth Analg 2013;116(3):685–93.
18. Crombie IK, Davies HT, Macrae WA. Cut and thrust: antecedent surgery and trauma among patients attending a chronic pain clinic. Pain 1998;76(1–2):167–71.
19. Cron DC, Englesbe MJ, Bolton CJ, Joseph MT, Carrier KL, Moser SE, Waljee JF, Hilliard PE, Kheterpal S, Brummett CM. Preoperative opioid use is independently associated with increased costs and worse outcomes after major abdominal surgery. Ann Surg 2017;265(4):695–701.
20. De Kock M. Expanding our horizons: transition of acute postoperative pain to persistent pain and establishment of chronic postsurgical pain services. Anesthesiology 2009;111(3):461–3.
21. De Kock M, Lavand'homme P, Waterloos H. The short-lasting analgesia and long-term antihyperalgesic effect of intrathecal clonidine in patients undergoing colonic surgery. Anesth Analg 2005;101(2):566–72.
22. De Kock M, Loix S, Lavand'homme P. Ketamine and peripheral inflammation. CNS Neurosci Ther 2013;19(6):403–10.
23. Edwards RR. Individual differences in endogenous pain modulation as a risk factor for chronic pain. Neurology 2005;65(3):437–43.
24. Fletcher D, Martinez V. Opioid-induced hyperalgesia in patients after surgery: a systematic review and a meta-analysis. Br J Anaesth 2014;112(6):991–1004.
25. Fletcher D, Stamer UM, Pogatzki-Zahn E, Zaslansky R, Tanase NV, Perruchoud C, Kranke P, Komann M, Lehman T, Meissner W, euCPSP group for the Clinical Trial Network group of the European Society of Anaesthesiology. Chronic postsurgical pain in Europe: an observational study. Eur J Anaesthesiol 2015;32(10):725–34.
26. Granot M. Can we predict persistent postoperative pain by testing preoperative experimental pain? Curr Opin Anaesthesiol 2009;22(3):425–30.
27. Grigoras A, Lee P, Sattar F, Shorten G. Perioperative intravenous lidocaine decreases the incidence of persistent pain after breast surgery. Clin J Pain 2013;28(7):567–72.
28. Hayes C, Browne S, Lantry G, Burstal R. Neuropathic pain in the acute pain service: a prospective study. Acute Pain 2002;4:45–8.
29. Hina N, Fletcher D, Poindessous-Jazat F, Martinez V. Hyperalgesia induced by low-dose opioid treatment before orthopaedic surgery: an observational case-control study. Eur J Anaesthesiol 2015;32(4):255–61.
30. Johansen A, Romundstad L, Nielsen CS, Schirmer H, Stubhaug A. Persistent postsurgical pain in a general population: prevalence and predictors in the Tromso study. Pain 2012;153(7):1390–6.
31. Joly V, Richebe P, Guignard B, Fletcher D, Maurette P, Sessler DI, Chauvin M. Remifentanil-induced postoperative hyperalgesia and its prevention with small-dose ketamine. Anesthesiology 2005;103(1):147–55.
32. Joris JL, Georges MJ, Medjahed K, Ledoux D, Damilot G, Ramquet CC, Coimbra CI, Kohnen LP, Brichant JF. Prevalence, characteristics and risk factors of chronic postsurgical pain after laparoscopic colorectal surgery: retrospective analysis. Eur J Anaesthesiol 2015;32(10):712–7.
33. Karanikolas M, Aretha D, Tsolakis I, Monantera G, Kiekkas P, Papadoulas S, Swarm RA, Filos KS. Optimized perioperative analgesia reduces chronic phantom limb pain intensity, prevalence, and frequency: a prospective, randomized, clinical trial. Anesthesiology 2011;114(5):1144–54.
34. Katz J, Weinrib A, Fashler SR, Katznelson R, Shah BR, Ladak SS, Jiang J, Li Q, McMillan K, Mina DS, Wentlandt K, McRae K, Tamir D, Lyn S, de Perrot M, Rao V, Grant D, Roche-Nagle G, Cleary SP, Hofer SO, Gilbert R, Wijeysundera D, Ritvo P, Janmohamed T, O'Leary G, Clarke H. The Toronto General Hospital Transitional Pain Service: development and implementation of a multidisciplinary program to prevent chronic postsurgical pain. J Pain Res 2015;8:695–702.
35. Kehlet H, Jensen TS, Woolf CJ. Persistent postsurgical pain: risk factors and prevention. Lancet 2006;367(9522):1618–25.

36. Kharasch ED, Brunt LM. Perioperative opioids and public health. Anesthesiology 2016;124(4):960–5.
37. Latremoliere A, Woolf CJ. Central sensitization: a generator of pain hypersensitivity by central neural plasticity. J Pain 2009;10(9):895–926.
38. Lavand'homme P. Transition from acute to chronic pain after surgery. Pain 2017;158(Suppl. 1):S50–4.
39. Lavand'homme P, De Kock M. The use of intraoperative epidural or spinal analgesia modulates postoperative hyperalgesia and reduces residual pain after major abdominal surgery. Acta Anaesthesiol Belg 2006;57(4):373–9.
40. Lavand'homme PM, Grosu I, France MN, Thienpont E. Pain trajectories identify patients at risk of persistent pain after knee arthroplasty: an observational study. Clin Orthop Relat Res 2014;472(5):1409–15.
41. Lavand'homme PM, Roelants F, Waterloos H, De Kock MF. Postoperative analgesic effects of continuous wound infiltration with diclofenac after elective cesarean delivery. Anesthesiology 2007;106(6):1220–5.
42. Martinez V, Ben Ammar S, Judet T, Bouhassira D, Chauvin M, Fletcher D. Risk factors predictive of chronic postsurgical neuropathic pain: the value of the iliac crest bone harvest model. Pain 2012;153(7):1478–83.
43. Martinez V, Pichard X, Fletcher D. Perioperative pregabalin administration does not prevent chronic postoperative pain: systematic review with a meta-analysis of randomized trials. Pain 2017;158(5):775–83.
44. Martinez V, Szekely B, Lemarie J, Martin F, Gentili M, Ben Ammar S, Lepeintre JF, Garreau de Loubresse C, Chauvin M, Bouhassira D, Fletcher D. The efficacy of a glial inhibitor, minocycline, for preventing persistent pain after lumbar discectomy: a randomized, double-blind, controlled study. Pain 2013;154(8):1197–203.
45. Martinez V, Uceyler N, Ben Ammar S, Alvarez JC, Gaudot F, Sommer C, Bouhassira D, Fletcher D. Clinical, histological, and biochemical predictors of postsurgical neuropathic pain. Pain 2015;156(11):2390–8.
46. McNicol ED, Schumann R, Haroutounian S. A systematic review and meta-analysis of ketamine for the prevention of persistent post-surgical pain. Acta Anaesthesiol Scand 2014;58(10):1199–213.
47. Montes A, Roca G, Sabate S, Lao JI, Navarro A, Cantillo J, Canet J, Group GS. Genetic and clinical factors associated with chronic postsurgical pain after hernia repair, hysterectomy, and thoracotomy: a two-year multicenter cohort study. Anesthesiology 2015;122(5):1123–41.
48. Morris BJ, Mir HR. The opioid epidemic: impact on orthopaedic surgery. J Am Acad Orthop Surg 2015;23(5):267–71.
49. Nguyen LC, Sing DC, Bozic KJ. Preoperative reduction of opioid use before total joint arthroplasty. J Arthroplasty 2016;31(9 Suppl.):282–7.
50. Ortner CM, Granot M, Richebe P, Cardoso M, Bollag L, Landau R. Preoperative scar hyperalgesia is associated with post-operative pain in women undergoing a repeat Caesarean delivery. Eur J Pain 2013;17(1):111–23.
51. Petersen KK, Arendt-Nielsen L, Simonsen O, Wilder-Smith O, Laursen MB. Presurgical assessment of temporal summation of pain predicts the development of chronic postoperative pain 12 months after total knee replacement. Pain 2015;156(1):55–61.
52. Pogatzki-Zahn E, Segelcke D, Schug S. Postoperative pain – from mechanisms to treatment. Pain Rep 2017;2(2):e588.
53. Pogatzki-Zahn EM, Zahn PK. From preemptive to preventive analgesia. Curr Opin Anaesthesiol 2006;19(5):551–5.
54. Richebe P, Rivat C, Liu SS. Perioperative or postoperative nerve block for preventive analgesia: should we care about the timing of our regional anesthesia? Anesth Analg 2013;116(5):969–70.
55. Rivat C, Ballantyne J. The dark side of opioids in pain management: basic science explains clinical observation. Pain Rep 2016;1:e570.
56. Romundstad L, Breivik H, Roald H, Skolleborg K, Romundstad PR, Stubhaug A. Chronic pain and sensory changes after augmentation mammoplasty: long term effects of preincisional administration of methylprednisolone. Pain 2006;124(1–2):92–9.
57. Salengros JC, Huybrechts I, Ducart A, Faraoni D, Marsala C, Barvais L, Cappello M, Engelman E. Different anesthetic techniques associated with different incidences of chronic post-thoracotomy pain: low-dose remifentanil plus presurgical epidural analgesia is preferable to high-dose remifentanil with postsurgical epidural analgesia. J Cardiothorac Vasc Anesth 2012;24(4):608–16.
58. Schroer WC, Diesfeld PJ, LeMarr AR, Reedy ME. Benefits of prolonged postoperative cyclooxygenase-2 inhibitor administration on total knee arthroplasty recovery: a double-blind, placebo-controlled study. J Arthroplasty 2011;26(6 Suppl.):2–7.
59. Searle RD, Simpson MP, Simpson KH, Milton R, Bennett MI. Can chronic neuropathic pain following thoracic surgery be predicted during the postoperative period? Interact Cardiovasc Thorac Surg 2009;9(6):999–1002.
60. Singh K, Phillips FM, Kuo E, Campbell M. A prospective, randomized, double-blind study of the efficacy of postoperative continuous local anesthetic infusion at the iliac crest bone graft site after posterior spinal arthrodesis: a minimum of 4-year follow-up. Spine (Phila Pa 1976) 2007;32(25):2790–6.

61. Steyaert A, Forget P, Dubois V, Lavand'homme P, De Kock M. Does the perioperative analgesic/anesthetic regimen influence the prevalence of long-term chronic pain after mastectomy? J Clin Anesth 2016;33:20–5.
62. Treede RD, Rief W, Barke A, Aziz Q, Bennett MI, Benoliel R, Cohen M, Evers S, Finnerup NB, First MB, Giamberardino MA, Kaasa S, Kosek E, Lavand'homme P, Nicholas M, Perrot S, Scholz J, Schug S, Smith BH, Svensson P, Vlaeyen JW, Wang SJ. A classification of chronic pain for ICD-11. Pain 2015;156(6):1003–7.
63. van Gulik L, Ahlers SJ, van de Garde EM, Bruins P, van Boven WJ, Tibboel D, van Dongen EP, Knibbe CA. Remifentanil during cardiac surgery is associated with chronic thoracic pain 1 yr after sternotomy. Br J Anaesth 2013;109(4):616–22.
64. van Helmond N, Steegers MA, Filippini-de Moor GP, Vissers K, Wilder-Smith O. Hyperalgesia and Persistent Pain after breast cancer surgery: a prospective randomized controlled trial with perioperative COX-2 inhibition. PLoS One 2016;12:e0166601.
65. VanDenKerkhof EG, Hopman WM, Goldstein DH, Wilson RA, Towheed TE, Lam M, Harrison MB, Reitsma ML, Johnston SL, Medd JD, Gilron I. Impact of perioperative pain intensity, pain qualities, and opioid use on chronic pain after surgery: a prospective cohort study. Reg Anesth Pain Med 2012;37(1):19–27.
66. Watkins LR, Milligan ED, Maier SF. Glial proinflammatory cytokines mediate exaggerated pain states: implications for clinical pain. Adv Exp Med Biol 2003;521:1–21.
67. Wegener JT, van Ooij B, van Dijk CN, Karayeva SA, Hollmann MW, Preckel B, Stevens MF. Long-term pain and functional disability after total knee arthroplasty with and without single-injection or continuous sciatic nerve block in addition to continuous femoral nerve block: a prospective, 1-year follow-up of a randomized controlled trial. Reg Anesth Pain Med 2012;38(1):58–63.
68. Weinbroum AA. Postoperative hyperalgesia-A clinically applicable narrative review. Pharmacol Res 2017;120:188–205.
69. Wildgaard K, Iversen M, Kehlet H. Chronic pain after lung transplantation: a nationwide study. Clin J Pain 2010;26(3):217–22.
70. Wong K, Phelan R, Kalso E, Galvin I, Goldstein D, Raja S, Gilron I. Antidepressant drugs for prevention of acute and chronic postsurgical pain: early evidence and recommended future directions. Anesthesiology 2014;121(3):591–608.
71. Woolf CJ. Central sensitization: implications for the diagnosis and treatment of pain. Pain 2011;152(3 Suppl.):S2–15.
72. Wylde V, Lenguerrand E, Gooberman-Hill R, Beswick AD, Marques E, Noble S, Horwood J, Pyke M, Dieppe P, Blom AW. Effect of local anaesthetic infiltration on chronic postsurgical pain after total hip and knee replacement: the APEX randomised controlled trials. Pain 2015;156(6):1161–70.
73. Yarnitsky D, Granot M, Granovsky Y. Pain modulation profile and pain therapy: between pro- and antinociception. Pain 2014;155(4):663–5.

SECTION 6

Translating Research into Clinical Practice

CHAPTER 19

Multimodal Drug Therapies for Postoperative Pain Control in Adults

Stephan A. Schug

Postoperative pain control is necessary from a humanitarian point of view to reduce pain and suffering in patients after surgery. Beyond this ethical imperative, optimal postoperative pain control is also able to reduce perioperative morbidity and possibly even mortality, improve clinical outcomes, facilitate rehabilitation, and enable earlier discharge from hospital. Large surveys, however, have shown that postoperative pain is still often severe, with significant adverse consequences in many patients [12]. In view of the potential severity of postoperative pain, the use of opioids to treat it is common; there is no doubt that opioids are effective in relieving severe postoperative pain. However, their use is often associated with adverse events, which can be life-threatening such as opioid-induced ventilatory impairment (OIVI) or can otherwise delay postoperative recovery such as impaired gastrointestinal function (nausea, vomiting, and constipation) or provoke unpleasant experiences such as itching, confusion, or agitation. The occurrence of adverse events due to opioid administration has been shown to delay recovery and rehabilitation and increase length of stay and costs of hospital admission [28]. It has also been shown that attempts to control postoperative pain by more aggressive opioid analgesia result in a significant increase of episodes of OIVI in the postoperative period [40].

It was Kehlet who suggested around 1989 that good pain relief allowing return to normal function cannot be achieved by a single drug or method without significant adverse effects [18]. On the basis of this hypothesis, Kehlet suggested the concept of multimodal or balanced analgesia [19]. This was in analogy to the preceding development of balanced anesthesia by using different drugs to achieve different goals of intraoperative anesthesia such as loss of awareness, analgesia, and muscle relaxation. In this context, multimodal analgesia is defined as the combination of analgesics with different mechanisms or sites of action along the pain pathway [4,13]. Multimodal analgesia is used to achieve the following outcomes by synergistic or at least additive effects of combinations of analgesics:

- Improved analgesia
- Reduced opioid requirements ("opioid-sparing" effect)
- Reduced adverse effects of, in particular, opioids

A simple but impressive demonstration of the potential benefits of multimodal analgesia has been achieved in a study where patients after laparoscopic cholecystectomy had a morphine patient-controlled analgesia (PCA) to which placebo or a cyclooxygenase 2 (COX2)-specific anti-inflammatory drug was added [11]. This approach resulted in significant reduction of pain, opioid consumption, and number and severity of adverse effects of opioids (see Figure 19-1). The achievement of a statistically significant opioid-sparing

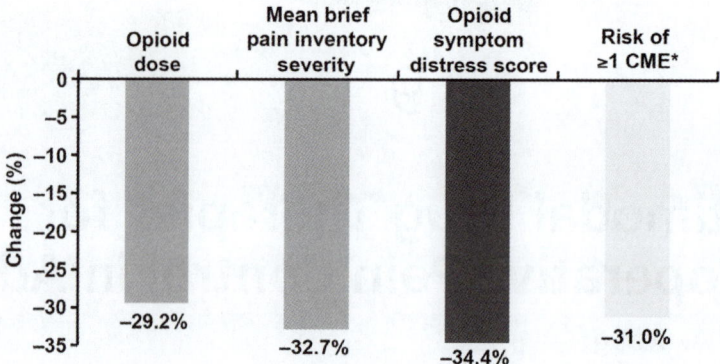

FIGURE 19-1 Effects of use of postoperative parecoxib/valdecoxib versus placebo on patient-controlled analgesia opioid consumption, pain intensity, and severity and numbers of adverse effects of opioids ($P < 0.01$ for all results). *CME, clinically meaningful effects. Calculated based on results of Ref. [11].

effect by itself would not be such an important treatment goal if there were no evidence that clinical opioid adverse effects, in particular nausea and vomiting [23], were significantly diminished [43]. In addition, opioid sparing might have further benefits, as there is increasing concern that exposure to opioid analgesics in the postoperative period carries potential risks of dependency, addiction, and abuse subsequently [8]; their increased postoperative use has been hypothesized to contribute to the current opioid epidemic in many countries, in particular, Canada, the United States, and Australia [15].

Looking at options for combining analgesics to achieve an additive or even synergistic effect, it is worthwhile to briefly discuss the pathophysiology of postoperative pain. Many of the earlier chapters in the present monograph explore multiple aspects of this pathophysiology; a detailed review has been recently published [31]. In principle, the initial nociceptive input from tissue injury caused by surgery is rapidly amplified by processes of a peripheral sensitization, mainly related to the inflammatory response to the initial injury. Subsequently central sensitization due to upregulation of spinal cord and brain nociceptive mechanisms develops in parallel to decreased inhibition. The result of combined peripheral and central sensitization is overall an amplification of the pain experience by a shift of the stimulus–response curve for pain to the left, leading to the development of hyperalgesia, as well as altered sensory processing resulting in allodynia. Counteracting peripheral sensitization by, for example, the use of anti-inflammatory medications or central sensitization by the use of centrally acting analgesics that reduce excitation (e.g., $\alpha 2\delta$ modulators or NMDA receptor antagonists) or increase inhibition (e.g., $\alpha 2$-agonists) will therefore partially reverse the sensitization processes and thereby reduce overall analgesic requirements. The reduction of sensitization by common analgesic drugs has been termed an "antihyperalgesic" action.

When looking at choices among analgesics, which work by different mechanisms or at various sites of action, it is worthwhile looking at the nociceptive pathways (see Figure 19-2). Here, options to interfere with transduction, i.e., the generation of action potentials by nociceptive neurons can be achieved with anti-inflammatory drugs and local anesthetics. The conduction or transmission of action potentials across the peripheral nervous system to the spinal cord can be reduced or even abolished by techniques of regional anesthesia at any point in this pathway including epidural analgesia acting at nerve roots before they enter the spinal cord. In the spinal cord, modulation of the nociceptive input can be influenced by opioids, nonsteroidal anti-inflammatory drugs (NSAIDs), N-methyl-D-aspartate

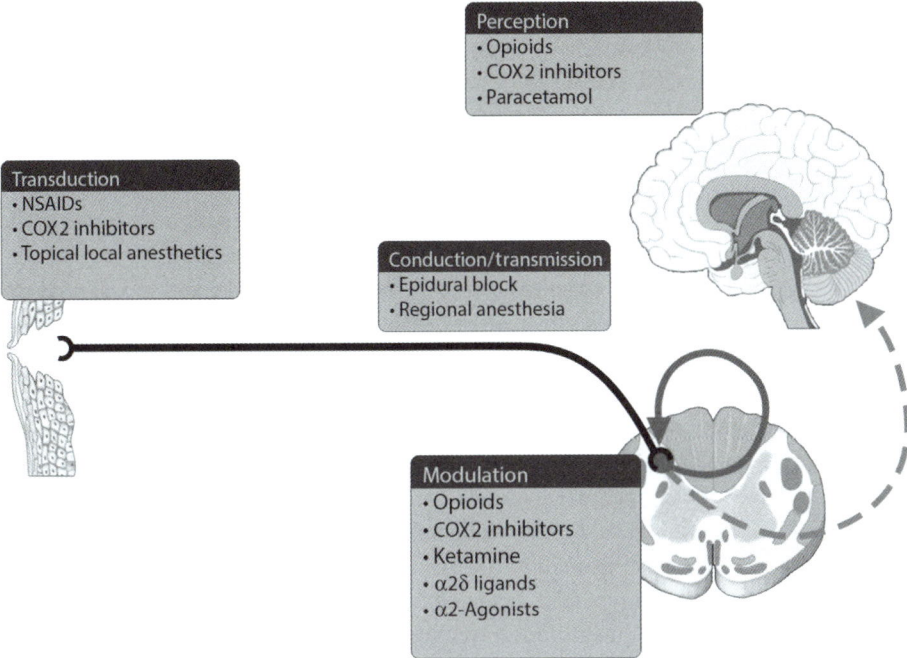

FIGURE 19-2 Sites of action of different medications along the pain pathway illustrating potential components of multimodal analgesia. NSAIDs, nonsteroidal anti-inflammatory drugs; COX2, cyclooxygenase 2.

(NMDA) receptor antagonists, α2δ ligands, and α2-agonists. Finally, perception of the pain in the brain is primarily influenced by opioids, although paracetamol and NSAIDs also have central sites of action.

SYSTEMIC MEDICATIONS AS COMPONENTS OF MULTIMODAL ANALGESIA

Nonopioid Analgesics

Nonopioid analgesics such as paracetamol, nonselective and COX2-selective NSAIDs, and dipyrone (metamizole) are important components of multimodal postoperative analgesia. With regard to efficacy, an excellent Cochrane review of the efficacy of these compounds given as a single dose in postoperative pain has been published [26]. Numbers needed to treat (NNTs) were 3.6 for 1000 mg of paracetamol, 1.5–2.5 for most selective and nonselective NSAIDs in appropriate therapeutic doses, and 1.6 for dipyrone (metamizole).

Paracetamol, as the weakest nonopioid analgesic, has an opioid-sparing effect when combined with opioids and only very limited effect on opioid side effects and is hence inferior in both respects to anti-inflammatory drugs and dipyrone [24]. However, the combination of paracetamol and NSAIDs is more effective than either compound alone [29]; such additive effects have been shown in particular for the combination of paracetamol and ibuprofen [2]. In addition, the perioperative administration of intravenous (IV) paracetamol significantly decreases postoperative nausea and vomiting (PONV) [1]. With regard to its adverse event profile, paracetamol shows a relatively benign effect in therapeutic doses [9].

Not surprisingly NSAIDs, which inhibit prostaglandin synthesis, thereby reducing peripheral sensitization, are superior to paracetamol in the postoperative setting [24]. The addition of NSAIDs to PCA with opioids results consistently in better analgesia, significant opioid sparing, and a reduced incidence of opioid side effects, in particular PONV. The efficacy of nonselective NSAIDs expressed as NNT is similar to those of COX2 selective agents in the perioperative period [26]. Use of the latter results in a significant reduction of adverse events, namely reduced gastrointestinal ulcers, reduced blood loss due to sparing of platelet function, and reduced bronchospasm in patients with NSAID-exacerbated respiratory disease [36]. Cardiovascular adverse events such as stroke and myocardial infarction are not increased by their short-term use [35], and lower-grade evidence suggests that there is also reduced risk of acute renal failure with COX2-selective compounds [20].

Dipyrone (metamizole) is a nonopioid analgesic that is not available in all countries. However, in countries where it is available such as Austria or Germany, guidelines recommend it as first-line treatment, and in Germany it is the most common nonopioid analgesic used for postoperative pain [30]. Its advantages are high efficacy comparable with NSAIDs [26] and a low rate of gastrointestinal, cardiovascular, or renal adverse effects [30]. The adverse effect of agranulocytosis is the reason that this drug is not registered in many countries, although repeated reviews and safety surveys suggest that this risk is extremely low, being orders of magnitude lower than the risks of adverse effects with NSAIDs [17].

Adjuvant Medications

The above account illustrates that nonopioid analgesics such as NSAIDs and related compounds are an essential component of successful multimodal analgesia. Moreover, research in the last two decades has shown that other types of medications initially used in other therapeutic areas are also useful in managing acute postoperative pain. Most of these adjuvant medications achieve their benefits by inhibiting central sensitization processes evoked by nociceptive input.

α2δ Ligands

Gabapentin and pregabalin are well-established medications for the treatment of neuropathic pain. Their effect is based on the reduction of intracellular calcium concentrations in nerve cells, thereby leading to a reduced release of excitatory amino acids, a major component of central sensitization. There is now good evidence that perioperative use of either of these agents improves analgesia at rest and with movement and reduces postoperative opioid consumption and diminishes PONV [25,39]. Contributing to the latter benefit may be an intrinsic antiemetic effect of gabapentin and pregabalin [14]. Most of the data suggest a beneficial effect in particular with a single preoperative dose lasting into the postoperative period, although data are also published on some studies have investigated extending their use into the postoperative period. In this context it is of note that sedation and visual disturbances are among the adverse effects of these compounds, in particular when extended into the postoperative period [25]. The increased risk for adverse drug effects illustrates that the attractiveness of multimodal analgesia must be tempered by the risk of additional adverse effects of coadministered drugs. Care must also be taken, as clinical observations indicate that these compounds, by their sedating actions, can increase the risk of opioid-induced respiratory depression [27].

There is no evidence for any other anticonvulsant medications to provide improved postoperative analgesia [36].

Antidepressants

Similar to α2δ ligands, antidepressants have an indication in neuropathic pain, here mainly because of augmenting activity in inhibitory nociceptive pathways. Although this inhibitory activity suggests a potential role in multimodal analgesia, the data are currently limited [36]. There is no evidence for an effect of tricyclic antidepressants, whereas there are some limited studies supporting serotonin and norepinephrine reuptake inhibitors (SNRIs) such as duloxetine and venlafaxine as potential components of multimodal analgesia.

NMDA Receptor Antagonists

The dissociative anesthetic ketamine has experienced a renaissance by its use in relatively low doses as an adjuvant in multimodal analgesia [16]. Ketamine is a noncompetitive antagonist at the NMDA receptor, thus offering a plausible rationale for an inhibitory effect on central sensitization. Perioperative low-dose IV ketamine has been shown to reduce opioid consumption, time to first request for postoperative analgesia, improved analgesia, and reduced PONV [22]. Its analgesic effect seems to be particularly pronounced in patients with severe pain, and therefore, it might have a role in major surgery such as thoracic, upper abdominal, and major orthopedic surgery. Another patient group in which ketamine could be particularly useful is patients with preexisting, opioid-induced tolerance or opioid-induced hyperalgesia [36]. A further potential indication is the treatment of acute neuropathic pain; this property may explain why ketamine is the only systemic drug with Level I evidence for a preventive effect on chronic postsurgical pain [6].

Magnesium, a functional NMDA receptor antagonist, has also been shown to have opioid-sparing effects and improves pain relief in the postoperative period [10].

α2-Agonists

Good evidence exists that administration of the α2-agonists clonidine or dexmedetomidine reduces postoperative pain intensity, as well as having an opioid-sparing effect and thereby reducing postoperative nausea [3]. The trade-off with the use of these substances as components of multimodal analgesia is again sedation, and also hypotension and bradycardia.

Systemic Local Anesthetics

After abdominal surgery, perioperative IV lidocaine infusions improve pain at rest and during movement, are opioid sparing, and reduce PONV as well as duration of ileus [38]. There is ongoing uncertainty about the optimal duration of such IV lidocaine infusions; most of the analyzed studies limit their use to the intraoperative and postanaesthesia care unit stay.

Corticosteroids

There is widespread perioperative use of corticosteroids, in particular dexamethasone, for the prevention of PONV. A meta-analysis showed that dexamethasone administration to surgical patients also reduces postoperative pain, opioid consumption, time to first analgesic request for rescue analgesia, and length of stay in the postanaesthesia care unit [41]. However, although these effects are statistically significant, they are small in magnitude. Perioperative corticosteroids might have additional benefits in the setting of enhanced recovery after surgery, as improvements in quality of recovery and decreased postoperative fatigue have been described [36].

There is no strong evidence to support the use of any other systemic adjuvants in the management of acute postoperative pain. This is in particular true for cannabinoids, which are currently so widely discussed in the setting of chronic and neuropathic pain [36].

REGIONAL ANALGESIC TECHNIQUES

The last 10 years have seen a dramatic increase in the use of regional anesthesia intraoperatively and the extension of these techniques by use of long-acting medications and adjuvants, or continuous catheter techniques into the postoperative period to provide analgesia [36]. This is in particular true for peripheral regional techniques, where developments of new blocks, ultrasound guidance, and availability of improved catheter technology have advanced this use significantly. Because the following chapter will survey regional analgesic techniques in depth, the present chapter will do so very briefly and focus on their integration within a multimodal regimen as opposed to primary use as sole agents.

Neuraxial Regional Analgesia

Epidural analgesia has been well known for many years to provide better pain relief than parenteral opioids [42]. In addition, the use of epidural analgesia has been shown to reduce the rate of a number of perioperative complications significantly, with particularly beneficial effects on pulmonary outcome, PONV, and improved bowel recovery [33]. These advantages have been shown in particular for open abdominal surgery and thoracic surgery. Without wanting to go into details in the context of this chapter, there has, at the same time, been an increasing concern about adverse effects of epidural analgesia, in particular in the context of increasing use of anticoagulants with extended duration of effect and the potential risk of epidural hematoma and neurologic compromise [36]. The use of epidural analgesia as a component of multimodal postoperative pain management requires, therefore, a careful benefit/risk analysis, although the advantages in multiple settings, in particular with regard to facilitation of enhanced recovery after major surgery, seem to be significant.

Intrathecal analgesia cannot be extended significantly into the postoperative period after the use of spinal microcatheters in this setting became controversial because of a significant risk of potential neurologic compromise. Intrathecal opioids, in particular morphine, have been shown to improve pain scores at rest and at movement for up to 24 hours with an opioid-sparing effect for up to 48 hours [32]. However, one has to realize that intrathecal opioid administration is still a form of opioid administration and typical opioid adverse effects such as nausea, vomiting, pruritus, and urinary retention will be increased. The increased risk of adverse effects may outweigh many benefits the opioid sparing accomplished by this technique. Last but not least, intrathecal morphine carries a potential risk of OIVI for extended duration after one injection, and therefore, safety procedures and monitoring guidelines need to be implemented to mitigate this effect.

Peripheral Regional Analgesia

As outlined earlier, the last 10 years have seen a dramatic increase in the use of peripheral regional analgesia for the treatment of postoperative pain.

This has been partially achieved by single injection peripheral nerve blocks with long-lasting local anesthetics such as bupivacaine, levobupivacaine, and ropivacaine and further extension of the duration of this effect by use of adjuvants to the local anesthetics, such as $\alpha 2$-agonists in the form of clonidine and dexmedetomidine and corticosteroids such as dexamethasone [36]. Extension of the duration of the block beyond 12 to 20 hours is, however, not achievable with single shot injections of currently available medications. There has been an increasing interest in the formulation of slow-release preparations for local anesthetics and in particular the development of bupivacaine encapsulated within liposomes. The currently available preparation for clinical use has been disappointing with regard to the duration of effect. Until recently it has only been officially registered for infiltration anesthesia, although trials with peripheral nerve blocks had been performed [36]. In the US, marketing approval for interscalene brachial plexus nerve block was granted in 2018.

The persisting unmet need for prolonged local anesthetic delivery explains the increasing interest in continuous peripheral nerve blocks by placement of a catheter adjacent to a peripheral nerve or plexus with repeated bolus administration or continuous infusion. These techniques improve analgesia, are opioid sparing, and reduce opioid-related adverse effects compared with systemic opioid analgesia [34]. Supportive data are published for many of the regional techniques, which are commonly used, as well as some interesting newer approaches such as paravertebral blocks and abdominal wall blocks [36]. These techniques have also been advanced due to the increasing use of ultrasound guidance in catheter insertion and the development of more advanced catheter technology and new infusion pumps with infusion protocols such as automated bolus dosing. On the other hand, recent recognition of toxicity of high concentrations of local anesthesia on articular chondrocytes has led to caution in adopting this technique for surgical procedures involving the joints.

CONCLUSION

The concept of multimodal analgesia is supported by strong recommendations based on high-quality evidence in most recent guidelines [7]. Although the preceding chapters in this volume suggest a large number of potential analgesic targets to be included in multimodal approach, it remains unclear which combinations of which compounds in which doses for which duration are best used in each circumstance. The answers to this question are difficult to obtain in view of the multiple combinations possible and the current lack of studies sufficient in quality and quantity, comparing different choices of multimodal analgesia. Most of the currently available literature looks at the addition of one component of multimodal analgesia to an opioid-based regimen and compares this to an opioid-only approach. Yet daily postoperative pain practice in most referral centers has moved beyond unimodal opioid therapy. The situation is further complicated by the fact that many relevant outcomes are procedure-specific. Although procedure-specific evidence-based guidelines have been published (www.postoppain.org), the lack of suitable background data reduces their usefulness and applicability. A limited number of studies have shown that combinations of more than two components of multimodal analgesia can be shown to have superiority over exclusive systemic opioid analgesia. These studies are not designed to answer the question as to which components of the multimodal approach are most important to the success of this approach. On the other hand, other trials have found that adding too many modalities to a multimodal approach may not necessarily always be beneficial.

Overall progress in the development of multimodal analgesia has led to the idea of opioid-free analgesia [5]. This has been seen to be of particular value in the setting of bariatric, i.e., obesity surgery in view of the significant respiratory risk associated with opioid analgesia in obese patients, who often have accompanying sleep-disordered breathing [37]. There are only limited data so far in the published literature, which show that it is possible to reduce opioid use to minimal amounts; this has been mainly demonstrated in case series with sometimes impressive results [21].

Future research efforts should aim to identify useful multimodal analgesic strategies, in a procedure-specific context, and compare different multimodal strategies for the same procedure.

PRACTICAL CLINICAL IMPLICATIONS

Currently available evidence on multimodal analgesia suggests that postoperative pain relief can be optimized and adverse effects of opioids reduced by adhering to the following three principles:

- Minimize use of systemic opioids
- Maximize the use of systemic nonopioids and adjuvants
- Use regional analgesic techniques whenever possible

With regard to the practical application of multimodal analgesia, it is therefore important to consider if a specific operation is amenable to regional analgesic techniques, including wound infiltration, local infiltration anesthesia into deeper tissues, wound catheters, single injection peripheral blocks with long-lasting local anesthetics and possibly adjuvants, and continuous regional analgesia catheter techniques or neuraxial techniques, i.e., epidural analgesia. With regard to systemic medications, it seems to make sense to currently recommend a single preoperative dose of pregabalin, at least before major surgery, and use of regular paracetamol in every patient and regular COX2-selective NSAIDs in all patients who lack renal contraindications. This should be carried out in combination with opioids on demand, either by parenteral PCA techniques or oral on-demand analgesia. In addition, systemic local anesthetics by perioperative infusion should be considered in major surgery, in particular if regional or neuraxial techniques are not used. There should be a low threshold for the additional initiation of a low-dose ketamine infusion when the aforementioned approaches provide insufficient analgesia and in particular in patients with preexisting opioid tolerance or acute neuropathic pain. Analgesia can be further improved by the opioid-sparing use of α2-agonists in particular in patients with withdrawal symptoms and agitation.

REFERENCES

1. Apfel CC, Turan A, Souza K, Pergolizzi J, Hornuss C. Intravenous acetaminophen reduces postoperative nausea and vomiting: a systematic review and meta-analysis. Pain 2013;154(5):677–89.
2. Bailey E, Worthington HV, van Wijk A, Yates JM, Coulthard P, Afzal Z. Ibuprofen and/or paracetamol (acetaminophen) for pain relief after surgical removal of lower wisdom teeth. Cochrane Database Syst Rev 2013;12:CD004624.
3. Blaudszun G, Lysakowski C, Elia N, Tramer MR. Effect of perioperative systemic alpha2 agonists on postoperative morphine consumption and pain intensity: systematic review and meta-analysis of randomized controlled trials. Anesthesiology 2012;116(6):1312–22.

4. Buvanendran A, Kroin JS. Multimodal analgesia for controlling acute postoperative pain. Curr Opin Anaesthesiol 2009;22(5):588–93.
5. Chaparro LE, Smith SA, Moore RA, Wiffen PJ, Gilron I. Pharmacotherapy for the prevention of chronic pain after surgery in adults. Cochrane Database Syst Rev 2013;7:CD008307.
6. Carr DB, Cohen RI. "Are perioperative opioids obsolete?" Proceedings of an IASP Acute Pain Special Interest Group Satellite Symposium September 25, 2016 Yokohama, Japan. PAIN Rep 2017;2(4):e604. doi:10.1097/PR9.0000000000000604.
7. Chou R, Gordon DB, de Leon-Casasola OA, Rosenberg JM, Bickler S, Brennan T, Carter T, Cassidy CL, Chittenden EH, Degenhardt E, Griffith S, Manworren R, McCarberg B, Montgomery R, Murphy J, Perkal MF, Suresh S, Sluka K, Strassels S, Thirlby R, Viscusi E, Walco GA, Warner L, Weisman SJ, Wu CL. Management of postoperative pain: a clinical practice guideline from the American Pain Society, the American Society of Regional Anesthesia and Pain Medicine, and the American Society of Anesthesiologists' Committee on Regional Anesthesia, Executive Committee, and Administrative Council. J Pain 2016;17(2):131–57.
8. Clarke H, Soneji N, Ko DT, Yun L, Wijeysundera DN. Rates and risk factors for prolonged opioid use after major surgery: population based cohort study. BMJ 2014;348:g1251.
9. Dart RC, Bailey E. Does therapeutic use of acetaminophen cause acute liver failure? Pharmacotherapy 2007;27(9):1219–30.
10. De Oliveira Jr GS, Castro-Alves LJ, Khan JH, McCarthy RJ. Perioperative systemic magnesium to minimize postoperative pain: a meta-analysis of randomized controlled trials. Anesthesiology 2013;119(1):178–90.
11. Gan TJ, Joshi GP, Zhao SZ, Hanna DB, Cheung RY, Chen C. Presurgical intravenous parecoxib sodium and follow-up oral valdecoxib for pain management after laparoscopic cholecystectomy surgery reduces opioid requirements and opioid-related adverse effects. Acta Anaesthesiol Scand 2004;48(9):1194–207.
12. Gerbershagen HJ, Aduckathil S, van Wijck AJ, Peelen LM, Kalkman CJ, Meissner W. Pain intensity on the first day after surgery: a prospective cohort study comparing 179 surgical procedures. Anesthesiology 2013;118(4):934–44.
13. Gritsenko K, Khelemsky Y, Kaye AD, Vadivelu N, Urman RD. Multimodal therapy in perioperative analgesia. Best Pract Res Clin Anaesthesiol 2014;28(1):59–79.
14. Guttuso Jr T. Gabapentin's anti-nausea and anti-emetic effects: a review. Exp Brain Res 2014;232(8):2535–9.
15. Häuser W, Schug S, Furlan AD. The opioid epidemic and national guidelines for opioid therapy for chronic noncancer pain: a perspective from different continents. Pain Rep 2017;2(3):e599.
16. Hocking G, Visser EJ, Schug SA. Ketamine: does life begin at 40? Pain Clin Updates (IASP) 2007;15(3):1–6.
17. Ibanez L, Vidal X, Ballarin E, Laporte JR. Agranulocytosis associated with dipyrone (metamizol). Eur J Clin Pharmacol 2005;60(11):821–9.
18. Kehlet H. Surgical stress: the role of pain and analgesia. Br J Anaesth 1989;63(2):189–95.
19. Kehlet H, Dahl JB. The value of "multimodal" or "balanced analgesia" in postoperative pain treatment. Anesth Analg 1993;77(5):1048–56.
20. Lafrance JP, Miller DR. Selective and non-selective non-steroidal anti-inflammatory drugs and the risk of acute kidney injury. Pharmacoepidemiol Drug Saf 2009;18(10):923–31.
21. Lam KK, Mui WL. Multimodal analgesia model to achieve low postoperative opioid requirement following bariatric surgery. Hong Kong Med J 2016;22(5):428–34.
22. Laskowski K, Stirling A, McKay WP, Lim HJ. A systematic review of intravenous ketamine for postoperative analgesia. Can J Anaesth 2011;58(10):911–23.
23. Marret E, Kurdi O, Zufferey P, Bonnet F. Effects of nonsteroidal antiinflammatory drugs on patient-controlled analgesia morphine side effects: meta-analysis of randomized controlled trials. Anesthesiology 2005;102(6):1249–60.
24. Maund E, McDaid C, Rice S, Wright K, Jenkins B, Woolacott N. Paracetamol and selective and non-selective non-steroidal anti-inflammatory drugs for the reduction in morphine-related side-effects after major surgery: a systematic review. Br J Anaesth 2011;106(3):292–7.
25. Mishriky BM, Waldron NH, Habib AS. Impact of pregabalin on acute and persistent postoperative pain: a systematic review and meta-analysis. Br J Anaesth 2015;114(1):10–31.
26. Moore RA, Derry S, McQuay HJ, Wiffen PJ. Single dose oral analgesics for acute postoperative pain in adults. Cochrane Database Syst Rev 2011;9:CD008659.
27. Myhre M, Diep LM, Stubhaug A. Pregabalin has analgesic, ventilatory, and cognitive effects in combination with remifentanil. Anesthesiology 2016;124(1):141–9.
28. Oderda GM, Evans RS, Lloyd J, Lipman A, Chen C, Ashburn M, Burke J, Samore M. Cost of opioid-related adverse drug events in surgical patients. J Pain Symptom Manage 2003;25(3):276–83.

29. Ong CK, Seymour RA, Lirk P, Merry AF. Combining paracetamol (acetaminophen) with nonsteroidal anti-inflammatory drugs: a qualitative systematic review of analgesic efficacy for acute postoperative pain. Anesth Analg 2010;110(4):1170-9.
30. Pogatzki-Zahn E, Chandrasena C, Schug SA. Nonopioid analgesics for postoperative pain management. Curr Opin Anaesthesiol 2014;27(5):513-9.
31. Pogatzki-Zahn EM, Segelcke D, Schug SA. Postoperative pain—from mechanisms to treatment. Pain Rep 2017;2(2):e588.
32. Popping D, Elia N, Marret E, et al. Opioids added to local anesthetics for single-shot intrathecal anesthesia in patients undergoing minor surgery: a met-analysis of randomised trials. Pain 2012;153:784-93.
33. Popping DM, Elia N, Van Aken HK, Marret E, Schug SA, Kranke P, Wenk M, Tramer MR. Impact of epidural analgesia on mortality and morbidity after surgery: systematic review and meta-analysis of randomized controlled trials. Ann Surg 2014;259(6):1056-67.
34. Richman JM, Liu SS, Courpas G, Wong R, Rowlingson AJ, McGready J, Cohen SR, Wu CL. Does continuous peripheral nerve block provide superior pain control to opioids? A meta-analysis. Anesth Analg 2006;102(1):248-57.
35. Schug SA, Joshi GP, Camu F, Pan S, Cheung R. Cardiovascular safety of the cyclooxygenase-2 selective inhibitors parecoxib and valdecoxib in the postoperative setting: an analysis of integrated data. Anesth Analg 2009;108(1):299-307.
36. Schug SA, Palmer GM, Scott DA, Halliwell R, Trinca J. Acute pain management: scientific evidence. Melbourne: ANZCA & FPM; 2015.
37. Schug SA, Raymann A. Postoperative pain management of the obese patient. Best Pract Res Clin Anaesthesiol 2011;25(1):73-81.
38. Sun Y, Li T, Wang N, Yun Y, Gan TJ. Perioperative systemic lidocaine for postoperative analgesia and recovery after abdominal surgery: a meta-analysis of randomized controlled trials. Dis Colon Rectum 2012;55(11):1183-94.
39. Tiippana EM, Hamunen K, Kontinen VK, Kalso E. Do surgical patients benefit from perioperative gabapentin/pregabalin? A systematic review of efficacy and safety. Anesth Analg 2007;104(6):1545-56 [table of contents].
40. Vila Jr H, Smith RA, Augustyniak MJ, Nagi PA, Soto RG, Ross TW, Cantor AB, Strickland JM, Miguel RV. The efficacy and safety of pain management before and after implementation of hospital-wide pain management standards: is patient safety compromised by treatment based solely on numerical pain ratings? Anesth Analg 2005;101(2):474-80 [table of contents].
41. Waldron NH, Jones CA, Gan TJ, Allen TK, Habib AS. Impact of perioperative dexamethasone on postoperative analgesia and side-effects: systematic review and meta-analysis. Br J Anaesth 2013;110(2):191-200.
42. Wu CL, Cohen SR, Richman JM, Rowlingson AJ, Courpas GE, Cheung K, Lin EE, Liu SS. Efficacy of postoperative patient-controlled and continuous infusion epidural analgesia versus intravenous patient-controlled analgesia with opioids: a meta-analysis. Anesthesiology 2005;103(5):1079-88 [quiz 1109-010].
43. Zhao SZ, Chung F, Hanna DB, Raymundo AL, Cheung RY, Chen C. Dose-response relationship between opioid use and adverse effects after ambulatory surgery. J Pain Symptom Manage 2004;28(1):35-46.

CHAPTER 20

Regional Anesthesia and Analgesia for Postoperative Pain Control in Adults

Dermot P. Maher and Jacques E. Chelly

Regional anesthesia (RA) usually refers to neuraxial blocks or peripheral nerve blocks (PNBs) and field blocks, alone or in combination. In this chapter, the focus will be on PNBs and field blocks; the prior chapter has briefly surveyed key issues related to neuraxial blocks, e.g., anticoagulant use. The importance of RA is best illustrated in that RA and acute pain medicine have jointly evolved as an independent subspecialty of anesthesiology with an accredited clinical training fellowship and medical licensing board recognition in the United States. Evidence supports that the use of RA is associated with improved outcomes, including physiologic and financial, compared with general anesthesia (GA).

From 1994 to 2014, total surgical volumes in America increased approximately 114%, mostly because of growth in the number of outpatient surgical procedures, whereas the average length of stay (LOS) in the hospital decreased from 6.7 to 5.5 days [6]. The trend toward outpatient surgery can be attributed to many factors including increasing reliance on minimally invasive surgical techniques and increased use of RA for intraoperative analgesia and/or perioperative pain control. RA reduces many of the side effects commonly associated with GA and/or opioids.

BENEFITS OF REGIONAL ANESTHESIA

Overall Mortality

The use of epidurals in patients with multiple rib fractures (but not hip fractures) has been shown to reduce overall mortality [31,43,89]. Additionally, there is no clear evidence to support that PNBs and/or field blocks reduce overall mortality.

Cardiovascular Dysfunction

Although largely dependent on the patient's preoperative cardiac status, the risk of perioperative cardiovascular events is influenced by the effectiveness of pain control [68]. The use of epidurals has been associated with fewer cardiovascular events compared with GA [54,68]. Decreased postoperative bleeding, with potentially reduced blood transfusion requirements, has been reported with the use of continuous femoral blocks following total knee replacement [19].

Cognitive Dysfunction and Neurologic Outcomes

The use of RA minimizes the need for GA. Meta-analyses comparing RA with GA have failed to demonstrate that RA is associated with a lower incidence of postoperative cognitive dysfunction (POCD) [23,53,64]. Age appears to be a more predictive risk factor [59]. However, it is important to recognize that POCD is often poorly defined. For example, an "RA cohort" may actually have received a combination of RA and GA [69].

The incidence of cerebrovascular accidents (CVAs) is equivalent between RA and GA following noncardiac and nonvascular surgery [30,31]. The incidence of a CVA or death in the first 30 days following a carotid endarterectomy is equivalent for subjects receiving GA or RA in the form of a superficial and/or deep cervical plexus block.

The use of continuous lumbar plexus for hip surgery has been associated with a reduction of opioid-related cognitive effects [52].

Pulmonary Dysfunction

The use of RA decreases the need for deep sedation, airway instrumentation with endotracheal intubation or a laryngeal mask airway, and control of ventilation. This simplification can be beneficial in managing patients with preexisting pulmonary disease including chronic obstructive pulmonary disease (COPD). RA decreases the incidence of postoperative unplanned intubation, pneumonia, and the need for prolonged mechanical ventilation [34]. However, in otherwise healthy subjects undergoing hip fracture surgery, the incidence of postoperative pneumonia or other respiratory complications is comparable between RA and GA [31]. In patients undergoing a thoracotomy or upper abdominal surgery, the use of truncal RA, including paravertebral blocks and intercostal nerve blocks, is associated with decreased pain and improved postoperative pulmonary mechanics [9,29,45].

Functional Outcomes

Following shoulder surgery, a single shot interscalene block is associated with decrease in pain with or without motion for the first 6 and 8 hours, respectively [1]. Compared with GA, the use of properly titrated RA allows earlier mobilization, functional recovery, and discharge from the hospital following either a total knee arthroplasty (TKA) or total hip arthroplasty (THA) [15,35,49].

Immunologic Outcomes

Surgical stress and opioid analgesics have the potential to decrease cell-mediated immune function in the perioperative period [16]. The use of PNBs has not been found to be associated with a lower rate of surgical site infections following a THA or TKA surgery in part because of impractically large study sample size requirements to detect changes in a low-incidence event [47]. However, preclinical and pilot clinical evidence suggests a possible benefit of RA over GA with regard to decreased recurrence of cancer [25,51]. Prospective studies are ongoing to confirm these findings and, if positive, establish a possible mechanism [71].

Opioid Analgesic Use

The use of femoral nerve blocks for TKA, lumbar plexus block for THA, and pelvic fracture and interscalene blocks for shoulder surgery has been shown to decrease opioid consumption

[1,15,65] and a reduction in opioid side effects such as nausea, vomiting, pruritus, and sedation along with superior analgesia compared to opioids alone [70]. The opioid-sparing effect of RA is a major benefit because it is now established that 15% to 20% of surgical patients receiving opioids for the treatment of perioperative pain develop chronic opioid use [44,78].

Economic Outcomes/Time to Discharge

The use of RA is associated with more rapid time to discharge after surgery in both ambulatory and hospital settings. In the ambulatory setting, the use of interscalene blocks for rotator cuff repair was associated with more frequent bypassing of stays in the postanesthesia care unit (PACU) and earlier (mean 2.5 hours) discharge compared with GA [32,85]. The use of a minimally invasive surgical approach combined with RA, including continuous lumbar plexus block, for TKA has allowed major joint replacement to be performed as an outpatient procedure [57]. The cost savings associated with this approach offset those of providing an acute pain service to optimize clinical analgesic management [79]. In the absence of defined reimbursement schedules for such services, however, it is difficult to determine their future in the context of "bundled reimbursement" in which a single lump sum is provided to the institution to cover all expenses related to the inpatient stay and follow-up of patients undergoing major joint replacement.

Patient Satisfaction

Patients report greater satisfaction with their care in the setting of PNBs compared with patient-controlled analgesia delivering an opioid [15]. Nonrandomized trials suggest that patient satisfaction is very high among patients who receive PNBs [42,50]. In the outpatient setting, the use of interscalene blocks was associated with greater patient satisfaction compared with GA [32]. It is unclear whether this increase in patient satisfaction is due to a reduction in opioid-related side effects, denser analgesia, or another described benefit of PNBs.

Enhanced Recovery After Surgery (ERAS)

Enhanced recovery after surgery (ERAS) represents a multifaceted approach to optimize surgical outcome [56]. The present recommendations include RA, particularly epidurals when feasible, to facilitate recovery after surgery [74]. Further research is needed to evaluate the benefits of PNBs and field blocks in this context.

INDICATIONS FOR REGIONAL ANESTHESIA

RA may be indicated for both surgical anesthesia and/or postoperative analgesia in hospitalized and ambulatory patients. Although spinals and epidurals are mostly indicated for anesthesia for thoracic, lower extremity and lower abdominal, and pelvic (including obstetric) procedures, the use of PNBs techniques is becoming more extensively practiced for abdominal and thoracic surgery. PNBs have been advocated for dental, neck, and breast surgery, upper and lower extremity surgery, and pelvic and selective urology procedures, especially in frail or unstable patients in whom systemic anesthesia should be minimized. Analysis of surgical and insurance databases suggests that even for procedures which would be highly amenable to RA, such as major joint replacement, PNBs are used only in a minority of appropriate indications [21]. However, data suggest that the use of PNBs for THA and TKA is increasing, along with a simultaneous decrease in neuraxial techniques [22,58].

RA has been shown to decrease postoperative nausea and vomiting (PONV), allow bypassing the phase I recovery unit, and facilitate rapid discharge from the hospital [60,76]. Beyond orthopedic surgery, RA has been successfully used in thoracic, gynecologic, and general surgical inpatient and outpatient procedures [5,7,63].

The use of RA is gaining momentum in the context of trauma in the emergency department and military scenarios [13,14]. In many emergency department and trauma scenarios, hemodynamic stability and continuous mentation assessment afforded by RA are optimal for patient care [27]. Concerns regarding potential masking of the signs and symptoms of a progressing compartment syndrome are not warranted based on current evidence.

In the past few years, an increased number of field blocks have been introduced including the transversus abdominis plane (TAP), rectus sheath block, quadratus lumborum, adductor canal, and (pectoral) serratus anterior block. The practical daily use of these blocks has been greatly facilitated by ultrasound imaging. These field blocks are based on the use of large volume and concentrated solutions because, in contrast to peripheral nerve blockade techniques, the performance of field blocks does not require the visualization of a tiny, threadlike nerve or plexus but rather planes separating large muscles.

The use of neuraxial anesthesia in the management of obstetric patients is the *sine qua non* in developed countries. The use of TAP blocks in patients with contraindications to neuraxial opioids has been demonstrated to provide excellent analgesia [2]. The use of PNBs for nongynecologic procedures during pregnancy is believed to be safe.

CONTRAINDICATIONS TO REGIONAL ANESTHESIA

Most contraindications for PNBs are relative and may include factors such as a lack of patient cooperation. Bleeding disorders and thrombolytic therapy increase the risk of major bleeding and nerve compression following PNBs, especially in continuous techniques. The use of indwelling catheters is contraindicated in the setting of active bacteremia.

LOCAL ANESTHETIC SYSTEMIC TOXICITY (LAST) AND ASSOCIATED COMPLICATIONS

The performance of an interscalene block has been associated with inadvertent intrathecal injection and with a rare but devastating spinal cord compression syndrome [10].

Local anesthetic systemic toxicity (LAST) is the result of supratherapeutic concentration of local anesthetics. The most concerning manifestations of LAST affect cardiac and central nervous system (CNS) [81]. In most cases, the development of LAST is a function of the dose at which the local anesthetic is administered, the rate of administration, the site-specific vascular uptake, and the rate of local anesthetic metabolism and excretion. In some cases, LAST results from direct intravascular injection of local anesthetic.

The CNS manifestations of LAST are concentration-dependent [75]. At low serum local anesthetic concentrations, predominant features include restlessness, disorientation, and depression. Neurologic symptoms associated with relatively low concentrations of local anesthetics are treated with the administration of benzodiazepines to prevent the development of seizures. At higher systemic concentrations of local anesthetics, tonic–clonic seizures may develop and require supportive therapeutic treatment. Acidosis resulting from the seizure may further exacerbate local anesthetic toxicity, causing decreased clearance of offending local anesthetic from neural tissue. Finally, very high levels of local anesthetics may produce CNS depression, respiratory arrest, and coma.

The cardiovascular manifestations of LAST include a dose-dependent decrease in myocardial contractility, cardiac conduction rate, and electrical excitability [55]. LAST manifests clinically as bradycardia, decreased cardiac output, and systemic hypotension. Possible ECG changes are QT prolongation, QRS prolongation, and arrhythmias including ventricular fibrillation. Local anesthetics also could decrease the function of cardiac pacemaker cells, resulting in bradyrhythmias. The development of cardiac manifestations of LAST is believed to be frequently, but not always, preceded by CNS symptoms. Treatment of cardiac manifestations of LAST is supportive and may include temporary mechanical cardiopulmonary bypass. As sympathomimetic rescue medications may be proarrhythmic, support of blood pressure with epinephrine should only be done with close monitoring, strict limitation of dose (less than 1 μg/kg of epinephrine), and readiness to defibrillate and manage deteriorating cardiac arrhythmias.

The treatment of LAST is similar to other advanced cardiac life support (ACLS) protocols with several important differences [86]. In addition to a reduced dose of epinephrine, the use of vasopressin, calcium channel blockers, and β-blockers is contraindicated. Seizure prophylaxis should be instituted early in suspected cases of LAST. Alerting a cardiopulmonary bypass team of the situation is also prudent in case of severe deterioration of cardiac function. The development of intralipid has been instrumental in the resuscitation of patients with LAST. A bolus of 1.5 mL/kg should be administered over 1 minute. Additional boluses may also be administered if the patient has persistent cardiovascular colipase. The initial bolus should be followed by continuous infusion of 0.25 mL/kg per minute, which can be doubled if the patient remains hypotensive. The infusion should continue for at least 10 minutes after adequate circulatory stability is maintained. The maximum dose of intralipid that can be administered in a 30 minutes period is 10 mL/kg. ACLS protocols should be continued during the intralipid infusion.

Peripheral nerve injury (PNI) is most often associated with transient neurologic symptoms that manifest in the days to weeks following either RA or GA. The pathogenesis of PNI is multifactorial and may include direct nerve trauma, localized alterations in blood flow, direct local anesthetic neurotoxicity, patient factors, and surgical factors [82]. Direct needle trauma to a nerve or the elicitation of paresthesias is neither necessary nor sufficient to cause PNI [37,62]. Acquired neuropathies may predispose subjects to PNI from nerve trauma [40].

COMPLICATIONS OF SPECIFIC BLOCKS

Following interscalene and, less frequently, supraclavicular blocks, a hemidiaphragmatic paresis (HDP) is routinely observed as a consequence of the normal anatomical coursing of the phrenic nerve through the anesthetized area. HDP is characterized by dyspnea and a lack of inspiratory effort due to blockade of the phrenic nerve [24]. It is especially troublesome in patients with preexisting pulmonary disease [61,62]. The incidence of HDP following an interscalene block is 100%, 34% following a supraclavicular block, and only 3% in infraclavicular blocks [66].

Pneumothorax is another important cause of dyspnea that can be due to passage of a needle through the pleura allowing air into the thoracic cavity. The incidence of a pneumothorax following an upper extremity block is believed to be approximately 1 in 1000 and has been observed following interscalene, supraclavicular, or infraclavicular blocks [3].

Major bleeding, including retroperitoneal hematoma, and vascular compression have been reported with the use of various PNBs including sciatic, lumbar plexus, and femoral nerve blocks and axillary block. Major risk factors include trauma caused by the needle during the performance of the block and coagulopathy.

USE OF ADDITIVES

Supplementation of local anesthetic solutions has been advocated to prolong the duration of single injection RA techniques. Sodium bicarbonate and epinephrine are two long-standing examples. The latter has been shown to prolong the duration of upper extremity blocks but to have no benefit on lower extremity blocks. Epinephrine's effects also depend on the type of local anesthetic solution used. It prolongs the analgesia observed when epinephrine is added to short-acting but not long-acting local anesthetics [46]. Epinephrine, being a vasoconstrictor, is believed to delay the absorption and systemic redistribution of local anesthetics [8,84]. The addition of sodium bicarbonate raises the percent of free-base local anesthetic, resulting in shortened latency, increased intensity, and prolonged analgesic duration [39]. While sodium bicarbonate does not appear to increase the toxicity of local anesthetics, clinically meaningful gains in the performance of local anesthetics are seldom realized.

Recently, other additives such as buprenorphine, steroids, and $\alpha 2$-adrenergic agonists (clonidine and dexmedetomidine) have been advocated for use alone and/or in combination. All of these medications prolong both the afferent sensory and efferent motor blocks. It is unclear whether perineural administration will result in more pronounced analgesic effects compared with systemic administration. A meta-analysis examined clonidine doses between 30 and 300 μg and found a prolongation of PNBs by an average of 122 minutes [67]. Clonidine has been noted to cause sedation, bradycardia, orthostatic hypotension, and fainting [67]. Similar data have been reported in a meta-analysis of 32 studies regarding the addition of 50 to 60 μg of dexmedetomidine [83]. Because peripheral opioid receptors have been identified, the addition of 0.1 to 0.3 mg of buprenorphine to local anesthetic solutions prolongs the duration of PNBs by approximately 8 hours, but it is associated with an increased incidence of PONV [73]. Two meta-analyses of 12 and 29 studies have examined the soluble corticosteroid dexamethasone and found that 4 to 10 mg administered with local anesthetic was associated with an average increase in PNB analgesic duration of 233 to 431 minutes with greater prolongation observed when combined with long-lasting local anesthetics (e.g., bupivacaine, ropivacaine) [4,38]. The effects of perineural steroid on PONV are not as clear [38].

Although many local anesthetics have been developed, most PNBs are performed using either lidocaine or mepivacaine for shorter duration blocks and either bupivacaine, ropivacaine, or levobupivacaine for longer duration blockade. Although interesting, the widespread use of the rapid-onset local anesthetic chloroprocaine remains uncommon. Combination of shorter- and longer-lasting local anesthetics, although studied, is a practice that seems to be less and less advocated. With respect to the pharmacology of local anesthetics, it is important to recognize that the duration of blocks has been found to be age-dependent; shorter in young adults than that in the elderly.

In late 2011, liposomal bupivacaine was introduced to prolong the duration of action of bupivacaine. At this point, the solution is approved for field blocks including TAP but only very recently (2018 in the US) for interscalene block alone among PNBs. Additional data are required to establish the short- and long-term benefits of such the formulation, especially because of the high cost of acquisition [33,40]. Thus, some controversy still exists about the cost to benefit ratio of liposomal bupivacaine versus bupivacaine.

The dose, volume, and concentration of local anesthetics administered for RA depend on the indication (anesthesia vs. analgesia), the need to preserve motor function, the relative toxicity of the medication, the mode of administration (single vs. continuous), the technique (neuraxial vs. peripheral nerve blockade vs. field blocks), and the use of additives. Surgical anesthesia with PNBs requires higher volumes and concentrations compared with perioperative pain control. In the case of a continuous infusion, it is important to consider the need for the preservation of motor function when choosing the rate and concentration. Thus, a rate of 3 mL per hour of 0.1% of ropivacaine is indicated for a continuous sciatic block following TKA. In contrast, 0.2% ropivacaine at a rate of 8 to 10 mL per hour may be required in the case of continuous paravertebral block following multiple rib fractures.

Increased volume and concentration characterize the use of local anesthetics in field blocks when compared with peripheral nerve blockade and continuous anesthetic infusions.

SINGLE INJECTION VERSUS CONTINUOUS PERIPHERAL NERVE BLOCK CATHETERS

Continuous peripheral nerve block catheters (CPNBCs) are indicated if postoperative pain is anticipated for at least 24 hours [41]. Catheters have been used in inpatient and outpatient settings and in pediatric populations with relatively few complications. Compared with single injection PNBs, the use of CPNBCs is associated with prolonged pain control, decreased postoperative opioid analgesic requirements, decreased PONV, and greater patient satisfaction [11]. Evidence for the use of CPNBC is limited to the treatment of cancer-related pain, complex regional pain syndrome, ulcer-derived pain, phantom limb pain, and pain requiring treatment with intercostal or paravertebral blocks [41].

CPNBCs use a catheter inserted proximal to a target nerve or plexus and can be used to apply local anesthetics and adjuvants continuously or on an as needed basis [41]. This is in contrast to wound infusion catheters placed directly into a surgical incision. Evidence suggests optimal placement can be achieved with ultrasound guidance using the "in plane" approach [18]. Catheters may then be fixed in place using adhesives or using a subcutaneous tunneling technique. The total dose of the infused local anesthetic, rather than either the volume or concentration, is the primary determinant of the degree of analgesia afforded by CPNBCs. The use of adjuvants, including epinephrine and opioids, in catheter solutions to improve analgesic outcomes is not conclusively supported by existing literature. There is also a paucity of literature to suggest optimal basal rates, bolus volumes, or lockout periods [17,18,41].

The complication rate of CPNBCs is believed to be comparable with that of single-shot PNBs [72]. The most common complications resulting in block failure are leaking displacement of the catheter away from the intended neural target, which occurs in approximately 30% of cases. The displacement of the catheter can be greatly reduced by the optimal fixation technique including subcutaneous tunneling, adhesive tape, and liquid adhesives [12,20,80].

The most troubling complication is postoperative neurologic symptoms (PONS), which could be multifactorial and attributed to the surgery itself, positioning, or use of tourniquets. The reported incidence of PONS after several months following CPNBC placement ranges from 0% to 1.9% [41]. Other serious complications, such as catheter infections, abscesses, or fulminant septicemia, are rare even when catheters are used in the ambulatory setting [18,41]. Although catheter complications are relatively common, clinically relevant sequelae are rare. There is concern that the use of CPNBCs may predispose patients to a greater risk of postoperative falls, especially when used for lower extremity pain control.

PERIPHERAL NERVE BLOCKS VERSUS EPIDURAL ANALGESIA

PNBs have been compared with epidural anesthesia for the treatment of intraoperative and postoperative THA, TKA, and thoracic surgery [26,28,88]. Analgesia has proven similar between the two regimens. However, motor blockade was greater in the PNB group, and side effects were more frequent in the epidural group, such as hypotension, urinary retention, and PONV [28,88]. Postoperative opioid consumption appears to be equivalent between PNBs versus epidurals [26].

TRANSITION FROM ACUTE TO CHRONIC PAIN

Chronic postsurgical pain (CPSP) is pain that lasts beyond the expected period of tissue inflammation and healing [87]. The pathogenesis, clinical features, and CPSP are described in multiple chapters of the present volume. Perioperative pain intensity has not uniformly been identified as a risk factor for the development of CPSP [77]. To date, the use of neither PNBs nor epidural anesthesia has reliably demonstrated an ability to decrease the incidence of CPSP [87,36].

The safe use of PNBs in patients with preexisting neurologic disease has not been definitively established but is believed to be safe in the setting of hereditary neuropathies including Charcot–Marie–Tooth disease and CNS disorders such as multiple sclerosis, postpolio syndrome, and amyotrophic lateral sclerosis [48]. PNBs are contraindicated in acquired neuropathies, such as diabetic peripheral neuropathy and chemotherapy-induced neuropathy, and inflammatory neuropathies, such as Guillain–Barre syndrome and postsurgical inflammatory neuropathy [48].

CONCLUSIONS AND FUTURE DIRECTIONS

The treatment of pain after surgery continues to evolve and develop, facilitating the performance of a growing list of surgical procedures accomplished increasingly in outpatients. The benefits of PNBs with regard to pain and physiology are numerous but must be balanced against the risks associated with these practices. The field continues to refine existing technology and incorporate new advances in ultrasound imaging, nonpharmacologic cryo- and thermoablative therapies, and the use of novel local anesthetics and other medications, including new formulations of existing agents. Training is becoming formalized and guided by national and international professional society standards. In appropriately selected patients, the use of PNBs may confer benefits not possible with GA, allowing for improve the patient experience and outcomes after surgery.

REFERENCES

1. Abdallah FW, Halpern SH, Aoyama K, Brull R. Will the real benefits of single-shot interscalene block please stand up? A systematic review and meta-analysis. Anesth Analg 2015;120(5):1114–29.
2. Abdallah FW, Halpern SH, Margarido CB. Transversus abdominis plane block for postoperative analgesia after Caesarean delivery performed under spinal anaesthesia? A systematic review and meta-analysis. Br J Anaesth 2012;109(5):679–87.
3. Abell DJ, Barrington MJ. Pneumothorax after ultrasound-guided supraclavicular block: presenting features, risk, and related training. Reg Anesth Pain Med 2014;39(2):164–7.
4. Albrecht E, Kern C, Kirkham KR. A systematic review and meta-analysis of perineural dexamethasone for peripheral nerve blocks. Anaesthesia 2015;70(1):71–83.
5. Allen RH, Micks E, Edelman A. Pain relief for obstetric and gynecologic ambulatory procedures. Obstet Gynecol Clin North Am 2013;40(4):625–45.
6. Analysis of American Hospital Association annual survey data. 2014. http://www.aha.org/research/reports/tw/chartbook/ch3.shtml2014.
7. Argenson JN, Husted H, Lombardi Jr A, Booth RE, Thienpont E. Global forum: an international perspective on outpatient surgical procedures for adult hip and knee reconstruction. J Bone Jt Surg Am 2016;98(13):e55.
8. Bailard NS, Ortiz J, Flores RA. Additives to local anesthetics for peripheral nerve blocks: evidence, limitations, and recommendations. Am J Health Syst Pharm 2014;71(5):373–85.
9. Ballantyne JC, Carr DB, deFerranti S, et al. The comparative effects of postoperative analgesic therapies on pulmonary outcome: cumulative meta-analyses of randomized, controlled trials. Anesth Analg 1998;86(3):598–612.
10. Benumof JL. Permanent loss of cervical spinal cord function associated with interscalene block performed under general anesthesia. Anesthesiology 2000;93(6):1541–4.
11. Bingham AE, Fu R, Horn JL, Abrahams MS. Continuous peripheral nerve block compared with single-injection peripheral nerve block: a systematic review and meta-analysis of randomized controlled trials. Reg Anesth Pain Med 2012;37(6):583–94.
12. Borgeat A, Kalberer F, Jacob H, Ruetsch YA, Gerber C. Patient-controlled interscalene analgesia with ropivacaine 0.2% versus bupivacaine 0.15% after major open shoulder surgery: the effects on hand motor function. Anesth Analg 2001;92(1):218–23.
13. Buckenmaier 3rd CC, Shields CH, Auton AA, et al. Continuous peripheral nerve block in combat casualties receiving low-molecular weight heparin. Br J Anaesth 2006;97(6):874–7.
14. Buckenmaier CC, McKnight GM, Winkley JV, et al. Continuous peripheral nerve block for battlefield anesthesia and evacuation. Reg Anesth Pain Med 2005;30(2):202–5.
15. Chan EY, Fransen M, Parker DA, Assam PN, Chua N. Femoral nerve blocks for acute postoperative pain after knee replacement surgery. Cochrane Database Syst Rev 2014;(5):Cd009941.
16. Chelly JE, Ben-David B, Williams BA, Kentor ML. Anesthesia and postoperative analgesia: outcomes following orthopedic surgery. Orthopedics 2003;26(8 Suppl.):s865–71.
17. Chelly JE, Gebhard R, Greger J, Al Samsam T. Regional anesthesia for outpatient orthopedic surgery. Minerva Anestesiol 2001;67(9 Suppl. 1):227–32.
18. Chelly JE, Ghisi D, Fanelli A. Continuous peripheral nerve blocks in acute pain management. Br J Anaesth 2010;105(Suppl. 1):i86–96.
19. Chelly JE, Greger J, Gebhard R, et al. Continuous femoral blocks improve recovery and outcome of patients undergoing total knee arthroplasty. J Arthroplasty 2001;16(4):436–45.
20. Chelly JE, Williams BA. Continuous perineural infusions at home: narrowing the focus. Reg Anesth Pain Med 2004;29(1):1–3.
21. Cozowicz C, Poeran J, Memtsoudis SG. Epidemiology, trends, and disparities in regional anaesthesia for orthopaedic surgery. Br J Anaesth 2015;115(Suppl. 2):ii57–67.
22. Cozowicz C, Poeran J, Zubizarreta N, Mazumdar M, Memtsoudis SG. Trends in the use of regional anesthesia: neuraxial and peripheral nerve blocks. Reg Anesth Pain Med 2016;41(1):43–9.
23. Davis N, Lee M, Lin AY, et al. Postoperative cognitive function following general versus regional anesthesia: a systematic review. J Neurosurg Anesthesiol 2014;26(4):369–76.
24. El-Boghdadly K, Chin KJ, Chan VWS. Phrenic nerve palsy and regional anesthesia for shoulder surgery: anatomical, physiologic, and clinical considerations. Anesthesiology 2017;127(1):173–91.
25. Exadaktylos AK, Buggy DJ, Moriarty DC, Mascha E, Sessler DI. Can anesthetic technique for primary breast cancer surgery affect recurrence or metastasis? Anesthesiology 2006;105(4):660–4.
26. Fowler SJ, Symons J, Sabato S, Myles PS. Epidural analgesia compared with peripheral nerve blockade after major knee surgery: a systematic review and meta-analysis of randomized trials. Br J Anaesth 2008;100(2):154–64.

27. Gadsden J, Warlick A. Regional anesthesia for the trauma patient: improving patient outcomes. Local Reg Anesth 2015;8:45–55.
28. Gerrard AD, Brooks B, Asaad P, Hajibandeh S, Hajibandeh S. Meta-analysis of epidural analgesia versus peripheral nerve blockade after total knee joint replacement. Eur J Orthop Surg Traumatol 2017;27(1):61–72.
29. Gottschalk A, Cohen SP, Yang S, Ochroch EA. Preventing and treating pain after thoracic surgery. Anesthesiology 2006;104(3):594–600.
30. Grau AJ, Eicke M, Burmeister C, Hardt R, Schmitt E, Dienlin S. Risk of ischemic stroke and transient ischemic attack is increased up to 90 days after non-carotid and non-cardiac surgery. Cerebrovasc Dis 2017;43(5–6):242–9.
31. Guay J, Parker MJ, Gajendragadkar PR, Kopp S. Anaesthesia for hip fracture surgery in adults. Cochrane Database Syst Rev 2016;2:Cd000521.
32. Hadzic A, Williams BA, Karaca PE, et al. For outpatient rotator cuff surgery, nerve block anesthesia provides superior same-day recovery over general anesthesia. Anesthesiology 2005;102(5):1001–7.
33. Hamilton TW, Athanassoglou V, Trivella M, et al. Liposomal bupivacaine peripheral nerve block for the management of postoperative pain. Cochrane Database Syst Rev 2016;(8):Cd011476.
34. Hausman Jr MS, Jewell ES, Engoren M. Regional versus general anesthesia in surgical patients with chronic obstructive pulmonary disease: does avoiding general anesthesia reduce the risk of postoperative complications? Anesth Analg 2015;120(6):1405–12.
35. Hebl JR, Dilger JA, Byer DE, et al. A pre-emptive multimodal pathway featuring peripheral nerve block improves perioperative outcomes after major orthopedic surgery. Reg Anesth Pain Med 2008;33(6):510–7.
36. Heesen M, Klimek M, Rossaint R, Imberger G, Straube S. Paravertebral block and persistent postoperative pain after breast surgery: meta-analysis and trial sequential analysis. Anaesthesia 2016;71(12):1471–81.
37. Hogan QH. Pathophysiology of peripheral nerve injury during regional anesthesia. Reg Anesth Pain Med 2008;33(5):435–41.
38. Huynh TM, Marret E, Bonnet F. Combination of dexamethasone and local anaesthetic solution in peripheral nerve blocks: a meta-analysis of randomised controlled trials. Eur J Anaesthesiol 2015;32(11):751–8.
39. Ikuta PT, Raza SM, Durrani Z, Vasireddy AR, Winnie AP, Masters RW. pH adjustment schedule for the amide local anesthetics. Reg Anesth 1989;14(5):229–35.
40. Ilfeld BM, Viscusi ER, Hadzic A, et al. Safety and side effect profile of liposome bupivacaine (Exparel) in peripheral nerve blocks. Reg Anesth Pain Med 2015;40(5):572–82.
41. Ilfeld BM. Continuous peripheral nerve blocks: an update of the published evidence and comparison with novel, alternative analgesic modalities. Anesth Analg 2017;124(1):308–35.
42. Ironfield CM, Barrington MJ, Kluger R, Sites B. Are patients satisfied after peripheral nerve blockade? Results from an International Registry of Regional Anesthesia. Reg Anesth Pain Med 2014;39(1):48–55.
43. Johnson RL, Kopp SL, Burkle CM, et al. Neuraxial vs general anaesthesia for total hip and total knee arthroplasty: a systematic review of comparative-effectiveness research. Br J Anaesth 2016;116(2):163–76.
44. Johnson SP, Chung KC, Zhong L, et al. Risk of prolonged opioid use among opioid-naive patients following common hand surgery procedures. J Hand Surg Am 2016;41(10):947–57.e3.
45. Joshi GP, Bonnet F, Shah R, et al. A systematic review of randomized trials evaluating regional techniques for postthoracotomy analgesia. Anesth Analg 2008:1026–40.
46. Kirksey MA, Haskins SC, Cheng J, Liu SS. Local anesthetic peripheral nerve block adjuvants for prolongation of analgesia: a systematic qualitative review. PLoS One 2015;10(9):e0137312.
47. Kopp SL, Berbari EF, Osmon DR, et al. The impact of anesthetic management on surgical site infections in patients undergoing total knee or total hip arthroplasty. Anesth Analg 2015;121(5):1215–21.
48. Kopp SL, Jacob AK, Hebl JR. Regional anesthesia in patients with preexisting neurologic disease. Reg Anesth Pain Med 2015;40(5):467–78.
49. Liu Q, Chelly JE, Williams JP, Gold MS. Impact of peripheral nerve block with low dose local anesthetics on analgesia and functional outcomes following total knee arthroplasty: a retrospective study. Pain Med 2015;16(5):998–1006.
50. Luber MJ, Greengrass R, Vail TP. Patient satisfaction and effectiveness of lumbar plexus and sciatic nerve block for total knee arthroplasty. J Arthroplasty 2001;16(1):17–21.
51. Maher DP, White PF. Proposed mechanisms for association between opioid usage and cancer recurrence after surgery. J Clin Anesth 2016;28:36–40.
52. Marino J, Russo J, Kenny M, Herenstein R, Livote E, Chelly JE. Continuous lumbar plexus block for postoperative pain control after total hip arthroplasty. A randomized controlled trial. J Bone Jt Surg Am 2009;91(1):29–37.

53. Mason SE, Noel-Storr A, Ritchie CW. The impact of general and regional anesthesia on the incidence of post-operative cognitive dysfunction and post-operative delirium: a systematic review with meta-analysis. J Alzheimers Dis 2010;22(Suppl. 3):67–79.
54. Matot I, Oppenheim-Eden A, Ratrot R, et al. Preoperative cardiac events in elderly patients with hip fracture randomized to epidural or conventional analgesia. Anesthesiology 2003;98(1):156–63.
55. McCutchen T, Gerancher JC. Early intralipid therapy may have prevented bupivacaine-associated cardiac arrest. Reg Anesth Pain Med 2008;33(2):178–80.
56. McEvoy MD, Scott MJ, Gordon DB, et al. American Society for Enhanced Recovery (ASER) and Perioperative Quality Initiative (POQI) joint consensus statement on optimal analgesia within an enhanced recovery pathway for colorectal surgery: part 1-from the preoperative period to PACU. Perioper Med 2017;6:8.
57. Mears DC, Mears SC, Chelly JE, Dai F, Vulakovich KL. THA with a minimally invasive technique, multimodal anesthesia, and home rehabilitation: factors associated with early discharge? Clin Orthop Relat Res 2009;467(6):1412–7.
58. Memtsoudis SG, Danninger T, Rasul R, et al. Inpatient falls after total knee arthroplasty: the role of anesthesia type and peripheral nerve blocks. Anesthesiology 2014;120(3):551–63.
59. Moller JT, Cluitmans P, Rasmussen LS, et al. Long-term postoperative cognitive dysfunction in the elderly ISPOCD1 study. ISPOCD investigators. International Study of Post-Operative Cognitive Dysfunction. Lancet 1998;351(9106):857–61.
60. Moore JG, Ross SM, Williams BA. Regional anesthesia and ambulatory surgery. Curr Opin Anaesthesiol 2013;26(6):652–60.
61. Neal JM, Brull R, Horn JL, et al. The second American Society of Regional Anesthesia and pain medicine evidence-based medicine assessment of ultrasound-guided regional anesthesia: executive summary. Reg Anesth Pain Med 2016;41(2):181–94.
62. Neal JM. Ultrasound-guided regional anesthesia and patient safety: update of an evidence-based analysis. Reg Anesth Pain Med 2016;41(2):195–204.
63. Oliver JA, Oliver LA. Beyond the caudal: truncal blocks an alternative option for analgesia in pediatric surgical patients. Curr Opin Anaesthesiol 2013;26(6):644–51.
64. Paredes S, Cortinez L, Contreras V, Silbert B. Post-operative cognitive dysfunction at 3 months in adults after non-cardiac surgery: a qualitative systematic review. Acta Anaesthesiol Scand 2016;60(8):1043–58.
65. Paul JE, Arya A, Hurlburt L, et al. Femoral nerve block improves analgesia outcomes after total knee arthroplasty: a meta-analysis of randomized controlled trials. Anesthesiology 2010;113(5):1144–62.
66. Petrar SD, Seltenrich ME, Head SJ, Schwarz SK. Hemidiaphragmatic paralysis following ultrasound-guided supraclavicular versus infraclavicular brachial plexus blockade: a randomized clinical trial. Reg Anesth Pain Med 2015;40(2):133–8.
67. Popping DM, Elia N, Marret E, Wenk M, Tramer MR. Clonidine as an adjuvant to local anesthetics for peripheral nerve and plexus blocks: a meta-analysis of randomized trials. Anesthesiology 2009;111(2):406–15.
68. Popping DM, Elia N, Van Aken HK, et al. Impact of epidural analgesia on mortality and morbidity after surgery: systematic review and meta-analysis of randomized controlled trials. Ann Surg 2014;259(6):1056–67.
69. Rasmussen LS, Larsen K, Houx P, Skovgaard LT, Hanning CD, Moller JT. The assessment of postoperative cognitive function. Acta Anaesthesiol Scand 2001;45(3):275–89.
70. Richman JM, Liu SS, Courpas G, et al. Does continuous peripheral nerve block provide superior pain control to opioids? A meta-analysis. Anesth Analg 2006;102(1):248–57.
71. Royds J, Khan AH, Buggy DJ. An update on existing ongoing prospective trials evaluating the effect of anesthetic and analgesic techniques during primary cancer surgery on cancer recurrence or metastasis. Int Anesthesiol Clin 2016;54(4):e76–83.
72. Saporito A, Anselmi L, Sturini E, Borgeat A, Aguirre JA. Is outpatient continuous regional analgesia more effective and equally safe than single-shot peripheral nerve blocks after ambulatory orthopedic surgery? A systematic review of randomized, double-blinded, placebo-controlled trials. Minerva Anestesiol 2017;83(9):972–81.
73. Schnabel A, Reichl SU, Zahn PK, Pogatzki-Zahn EM, Meyer-Friessem CH. Efficacy and safety of buprenorphine in peripheral nerve blocks: a meta-analysis of randomised controlled trials. Eur J Anaesthesiol 2017;34(9):576–86.
74. Scott MJ, McEvoy MD, Gordon DB, et al. American society for enhanced recovery (ASER) and perioperative quality initiative (POQI) joint consensus statement on optimal analgesia within an enhanced recovery pathway for colorectal surgery: part 2-From PACU to the transition home. Perioper Med 2017;6:7.
75. Spence AG. Lipid reversal of central nervous system symptoms of bupivacaine toxicity. Anesthesiology 2007;107(3):516–7.
76. Stein BE, Srikumaran U, Tan EW, Freehill MT, Wilckens JH. Lower-extremity peripheral nerve blocks in the perioperative pain management of orthopaedic patients: AAOS exhibit selection. J Bone Jt Surg Am 2012;94(22):e167.

77. Sun EC, Bateman BT, Memtsoudis SG, Neuman MD, Mariano ER, Baker LC. Lack of association between the use of nerve blockade and the risk of postoperative chronic opioid use among patients undergoing total knee arthroplasty: evidence from the Marketscan database. Anesth Analg 2017;125(3):999–1007.
78. Sun EC, Darnall BD, Baker LC, Mackey S. Incidence of and risk factors for chronic opioid use among opioid-naive patients in the postoperative period. JAMA Intern Med 2016;176(9):1286–93.
79. Tighe P, Buckenmaier 3rd CC, Boezaart AP, et al. Acute pain medicine in the United States: a status report. Pain Med 2015;16(9):1806–26.
80. Tuominen M, Haasio J, Hekali R, Rosenberg PH. Continuous interscalene brachial plexus block: clinical efficacy, technical problems and bupivacaine plasma concentrations. Acta Anaesthesiol Scand 1989;33(1):84–8.
81. Vasques F, Behr AU, Weinberg G, Ori C, Di Gregorio G. A review of local anesthetic systemic toxicity cases since publication of the American Society of Regional Anesthesia recommendations: to whom it may concern. Reg Anesth Pain Med 2015;40(6):698–705.
82. Verlinde M, Hollmann MW, Stevens MF, Hermanns H, Werdehausen R, Lirk P. Local anesthetic-induced neurotoxicity. Int J Mol Sci 2016;17(3):339.
83. Vorobeichik L, Brull R, Abdallah FW. Evidence basis for using perineural dexmedetomidine to enhance the quality of brachial plexus nerve blocks: a systematic review and meta-analysis of randomized controlled trials. Br J Anaesth 2017;118(2):167–81.
84. Weber A, Fournier R, Van Gessel E, Riand N, Gamulin Z. Epinephrine does not prolong the analgesia of 20 mL ropivacaine 0.5% or 0.2% in a femoral three-in-one block. Anesth Analg 2001;93(5):1327–31.
85. Williams BA, Kentor ML, Williams JP, et al. PACU bypass after outpatient knee surgery is associated with fewer unplanned hospital admissions but more phase II nursing interventions. Anesthesiology 2002;97(4):981–8.
86. Wolfe JW, Butterworth JF. Local anesthetic systemic toxicity: update on mechanisms and treatment. Curr Opin Anaesthesiol 2011;24(5):561–6.
87. Wu CL, Raja SN. Treatment of acute postoperative pain. Lancet 2011;377(9784):2215–25.
88. Zaric D, Boysen K, Christiansen C, Christiansen J, Stephensen S, Christensen B. A comparison of epidural analgesia with combined continuous femoral-sciatic nerve blocks after total knee replacement. Anesth Analg 2006;102(4):1240–6.
89. Zaw AA, Murry J, Hoang D, et al. Epidural analgesia after rib fractures. Am Surg 2015;81(10):950–4.

CHAPTER 21

Pre- and Postsurgical Psychological Assessment and Management of Pain

Ronald J. Kulich, Emily A. Walsh, and Ana-Maria Vranceanu

This chapter addresses psychosocial determinants of pain-related outcomes after surgery in adults. We describe psychosocial risk factors for adverse outcomes after surgery. We offer guidance on self-report measures that may be useful to identify individuals at risk versus those who may recover uneventfully on their own and survey evidence for the efficacy of psychosocial interventions to treat those at risk. We summarize barriers to delivering psychosocial interventions and propose strategies to overcome these barriers. Furthermore, emphasizing chronic postsurgical pain (CPSP) because of its theoretical and practical importance, we complement other chapters in this volume by describing evidence-based psychosocial approaches to decrease the risk of CPSP, including novel technologic approaches that circumvent barriers to care.

ASSESSMENT AND IDENTIFICATION OF RISK FACTORS

Multiple psychological risk factors have been identified as predictors of adverse pain-related outcomes after surgery. Block and Sarwer [4] provided a template for clinicians, offering detailed protocols for assessment, which can be modified to fit specific patient concerns and medical practice [4]. Adverse pain-related outcomes after surgery involve multiple factors including medical, psychological, functional, social, and economic influences. The main psychosocial risk factors are emotional (e.g., depression and anxiety), coping ability (e.g., pain catastrophizing, pain anxiety), medication-related (e.g., opioid misuse, substance use disorder), and situational (e.g., familial, economic, and medical stress) [54,57]. These risks overlap and are interrelated, making it a challenge to isolate any single one [28,47]. Preoperative pain level and history of chronic pain, anxiety, fear of surgery, pain catastrophizing, early trauma/posttraumatic stress disorder (PTSD), depression, substance misuse and abuse, opioid use, fear avoidance and impaired function, impaired sleep, and catastrophizing all have predictive value for adverse outcomes including CPSP [2,6,19,32,34–36,43,45,50] (see below). For some surgical procedures, particularly cardiac operations, presurgical depression is particularly predictive [2,5,24,29,48]. Approximately 23% to 45% of cardiac surgical patients suffer from depressive symptoms or clinical depression [12], suggesting the importance of behavioral interventions in this population. Intake of antidepressant medication also is a risk factor for adverse pain-related outcomes, although antidepressants are often used for conditions other than depression [35]. In a review of studies on total joint arthroplasties, Dowsey et al. [14] reported that the incidence of preoperative psychological distress was between 30% and 60%, and level of distress was associated with increased postsurgical pain, worse postoperative functional outcomes, increased analgesic intake, increased hospital admissions, and long-term mortality [14]. Psychological factors influence postoperative course even after minor operations. Presurgical depression predicts recovery after elective hand surgery [57], and pain anxiety affects the level of postoperative pain in dermatologic surgery [8]. Dental surgery outcomes are well known to be affected by psychological factors [37]. Severity of pain immediately after wisdom tooth extraction is a risk factor for PTSD, suggesting the importance of assessment and management of the patient's "individual predisposition to anxiety or trauma-related symptoms to reduce the risk of iatrogenic psychological harm" [37]. These and other studies suggest that the experience of pain and other stressful issues related to surgery may retraumatize the patient [30].

Impaired presurgical physical functioning is also a predictor of poor outcome after many types of surgery [53]. Early postoperative fear of movement as well as early presurgical depression predicts pain, disability, and self-reported physical health 6 months postspine surgery [2], supporting efforts for preoperative assessment and rehabilitation in such individuals. Several additional psychological variables also warrant attention. Somatization, multiple pain sites, prior surgical interventions, and patient expectations also have been demonstrated to predict and to report increased pain and poor overall outcomes, with much of these data coming from spinal surgery studies [4,60]. Opioid and other substance use disorders have received increasing attention in Europe, Australia, and North America. There is evidence that preoperative use of opioids predicts moderate to severe postoperative pain, particularly in the context of younger age and in the presence of psychological risk factors [20,23,24,35,53]. Higher preoperative pain scores not only predict higher postoperative scores but also greater postoperative opioid doses [17]. One cannot assume that these individuals using higher doses of opioids after surgery suffer from opioid use disorders, although we do know that high-dose chronic opioid therapy may predict poorer long-term outcomes of many surgical or nonsurgical treatments [13]. When substance use disorder is identified in an individual patient, the opportunity exists for referral and close collaboration with addiction medicine clinicians. In instances where cognitive impairment is present for reasons other than substance use, geriatric mental health assessment may lead to interventions that enhance postoperative course and even improve survival [10,40]. To facilitate identification and assessment of substance use, standardized brief screening questionnaires are widely available and already in regular use by most primary care practices, e.g., the AUDIT-C for alcohol use and the SOAPP-R for assessing risk during chronic opioid therapy. When a patient presents taking high doses of opioids preoperatively but does not meet criteria for substance use disorder, structured tapering programs can be offered before or after surgery, depending on the patient's particular medical and psychiatric needs [3,23].

QUESTIONNAIRES FOR SCREENING AND TREATMENT PLANNING

Because multiple psychological factors influence the experience of pain after surgery, the selection of a specific assessment measure may be problematic. Scott and McCracken argue that use of one instrument covering all domains can lead to problems with incremental validity or problems with construct overlap with each new psychological factor

[47]. Although a thorough psychological assessment is important and may be possible for planned procedures such as bariatric surgery, this may not be feasible for other planned or emergency surgical procedures. Nonetheless, we encourage measures previously validated in the chronic pain population, and a number of resources are available to determine the best questionnaires for the population being assessed. At a minimum, we recommend using a measure of emotional functioning, a measure of coping, and a measure of opioid risk or misuse and general substance use disorder risk.

PSYCHOSOCIAL TREATMENTS

Although there is robust scientific literature on the use of psychological interventions with chronic pain conditions, studies that address the application of such treatments perioperatively are fewer. In reviewing the research gaps addressed in a multisociety practice guideline for acute postoperative pain management, Gordon et al. comment that "evidence is available for many of the non-pharmacological and biobehavioral interventions including cognitive and physical agents" [16]. Although it is uncertain which cognitive methods are most effective, none appear to be associated with significant harm. Extrapolating from the extensive literature on the behavioral management of chronic pain is necessary, with the caveat that such generalization may not be valid. A patient undergoing a minor dental procedure likely differs from one undergoing a spinal fusion, both in terms of patient characteristics, expectations for, and the experience of the procedure. Hence, there is a need to individualize behavioral interventions, tying the treatment to the particular problems presented by the patient. Below we summarize skill-based interventions and modules that have support in prior research and can be incorporated pre- and postsurgery to prevent CPSP in at risk individuals.

Relaxation or Mindfulness

Relaxation or mindfulness approaches may reduce pre- and postsurgical pain as shown by Vranceanu et al. in hand surgery patients [56]. Acceptance therapy techniques, often considered a subset of cognitive therapy, also may help to foster psychological "flexibility" in pre- and postsurgical patients. For example, patients often struggle to control their symptoms, spending much time worrying or catastrophizing about their symptoms and their medical care [21]. Such patients may benefit from being taught to accept symptoms of anxiety or pain without fighting or engaging in a defensive response to them.

Hypnosis

Hypnosis has a long history of clinical use in acute and postsurgical settings where patient anxiety symptoms predominate. Montgomery et al. have presented supporting data from a meta-analysis of hypnosis for CPSP [39]. More recently, Kendrick et al. offered recommendations from a review of recent studies on hypnosis for acute procedural pain [29]. Although most studies lacked adequate controls, the authors concluded that hypnosis decreased pain and, for minor surgical procedures, was at least as effective as adjunctive psychological therapies. The literature also suggests incremental benefit from multiple treatment sessions before surgery, similar to other behavioral interventions.

Treatment of Depression

The role of treating depression to reduce CPSP was studied by Doering et al., who found that cognitive–behavioral therapy (CBT) for depressive symptoms decreased pain interference ($P = 0.02$) and pain severity ($P = 0.03$) [12]. Their treatment model was relatively intensive and home-based for patients recovering from surgery, including eight 1-hour sessions with an advanced practice nurse who had received training in a standardized protocol from the Beck Institute in Pennsylvania. Although support for behavioral interventions for depression is well established, few controlled studies have directly targeted affective symptoms in patients undergoing surgical procedures.

Opioid Management and Tapering

The adverse acute and chronic effects of opioid therapy and issues of dose escalation postsurgery have been well established. Katz et al. described an intensive multidisciplinary program to prevent surgical pain and address opioid risks, combining behavioral and acceptance therapies, rehabilitative therapies, and medical therapies [27]. In a follow-up report, the same group compared 91 patients receiving perioperative acceptance and commitment therapy ("ACT") with 252 in a "no ACT group." Although both groups showed reductions in pain, opioid use, pain interference, pain catastrophizing, and anxiety, additional gains were found in the ACT group for more complex patients [27]. From a clinical and cost standpoint, this study suggests that it is reasonable to screen for individuals with psychological comorbidities who might best benefit from ACT. Whether ACT is better than other behavioral approaches or adds to the effect of an interdisciplinary program remains unclear.

When considering the role of behavioral interventions to decrease opioid consumption for postsurgical pain, it is again necessary to extrapolate from outcome studies that address other pain conditions. Berna et al. reviewed opioid tapering programs for patients who do not meet criteria for substance use disorder, i.e., the majority of those encountered in a postsurgical setting [3]. They were able to identify only two randomized clinical trials involving behavioral treatment for preoperative tapering of opioids, both with small sample sizes. Extrapolating from the robust scientific literature on behavioral management of chronic pain, they concluded that there is a potential role for behavioral treatment components for the nonaddicted patient with persistent pain, provided as part of a structured template for opioid tapering [23]. Referring to a similar template for opioid tapering, Huxtable et al. underscored "the importance of providing the patient with a consistent message about management along with explicit behavioural limits," a statement consistent with the aforementioned literature on behavioral treatment [23].

Treatments Directed at Physical Functioning

Archer and colleagues evaluated comprehensive behavioral treatment interventions for pre- and postsurgical patients, with a particular focus on the relationship of function and postsurgical outcomes [1,2]. Higher presurgical levels of function correlated with lower levels of postsurgical pain intensity, a conclusion now consistent with animal studies wherein exercise training reduced postsurgical pain behaviors in rats [9]. Archer and colleagues studied 86 adults undergoing lumbar laminectomies. Patients were recruited from 499 subjects screened preoperatively to select those with high fear of movement as measured by the Tampa Scale for kinesiophobia. The latter group were randomized to CBT and rehabilitation or an education program offered for 6 weeks after surgery. The program was relatively intensive and focused on reducing pain and disability by reducing fear of movement and increased self-efficacy. The treatment was individualized, encouraging attainment of patient-specific functional activity goals despite pain. Participants reported decreased pain and disability, as well as increased general health and physical performance compared with the education-only group. These results were maintained at the 3-month follow-up [1]. Implementing the aforementioned interventions for all surgical patients may prove costly and labor-intensive but potentially worthwhile for those patients at increased risk for adverse postsurgical outcomes. Others working to apply similar intensive models of care are using technology to reduce cost and decrease one-on-one time, e.g., in the patient's home environment (see below).

BARRIERS

Although the assessment of psychological variables is generally accepted as the standard of care when addressing chronic pain conditions, this is not the case with presurgical assessment. Postsurgical factors such as excessive duration of analgesic prescribing or patient nonadherence to medications are additional challenges. Barriers to presurgery assessment occur at the patient level (e.g., stigma), provider level (e.g., challenges with communicating psychosocial factors), and system level (e.g., access to resources, cost) [55]. We limit the present comments to several factors that have received most attention in prior research.

Access to Resources

Access to resources may be limited, and the knowledge base of the psychologist and most other mental health providers may be lacking. Surgeons typically do not practice within teams that include psychological services, although there are exceptions to this in acute care medical center settings [55]. Most specialists practice in relative isolation. For example, dentists or oral surgeons perform many surgical procedures and cumulatively prescribe large amounts of opioids for acute pain yet do so in a practice model that does not involve interdisciplinary evaluation and management. Efforts are underway to educate dentists by reinforcing the use of risk screening questionnaires and provide guidance as to counseling and referral, particularly with respect to substance use disorder risk [32,41].

Patient Adherence

Patient adherence is another opportunity for improved postsurgical pain management. For every prescription written, 48% to 66% are picked up from the pharmacy, 25% to 30% are taken properly, and 15% to 20% are refilled as prescribed [13]. Particularly with concurrent serious conditions such as cancer or cardiac disease, severely ill patients are significantly less likely to be adherent to medical and mental health regimens, leading to increased postsurgical pain and poor health care outcomes [18]. Cheatle and Dhingra reviewed strategies for assessment and managing adherence with various pain conditions, although the supporting scientific literature on the subject remains weak [7]. Dozens of variables impact patient adherence, and most can be categorized as psychosocial [25]. Given the quantity of factors and the likelihood that many overlap, there has been an increasing focus on customizing behavioral interventions to target a particular patient's needs, e.g., the clinician may address specific patient misunderstandings or fears about the particular planned operation, concerns over medication effects and side effects, and expectations about surgical outcome.

Stigma

Stigma associated with undergoing psychological assessments and interventions may also be a barrier to accessing such services, as can the cost and administrative burdens needed to secure insurance coverage. With respect to stigma, there is a risk of "blaming the patient" for ultimate negative outcome of surgery [47,50]. From the patient and family's perspective, involvement of a mental health provider runs the risk of their feeling that his/her clinicians believe "it's all in my head." Indeed, the patient may have a realistic fear that stigma will lead to reluctance or deferral of a potentially helpful operation or failure to receive sufficient analgesics pre- or postsurgery. Individual, family, and cultural barriers also must be recognized and addressed directly and compassionately (including early introduction to the mental health provider) at the earliest phase of patient care.

Cost

Cost and related financial coverage barriers have long been impediments to obtaining psychological assessment and services, particularly in cases where a patient does not present with a documented psychiatric disorder. Failed adherence to medical recommendations was attributed to cost by 22% of patients [13]; even lower adherence rates are reported for mental health services recommended in the context of pain care [15].

Provider-Related Barriers

Provider-related barriers such as not appreciating the role of biopsychosocial factors or learning to assess and treat them can perpetuate stigma, undermine compassion, and perpetuate patients' emotional and coping difficulties. Operating, reoperating, or prescribing medications is often preferred to uncomfortable discussions aimed at uncovering psychosocial factors. Indeed, surgeons are unlikely to screen for psychological factors or provide referrals for psychosocial treatments [55].

PSYCHOSOCIAL FACTORS AND CPSP

Earlier chapters in this volume have pointed out that CPSP is common, challenging to treat, and costly [11,13], with prevalence rates in the general postsurgical population as high as 10% to 20% [11,13]. The International Association of Study of Pain (IASP), together with the European Pain Federation (EFIC) designated 2017 as the Global Year Against Pain After Surgery to increase awareness of acute and chronic pain after surgery among policy makers, health care organizations, health care professionals, and the general public. Overall, such recognition aimed to advance basic and clinical pain research, translate new findings and existing evidence into clinical practice, and provide enduring educational resources that will ultimately benefit patients with pain.

CPSP is a particular focus of these current efforts, as it was in the first and present edition of this volume. Multiple biopsychosocial factors are associated with risk for CPSP; many are similar to those associated with the development of chronic pain after trauma or acute painful illnesses such as herpes zoster. First, presurgical psychosocial factors (e.g., depression and anxiety) are predictors of pain and disability after elective surgery [57]. Second, ineffective coping skills including catastrophic thinking about pain and pain intensity have been found to predict both pain and disability after orthopedic surgery for trauma [54]. Third, postsurgical prescribing of higher dose opioids has been associated with persistent pain and worsened disability among those who continue to take opioid at 1 to 2 months after surgery [22]. Within the United States, the problem has been further complicated by secondary issues related to the continuation of opioids long after the operation and the related risks associated with substance use, including sharing, pilfering, and/or diversion by family members or friends. Addressing these pre- and postsurgical factors is an important component of a necessary multidimensional strategy both to reduce the occurrence of CPSP as well as substance use disorder. Surgeons who manage patients with either CPSP or substance use disorder are not typically trained to, nor comfortable in discussing psychosocial issues with patients [48] although recent guidelines and policies emphasize the importance of a "multidisciplinary" or "multimodal" focus for patient assessment and care [16]. Evidence-based, postsurgical opioid prescribing guidelines including information about how to taper off of opioids are imperative. Surgeons should understand that patients who require higher doses and more prolonged courses of opioids are typically those with psychosocial comorbidities. The US multiorganization "Guidelines on the Management of Postoperative Pain" strongly recommend that "clinicians conduct a preoperative evaluation including assessment of medical and psychiatric comorbidities, concomitant medications, history of chronic pain, substance abuse, and previous postoperative treatment regimens and responses...." Regrettably, routine bedside clinical practice is only now approaching this aspiration [16].

FUTURE DIRECTIONS AND NOVEL APPROACHES

Given the patient, provider, and system barriers described earlier, comprehensive labor- and time-intensive psychological treatment approaches may not be feasible for more than a small fraction of patients undergoing surgery. Therefore, several brief approaches have been developed as less costly and labor-intensive alternatives.

Vranceanu et al. [55,59] have shown that a 60-second, personalized mindfulness intervention (http://www.pixelthoughts.co) is feasible to administer, accepted, and usable by patients with orthopedic surgical pain. Its use is associated with decreased pain intensity and emotional distress in surgical outpatients. Furthermore, Vranceanu et al. have developed a four-session "Cognitive Behavioral Relaxation Response Intervention" that is associated with decreased pain, improved coping, and decreased disability in orthopedic patients with acute fractures or postoperative pain [57]. The intervention, currently labeled "Toolkit for Optimal Recovery" is currently being tested in a large randomized controlled trial in which the program is delivered via live video using a secure platform [33]. Preliminary analyses show high feasibility and acceptability and statistically and clinically significant improvement in coping and decreased pain and disability [58,59] This intervention may lower barriers described earlier, including patient stigma and cost. It provides relaxation and mindfulness skills (e.g., breath awareness and body scan), cognitive–behavioral skills (adaptive thinking and problem solving), and activity pacing, while also challenging myths associated with recovery after surgery (e.g., "One should be pain free after surgery", "Pain means there is something wrong"). Pain education videos delivered to patients immediately after surgery can convey educational information on expectations of recovery, dangers of opioids, and normalizing potential coping and emotional difficulties postsurgery, while also bypassing some of the barriers to care through empowering patients to ask for skills training rather than waiting for provider referrals. Fischenbauer et al. developed such a postsurgery video for patients undergoing orthopedic surgery [58,61].

Other technologic advances also provide an opportunity for cost-effective behavioral assessment and management of postoperative pain. Interactive, inexpensive digital activity trackers can systematically monitor patient behavior, evaluate sleep, and analyze physiological data, reinforce activity levels, and provide a vehicle for addressing fear avoidance of activity. The major leading digital tracking company has sold more than 38 million devices worldwide with as many as 16 million active users [49]. Commercially available devices were first introduced with patients suffering from pain disorders such as fibromyalgia [51]. Kurti et al. found that sedentary adults over age 50 increased their steps by 108% to 183% when using a simple activity tracking device, with the highest rates for those receiving incentives to increase activity [31]. A trend toward their more routine postsurgical use quickly ensued, with commercial digital trackers now being used in patients after total knee arthroplasty, gastrointestinal surgery, lumbar spine surgery, and transforaminal interbody fusion surgery [38,42,44,46,52]. These behavioral assessment and interactive treatment modalities may provide the cost-effective methods to address and implement behavior change including improved patient adherence in the future.

REFERENCES

1. Archer KR, Devin CJ, Vanston SW, Koyama T, Phillips SE, George SZ, McGirt MJ, Spengler DM, Aaronson OS, Cheng JS, Wegener ST. Cognitive-behavioral-based physical therapy for patients with chronic pain undergoing lumbar spine surgery: a randomized controlled trial. J Pain 2016;17(1):76–89.
2. Archer KR, Seebach CL, Mathis SL, Riley 3rd LH, Wegener ST. Early postoperative fear of movement predicts pain, disability, and physical health six months after spinal surgery for degenerative conditions. Spine J 2014;14(5):759–67.
3. Berna C, Kulich RJ, Rathmell JP. Tapering long-term opioid therapy in chronic noncancer pain: evidence and recommendations for everyday practice. Mayo Clin Proc 2015;90(6):828–42.
4. Block A, Sarwer D. Presurgical psychological screening: understanding patients. In: Improving outcomes. American Psychological Association; 2013.
5. Caumo W, Schmidt AP, Schneider CN, Bergmann J, Iwamoto CW, Adamatti LC, Bandeira D, Ferreira MB. Preoperative predictors of moderate to intense acute postoperative pain in patients undergoing abdominal surgery. Acta Anaesthesiol Scand 2002;46(10):1265–71.
6. Chan EY, Blyth FM, Nairn L, Fransen M. Acute postoperative pain following hospital discharge after total knee arthroplasty. Osteoarthritis Cartilage 2013;21(9):1257–63.
7. Cheatle M, Fine PG. Facilitating treatment adherence in pain medicine. Oxford University Press; 2017.
8. Chen YW, Hsieh PL, Chen YC, Hung CH, Cheng JT. Physical exercise induces excess hsp72 expression and delays the development of hyperalgesia and allodynia in painful diabetic neuropathy rats. Anesth Analg 2013;116(2):482–90.
9. Chen YW, Lin MF, Chen YC, Hung CH, Tzeng JI, Wang JJ. Exercise training attenuates postoperative pain and expression of cytokines and N-methyl-D-aspartate receptor subunit 1 in rats. Reg Anesth Pain Med 2013;38(4):282–8.
10. Cooney MF. Postoperative pain management: clinical practice guidelines. J Perianesth Nurs 2016;31(5):445–51.
11. Dobrogowski J, Przeklasa-Muszyńska A, Wordliczek J. Persistent post-operative pain. Folia Med Cracov 2008;49(1–2):27–37.
12. Doering LV, McGuire A, Eastwood JA, Chen B, Bodan RC, Czer LS, Irwin MR. Cognitive behavioral therapy for depression improves pain and perceived control in cardiac surgery patients. Eur J Cardiovasc Nurs 2016;15(6):417–24.
13. Dowell D, Haegerich T, Chou R. CDC guideline for prescribing opioids for chronic pain. MMWR Recomm Rep 2016;65(1):1–50.
14. Dowsey MM, Castle DJ, Knowles SR, Monshat K, Salzberg MR, Choong PF. The effect of mindfulness training prior to total joint arthroplasty on post-operative pain and physical function: study protocol for a randomised controlled trial. Trials 2014;15:208.

15. Gatchel RJ, McGeary DD, McGeary CA, Lippe B. Interdisciplinary chronic pain management: past, present, and future. Am Psychol 2014;69(2):119–30.
16. Gordon DB, de Leon-Casasola OA, Wu CL, Sluka KA, Brennan TJ, Chou R. Research gaps in practice guidelines for acute postoperative pain management in adults: findings from a review of the evidence for an American Pain Society clinical practice guideline. J Pain 2016;17(2):158–66.
17. Grant D, Schoenleber S, McCarthy A, Neiss G, Yorgova P, Rogers K, Gabos P, Shah S. Are we prescribing out patients too much pain medication? Best predictors of narcotic usage after spinal surgery for scoliosis. J Bone Joint Surg 2016;98(18):1555–62.
18. Grassi L, Caruso R, Sabato S, Massarenti S, Nanni MG, The UniFe Psychiatry Working Group C. Psychosocial screening and assessment in oncology and palliative care settings. Front Psychol 2014;5:1485.
19. Grosen K, Drewes AM, Pilegaard HK, Pfeiffer-Jensen M, Brock B, Vase L. Situational but not dispositional pain catastrophizing correlates with early postoperative pain in pain-free patients before surgery. J Pain 2016;17(5):549–60.
20. Grosu I, de Kock M. New concepts in acute pain management: strategies to prevent chronic postsurgical pain, opioid-induced hyperalgesia, and outcome measures. Anesthesiol Clin 2011;29(2):311–27.
21. Hann K, McCracken L. A systematic review of randomized controlled trials of acceptance and commitment therapy for adults with chronic pain: outcome domains, design quality, and efficacy. J Contextual Behav Sci 2014;3(4):217–27.
22. Helmerhorst GT, Vranceanu AM, Vrahas M, Smith M, Ring D. Risk factors for continued opioid use one to two months after surgery for musculoskeletal trauma. J Bone Joint Surg Am 2014;96(6):495–9.
23. Huxtable CA, Roberts LJ, Somogyi AA, MacIntyre PE. Acute pain management in opioid-tolerant patients: a growing challenge. Anaesth Intensive Care 2011;39(5):804–23.
24. Ip HY, Abrishami A, Peng PW, Wong J, Chung F. Predictors of postoperative pain and analgesic consumption: a qualitative systematic review. Anesthesiology 2009;111(3):657–77.
25. Kardas P, Lewek P, Matyjaszczyk M. Determinants of patient adherence: a review of systematic reviews. Front Pharmacol 2013;4:91.
26. Katz J, Seltzer Z. Transition from acute to chronic postsurgical pain: risk factors and protective factors. Expert Rev Neurother 2009;9(5):723–44.
27. Katz J, Weinrib A, Fashler SR, Katznelson R, Shah BR, Ladak SS, Jiang J, Li Q, McMillan K, Mina DS, Wentlandt K, McRae K, Tamir D, Lyn S, de Perrot M, Rao V, Grant D, Roche-Nagle G, Cleary SP, Hofer SO, Gilbert R, Wijeysundera D, Ritvo P, Janmohamed T, O'Leary G, Clarke H. The Toronto General Hospital Transitional Pain Service: development and implementation of a multidisciplinary program to prevent chronic postsurgical pain. J Pain Res 2015;8:695–702.
28. Kendrick C, Sliwinski J, Yu Y, Johnson A, Fisher W, Kekecs Z, Elkins G. Hypnosis for acute procedural pain: a critical review. Int J Clin Exp Hypn 2016;64(1):75–115.
29. Kinjo S, Sands LP, Lim E, Paul S, Leung JM. Prediction of postoperative pain using path analysis in older patients. J Anesth 2012;26(1):1–8.
30. Kleiman V, Clarke H, Katz J. Sensitivity to pain traumatization: a higher-order factor underlying pain-related anxiety, pain catastrophizing and anxiety sensitivity among patients scheduled for major surgery. Pain Res Manag 2011;16(3):169–77.
31. Kurti AN, Dallery J. Internet-based contingency management increases walking in sedentary adults. J Appl Behav Anal 2013;46(3):568–81.
32. Lange JF, Kaufmann R, Wijsmuller AR, Pierie JP, Ploeg RJ, Chen DC, Amid PK. An international consensus algorithm for management of chronic postoperative inguinal pain. Hernia 2015;19(1):33–43.
33. Lenn J. Rethinking recovery after orthopaedic injury. AAOS Now: Orthopaedic Research and Education Foundation; 2017.
34. Lewis GN, Rice DA, McNair PJ, Kluger M. Predictors of persistent pain after total knee arthroplasty: a systematic review and meta-analysis. Br J Anaesth 2015;114(4):551–61.
35. Liu SS, Buvanendran A, Rathmell JP, Sawhney M, Bae JJ, Moric M, Perros S, Pope AJ, Poultsides L, Della Valle CJ, Shin NS, McCartney CJ, Ma Y, Shah M, Wood MJ, Manion SC, Sculco TP. Predictors for moderate to severe acute postoperative pain after total hip and knee replacement. Int Orthop 2012;36(11):2261–7.
36. Macrae WA. Chronic post-surgical pain: 10 years on. Br J Anaesth 2008;101(1):77–86.
37. Meissner W, Coluzzi F, Fletcher D, Huygen F, Morlion B, Neugebauer E, Perez AM, Pergolizzi J. Improving the management of post-operative acute pain: priorities for change. Curr Med Res Opin 2015;31(11):2131–43.
38. Mobbs RJ, Phan K, Maharaj M, Rao PJ. Physical activity measured with accelerometer and self-rated disability in lumbar spine surgery: a prospective study. Global Spine J 2016;6(5):459–64.

39. Montgomery GH, David D, Winkel G, Silverstein JH, Bovbjerg DH. The effectiveness of adjunctive hypnosis with surgical patients: a meta-analysis. Anesth Analg 2002;94(6):1639–45 [table of contents].
40. Owczuk R. Guidelines for general anaesthesia in the elderly of the committee on quality and safety in anaesthesia, Polish Society of Anaesthesiology and Intensive Therapy. Anaesthesiol Intensive Ther 2013;45(2):57–61.
41. Parish CL, Pereyra MR, Pollack HA, Cardenas G, Castellon PC, Abel SN, Singer R, Metsch LR. Screening for substance misuse in the dental care setting: findings from a nationally representative survey of dentists. Addiction 2015;110(9):1516–23.
42. Phan K, Mobbs RJ. Long-term objective physical activity measurements using a wireless accelerometer following minimally invasive transforaminal interbody fusion surgery. Asian Spine J 2016;10(2):366–9.
43. Pinto P, McIntyre T, Araujo-Soares V, Ferro R, Almeida A. The role of pain catastrophizing in the provision of rescue analgesia by health care providers following major joint arthroplasty. Pain Physician 2014;17(6):515–24.
44. Rao PJ, Phan K, Maharaj MM, Pelletier MH, Walsh WR, Mobbs RJ. Accelerometers for objective evaluation of physical activity following spine surgery. J Clin Neurosci 2016;26:14–8.
45. Riddle DL, Wade JB, Jiranek WA, Kong X. Preoperative pain catastrophizing predicts pain outcome after knee arthroplasty. Clin Orthop Relat Res 2010;468(3):798–806.
46. Roe C, Preede L, Dalen H, Bautz-Holter E, Nyquist A, Sandvik L, Saebu M. Does adapted physical activity-based rehabilitation improve mental and physical functioning? A randomized trial. Eur J Phys Rehabil Med 2016. https://www.minervamedica.it/en/journals/europa-medicophysica/article.php?cod=R33Y9999N00A16051202.
47. Scott W, McCracken L. Psychological assessment to identify patients at risk of postsurgical pain: the need for theory and pragmatism. Br J Anaesth 2016;117(5):546–8.
48. Sinikallio S, Aalto T, Airaksinen O, Herno A, Kroger H, Viinamaki H. Depressive burden in the preoperative and early recovery phase predicts poorer surgery outcome among lumbar spinal stenosis patients: a one-year prospective follow-up study. Spine (Phila Pa 1976) 2009;34(23):2573–8.
49. Statista. Number of Fitbit devices sold worldwide from 2010 to 2016: Statista. 2017. https://www.statista.com/statistics/472600/fitbit-active-users/.
50. Sullivan M, Tanzer M, Stanish W, Fallaha M, Keefe FJ, Simmonds M, Dunbar M. Psychological determinants of problematic outcomes following Total Knee Arthroplasty. Pain 2009;143(1–2):123–9.
51. Sundararaman LV, Edwards RR, Ross EL, Jamison RN. Integration of mobile health technology in the treatment of chronic pain: a critical review. Reg Anesth Pain Med 2017;42(4):488–98.
52. Symer MM, Abelson JS, Milsom J, McClure B, Yeo HL. A mobile health application to track patients after gastrointestinal surgery: results from a pilot study. J Gastrointest Surg 2017;21(9):1500–5.
53. Thomazeau J, Rouquette A, Martinez V, Rabuel C, Prince N, Laplanche JL, Nizard R, Bergmann JF, Perrot S, Lloret-Linares C. Acute pain Factors predictive of post-operative pain and opioid requirement in multimodal analgesia following knee replacement. Eur J Pain 2016;20(5):822–32.
54. Vranceanu AM, Bachoura A, Weening A, Vrahas M, Smith RM, Ring D. Psychological factors predict disability and pain intensity after skeletal trauma. J Bone Joint Surg Am 2014;96(3):e20.
55. Vranceanu AM, Beks RB, Guitton TG, Janssen SJ, Ring D. How do orthopaedic surgeons address psychological aspects of illness? Arch Bone Jt Surg 2017;5(1):2–9.
56. Vranceanu AM, Hageman M, Strooker J, ter Meulen D, Vrahas M, Ring D. A preliminary RCT of a mind body skills based intervention addressing mood and coping strategies in patients with acute orthopaedic trauma. Injury 2015;46(4):552–7.
57. Vranceanu AM, Jupiter JB, Mudgal CS, Ring D. Predictors of pain intensity and disability after minor hand surgery. J Hand Surg Am 2010;35(6):956–60.
58. Vranceanu AM, Zale E, Funes C, Lin A, Ring D. The Virtual Toolkit for Optimal Recovery; A randomized controlled trial. Presentation at the Society of Behavioral Medicine, April 11th-14th, 2018, New Orleans, LA.
59. Westenberg R, Zale E, Henhuis T, Ozkan S, Lee S, Chen N, Ring D, Vranceanu AM. Does a brief mindfulness exercise improve outcomes in upper extremity patients? A randomized controlled trial. Clin Orthop Relat Res 2018;476(4):790–8.
60. Wilhelm M, Reiman M, Goode A, Richardson W, Brown C, Vaughn D, Cook C. Psychological predictors of outcomes with lumbar spinal fusion: a systematic literature review. Physiother Res Int 2017;22(2).
61. YouTube. Pain relief. 2017. https://youtu.be/Tt52qS5Zttk.

CHAPTER 22

Children's Pain After Surgery

Renee C.B. Manworren and G. Allen Finley

Dr. Joanne Eland was a pioneer for eliminating the disparities in recognition and treatment of children's pain. In 1977, her research compared the treatment of pain after equivalent operative procedures performed on adults and children [11]. This seminal publication was the first to describe medical maltreatment of children as a result of pain-processing myths and treatment fears. Of 25 children (4 to 8 years old), only 12 received any analgesics after surgery and those 12 received a total of 24 analgesic doses. The treatment disparity is self-evident when you compare her findings from a group of 18 adults who received 372 opioid doses and 299 nonopioid analgesics after surgery. Dr. Eland continued to advocate for children by disseminating knowledge to debunk myths and break down barriers to ensure optimal and equitable treatment of children's pain. She was a strong voice for developmentally nonverbal, preverbal, marginalized, and ignored children suffering with pain. Her message remains powerful, as it is echoed by those of us inspired by Dr. Eland to treat the pain of others with enduring human kindness.

This chapter is dedicated to her memory and legacy.

Ironically in 1985—nearly a decade after Dr. Eland's seminal paper—one of the authors (R.C.B.M.) witnessed first-hand the continued dramatic disparity in the recognition and treatment of children's pain through the experience of advocating for adequate analgesia for her own daughter after open-heart surgery. She had entrusted the care of her fragile infant to intelligent, educated, and caring health care professionals who did not prioritize treatment of pain after surgery. We must continue to advocate and pursue rigorous scientific inquiry and knowledge translation to optimize pain treatment and relieve the suffering of our vulnerable patients—the world's children and our future. In this chapter, we survey the tools at our disposal, highlight the clinical challenges that remain, and call for the vigorous pursuit of knowledge to overcome barriers to state-of-the-art and humane treatment of children's pain after surgery.

SCOPE OF THE PROBLEM

An estimated 4 million children undergo surgery each year in the United States, but only 300,000 are hospitalized for their procedure [48,49]. Despite advances in surgical techniques including minimally invasive approaches, at least 60% of children who have surgery are likely to report moderate to severe pain [22] and more than 5% will have persistent pain after surgery [13,23,41,38]. Clinical practice guidelines for the treatment of children's pain after surgery have been developed by the American Pain Society, American Academy of Pediatrics, American Society of Anesthesiologists, Association of Paediatric Anaesthetists of Great Britain and

Ireland, Royal College of Nursing, and others around the world [9]. These guidelines provide recommendations for assessing and treating children's pain after surgery. They also describe a dearth of good quality evidence to support many recommendations, disparities in the quantity and quality of evidence for assessing and treating pain after surgery in children as compared with adults, and the need for research focused on children's pain after surgery. This chapter will highlight some established care practices and challenge the foundational knowledge supporting certain approaches to pain management after pediatric surgery.

ASSESSMENT

Tissue injury inflicted by even the most minimally invasive surgical technique typically produces pain. However, objective bedside measures of tissue damage that correlate with human pain experiences do not yet exist. Therefore, recognition and assessment of pain continues to rely primarily on patient self-report. Developmentally appropriate methods to elicit self-report of pain presence, location, and intensity have been validated as reliable measures of children's pain after surgery. Simple numeric rating scales (NRSs) of pain intensity are valid for use with most children 8 years of age and older who can understand numeric rank and order [9]. Children's self-reported pain ratings using NRS, visual analogue scale (VAS), and the Faces pain scale-revised (FPS-R) correlate, although children tend to report higher pain ratings when pain is assessed with the NRS [46,52]. Pictorial adaptations of the VAS with faces, such as the Wong-Baker FACES scale, Oucher, and FPS-R, have been validated for children as young as 3 to 4 years of age to facilitate their self-report of pain intensity [46]. Children 6 to 16 years of age prefer the FPS-R to the NRS for reporting pain intensity in clinical settings [32]. Health care professionals have expressed a preference for pain assessment tools based on a 0 to 10 scale and use of a common metric to make pain scores easier to compare and interpret [51]. However, the developmental appropriateness, need, and interpretable meaning of offering 11 choices of pain intensity to a child are questionable, especially considering that the faces scales continue to offer only six choices but were renumbered to provide only the even number choices of the 0 to 10 metric.

Pain measurement after surgery is generally limited to assessing the intensity of children's pain; however, pain assessment after surgery should emphasize the multidimensional nature of pain. Pain is a biopsychosocial phenomenon with sensory, cognitive, developmental, behavioral, emotional, spiritual, and cultural dimensions. Each individual able to self-report pain learns the meaning of pain through tissue injury experiences, such as surgery. Pain assessment tools anchored with smiling and crying faces, such as the Wong-Baker FACES pain scale, have been criticized as potentially confounding a measure of pain intensity with a measure of pain affect [46]. However, the affective dimension of pain is also important for assessing and treating pain after surgery. Unfortunately, health care professionals and parents continue to marginalize children's self-reports of pain when intensity assessed using validated, developmentally matched pain assessment tools is incongruent with apparent or expected tissue damage, behavior, and/or function. The subjectivity of pain assessment remains a significant barrier to optimal recognition and treatment of children's pain after surgery.

Inability to self-report pain (e.g., in infants, young children, and individuals with deficits that impair communication) does not prevent or negate the experience of pain after surgery. There is ample evidence that even extremely premature neonates experience pain after surgery and that infants are actually more sensitive to painful stimuli and have reduced pain tolerance than children and adults [12,17,19,20,42]. Pain perception depends on complex neuronal interactions that include nociceptive transmission, modulation, and suppression. Inflammation after surgery may intensify nociceptive input and elicit a neuroplastic response, causing physical changes to individual neurons, interneuron communication, and remapping at the cortical and whole-brain level [6,15,16,40,53]. Noxious stimuli experienced during the neonatal period may trigger long-term epigenetic changes that affect neurodevelopment and pain reactivity. Neuroplasticity from early or repeated exposure to pain after surgery may result in a maladaptive reorganization of the peripheral and central nervous system, brain microstructure and function, stress responses including stress-sensitive behaviors, and neurodevelopment. Postsurgical infants and children who are unable to self-report are more vulnerable to pain given their frequent exposures, insufficient cognitive ability to evaluate the meaning of their pain experience, and inability to prevent pain and seek pain management interventions and treatments.

Valid and reliable pain assessment tools provide a proxy measure of pain after surgery for infants, preverbal children, and other children unable to provide self-report [18]. These tools are indirect measures of pain that quantify behavioral and physiologic responses to pain-related distress. Responses to pain are influenced by contextual factors, such as site and technique of surgery, severity of illness, physiologic stability, gestational age, temperament, and developmental ability to control behavior. Therefore, scores from these pain assessment tools are proxy measures that must be interpreted based on expected or potential tissue damage.

New approaches to pain assessment after surgery include patient-reported outcomes measurement information systems (e.g., PROMIS) and the use of mobile apps. These psychometrically sound, validated, person-centered measures are designed to enhance communication and help assess, evaluate, and monitor physical, social, and emotional symptoms of health and function [24,31,44]. Self-report and proxy PROMIS pain measures are available for children 8 to 17 and 5 to 17 years of age, respectively [31]. Apps to monitor pain and function after surgery are commercially available, but health care professionals for the most part have been minimally involved in the development, testing, and validation of currently available pain assessment and management apps [24,44].

Despite valid and reliable pain assessment tools for children and improvements in pain assessment practices, moderate to severe pain that delays functional recovery after surgery is common. Moreover, there are no objective, validated measures of functional recovery from surgery, and self-report measures lack rigorous validation [30,37]. Therefore, the content of procedure-specific pediatric pain assessment tools and/or the translation of clinical assessment research are insufficient for providing meaningful, procedure- and person-specific measurement of children's pain after surgery. The same point is made concerning pain after surgery in adults, in other chapters and the introduction to this volume. Objective biomarkers are needed and must continue to be pursued through rigorous scientific inquiry. Hopefully, objective measures that are sensitive to individual variability in pain sensitivity, pain history, and analgesic response will help overcome the psychosocial and developmental barriers to optimal pain treatment of children after surgery. Further evidence of the need for more sensitive and specific objectives measures to assess pain in children after surgery will be presented below in the treatment section of this chapter.

TREATMENT

Effective pain management after surgery requires ongoing assessment of pain presence, intensity, and response to treatment. Although guidelines may recommend starting doses of drugs for pain control, individual variation is huge, and the clinical practice of using predetermined cut points on NRS, VAS, or Faces pain scales puts children at risk for oversedation, respiratory depression, and poor pain management after surgery [35]. The accepted minimal clinically significant difference in pain scores currently associated with pain relief in school-aged children is only 1 number change on the 0 to 10 metric. The magnitude of this single number change will rarely represent a reduction in pain from severe or moderate to mild or complete pain relief [2,50].

Nonpharmacologic and Biobehavioral Treatments

Systematic reviews, clinical trials, and descriptive studies provide some support for age and developmentally appropriate nondrug and biobehavioral interventions such as skin-to-skin care, sucrose or other sweet solutions, breastfeeding, music, distraction, intraoperative suggestion, guided imagery, hypnosis, relaxation, massage, thermal therapies (for example, ice, cold, and heat application), transcutaneous electrical nerve stimulation (TENS), acupuncture, and other interventions to treat brief procedural pain in children [4,5,10,21,36,43,54]. Evidence for these interventions is inconsistent, and the models studied rarely include pain after surgery. However, reports of harm or increased risk of adverse effects from these interventions are also rare [9].

Evidence suggests differences in the efficacy of specific nonpharmacologic and biobehavioral interventions when used with adults and children, again reinforcing the old adage that children are not just little adults [9]. Overall, most trials that evaluated outcomes related to anxiety or emotional well-being report a positive effect from nonpharmacologic and biobehavioral interventions in both adults and children. Some nonpharmacologic and biobehavioral interventions help children cope with pain, manage pain-related fear and anxiety, and decrease pain-related behaviors. However, there is little evidence that nonpharmacologic and biobehavioral interventions are adequate as an *alternative* to appropriate pharmacologic analgesics to manage children's pain after surgery. This may explain why nondrug therapies have not been routinely adopted in clinical practice. More research is required to understand their role in combination with multimodal pharmacologic therapy.

Pharmacologic Treatment

Earlier chapters in this volume as well as many monographs present the current understanding of the pathophysiologic mechanisms of postoperative pain. Traditionally, pain after surgery has been considered acute and nociceptive as opposed to chronic and neuropathic [34]. Recent translational research and treatment trends, however, advocate for postoperative use of medications that were previously reserved for chronic and/or neuropathic pain management, such as ketamine, gabapentin, and pregabalin [9]. These trends have been stimulated by desires for a more mechanism-based approach to analgesia, to decrease opioid use after surgery with its side effects and to reduce the occurrence of persistent pain after surgery. Chronic neuropathic pain is frequently caused by peripheral nerve injury and characterized by dysesthesias, allodynia (pain from a normally nonpainful stimulus), and hyperalgesia (increased pain intensity from a painful stimulus). However, injury from surgical procedures can also precipitate mechanical allodynia and thermal hyperalgesia. Current evidence suggests that hyperalgesia is a consequence of somatosensory stimulation and perturbation of the nociceptive system with peripheral and/or central sensitization [34]. Clinically, sensitization, or the increased responsiveness of nociceptive neurons to their normal input and/or recruitment of a response to subthreshold afferent input, may only be inferred from observations of hyperalgesia or allodynia. These definitions may change as our knowledge of pain mechanisms advances.

Acetaminophen, NSAIDS, opioids, local anesthetics, and combinations of these medications are routinely used to treat children's pain after surgery, even though few systematic reviews, trials, and descriptive studies of drugs used to treat pain after surgery include pediatric patients [9]. For drug classes with well-understood analgesic properties and mechanisms of action (e.g., μ-opioid agonists or local anesthetics), clinical effectiveness in children more than 2 years of age is considered comparable with that of adults [3]. However, pediatric efficacy and safety studies are needed when the mechanism of action or efficacy of the drug is not well established and for patients under 2 years of age.

Has multimodal analgesia including nonanalgesic pharmacologic interventions resulted in reliable and desired self-report and objective outcomes, such as decreased pain intensity, improved function, and reduced need for opioids or rescue drugs? Will this multimodal approach prevent persistent pain after surgery? Do the benefits from these additional medications outweigh the risks of adverse effects and the dangers of polypharmacy? More research is needed to determine the benefits and risks of multimodal therapy to treat children's pain after surgery, including the early postoperative use of medications previously reserved for chronic and neuropathic pain.

In an effort to optimize pain relief for children, clinical practice guidelines and standardized protocols have been developed and tested [28,35]. Like randomized controlled trials, standardized protocols are as effective as a normal distribution would predict. But what about the extremes of the bell curve [26,28]? How should the health care professional approach these vulnerable children and address their pain management needs after surgery? For example, codeine was once the most widely used opiate analgesic to treat pain after surgery in North America and some other areas. Recent recognition of the potential for ultrarapid metabolizers to convert codeine to lethal blood levels of morphine and the ineffectiveness of codeine in null metabolizers has led to widespread efforts to eliminate the use of this analgesic in all children [14], not just those at the extremes of the pharmacogenetic spectrum. Perhaps, as genetic testing increasingly informs personalized medical care, precision medicine approaches will move care from standardized protocols to safe and effective treatment of pain for all children after surgery.

The safety profiles of pharmacologic treatments are especially important, as hospital lengths of stay have decreased and inpatient procedures have moved to the outpatient setting. This trend has shifted care of children's pain after surgery to parents and guardians in unmonitored settings. As expectations for adequate pain control have risen following discharge to home after surgery, opioid prescribing has increased to manage the severe pain children may experience at home [14]. Although there is no clear relationship between short-term postoperative medical use of opioids in children and adolescents and later substance abuse disorders, it is possible that increased opioid misuse, abuse, and addiction may be unintended long-term consequences of the increased amount of opioids prescribed. Furthermore, reported discrepancies between the amounts prescribed and the smaller amounts actually administered for pain after surgery, in both children and adults, are concerning [1,14,25,27,33,39,45].

Parents may be knowledgeable about their children's responsiveness to treatments for common acute pain events, such as bumps and bruises; however, research indicates that parents still routinely undertreat their children's pain at home after surgery [8]. Research on the care of children's pain at home after surgery is difficult and imperfect, typically relying on proxy measures of pain and analgesic use without secondary validation [1,25,27,33,45]. More research and new methods to study children's pain and pain management at home after surgery are needed [8,25].

Despite decades of exciting basic and clinical advances in understanding and treating children's pain, many if not most children still suffer unnecessary pain after surgery or trauma. There remains an unmet need for innovative and effective approaches to implementing the knowledge we already possess, as well as creating new knowledge to expand our understanding and repertoire of management techniques [7,39,47].

REFERENCES

1. Abou-Karam M, Dubé S, Kvann HS, Mollica C, Racine D, Bussières JF, Lebel D, Nguyen C, Thibault M. Parental report of morphine use at home after pediatric surgery. J Pediatr 2015;167:599–604.e12.
2. Bailey B, Daoust R, Doyon-Trottier E, et al. Validation and properties of the verbal numeric scale in children with acute pain. Pain 2010;149:216–21.
3. Berde CB, Walco GA, Krane EJ, Anand KJS, Aranda JV, Craig KD, Dampier CD, Finkel JC, Grabois M, Johnston C, Lantos J, Lebel A, Maxwell LG, McGrath P, Oberlander TF, Schanberg LE, Stevens B, Taddio A, von Baeyer CL, Yaster M, Zempsky WT. Pediatric analgesic clinical trial designs, measures, and extrapolation: report of an FDA scientific workshop. Pediatrics 2012;129:354–64.
4. Bueno M, Stevens B, de Camargo PP, Toma E, Krebs VLJ, Kimura AF. Breast milk and glucose for pain relief in preterm infants: a noninferiority randomized controlled trial. Pediatrics 2012. doi:10.1542/peds.2011-2024.
5. Bueno M, Yamada J, Harrison D, et al. A systematic review and meta-analyses of nonsucrose sweet solutions for pain relief in neonates. Pain Res Manag 2013;18(3):153–61.
6. Burke NN, Finn DP, McGuire BE, Roche M. Psychological stress in early life as a predisposing factor for the development of chronic pain: clinical and preclinical evidence and neurobiological mechanism. J Neurosci Res 2016. doi: 10.1002/jnr.23802.
7. Chorney JM, McGrath P, Finley GA. Pain as the neglected adverse event. CMAJ 2010;182(7):732.
8. Chorney JM, Twycross A, Mifflin K, Archibald K, Can We Improve Parents' Management of their Children's Postoperative Pain at Home? Pain Res Manag 2014;19(4):e115–23. doi:10.1155/2014/938352.
9. (a) Chou R, Gordon DB, de Leon-Casasola OA, et al. Management of postoperative pain: a clinical practice guideline from the American Pain Society, the American Society of Regional Anesthesia and Pain Medicine, and the American Society of Anesthesiologists' Committee on Regional Anesthesia, Executive Committee, and Administrative Council. J Pain 2016;17(2):131–57. (b) The assessment and management of acute pain in infants, children, and adolescents. Pediatrics 2001;108(3):793–7. (c) Apfelbaum JL. Practice guidelines for acute pain management in the perioperative setting: an updated report by the American Society of Anesthesiologists Task Force on Acute Pain Management. Anesthesiology 2012;116(2):248–73. (d) Association of Paediatric Anaesthetists of Great Britain and Ireland. Good practice in postoperative and procedural pain management, 2nd edition. Paediatr Anaesth 2012;(Suppl. 1):1–79.
10. Davidson F, Snow S, Hayden J, Chorney J. Psychological interventions in managing post- operative pain in children: a systematic review. J Pain 2016;157(9):1872–86 [PMID:27355185].
11. Eland JM, Anderson JE. The experience of pain in children. In: Jacox AK, editor. Pain: a source book for nurses and other health professionals. Boston: Little, Brown; 1977. p. 453–73.
12. Fitzgerald M, Beggs S. The neurobiology of pain: developmental aspects. Neuroscientist 2001;7(3):246–57.
13. Fortier MA, Chou J, Maurer EL, et al. Acute to chronic postoperative pain in children: preliminary findings. J Pediatr Surg 2011;46:1700–5.
14. George JA, Park PS, Hunsberger J, Shay JE, Lehmann CU, White ED, Lee BH, Yaster M. An analysis of 34,218 pediatric outpatient controlled substance prescriptions. Anesth Analg 2016;122:807–13.
15. Grunau RE. Neonatal pain in very preterm infants: long-term effects on brain, neurodevelopment and pain reactivity. Rambam Maimonides Med J 2013;4(4):e0025. doi:10.5041/RMMJ.10132 [eCollection 2013].

16. Hatfield LA. Neonatal pain: what's age got to do with it? Surg Neurol Int 2014;5(Suppl. 13):S479–89. doi:10.4103/2152-7806.144630 [eCollection 2014].
17. Hermann C, Hohmeister J, Demirakca S, Zohsel K, Flor H. Long-term alteration of pain sensitivity in school-aged children with early pain experiences. Pain 2006;125(3):278–85.
18. Herr K, Coyne PJ, Manworren RCB, McCaffery M, Merkel S. Pain assessment in the patients unable to self-report: position statement update. Pain Manag Nurs 2011;12(4):230.
19. Hohmeister J, Demirakca S, Zohsel K, Flor H, Hermann C. Responses to pain in school-aged children with experience in a neonatal intensive care unit: cognitive aspects and maternal influences. Eur J Pain 2009;13(1):94–101.
20. Hohmeister J, et al. Cerebral processing of pain in school-aged children with neonatal nociceptive input: an exploratory fMRI study. Pain 2010;150(2):257–67.
21. Johnston C, Campbell-Yeo M, Fernandes A, Inglis D, Streiner D, Zee R. Skin-to-skin care for procedural pain in neonates. Cochrane Database Syst Rev 2014;1:CD008435. doi:10.1002/14651858.CD008435.pub2.
22. Kozlowski LJ, Kost-Byerly S, Colantuoni E, et al. Pain prevalence, intensity, assessment and management in a hospitalized pediatric population. Pain Manag Nurs 2014;15:22–35.
23. Kristensen AD, Ahlburg P, Lauridsen MC, Jensen TS, Nikolajsen L. Chronic pain after inguinal hernia repair in children. Br J Anaesth 2012;109(4):603–8.
24. Lalloo C, Jibb LA, Rivera J, et al. "There's a Pain App for That": review of patient-targeted smartphone applications for pain management. Clin J Pain 2015;31:557–63.
25. Manworren RCB, Gilson AM. Nurses' role in preventing prescription opioid diversion. Am J Nurs 2015;115(8):34–40. http://journals.lww.com/ajnonline/Abstract/2015/08000/CE___Nurses__Role_in_Preventing_Prescription.21.aspx
26. Manworren RCB, Jeffries L, Pantaleao A, Seip R, Zempsky WT, Ruaño G. Pharmacogenetic testing for analgesic adverse effects: pediatric case series. Clin J Pain 2016;32(2):109–15. doi:10.1097/AJP.0000000000000236. http://www.ncbi.nlm.nih.gov/pubmed/25803758.
27. Manworren RCB, Karamessinis L, Cooper J. Home management of children's pain after laparoscopic appendectomy: unexpected findings [abstract]. J Pain 2013;14(4):S38.
28. Manworren RCB, McElligott CD, Deraska PV, Santanelli J, Blair S, Ruscher KA, Weiss R, Rader C, Finck C, Bourque M, Campbell B. Efficacy analysis of analgesic treatments to manage children's post-operative pain after laparoscopic appendectomy: retrospective medical record review. AORN J 2016;103(3):317.e1–e11. http://www.ncbi.nlm.nih.gov/pubmed/26924376.
29. McCabe SE, Veliz P, Schulenberg JE. Adolescent context of exposure to prescription opioids and substance use disorder symptoms at age 35: a national longitudinal study. Pain 2016;157(10):2173–8.
30. McGrath PJ, Walco GA, Turk DC, Dworkin RH, Brown MT, Davidson K, Eccleston C, Finley GA, Goldschneider K, Haverkos L, Hertz SH, Ljungman G, Palermo T, Rappaport BA, Rhodes T, Schechter N, Scott J, Sethna N, Svensson OK, Stinson J, von Baeyer CL, Walker L, Weisman S, White RE, Zajicek A, Zeltzer L. Core outcome domains and measures for pediatric acute and chronic/recurrent pain clinical trials: PedIMMPACT recommendations. J Pain 2008;9:771–83.
31. Northwestern University. PROMIS (patient-reported outcomes measurement information system), National Institutes of Health grant U2C CA186878 01. 2016. http://www.healthmeasures.net/resource-center/about-us.
32. Pagé MG, Katz J, Stinson J, et al. Validation of the numerical rating scale for pain intensity and unpleasantness in pediatric acute postoperative pain: sensitivity to change over time. J Pain 2012;13:359–69.
33. Pantaleo A, Cooper J, Karamessinis L, Manworren RCB. Monitoring home pain management after laparoscopic appendectomy [abstract]. J Pain 2015;16(4):S3.
34. Part III: Pain terms, a current list with definitions and notes on usage (pp. 209–214), Classification of chronic pain, 2nd ed. In: Merskey H, Bogduk N, editors. Task Force on Taxonomy. Seattle: IASP Press; 1994.
35. Pasero C, Quinlan-Colwell A, Rae D, et al. American Society for Pain Management Nursing position statement: prescribing and administering opioid doses based solely on pain intensity. Pain Manag Nurs 2016;17:170–80.
36. Pillai Riddell RR, Racine NM, Gennis HG, Turcotte K, Uman LS, Horton RE, Ahola Kohut S, Hillgrove Stuart J, Stevens B, Lisi DM. Non-pharmacological management of infant and young child procedural pain (Review). Cochrane Database Syst Rev 2015(12):CD006275. doi:10.1002/14651858.CD006275.pub3.
37. Rabbitts JA, Aaron RV, Zempsky WT, Palermo TM. Validation of the youth acute pain functional ability questionnaire in children and adolescents undergoing inpatient surgery. J Pain 2017;18(10):1209–15. doi:10.1016/j.jpain.2017.05.004.

38. Rabbitts JA, Zhou C, Groenewald CB, Durkin L, Palermo TM. Trajectories of postsurgical pain in children: risk factors and impact of late pain recovery on long-term health outcomes after major surgery. Pain 2015;156(11):2383–9. doi:10.1097/j.pain.0000000000000281 [PMID:26381701].
39. Schechter NL, Finley GA, Bright NS, Laycock M, Forgeron PA. ChildKind: a global initiative to reduce pain in children. Pediatr Pain Lett 2010;12(3):27–30. http://childpain.org/ppl/issues/v12n3_2010/v12n3_schechter.pdf.
40. Seifert F, Maihöfner C. Functional and structural imaging of pain-induced neuroplasticity. Curr Opin Anaesthesiol 2011;24:515–23.
41. Sieberg CB, Simons LE, Edelstein MR, et al. Pain prevalence and trajectories following pediatric spinal fusion surgery. J Pain 2013;14(12):1694–702. doi:10.1016/j.jpain.2013.09.005.
42. Slater R, et al. Premature infants display increased noxious-evoked neuronal activity in the brain compared to healthy age-matched term-born infants. Neuroimage 2010;52(2):583–9.
43. Stevens B, Yamada J, Gy L, Ohlsson A. Sucrose for analgesia in newborn infants undergoing painful procedures. Cochrane Database Syst Rev 2013(1). doi:CD001069\r10.1002/14651858.CD001069.
44. Stinson J, Huguet A, McGrath P, et al. A qualitative review of the psychometric properties and feasibility of electronic headache diaries for children and adults: where we are and where we need to go. Pain Res Manag 2013;18:142–52.
45. Thibault M, Lebel D, Nguyen C. Opioids after discharge in pediatric patients. Anesth Analg 2016;122:2064.
46. Tomlinson D, von Baeyer CL, Stinson JN, et al, A systematic review of faces scales for the self-report of pain intensity in children. Pediatrics 2010;126:e1168–98.
47. Twycross A, Forgeron P, Chorney J, Backman C, Finley GA. Pain as the neglected patient safety concern: five years on. J Child Health Care 2016;20(4):537–41.
48. U.S. Department of Health and Human Services, Centers for Disease Control and Prevention. Ambulatory surgery in the United States. 2006. National Health Statistics Reports. http://www.cdc.gov/nchs/data/nhsr/nhsr011.pdf.
49. U.S. Department of Health and Human Services, Centers for Disease Control and Prevention: National Health Statistics Reports. Health, United States, 2015. DHHS Publication No. 2016-1232. http://www.cdc.gov/nchs/hus.htm.
50. Voepel-Lewis T, Burke CN, Jeffreys N, et al. Do 0-10 numeric rating scores translate into clinically meaningful pain measures for children? Anesth Analg 2011;112:415–21.
51. von Baeyer CL. Children's self-report of pain intensity: what we know, where we are headed. Pain Res Manag 2009;14(1):39–45.
52. vonBaeyer CL, Spagrud LJ, McCormick JC, et al, Three new datasets supporting use of the Numerical Rating Scale (NRS-11) for children's self- reports of pain intensity. Pain 2009;143:223–7.
53. Walker SM. Translational studies identify long-term impact of prior neonatal pain experience. Pain 2017;158:S29–42.
54. Wilkinson DJC, Savulescu J, Slater R. Sugaring the pill: ethics and uncertainties in the use of sucrose for newborn infants. Arch Pediatr Adolesc Med 2012;166(7):629–33.

CHAPTER 23

Postoperative Pain Control for Older Persons

Babita Ghai, Jeetinder Kaur Makkar, and Dipika Bansal

Acute postoperative pain is experienced in 80% of patients of whom less than half report adequate analgesia [3,18]. Data sampled from developed countries such as the United States and the Netherlands indicate that 41% to 69% of persons report experiencing moderate to severe postoperative pain [18,53].

Extensive literature is available on the challenges involved in aiming for and achieving optimal postoperative pain control; much of this literature is reviewed in other chapters of this volume. Relatively few studies relate this issue in older persons [6]. Older persons (≥65 years) are the fastest growing segment of the population worldwide, constituting a sixth or a seventh of the total population of the United Kingdom and United States, a figure that is projected to reach one in four by 2050 [43,56]. The likelihood of undergoing a surgical procedure is 1.6 to 3 times higher in older versus younger adults [33]. Furthermore, medical (e.g., oncologic) and surgical advances have contributed to improvement in quality of life and longer survival [44]. By 2025, people aged >75 years will compose 10% of the total population and many will require surgical care [47].

Despite concurrent advances in analgesic techniques and agents, many older persons still experience unacceptable levels of postoperative pain [9]. Improving this situation is crucial, as inadequate pain control after surgery may have significant functional, cognitive, emotional, and societal consequences and also increase the risk of chronic postsurgical pain (CPSP) [12,16].

AGING AND PHYSIOLOGY

Aging is individualized, is progressive, and involves multiple changes occurring at molecular, structural, and functional levels [16]. Broadly speaking, older persons have limited physiologic reserves and compromised compensatory mechanisms. The functional and behavioral consequences of these changes are difficult to predict. Postoperative pain management in older patients is complicated by age-related physiologic changes; potential alterations in pharmacokinetics and pharmacodynamics of analgesics; a diversity of pain perception and assessment methods; frequent comorbidities including the possibility of cognitive impairment; and drug interactions because of polytherapy [12].

PHARMACOKINETIC AND PHARMACODYNAMIC CHANGES

Aging is associated with reduced muscle mass, increased body fat, and reduced body water. These changes increase the volume of distribution (Vd) of lipophilic analgesics such as lidocaine and fentanyl, which in turn can delay the onset of action and elimination rate, thereby prolonging their duration of action [16]. Conversely, the Vd of hydrophilic analgesics such as morphine and hydromorphone decreases, resulting in higher plasma levels after similar doses. These higher plasma levels may increase the analgesic effect along with undesired side effects.

Aging is associated with gradual deterioration of functional capacities of all organ systems. Reduced hepatic function diminishes first-pass metabolism of drugs such as lidocaine and opioids. This decrease in metabolism increases their bioavailability compared with similar doses in younger persons. Chronic hepatic disease typically necessitates a reduction in drug doses or prolongation of interdose interval to avoid sudden rises in blood concentrations after bolus administration and prolonged high levels, with heightened risk of adverse drug effects [38,48].

Age-related reduction in renal drug clearance leads to accumulation of drugs and metabolites that are renally excreted and hence prolongs their effects [16]. The amount and frequency of dosing may require adjustment to accumulation to toxic levels, especially for drugs such as morphine, which have renally excreted bioactive metabolites [29,38,48].

Older persons may be more susceptible to the adverse effects of centrally acting drugs such as antidepressants, antiepileptic drugs, and antipsychotics, which are used as analgesics or concurrently administered with analgesics [55]. It has been suggested that older persons do not become tolerant to the effects of opioids as quickly as younger patients [7]. Hence, drug kinetic and dynamic changes with aging give rise to predictable changes that must be anticipated and monitored with vigilance.

AGING AND NOCICEPTION

Aging brings neuroanatomical, physiologic, and biochemical variations in the nociceptive pathways. These include selective loss of myelinated peripheral nerve fibers, signs of axonal involution, and reduced nerve conduction velocity and endoneural blood flow [57]. There is age-related decline in GABA and serotonin receptors, whereas receptor affinity is increased resulting in greater therapeutic efficacy as well as adverse events. These changes may lead to declines in pain threshold and pain tolerance [55].

CLINICAL EVALUATION

A targeted pain history is required as part of the postoperative pain control plan to document preexisting pain and other comorbidities relevant to postoperative treatment [22,25,41]. Preoperative cognitive, renal, and hepatic functions must be assessed owing to their importance for pharmacokinetics and pharmacodynamics. Medication history may reveal drugs that alter cardiac or ventilatory function. Preoperative opioid use may result in tolerance to its analgesic effects, by definition requiring higher doses to achieve the desired effect perioperatively compared with opioid-naïve patients [16,25]. Physical examination regarding patient's ability to move, communicate, and display satisfactory short-term memory allows identification and documentation of focal or diffuse neurologic deficits including those that may be provoked by anesthetic agents. Appropriate laboratory investigations must be performed to document baseline vital organ functioning relevant to pain and pain-related dysfunction [25].

PAIN ASSESSMENT

Barriers to Pain Assessment

Misconceptions, lack of communication, and cognitive impairment are three major barriers to adequate pain assessment in older persons [22]. One persistent misconception is the belief that pain is an expected and natural consequence of aging. Furthermore, older persons are assumed to experience less pain than their younger counterparts [9]. However, pain perception does not decrease with age [5]. An older person may interpret pain as heralding severe pathology including impending death or as provoking yet more pain due to additional blood sampling, invasive diagnostic investigations, and prolonged hospitalization [24]. Thus, they may act stoically and not show pain behaviors. Postoperative delirium and/or dementia can occur in 10% to 70% patients, which may both indicate poor pain control and impede effective pain control if pain intensity or improvement is reported inconsistently [49].

Assessment Instruments

Pain can be assessed by self-report, behavioral, and physiologic measures. Self-reporting is the gold standard and should be used in elderly capable of understanding the task and communicating effectively. Evaluation of pain-reporting ability, measurement, and documentation of pain is essential. Dynamic pain relief (i.e., the ability of patient to cough or otherwise move without being stopped by pain) should be taken as an endpoint of analgesic adequacy [16]. Frequent reassessment of pain may be required as the postoperative analgesic regimen is titrated and side effects, identified and dealt with.

Various unidimensional scales such as verbal descriptive scale (VDS), numerical rating scale (NRS), and faces pain scale (FPS) have acceptable validity and reliability in elderly. NRS and VDS are preferred by older adults [14,47]. Use of NRS is a good first choice for this population. For patients with mild dementia, VDS is a better measure [17]. Both the VDS and FPS [23] have acceptable validity and reliability in elderly. Although the visual analogue scale (VAS) is relatively easy to use, difficulties have been reported with its use by older adults, leading to reduced validity and a high rate of unscorable data [23].

Self reported pain assessment tools should be attempted at first even in severely demented patients. Observer assessment should be used only if self-reported tools are found unsuccessful. Several observer-based tools use behavioral signs as pain proxies. Most structured tools rely on six major domains of pain: facial expression, body language and negative vocalization, changes in interpersonal interactions, changes in activity patterns, and mental status changes. However, interpreting these tools may be challenging because of their overlap with common behavioral symptoms such as anxiety, depression or disorientation [27]. Thus, validation of such tools remains problematic in severely demented patients. A recent systematic review of eight reviews reported 28 different behavioral pain assessment tools developed for use in cognitively impaired elderly patients. However, their validity, reliability, and clinical testing are incompletely characterized [32].

TREATMENT

An individualized approach tailored to the patient and context is optimal. The postoperative pain plan should be developed preoperatively through shared decision-making with the patient and family in written or electronic form for all care providers to access [41]. It should be multimodal and opioid-sparing [12,41], using nonpharmacologic and pharmacologic modalities including integrative techniques as feasible [12,24].

Multimodal Analgesia

As described in several other chapters in this volume, multimodal analgesia ("balanced analgesia") works on the principle of using an array of techniques and/or drugs having different sites/mechanisms of action to minimize doses of each component and thereby achieve a high benefit-to-risk ratio [30]. These regimens should take into consideration the presence of any preexisting medical conditions, type of surgery, effects and side effects of individual medications to be administered postoperatively, and the patient's previous experience with analgesic drugs for acute pain management [8]. A specific version of this technique has yielded improved outcomes following day surgical procedures as well as complex operations in older patients [21]. It is based on choosing acetaminophen and/or nonsteroidal anti-inflammatory drugs (NSAIDs) for low-intensity pain and adding opioids and/or local analgesic techniques for moderate to high intensity pain [9]. The best outcomes are achieved with pain management initiated preoperatively and continued in for 3 to 7 days postoperatively [59].

Nonpharmacologic Modalities

Modalities such as transcutaneous electrical nerve stimulation (TENS), acupuncture, music therapy, massage, hot or cold packs, etc., are safe adjuvant therapies, albeit with limited evidence of effectiveness when pain is moderate to severe [12]. Psychosocial therapies such as self-management education and cognitive–behavioral therapy are also useful postoperatively [12]. TENS applied at specific acupuncture points is reported to be effective in reducing postoperative opioid requirement in elderly patients after total hip arthroplasty [31].

Pharmacologic Therapies

General Considerations

As described earlier, physiologic changes in older persons increase their sensitivity to the effects and side effects of analgesic medications, resulting in a need for downward dose adjustment. However, the analgesic dosages should always be titrated to the individual's response. It is advisable "to start low and go slow" with close monitoring during incremental dosing [9,16]. Use of the intramuscular (IM) route for opioid administration may be risky in older persons because of muscle wasting and increased fatty tissue [38,48]. Not only should the IM route be avoided but in general it is best to switch to the most noninvasive feasible route of drug delivery, i.e., oral administration [9].

Nonopioid Analgesics

This analgesic group includes acetaminophen, NSAIDs, and coxibs. Nonopioid analgesics are considered appropriate alone for treating mild to (some cases of) moderate postoperative pain and in combination with opioids and/or local anesthetic techniques for moderate to severe postoperative pain [2].

Besides their opioid-sparing effect [51], benefits of using nonopioid analgesics in postoperative older patients compared with opioids are that the former do not produce respiratory depression, sedation, or slow gastric motility. A major limitation is their ceiling effect with increasing doses.

Acetaminophen/Paracetamol

Acetaminophen (paracetamol) is the first-line drug for postoperative pain treatment. It is used alone for mild-to-moderate pain in the elderly [9]. Its use with NSAIDs decreases the opioids requirement by 20% [9]. The maximum recommended safe dosage over 24 hours is 4 g in healthy older adults and 2 to 3 g in frail elderly because of their increased risk for hepatotoxicity [1]. Its onset of action is 5 minutes and peak plasma concentrations are attained within 15 minutes of intravenous administration of drug [9,34,39]. Dose adjustment is not generally required for mild-to-moderate renal impairment [13]. Caution is dictated, however, when using it in patients with liver disease. The most serious adverse effect of acute overdose is dose-dependent hepatic necrosis.

NSAIDs

NSAIDs inhibit prostaglandin synthesis both at peripheral and central sites by inhibiting cyclooxygenase (COX) isoenzymes. Intravenous formulations of NSAIDs are a standard part of multimodal analgesia [16,25,28,37], as well as decreasing opioid requirements in patients with moderate to severe postoperative pain [22]. Although increased incidence of adverse events and side effects warrants cautious use in elderly, short-term administration of NSAIDs during the immediate postoperative period is shown to be generally safe, particularly in otherwise persons undergoing procedures not associated with risk of bleeding or renal dysfunction [58]. Because older age, male gender, appreciable blood loss, the use of pressors, and presence of diabetes mellitus and other risk factors have been identified as predictors of postoperative (usually reversible) renal insufficiency, it is advisable to use the lowest effective dose for the shortest duration and have a low threshold to investigate and address side effects including gastrointestinal bleeding, nephrotoxicity, and delirium.

Opioid Analgesics

Opioids are a cornerstone for management of moderate to severe postoperative pain [2,16]. In appropriately selected subjects, they provide a safe and effective means of analgesia. Unlike NSAIDs and acetaminophen, opioids do not have ceiling effect and can provide profound pain relief by gradual escalation of dose. The parenteral route is commonly used postoperatively: intravenous administration by nurse-administered bolus or patient-controlled analgesia (PCA). Epidural opioids are also commonly given for the initial 24 to 48 hours postoperatively. The basic principle of safe opioid administration in elderly is to decrease the usual starting dose by 25% to 50% with upward titration based on patient's response with vigilant monitoring of side effects particularly respiratory depression but also sedation, nausea and vomiting, urinary retention, and constipation [2,16]. There is major interindividual variation in analgesic response to, and dosage requirements for, postoperative opioids. Ongoing opioid consumption must be scrutinized and individualized.

Furthermore, a clear plan for opioid tapering should be in place to avoid unnecessarily prolonged therapy postdischarge. Morphine, hydromorphone, and fentanyl are the most commonly used opioids for postoperative pain management [19].

Morphine

The principal pharmacokinetic changes of morphine in older persons include a decrease in Vd, clearance and protein binding, thus prolonging elimination half-life (~4.9 hours) [45]. Hence, elderly patients frequently experience more complete and longer-lasting pain relief with standard, default doses given to younger adults, and the use of smaller starting doses must be considered for older patients. For example, a "younger" elderly patient aged 65 years might safely have his/her moderate to severe acute pain titrated using bolus doses of 2 to 3 mg every 5 minutes in the PACU [4]. However, in "older" elderly patients (≥90 years), bolus dosing should not exceed 1 mg and the interdose interval between two boluses should be lengthened [2].

A major active metabolite of morphine, morphine-6-glucuronide, also produces analgesia and sedation. It is produced in the liver and excreted renally and hence may accumulate in patients with renal compromise. In the absence of dosage reductions, patients with decreased renal function are at risk for opioid-related adverse effects. Sedation is a useful herald and marker of respiratory depression in medically monitored patients of all ages. Supplemental oxygen for at least first 48 hours after the surgery reduces the risk of postoperative hypoxia [2]. A previously held belief that this practice jeopardized patients with pulmonary disease who relied on their baseline hypoxia to stimulate ventilatory drive has largely been abandoned.

Hydromorphone

Hydromorphone, 7.5 to 10 times more potent than morphine, is an effective alternative to morphine for moderate to severe pain. It has a rapid onset of action (5 minutes after intravenous injection), although its maximum effect may not be achieved for as long as 20 minutes. Active metabolites of hydromorphone have neuroexcitatory effects but no analgesic action, in contrast to those of morphine. It is not metabolized by the cytochrome P450 pathway and is less subject to drug–drug interactions. It can be used short-term in patients with renal failure and after organ transplantation [26].

Fentanyl

Fentanyl is a synthetic μ (or morphine receptor)–selective opioid with many desirable physicochemical properties, including a high lipophilicity and predictable pharmacokinetics. Intravenous fentanyl has stood the test of time as a valuable formulation for perioperative pain management. It has fewer adverse hemodynamic effects and no clinically relevant active metabolites during acute use. Some patients treated long-term with transdermal fentanyl developed signs and symptoms of adverse excitatory effects of the metabolite norfentanyl. It remains the opioid of choice in patients with renal failure particularly those having acute pain and breakthrough cancer pain [54].

Tramadol

Tramadol is an atypical centrally acting opioid. It is effective for mild-to-moderate pain. Its use is associated with lesser degrees of constipation and respiratory depression compared with other opioids. The highest daily recommended dosage is 400 mg/day. It has an active metabolite, which is also an analgesic. This metabolite is excreted renally, and its elimination is also decreased in liver failure. Therefore, lower doses of the parent compound should be used in patients with hepatic or renal compromise [1]. It is also advisable to increase the duration between doses in patients >75 years. Caution is warranted in patients with a history of seizures, as lowering of the seizure threshold is an adverse effect. A "serotonin syndrome" with tachycardia and hypertension has been observed in some patients and patients concurrently taking serotonin reuptake inhibitors and the drug is contraindicated in patients taking monoamine oxidase (MAO) inhibitors. A slow upward titration of dose appears to result in less nausea and vomiting [2].

Opioid-Induced Adverse Effects

Because opioid-induced adverse effects are common and potentially lethal (i.e., hypoventilation) in the acute postoperative phase, patients must be monitored and treated with diligence. In this era of short-stay surgery, the most frequent and troublesome side effects involve the gastrointestinal system: nausea, vomiting, and constipation. Nausea may also occur because of slow gastric motility, increased vestibular sensitivity, or increased activity at the chemoreceptor trigger zone [2].

Constipation if unattended by may lead to fecal impaction and, as a result, nausea. During the recuperative phase, all patients including older people must be encouraged to advance their physical activity and fluid intake as prophylaxis for constipation. For optimal discharge planning (see below) any patient prescribed opioids (not just older patients) should be coprescribed a stimulant laxative, such as senna and a stool softener prophylactically [41]. Recently, other types of medications to treat constipation by blocking peripheral opioid receptors without interfering with opioids' central analgesic actions have become available for postoperative and chronic use.

Other opioid side effects commonly encountered in the acute postoperative phase include sedation, postural hypotension, pruritus, and urinary retention. Last but not least, the risk of respiratory depression has become recognized as extremely significant as postoperative PCA (see below) with opioids has become common, and increasing numbers of patients are monitored for postoperative ventilatory status. This risk—potentially lethal—affects patients of all ages but particularly (for reasons described earlier) older persons. Depending on the resources available in the particular setting, respiratory status should be monitored at a minimum by frequent assessment of sedation, a frequent harbinger of impending ventilator insufficiency, and in resource-rich settings, continuous capnography. The occurrence of unexpected, fatal respiratory compromise in patients lacking risk factors for same has led to the recognition that postoperative respiratory (or sedation) assessment must be provided to all patients, not just those with clear risk factors such as older age, obesity, obstructive sleep apnea, coadministration of benzodiazepines, etc.

Patient-Controlled Analgesia

PCA is a generally safe and effective mode of providing analgesia in older patients with intact cognition. The basic underlying principle is that only the patient can measure the pain intensity and how much analgesic is required to relieve it. Morphine, being cheap and effective, is the preferred drug for PCA. Bolus doses of 1 to 2 mg with a lockout period of 5 to 10 minutes and a 4-hour maximal dosage between 20 and 30 mg are commonly used [40]. Background infusions of morphine are strictly contraindicated in older patients because of age-related changes in pharmacokinetics and pharmacodynamics as described earlier.

Fentanyl PCA is preferred in renally compromised patients because of its rapid redistribution to inactive (e.g., adipose) tissues and consequent short duration of action. The bolus dose range varies from 10 to 50 μg with a lockout interval of 5 minutes [42].

Advantages of PCA include reduced incidence of confusion and pulmonary complications owing to the self-correcting nature of sedation as a limiting factor in self-overdosing [4]. However, use of PCA in older patients has some limitations, starting with their preference to call the nurse to address their needs for ongoing analgesia and lack of comfort in using the device. Patients who are confused preoperatively or have cognitive impairment are at risk of inadequate pain relief secondary to inappropriately infrequent self-dosing. As stressed earlier, the continuous infusion component available with many PCA devices should in general not be used in older persons.

Regional Analgesic Techniques

For operations whose anatomy lends them to regional anesthesia, methods that spatially target nociceptive afferent pathways as opposed to the entire body are a useful component of multimodal pain management for patients of all ages. Providing that local anesthetic blood levels do not approach toxic blood and brain concentrations, these methods rarely interfere with cognition and may actually benefit it by virtue of their analgesic and opioid-sparing effects.

Epidural Analgesia

Epidural analgesia can be administered as boluses, continuous background infusion, or patient-controlled epidural analgesia (PCEA). With progressing age, intervertebral foramina are increasingly filled with bony or fibrous tissue, reducing the volume and compliance of the epidural space. As a result, there is a greater cephalic spread with same volume of drug injected epidurally in older patients. Also, older persons are more sensitive to local anesthetics [52], and thus, it is advisable to use lower volumes in comparison with younger persons. Complications commonly associated with epidural analgesia such as hypotension (particularly in hypovolemic persons soon after surgery), respiratory depression, and motor blockade are more severe in older persons [52]. PCEA using a combination of local anesthetic with opioids can decrease the amount of local anesthetic administered and hence reduce the number of episodes of hypotension. As compared with intravenous PCA, use of PCEA provides better pain relief, bowel activity, and mental status and reduces the risk of postoperative cardiac complications [30,41].

Dilute concentrations of bupivacaine (0.05% to 0.15%) or ropivacaine (0.15% to 0.20%) provide a balance between analgesia and motor block or hypotension [36]. Clearly, a standard PCEA protocol cannot be recommended for postoperative pain control after all surgical procedures in all patients. That said, a default approach to PCEA after many larger procedures such as open abdominal or thoracic procedures in older patients is to provide a background infusion (3 to 6 mL/hour) of a local anesthetic with an opioid, supplemented with a bolus of 2 to 3 mL repeated no sooner than every 15 to 20 minutes [35]. Sensorimotor function and ventilator status should be monitored and treated postoperatively in all patients receiving epidural analgesia whether or not it is patient-controlled and regardless of their age.

Peripheral Nerve Blocks

Peripheral nerve blocks (PNBs) are used extensively in orthopedic and upper limb surgery in older persons. When applicable to the particular surgical anatomy and properly performed, this technique provides prolonged postoperative analgesia without the adverse effects of systemic opioids or epidural analgesia. As described earlier, increased sensitivity to local anesthetics and reduced clearance result in additional prolongation of motor and sensory blockade in the elderly [46]. Moderate to high quality evidence supports reduced pain on movement, decreased time to first mobilization, and cost reduction of analgesic regimen with PNBs for hip fracture [20]. Femoral nerve block is associated with more effective analgesia than PCA opioid alone and similar analgesic efficacy as epidural analgesia, in patients undergoing total knee arthroplasty, and with less nausea/vomiting than with either of the latter two techniques [10]. Similarly, sciatic nerve block in the psoas compartment was associated with prolonged postoperative analgesia in high-risk older patients [15]. One may speculate that the recent availability of long-acting liposomal preparations of local anesthetic may allow a one-shot block to confer some of the benefits available previously only by using a 1- to 2-day infusion of local anesthetic.

Other Local Anesthetic Techniques

Various other local anesthetic techniques (wound infiltration, topical analgesia, intra-articular and periarticular infiltration, transverse abdominis block, etc.) can be valuable components of multimodal analgesia [9] for all patients including older persons. Wound infiltration after carotid endarterectomy reduced postoperative opioid requirement and opioid-related side effects in an older population [11]. Intraoperative periarticular infiltration has been found to be helpful for 24 hours in pain control in adult patients undergoing total knee arthroplasty [50].

PAIN MANAGEMENT PLAN AT DISCHARGE

The discharge plan is an essential component of postoperative pain management. Documented, i.e., written, instructions should include advice from the surgeon and anesthesiologist, nursing staff, physiotherapists, and other members of the care team as appropriate (e.g., occupational therapist, pharmacist) to coordinate a smooth transition of patient from hospital to home. Clear communication individualized for patients and their primary health care providers should be established about all pain-related modalities. Particular clarity should be given to the medications the patient is receiving, e.g., their dose, schedule, how to monitor any specific side effects, and when and how to cease therapy as appropriate. The plan must integrate nonpharmacologic interventions as well. There should be clarity regarding specifics of when and whom to contact in case of uncontrolled or persistent pain.

The discharge plan must seek an optimal balance between pain control and resumption of activities of daily living. Patients and caregivers must be appropriately counseled regarding the avoidance of concurrent use of other centrally acting agents (e.g., alcohol) or drugs (e.g., benzodiazepines or drugs of abuse such as illicit opioids) in combination with prescribed opioids, as this can lead to accidental toxicity. Clear instructions must also address tapering and discontinuation of opioids and appropriate disposal of unused opioids and other medications.

No uniform recommendations have been promulgated regarding postdischarge weaning of opioids prescribed to patients with postoperative pain. However, opioid theft and abuse of postoperative prescription opioids left unused by patients after surgery clearly contributes to this major public health problem and is now prompting the emergence of numerous practice guidelines restricting opioid dosage, duration or both. After minor operations involving soft tissue (e.g., abscess drainage), or removal of orthopedic hardware, patients may be appropriately discharged on acetaminophen or NSAIDs. Generally, patients who have not received any preoperative long-term opioid therapy and have been prescribed with opioids for more than 1 to 2 weeks postoperation should be instructed to gradually taper the opioid dosage to prevent opioid abstinence symptoms. If the surgical procedure appears to be healing quickly and uneventfully, and/or to have removed the source of pain the patient had preoperatively, dose reductions to the tune of 20% to 25% of the discharge dose every few days to a week are usually tolerated by most patients. Patients who were chronically prescribed opioids before surgery require individualized planning to taper their opioid to the preoperative maintenance dose [12] or to zero if the operation succeeds in removing the source of the patient's preoperative pain.

SUMMARY

Recent advances in surgical techniques increasingly allow procedures to be performed in older patients who might not have been candidates for earlier, more invasive techniques. This opportunity, together with rising numbers of older persons worldwide, has increased the numbers of operations performed in this population and the number of older persons requiring pain control both perioperatively and later, at home. However, despite extensive research including observations of decreased capacity for endogenous pain modulation in older persons, elderly patients continue to suffer the adverse effects of poorly controlled pain after surgery.

Older patients typically experience multiple comorbidities such as cognitive changes along with age-related physiologic changes that affect pain and analgesic pharmacology. The likelihood of polytherapy and polypharmacy including drug interactions renders postoperative pain management all the more complex in older patients. It is not unsafe to treat pain after surgery in older patients—to the contrary. Yet until evidence-based consensus is reached as to how best to individualize the pain control plan for each older person, plans based on generalizing evidence from broader populations should be viewed with caution. An approach based on "start low and go slow" should be adopted, along with vigilance for the emergence of side effects.

REFERENCES

1. American Geriatrics Society Panel on Pharmacological Management of Persistent Pain in Older Persons: Pharmacological management of persistent pain in older persons. J Am Geriatr Soc 2009;57:1331–46.
2. American Pain Society. Principles of analgesic use for the treatment of acute pain and cancer pain, 7th ed. Glenview, IL: American Pain Society; 2016.
3. Apfelbaum JL, Chen C, Mehta SS, Gan TJ. Postoperative pain experience: results from a national survey suggest postoperative pain continues to be undermanaged. Anesth Analg 2003;97:534–40.
4. Aubrun F, Monsel S, Langeron O, Coriat P, Riou B. Postoperative titration of intravenous morphine in the elderly patient. Anesthesiology 2002;96:17–23.
5. Bettelli G. Anaesthesia for the elderly outpatient: preoperative assessment and evaluation, anaesthetic technique and postoperative pain management. Curr Opin Anaesthesiol 2010;23:726–31.
6. Brown D. A literature review exploring how healthcare professionals contribute to the assessment and control of postoperative pain in older people. J Clin Nurs 2004;13:74–90.

7. Buntin-Mushock C, Phillip L, Moriyama K, Palmer PP. Age-dependent opioid escalation in chronic pain patients. Anesth Analg 2005;100:1740–5.
8. Buvanendran A, Kroin JS. Multimodal analgesia for controlling acute postoperative pain. Curr Opin Anaesthesiol 2009;22:588–93.
9. Cao X, Elvir-Lazo OL, White PF, Yumul R, Tang J. An update on pain management for elderly patients undergoing ambulatory surgery. Curr Opin Anaesthesiol 2016;29:674–82.
10. Chan EY, Fransen M, Parker DA, Assam PN, Chua N. Femoral nerve blocks for acute postoperative pain after knee replacement surgery. Cochrane Database Syst Rev 2014;5:CD009941.
11. Cherprenet AL, Rambourdin-Perraud M, Laforêt S, Faure M, Guesmi N, Baud C, Rosset E, Schoeffler P, Dualé C. Local anaesthetic infiltration at the end of carotid endarterectomy improves postoperative analgesia. Acta Anaesthesiol Scand 2015;59:107–14.
12. Chou R, Gordon DB, de Leon-Casasola OA, Rosenberg JM, Bickler S, Brennan T, Carter T, Cassidy CL, Chittenden EH, Degenhardt E, Griffith S, Manworren R, McCarberg B, Montgomery R, Murphy J, Perkal MF, Suresh S, Sluka K, Strassels S, Thirlby R, Viscusi E, Walco GA, Warner L, Weisman SJ, Wu CL. Management of postoperative pain: a clinical practice guideline from the American Pain Society, the American Society of Regional Anesthesia and Pain Medicine, and the American Society of Anesthesiologists' Committee on Regional Anesthesia, Executive Committee, and Administrative Council. J Pain 2016;17:131–57.
13. Coldrey JC, Upton RN, Macintyre PE. Advances in analgesia in the older patient. Best Pract Res Clin Anaesthesiol 2011;25:367–78.
14. Cornelius R, Herr KA, Gordon DB, Kretzer K, Butcher HK. Evidence-based practice guideline: acute pain management in older adults. J Gerontol Nurs 2017;43:18–27.
15. Demirel I, Ozer AB, Duzgol O, Bayar MK, Karakurt L, Erhan OL. Comparison of unilateral spinal anesthesia and L_1 paravertebral block combined with psoas compartment and sciatic nerve block in patients to undergo partial hip prosthesis. Eur Rev Med Pharmacol Sci 2014;18:1067–72.
16. Falzone E, Hoffmann C, Keita H. Postoperative analgesia in elderly patients. Drugs Aging 2013;30:81–90.
17. Gagliese L, Weizblit N, Ellis W, Chan VW. The measurement of postoperative pain: a comparison of intensity scales in younger and older surgical patients. Pain 2005;117:412–20.
18. Gan TJ, Habib AS, Miller TE, White W, Apfelbaum JL. Incidence, patient satisfaction, and perceptions of post-surgical pain: results from a US national survey. Curr Med Res Opin 2014;30:149–60.
19. Garimella V, Cellini C. Postoperative pain control. Clin Colon Rectal Surg 2013;26:191–6.
20. Guay J, Parker MJ, Griffiths R, Kopp S. Peripheral nerve blocks for hip fractures. Cochrane Database Syst Rev 2017;5:CD001159.
21. Halaszynski TM. Pain management in the elderly and cognitively impaired patient: the role of regional anesthesia and analgesia. Curr Opin Anaesthesiol 2009;22:594–9.
22. Herr KA, Garand L. Assessment and measurement of pain in older adults. Clin Geriatr Med 2001;17:457–78.
23. Herr KA, Spratt K, Mobily PR, Richardson G. Pain intensity assessment in older adults: use of experimental pain to compare psychometric properties and usability of selected pain scales with younger adults. Clin J Pain 2004;20:207–19.
24. Hofland SL. Elder beliefs: blocks to pain management. J Gerontol Nurs 1992;18:s19–23.
25. Horgas AL, Yoon SL, Grall M, Boltz M, Capezuti E, Fulmer T, Zwicker D. Pain management in older adults. In: Evidence-based geriatric nursing protocols for best practice. Springer Publishing Company; 2012. p. 246–67.
26. Jeleazcov C, Ihmsen H, Saari TI, Rohde D, Mell J, Fröhlich K, Krajinovic L, Fechner J, Schwilden H, Schüttler J. Patient controlled analgesia with target-controlled infusion of hydromorphone in postoperative pain therapy. Anesthesiology 2016;124:56–68.
27. Jordan AI, Regnard C, Hughes JC. Hidden pain or hidden evidence? J Pain Symptom Manage 2007;33:658–60.
28. Karani R, Meier DE. Systemic pharmacologic postoperative pain management in the geriatric orthopaedic patient. Clin Orthop Relat Res 2004;425:26–34.
29. Klotz U. Pharmacokinetics and drug metabolism in the elderly. Drug Metab Rev 2009;41:67–76.
30. Koh JC, Song Y, Kim SY, Park S, Ko SH, Han DW. Postoperative pain and patient-controlled epidural analgesia-related adverse effects in young and elderly patients: a retrospective analysis of 2,435 patients. J Pain Res 2017;10:897–904.
31. Lan F, Ma YH, Xue JX, Wang TL, Ma DQ. Transcutaneous electrical nerve stimulation on acupoints reduces fentanyl requirement for postoperative pain relief after total hip arthroplasty in elderly patients. Minerva Anestesiol 2012;78:887–95.
32. Lichtner V, Dowding D, Esterhuizen P, Closs SJ, Long AF, Corbett A, Briggs M. Pain assessment for people with dementia: a systematic review of systematic reviews of pain assessment tools. BMC Geriatr 2014;14:138.
33. Liu JH, Etzioni DA, O'Connell JB, Maggard MA, Ko CY. The increasing workload of general surgery. Arch Surg 2004;139:423–8.

34. Liukas A, Kuusniemi K, Aantaa R, Virolainen P, Niemi M, Neuvonen PJ, Olkkola KT. Pharmacokinetics of intravenous paracetamol in elderly patients. Clin Pharmacokinet 2011;50:121–9.
35. Mann C, Pouzeratte Y, Boccara G, Peccoux C, Vergne C, Brunat G, Domergue J, Millat B, Colson P. Comparison of intravenous or epidural patient-controlled analgesia in the elderly after major abdominal surgery. Anesthesiology 2000;92:433–41.
36. Mann C, Pouzeratte Y, Eledjam JJ. Postoperative patient-controlled analgesia in the elderly: risks and benefits of epidural versus intravenous administration. Drugs Aging 2003;20:337–45.
37. McCartney CJ, Nelligan K. Postoperative pain management after total knee arthroplasty in elderly patients: treatment options. Drugs Aging 2014;31:83–91.
38. McCleane G. Pharmacological pain management in the elderly patient. Clin Interv Aging 2007;2:637–43.
39. McNicol ED, Ferguson MC, Haroutounian S, Carr DB, Schumann R. Single dose intravenous paracetamol or intravenous propacetamol for postoperative pain. Cochrane Database Syst Rev 2016;5:CD007126.
40. Mercadante S. Intravenous patient-controlled analgesia and management of pain in post-surgical elderly with cancer. Surg Oncol 2010;19:173–7.
41. Mohanty S, Rosenthal RA, Russell MM, Neuman MD, Ko CY, Esnaola NF. Optimal perioperative management of the geriatric patient: a best practices guideline from the American College of Surgeons NSQIP and the American Geriatrics Society. J Am Coll Surg 2016;222:930–47.
42. Momeni M, Crucitti M, De Kock M. Patient-controlled analgesia in the management of postoperative pain. Drugs 2006;66:2321–37.
43. Office for National Statistics. Overview of the UK population. March 2017. https://www.ons.gov.uk/peoplepopulationandcommunity/populationandmigration/populationestimates/articles/overviewoftheukpopulation/mar2017.
44. Oksuzyan A, Jeune B, Juel K, Vaupel JW, Christensen K. Changes in hospitalisation and surgical procedures among the oldest-old: a follow-up study of the entire Danish 1895 and 1905 cohorts from ages 85 to 99 years. Age Ageing 2013;42:476–81.
45. Owen JA, Sitar DS, Berger L, Brownell L, Duke PC, Mitenko PA. Age-related morphine kinetics. Clin Pharmacol Ther 1983;34:364–8.
46. Paqueron X, Boccara G, Bendahou M, Coriat P, Riou B. Brachial plexus nerve block exhibits prolonged duration in the elderly. Anesthesiology 2002;97:1245–9.
47. Pearce L, Bunni J, McCarthy K, Hewitt J. Surgery in the older person: training needs for the provision of multidisciplinary care. Ann R Coll Surg Engl 2016;98:367–70.
48. Pergolizzi J, Böger RH, Budd K, Dahan A, Erdine S, Hans G, Kress HG, Langford R, Likar R, Raffa RB, Sacerdote P. Opioids and the management of chronic severe pain in the elderly: consensus statement of an International Expert Panel with focus on the six clinically most often used World Health Organization Step III opioids (buprenorphine, fentanyl, hydromorphone, methadone, morphine, oxycodone). Pain Pract 2008;8:287–313.
49. Schenning KJ, Deiner SG. Postoperative delirium in the geriatric patient. Anesthesiol Clin 2015;33:505–16.
50. Seangleulur A, Vanasbodeekul P, Prapaitrakool S, Worathongchai S, Anothaisintawee T, McEvoy M, Vendittoli PA, Attia J, Thakkinstian A. The efficacy of local infiltration analgesia in the early postoperative period after total knee arthroplasty: a systematic review and meta-analysis. Eur J Anaesthesiol 2016;33:816–31.
51. Silvanto M, Lappi M, Rosenberg PH. Comparison of the opioid-sparing efficacy of diclofenac and ketoprofen for 3 days after knee arthroplasty. Acta Anaesthesiol Scand 2002;46:322–8.
52. Simon MJ, Veering BT, Stienstra R, van Kleef JW, Burm AG. The effects of age on neural blockade and hemodynamic changes after epidural anesthesia with ropivacaine. Anesth Analg 2002;94:1325–30.
53. Sommer M, de Rijke JM, van Kleef M, Kessels AG, Peters ML, Geurts JW, Gramke HF, Marcus MA. The prevalence of postoperative pain in a sample of 1490 surgical inpatients. Eur J Anaesthesiol 2008;25:267–74.
54. Tawfic QA, Bellingham G. Postoperative pain management in patients with chronic kidney disease. J Anaesthesiol Clin Pharmacol 2015;31:6–13.
55. Trifirò G, Spina E. Age-related changes in pharmacodynamics: focus on drugs acting on central nervous and cardiovascular systems. Curr Drug Metab 2011;12:611–20.
56. U.S. Census Bureau: May 2014. An aging nation: the older population in the United States. https://www.census.gov/prod/2014pubs/p25-1140.pdf.
57. Verdú E, Ceballos D, Vilches JJ, Navarro X. Influence of aging on peripheral nerve function and regeneration. J Peripher Nerv Syst 2000;5:191–208.
58. White PF, Tang J, Wender RH, Zhao M, Time M, Zaentz A, Yumul R, Sloninsky A, Naruse R, Kariger R, Webb T, Fermelia DE, Tsushima GK. The effects of oral ibuprofen and celecoxib in preventing pain, improving recovery outcomes and patient satisfaction after ambulatory surgery. Anesth Analg 2011;112:323–9.
59. White PF. Multimodal pain management – the future is now! Curr Opin Investig Drugs 2007;8:517–8.

CHAPTER 24

Methods and Measures to Improve the Quality of Pain After Surgery

Debra B. Gordon, Ruth Zaslansky, and Winfried Meissner

...Quality is never an accident: It is always the result of high intention, sincere effort, intelligent direction, and skillful execution; It represents the wise choice of many alternatives...

Will A. Foster
Gabel-Risdon Creamery Co, Detroit, Mich.

"Quality" is a nebulous concept, especially in the realm of health care. The overarching goals of health care quality are to minimize medical errors and adverse events and to improve outcomes [73]. Health care quality is frequently described in terms of the attributes and outcomes of care provided by practitioners and received by patients [3]. Quality in health care has been defined as "the degree to which health services for individuals and populations increase the likelihood of desired health outcomes and are consistent with current professional knowledge" [40, p. 21]. Yet, the definition of quality depends on both the perspective of the measurer and the purpose of measurement. For example, in a given instance of health care delivery, the patient, the clinician, and the payer may have very different perceptions of the quality of care.

The Structure–Process–Outcome model, first developed by Donabedian [14] and later adopted by many other investigators is a useful framework for conceptualizing quality (see Figure 24-1).

Structure is defined as the physical and organizational properties of the setting in which care is provided; *process* is what is done for patients; and *outcome* relates to what is accomplished for patients. According to this model, any examination of quality should include measurements in all three of these dimensions, even though outcomes are generally the most sought after validation of quality. A more specific definition emphasizes the technical aspects and characteristics of interactions between provider and patient [54]. Important attributes of the provider–patient interaction include communication, trust, empathy, sensitivity, and honesty [4]. *Technical quality* consists of "doing the right thing right" [13, p. 892], e.g., performing the right tests or providing the right services to accomplish the desired result. The indication for an intervention or treatment is increasingly recognized as an important variable in quality because even if an intervention meets the literal requirements for quality structure and process, it may not be indicated and results in overtreatment.

Pain care quality becomes even more difficult to define because pain itself is a highly individualized, subjective experience intertwined with emotion that does not easily lend itself to standardized evaluation or care. Furthermore, pain is managed in many different ways (e.g., pharmacologic, interventional, nonpharmacologic) and in many different phases of perioperative care by individuals and teams. High-quality pain management has been defined to include "appropriate assessment, including screening for the presence of pain, completion of a comprehensive initial assessment when pain is present, and frequent

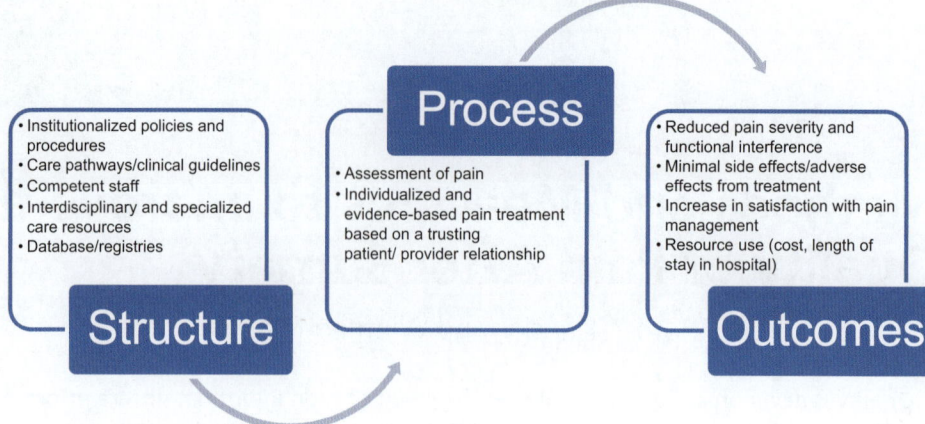

FIGURE 24-1 Elements of quality pain management.

reassessments of patient responses to treatment; interdisciplinary, collaborative care planning, including patient and family input; appropriate treatment that is efficacious, cost conscious, culturally and developmentally appropriate, and safe; and access to specialty care as needed" [21, p. 1575]. However, this definition lacks a description of desired outcomes and is indicative that there is currently no agreed upon definition as to what constitutes high-quality perioperative pain management [74]. There is also lack of consensus as to what should be the desired health outcomes as well as how and when to measure them and which thresholds should be used to judge quality [41,50].

Despite being ill-defined, current forces demand that acute pain care quality be systematically assessed, improved, and publicized. Quality pain management necessitates transformation in the health care system [28,29], as it relates to the way pain after surgery is understood, assessed, and treated. This chapter provides an overview of quality improvement (QI) and methods to redesign systems to facilitate implementation of best practices for acute perioperative pain management with the goal of improving outcomes. Strategies for quality measurement are also addressed.

APPROACHES TO IMPROVING QUALITY OF PAIN MANAGEMENT AFTER SURGERY

Several broad approaches have been used to cultivate health care quality. For many years, accreditation (of programs) and certification (of individuals) were the primary mechanisms used to foster quality. These relied, to a large extent, on structural and process parameters. In recent years, quality measurement and improvement have changed significantly with developments in clinical epidemiology, outcomes research, systems science, and information technology, accelerating the health care quality narrative.

Quality Improvement/Management (QI)

QI in health care is a compilation of methods adapted from industry and operations research to avert predictable human errors, eliminate unnecessary and harmful variations in practice, and improve the production of goods and services [3]. There are numerous approaches to QI, which share core principles. QI focuses on reducing variation in a production process, standardization, and continuous improvement in outcomes rather than on the identification and elimination of defects. QI enlists an entire organization to work toward a goal of continuous improvement in quality by carefully studying the process one is attempting to improve; QI also involves changing the responsibilities and power of frontline workers [37]. QI theory states that data can be collected to help understand a system's processes and uncover the root causes of inconsistencies or variations that contribute to quality problems. Unlike the earlier quality assurance model, there is no predetermined final yardstick of quality; instead, the goal is continuous improvement. The concept of QI was first applied to improving outcomes of analgesic treatment in pain by Mitchell Max [44], who noted the failure of education to change behaviors and outlined the need to address a set of background factors including redesign of drug ordering systems and regulations.

Contemporary approaches that are becoming more common to improve the quality of perioperative care include use of QI process initiatives such as standardizing multimodal analgesia within enhanced recovery after surgery (ERAS) pathways [65] or outside of them [67] and redesign of workflow and teams within a system such as integrated acute pain care services in the preoperative and postdischarge environments. We elaborate on these examples below.

ERAS Pathways

ERAS pathways provide a structured approach to reduce variation and improve quality that works well within a QI approach. These pathways of care comprise evidence-based, best-practice recommendations throughout the perioperative period, which, when consistently applied, may result in improved patient outcome although reports are mixed [34]. The concept of applying perioperative clinical pathways to facilitate postoperative rehabilitation by optimizing analgesia, early oral intake and ambulation, and avoidance of fluid overload was first proposed by Kehlet and colleagues [72]. ERAS regimens use a comprehensive perioperative care pathway, with multimodal opioid-sparing analgesia as a key component. Miller and colleagues [48] assessed the effect of implementing an ERAS pathway, including a standard multimodal pain management regimen for colorectal operations, on a variety of outcomes including pain intensity and opioid consumption. Pain intensity scores averaged across the 5-day hospitalization period were lower in ERAS-treated patients, and opioid consumption was lower compared with non-ERAS patients, whose analgesic regimens were not standardized. Tan and colleagues [65] address the challenge of assessing the effectiveness of multimodal pain management in the context of ERAS protocols because of the challenge of teasing out the relative importance of any component, including analgesia. The success of ERAS programs is most likely the result of a cumulative structured, evidence-based approach [58]. Yet, the authors of a 2011 Cochrane review questioned using ERAS as a standard of care because of the poor quality of studies [63]. Recently, Liu and colleagues [38] in a large multicenter, controlled study of ERAS colorectal resection and emergency hip fracture repair found benefits of ERAS upon length of hospital stay, complications, and mortality. The total intravenous morphine-equivalent dosage of opioid medication administered from hospitalization through the third postoperative day was significantly reduced as expected using multimodal analgesia. However, the proportion of time in which patients rated their current pain as "acceptable" was not significantly different.

Use of data to track trends has been shown to be a critical factor in ERAS programs. Moonesinghe and colleagues [49] recommend that ERAS measurement have three tiers, which are sensitive to the resources available to local hospitals. First, the "core" dataset comprises routine administrative data and is obtainable from routine hospital data collection processes. Second, the QI dataset is more comprehensive and focuses on processes including adherence to certain elements of the protocol and outcomes including patient experience such as analgesia, mobilization, and sleeping. Data collection is recommended at regular intervals throughout the year on a sample of patients (perhaps 20% per year) so that variation in processes can be tracked. Third, the "best practice" dataset is a comprehensive measurement and monitoring system that uses validated measures that can be applicable to any hospital or case mix including adherence to all aspects of the protocol and longer-term mortality and health-related quality of life. Comparing performance between health care organizations ostensibly creates a market demand for the systems with the best quality performance scores.

Clinical Practice Guidelines

Clinical Practice Guidelines provide a quality structure to aid in the development of pain treatment protocols by offering clinicians up-to-date, evidence-based guidance. As with many fields of health care, the greatest obstacle is not in the development of guidelines but in their dissemination and adoption in clinical practice. Additionally, once implemented, it is necessary to assess if the recommendations are effective in real life conditions [8]. Compliance with acute pain guidelines is highly variable and may be better in larger and university-affiliated hospitals [52], although a recent national survey in Germany found no differences between different types of hospital [47]. Resource availability, particularly staff with pain management expertise, and the existence of formal quality programs to monitor pain management are positive predictors of compliance with guidelines [32].

Workflow Redesign through Integrated Acute Pain Services

The concept of an "analgesic team" who would supervise and administer pain relief and be responsible for teaching and training in postoperative pain management was described in the mid-1970s. This concept evolved to establishing an Acute Pain Service ("APS") by Ready at the University of Washington in 1986 [59] and was further propagated by guidelines recommending a systems-level organization of acute pain therapies in other countries [42].

Surveys in Germany, Italy, Ireland, and the United States demonstrate that there is wide diversity in the structure of an APS across the globe, with little consensus as to what the service consists of in terms of personnel and roles [57]. Furthermore, there is also significant variability with regard to assigning specific physicians and/or nurses or other professionals (e.g., pharmacists) to the APS, standard protocols or practice parameters, quality management efforts, and use of multimodal and interventional approaches to acute pain management [16,56]. Some studies [62] have reported that patients managed by an APS report lower pain intensity, fewer side effects, and greater satisfaction with care when compared with patients treated by non–pain-specialized providers. However, an extensive evidence review performed for the 2016 multisociety postoperative pain guidelines [10] found insufficient evidence to determine optimal characteristics of an APS, only observational studies and several low-quality randomized trials that associated an APS with slightly increased costs, and insufficient evidence to demonstrate clear, clinically relevant differences in pain or other clinical outcomes under the care of an APS compared with routine care. As APS staff tend to focus on more "high-tech" approaches and may have limited staffing, their scope often benefits only a small number of patients within a hospital, while leaving less time available to carry out roles related to core activities of education and developing local guidelines [52,64]. Given this background and reports of unfavorable patient-reported outcomes ("PROs"), Erlenwein and colleagues [16] suggest a need to revisit the structure, organization, and quality of APSs.

Recent progress toward more proactive coordinated and team-based approaches has led to innovative models of perioperative care including the *perioperative surgical home* ("PSH") [69] and integrated services by pain specialists. The PSH is a physician-led care delivery model that emphasizes interprofessional teams, care coordination and improved patient experience with shared decision-making, "prehabilitation" of the patient before surgery, and effective transitions to reduce cost, complications, and readmissions [36]. *Integrated care* involves bringing together clinical service with organizational and administrative aspects of care to achieve continuity of care between all health care workers involved in the care network of patients [19]. Integrated care models have been shown to produce positive results with respect to knowledge transfer and personal confidence in treating acute pain [17] and in other areas of health care [19]. Though much has been written about integrated chronic pain care [15], less in known about how such integration can be achieved in acute care settings. Here, too, there is great variability in the structure, staffing, and scope of integrated pain care services. One example from the University of Washington emerged from collaboration between the APS and the preanesthesia clinic to routinely perform screening of all presurgical patients using predefined criteria for risk of difficulties in controlling perioperative pain (see Figure 24-2).

Each day, high-risk patients are flagged on an electronic list alerting the APS on a daily basis when these patients are admitted, to facilitate timely inpatient pain consultative care. The attending pain consultant is also available daily in the preanesthesia clinic to see select patients identified by the routine screening as benefiting from a preemptive pain care plan. Additionally, high-risk patients undergo additional behavioral health screening to afford the APS psychologist an opportunity to intervene preoperatively in a separate outpatient clinic visit with brief biobehavioral interventions to help reduce catastrophizing and improve coping skills. The psychologist then follows patients more closely through their hospitalization in team care and, if needed, in the postdischarge transitional pain care clinic. This is just one example of how redesign of workflow aimed to improve outcomes is evolving. Novel brief cognitive–behavioral interventions designed to expand access to low-cost efficient care and reduce pain catastrophizing and improve coping skills preoperatively appear promising but their impact on pain after surgery is yet to be determined [12,55]. In addition to risk screening for difficult-to-control postoperative pain, important processes for workflow redesign consideration include pain and opioid safety assessments. These assessments are critical in making decisions about initiating treatment and modifying them over time. Clarity about the "who, how, and when" of pain assessment is a critical process and structure issue for a system. Routine assessment and documentation of pain is a process measure that aimed to provide safety and guide quality care. The recommendation that nursing staff perform routine assessment and documentation of pain after surgery is universal; however, there is remarkably little evidence to link pain assessment to better outcomes [25]. Campaigns starting in the 1990s led by the American Pain Society to make pain "the fifth vital sign" [7] did much to increase the visibility of and attention to pain assessment, prompting routine screening for pain and development of organizational policies that demanded timely reassessment. In the United States, assessment of pain has been a prerequisite for organizational accreditation [33]. In France, Italy, Belgium, and Israel,

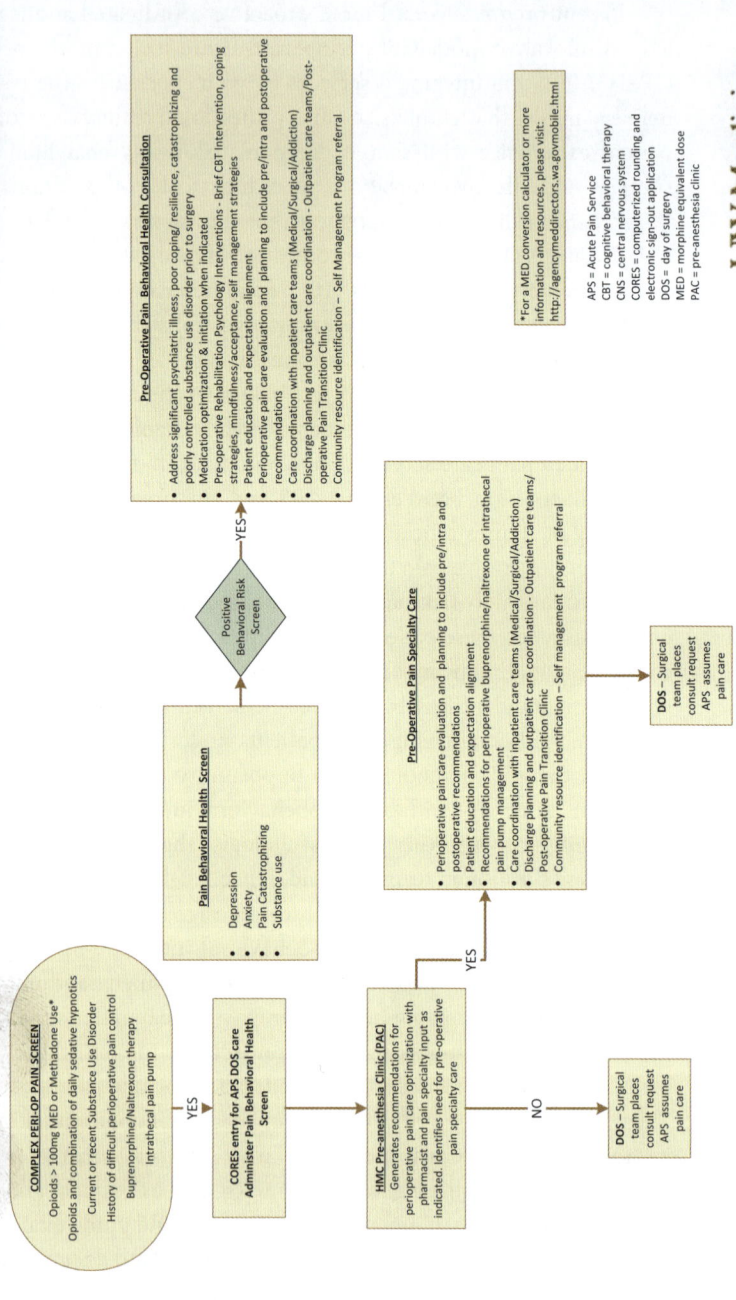

FIGURE 24-2 University of Washington Harborview Medical Center Perioperative Integrated Pain Care Pathway.

national regulations require that nurses assess pain, its effect, and treatments provided. Heikkilä and colleagues [27] suggest that documentation is inadequate in many health care systems, worldwide. However, even in wards where a high proportion of patients have their pain assessed and documented, this is not associated with improved PROs. This observation is supported by a body of evidence from the United States and Europe [7,18,26,51,72]. The reasons for these counterintuitive findings are not clear and could be multifactorial. Unidimensional scales such as pain intensity ratings undervalue the complexity of the pain experience. Postoperative pain is often measured at rest and may be low and not require intervention as opposed to pain measured during movement. Alternatively, staff may carry out the measurement mechanistically to fulfil the regulatory requirement, yet they do not communicate or use the findings to guide decision-making. Of note, effective January 2018, the United States' Joint Commission hospital accreditation standards [33] will include a new element of performance that medical staff be actively involved in pain assessment through participation in the establishment of protocols and quality metrics and reviewing performance data. Focus on pain intensity rating assessments in some hospitals has led to unwanted consequences, such as increased use of opioids and adverse effects [45,70], leading to mistrust in the process of assessment. Lastly, providers often mistrust the findings obtained from using what seems to be a simplistic method for evaluating pain that can be compounded by the discrepancy between subjective ratings of pain and observations of patient behavior by providers.

Though a variety of pain assessment questionnaires are available, research has not identified a single best tool or optimal frequency for assessing and reassessing postoperative pain [23]. A potential technique for better documenting the dynamic nature of pain is a **pain trajectory**. A trajectory is a representation of a patient's pain severity during the observation period. Compared with a single pain rating, trajectories draw attention to speed of onset of initial pain relief, stability of pain relief, and the overall amount of pain relief achieved [9,35]. To date, trajectories are used in the context of clinical studies not in the clinical routine. Future QI work is needed to more fully address which parameters should be assessed and approach pain management as a complex process that must go beyond assessment and documentation of simple pain ratings [24,68].

Patient-Reported Outcomes (PROs)

PROs are in demand in all areas of health care because most health care aims to reduce symptoms, minimize disability, and improve quality of life, and these are aspects that only patients can assess [2]. PROs allow for self-assessment of symptoms or of physical performance; they are key measures in areas for which externally observable outcomes are unavailable, or likely to be biased, as occurs in conditions associated with pain.

For pain after surgery, PRO measurement should be generally focused on the overarching goal of early functional recovery. Core outcome measures may include (1) patient report of pain severity, (2) pain interference with function (e.g., movement in or out of bed, or sleep), (3) presence and severity of adverse effects, and (4) how the patient perceives the treatment he/she received (e.g., satisfaction, wish for additional pain treatment, and receipt of information about treatment options). Outcome targets should, when possible, include pain no worse than "mild" [50] and minimal interference with function from pain or pain treatments. The United Kingdom Royal College of Anaesthetists [61] recommends quality measures of outcomes along with process measures that can be collected easily during daily acute pain ward rounds and can be applied both generally and to specific patient groups, such as elderly patients more than 80 years of age or after cesarean section. Existing literature on postoperative pain-related PROs predominately focuses on in-hospital short-term experiences leaving an important gap in assessing long-term problems arising from under-management of pain after surgery.

The American Pain Society Patient Outcome Questionnaire-revised (APS-POQ-R) [22] and the International Pain Outcomes Questionnaire (IPO-Q) [60] are two PRO instruments that have been developed specific to pain after surgery for the purposes of QI and benchmarking. Both are available in several languages, have preliminary psychometric validation, and are intended for use on the first postoperative day though they have been applied at other time points [43]. Although the factor analyses revealed slightly different domains, both questionnaires ask patients to evaluate pain intensity and relief, physical and emotional interference due to postoperative pain, treatment side effects, and perceptions of care including participation in decision-making and satisfaction with pain management. Both questionnaires include a process measure regarding use of nonpharmacologic methods, and the IPO-Q includes questions about the presence and severity of pain before surgery. The IPO-Q provides a uniform methodology for assessing PRO as a component of the PAIN OUT international perioperative pain registry, discussed below. Recent studies reveal challenges of using these questionnaires for international comparisons, and further work is required to clarify the validity of the different scales [9,75] when used with patients internationally [6].

PROs are being incorporated within perioperative pain registries, which are used as multicenter (national or international) mechanisms for providing clinicians with information about effectiveness and appropriateness of care in real-world conditions.

Patient Registries

Lack of evidence about appropriateness and effectiveness of pain interventions is regarded as one of the five major crises in pain management today [39]. Creating a database for outcomes in real-world patients may allow carrying out meaningful evaluations of the quality of clinical pain care [29]. The US National Pain Strategy [53] identifies an urgent need for such registries. Although this call to action is focused on chronic pain, it also applies to registries related to management of pain after surgery.

A patient registry is an organized system that uses observational study methods to collect uniform data to evaluate specified outcomes for a population defined by a particular disease, condition, or exposure and that serves one or more predetermined scientific, clinical, or policy purposes [20]. Patient registries provide a real-world view of clinical practice, PROs, safety, and comparative effectiveness. Registries can be used for QI by providing audit and feedback to providers about their daily practice. Measuring quality of clinical care through audit and feedback (assessing one's own performance over time) and benchmarking (comparing one's results with those of others) is widely used in medicine to change provider conduct and improve quality of care. Audit and feedback is based on the premise that professionals will modify their performance when they receive feedback that their practice is not in line with a desired target.

Quality Improvement in Postoperative Pain Management (QUIPS) and PAIN OUT are two established perioperative pain registries, with QUIPS performing on a national (Germany and Austria) level and PAIN OUT, internationally. QUIPS was created in 2005 [47] offering clinicians standardized and validated tools to assess perioperative pain management processes and PROs in adults. Clinicians can receive immediate web-based feedback and benchmarking of summarized PROs. QUIPS also provides a platform for discussion, "learning from the best," and research opportunities. QUIPS operates under the auspices of German Societies and Professional Associations of Anaesthesiology and Intensive Care and Surgery. The QUIPS repository consists of data from over 500,000 patients, recruited from over 200 medical centers. The data are being used to evaluate effectiveness of interventions to reduce pain after surgery [11] and as a means to raise awareness that pain related to surgery still represents a largely unrecognized clinical problem [46]. In 2007, the tool was adapted for use in children, "Quality Improvement in Postoperative Pain Management in Infants" (QUIPS Infant).

PAIN OUT was established with funding from the European Commission during the period 2009 to 2012. It continues as a not-for-profit academic project open to participants internationally. PROs are collected using the IPO-Q, described earlier. The IPO-Q is available in 18 languages, allowing patients to assess PROs using a standardized and uniform platform and to do so in their native language. The repository consists of more than 60,000 datasets from patients in Europe, Americas, Africa, and South East Asia. PAIN OUT offers tools for clinicians to receive feedback and benchmarking of PROs and to use this performance information as motivation to change practice. Experience shows that although clinicians may be interested to carry out improvement work in their hospital, it is challenging to do so without a structured program.

In a systematic Cochrane review, Jamtvedt and colleagues [31] assessed the effect of audit and feedback on the performance of health care professionals and found that when effective, the impact of audit and feedback was generally small to moderate. The effectiveness increased when the baseline adherence to the recommended practice was low and when the feedback was delivered more intensively, e.g., was given verbally to individual recipients. The Cochrane review does not support mandatory or unevaluated use of audit and feedback as an intervention to change practice. A more recent review [30] found that audit and feedback can effectively improve quality of care, but feedback appears most effective when it is delivered by a supervisor or respected colleague; is presented frequently; features both specific goals and action plans; and aims to decrease the targeted behavior and when baseline performance is lower and recipients are nonphysicians. To address concerns such as these, PAIN OUT is now developing a structured change management program that combines feedback and benchmarking with Plan-Do-Study-Act (PDSA) cycles. PDSA cycles are small, rapid cycle QI projects designed to test an intervention, measure impact, and test again [66].

In the United States, work is ongoing through the Stanford Collaborative Health Outcomes Information Registry (CHOIR) (https://choir.stanford.edu/) to adapt what has been done for chronic pain to acute pain and the perioperative arena. Although designed to capture outcomes of surgical procedures performed for chronic pain, the National Perioperative Outcomes for Intrathecal Pump, Spinal Cord Stimulator, and Peripheral Nerve Stimulator Procedures (NACOR) provides a unique national registry that directly imports electronic data from professional billing systems, anesthesia information management systems, anesthesia quality measurement systems, and hospital electronic systems [1]. The German Society for Anaesthesiology and Intensive Care established the Regional Anaesthesia Network, that collects data about risk profiles and complications associated with regional anesthesia and analgesia. The network includes providers from 25 medical centers in Germany. The process of collecting data fulfils two purposes: routine follow-up of patients receiving regional analgesia and cared for by acute pain service personnel, and quality feedback and benchmarking of institutional outcomes [5].

CONCLUSIONS

Quality pain management after surgery remains a moving target. There is, as yet, no consensus as to the definition of "good quality" in perioperative pain management. The reasons are multifactorial but due to, in part, different perspectives of the stakeholders involved. Descriptions of quality, the health care environment and other forces impacting the delivery, measurement and methods to improve quality pain management continue to evolve. Focusing on structures, such as APSs, and processes, such as routine assessment and recording of pain, has not thus far produced the anticipated results. The experience gained with implementing these approaches attests that significant knowledge gaps exist as to how to achieve optimal organizational care delivery models and measures. However, it seems clear that clinicians in organizations in which surgery is performed should continue to create structures and processes aimed at improving safe and effective (quality) perioperative pain care. An interdisciplinary approach using measurement-driven models of care to guide QI efforts in perioperative pain control seems prudent. Parameters eventually selected as quality indicators should be associated with patients' overall outcome after surgery. It is yet to be determined whether emerging organizational models of care and translation of new research findings into practice will result in improved outcomes.

REFERENCES

1. Albrecht CR, Gabriel RA, Dutton RP, Kaye AD, Michna E, Urman RD. National perioperative outcomes for intrathecal pump, spinal cord stimulator, and peripheral nerve stimulator procedures. Pain Physician 2015;18(6):547–54.
2. Black N. Patient reported outcome measures could help transform healthcare. BMJ 2013;346:f167. doi:10.1136/bmj.f167.
3. Blumenthal D. Total quality management and physicians' clinical decisions. JAMA 1993;269:2775–8.
4. Blumenthal D. Quality of health care. Part 1: what is it? N Engl J Med 1996;335(12):891–3.
5. Bomberg H, Bayer I, Wagenpfeil S, Kessler P, Wulf H, Standl T, Gottschalk A, Döffert J, Hering W, Birnbaum J, Spies C, Kutter B, Winckelmann J, Liebl-Biereige S, Meissner W, Vicent O, Koch T, Sessler DI, Volk T, Raddatz A. Prolonged catheter use and infection in regional anesthesia: a retrospective registry analysis. Anesthesiology 2018. doi:10.1097/ALN.0000000000002105.
6. Botti M, Khaw D, Jørgensen EB, Rasmussen B, Hunter S, Redley B. Cross-cultural examination of the structure of the revised American Pain Society patient outcome questionnaire (APS-POQ-R). J Pain 2015; 16:727–40.
7. Campbell JN. The fifth vital sign revisited. Pain 2016;157:3–4.
8. Chapman CR, Stevens DA, Lipman AG. Quality of postoperative pain management in American versus European institutions. J Pain Palliat Care Pharmacother 2013;27:350–8.
9. Chapman CR, Donaldson GW, Davis JJ, Bradshaw DH. Improving individual measurement of postoperative pain: the pain trajectory. J Pain 2011;12(2):257–62.
10. Chou R, Gordon DB, de Leon-Casasola OA, Rosenberg JM, Bickler S, Brennan T, Carter T, Cassidy CL, Chittenden EH, Degenhardt E, Griffith S, Manworren R, McCarberg B, Montgomery R, Murphy J, Perkal MF, SureshSluka SK, Strassels S, Thirlby R, Viscusi E, Walco GA, Warner L, Weisman SJ, Wu CL. Management of postoperative pain: a clinical practice guideline from the American Pain Society, the American Society of Regional Anesthesia and Pain Medicine, and the American Society of Anesthesiologists' Committee on Regional Anesthesia, Executive Committee, and Administrative Council. J Pain 2016;17(2):131–57.
11. Cruz JJ, Diebolder H, Dogan A, Mothes A, Rengsberger M, Hartmann M, Meissner W, Runnebaum IB. Combination of pre-emptive port-site and intraoperative intraperitoneal ropivacaine for reduction of postoperative pain: a prospective cohort study. Eur J Obstet Gynecol Reprod Biol 2014;179:11–6.
12. Darnall BD. Pain psychology and pain catastrophizing in the perioperative setting. A review of impacts, interventions and unmet needs. Hand Clin 2016;32:33–9.
13. Donabedian A. The quality of care. How can it be assessed? JAMA 1988;260(12):1743–8.

14. Donabedian A. Promoting quality through evaluation of the process of patient care. Med Care 1968;6:181–202.
15. Driscoll MA, Kerns RD. Integrated, team-based chronic pain management: bridges from theory and research to high quality patient care. Adv Exp Med Biol 2016;904:131–47. doi:10.1007/978-94-017-7537-3_10.
16. Erlenwein J, Koschwitz R, Pauli-Magnus D, Quintel M, Meissner W, Petzke F, Stamer U. A follow-up on Acute Pain Services in Germany compared to international survey data. Eur J Pain 2015;20:874–83.
17. Feldman K, Berall A, Karuza J, Sendervoich H, Perri GA, Grossman D. Knowledge translation: an interprofessional approach to integrating a pain consult team within an acute care unit. J Interprof Care 2016;39(6):816–8.
18. Fletcher D, Fermanian C, Mardaye A, Aegerter P, Pain and Regional Anesthesia Committee of the French Anesthesia and Intensive Care Society (SFAR). A patient-based national survey on postoperative pain management in France reveals significant achievements and persistent challenges. Pain 2008;137(2):441–51.
19. Garralsa E, Hasselaar J, Carrasco JM, Beek KV, Siouta N, Ccikos A, Menten J, Centeno C. Integrated palliative care in the Spanish context: a systematic review of the literature. BMC Palliat Care 2016;15:49. doi:10.1186/s12904-016-0120-9.
20. Gliklich RE, Levy D, Karl J, Leavy MB, Taylor T, Campion DM. Registry of patient registries (RoPR): project overview. Effective health care program research report No. 40. (Prepared by Outcome DEcIDE Center under Contract No. HHSA 290-2005-0035-1.) AHRQ Publication No. 12-EHC058-EF. Rockville, MD: Agency for Healthcare Research and Quality; 2012. effectivehealthcare.ahrq.gov/reports/final.cfm.
21. Gordon DB, Dahl JL, Miaskowski C, BcCarber B, Todd KH, Paice JA, Lipman AG, Bookbinder M, Sanders SH, Turk DC, Carr DB. American Pain Society recommendations for improving the quality of acute and cancer pain management. Arch Intern Med 2005;165:1574–80.
22. Gordon DB, Polomano R, Pellino TA, Turk DC, McCracken L, Sherwood G, Farrar J, Paice J, Wallace M, Strassels S. Psychometrics of the revised American Pain Society Patient Outcome Questionnaire (APS-POQ) for quality improvement of acute and cancer pain management. J Pain 2010;11(11):1172–86.
23. Gordon DB, DeLeon-Casasola OA, Wu CL, Sluka K, Brennan T, Chou R. Research gaps on practice guidelines for acute perioperative pain management in adults: findings from a review of the evidence for an American Pain Society clinical practice guideline. J Pain 2016;17(2):158–66.
24. Gordon DB. Acute pain assessment tools: let us move beyond simple pain ratings. Curr Opin Anaesthesiol 2015;28(5):565–9.
25. Gould TH, Crosby DL, Harmer M, et al. Policy for controlling pain after surgery: effect of sequential changes in management. BMJ 1992;305:1187–93.
26. Hadjistavropoulos T, MacNab Y, Lints-Martindale A, Martin R, Hadjistavropoulos H. Does routine pain assessment result in better care? Pain Res Manag 2009;14:211–6.
27. Heikkilä K, Peltonen LM, Salanterä S. Postoperative pain documentation in a hospital setting: a topical review. Scand J Pain 2016;11:77–89
28. Institute of Medicine (IOM). Crossing the quality chasm. Crossing the quality chasm: a new health system for the 21st century. Washington, DC: National Academy Press; 2001.
29. Institute of Medicine (U.S.). Relieving pain in America: a blueprint for transforming prevention, care, education, and research. Washington, DC: National Academies Press; 2011.
30. Ivers NM, Grimshaw JM, Jamtvedt G, Flottorp S, O'Brien MA, French SD, Young J, Odgaard-Jensen J. Growing literature, stagnant science? Systematic review, meta-regression and cumulative analysis of audit and feedback interventions in health care. J Gen Intern Med 2014;29(11):1534–41.
31. Jamtvedt G, Young JM, Kristoffersen DT, O'Brien MA, Oxman AD. Audit and feedback: effects on professional practice and health care outcomes. Cochrane Database Syst Rev 2006;2:CD000259.
32. Jiang HJ, Lagasse RS, Ciccone K, et al. Factors influencing hospital implementation of acute pain management practice guidelines. J Clin Anesth 2001;13(4):268–76.
33. Joint Commission. Joint Commission enhances pain assessment and management requirements for accredited hospitals. Joint Comm Perspect 2017;37:7. http://www.jcrinc.com/the-joint-commission-perspectives/.
34. Kaplan JA, Finlayson E, Auerbach AD. Impact of multimodality pain regimens on elective colorectal surgery outcomes. Am Surg 2017;83(4):414–20.
35. Kannampallil T, Galanter WL, Falck S, Gaunt MJ, Gibbons RD, McNutt R, Odwazny R, Schiff G, Vaida AJ, Wilkie DJ, Lambert BL. Characterizing the pain score trajectories of hospitalized adult medical and surgical patients: a retrospective cohort study. Pain 2016;157(12):2739–46.
36. Kash BA, Zhang U, Cline KM, Menser T, Miller TR. The perioperative surgical home (PHS): a comprehensive review of US and non-US studies shows predominately positive. Milbank Q 2014;92(4):796–821.
37. Kritchevsky SB, Simmons BP. Continuous quality improvement: concepts and applications for physician care. JAMA 1991;266:1817–23.

38. Liu VX, Rosas E, Hwang J, Cain E, Foss-Durant A, Clopp M, Huang M, Lee DC, Mustille A, Kipnis P, Parodi S. Enhanced recovery after surgery program implementation in 2 surgical populations in an integrated health care delivery system. JAMA Surg 2017;152(7):e171032. doi:10.1001/jamasurg.2017.1032.
39. Loeser JD. Five crises in pain management. IASP. Pain Clin Updates 2012;xx(1):1–4.
40. Lohr KN. Medicare. A strategy for quality assurance. Washington, DC: National Academy Press; 1990.
41. Malhotra A, Mackey S. Outcomes in pain medicine: a brief review. Pain Ther 2012;1(1):5.
42. Maier C, Kibbel K, Mercker S, Wulf H. Postoperative pain therapy at general nursing stations: an analysis of eight year's experience at an anesthesiological acute pain service. Anaesthesist 1994;43:385–97.
43. Mandell MS, Smith AR, Dew MA, Gordon DB, Holtzman SD, Howell T, MiMartini A, Zeeshan B, Simpson MA, Ladner DP, Freise CE, McCluskey SA, Fisher RA, Guarrera JV, Olthoff KM, Pomfret EA. Early postoperative pain and its predictors in adult to adult living donor liver transplantation cohort study. Transplantation 2016;100(11):2362–71.
44. Max M. Improving outcomes of analgesic treatment: is education enough? 1990;113(11):885–9.
45. Mehendale AW, Goldman MP, Mehendale RP. Opioid overuse pain syndrome (OOPS): the story of opioids, Prometheus unbound. J Opioid Manag 2013;9(6):421–38.
46. Meissner W, Komann M, Erlenwein J, Stamer U, Scherag A. The quality of postoperative pain therapy in German hospitals. Dtsch Arztebl Int 2017;114(10):161–7.
47. Meissner W, Mescha S, Rothaug J, Zwacka S, Goettermann A, Ulrich K, Schleppers A. A Quality improvement in postoperative pain management: results from the QUIPS project. Dtsch Arztebl Int 2008;105:865–70.
48. Miller TE, Thacker JK, White WD, Mantyh C, Migaly J, Jin J, Roche AM, Eisenstein EL, Edwards R, Anstrom KJ, Moon RE, Gan TJ, Enhanced Recovery Study Group. Reduced length of hospital stay in colorectal surgery after implementation of an enhanced recovery protocol. Anesth Analg 2014;118(5):1052–61.
49. Moonesinghe SR, Grocott MP, Bennett-Guerrero E, Bergamaschi R, Gottumukkala V, Hopkins TJ, McCluskey S, Gan TJ, Mythen MM, Shaw AD, Miller TE, Perioperative Quality Initiative (POQI) I Workgroup. American Society for Enhanced Recovery (ASER) and Perioperative Quality Initiative (POQI) joint consensus statement on measurement to maintain and improve quality of enhanced recovery pathways for elective colorectal surgery. Perioper Med (Lond) 2017;6:6.
50. Moore RA, Straube S, Aldington D. Pain measures and cut-offs - 'no worse than mild pain' as a simple, universal outcome. Anaesthesia 2013;68(4):400–12.
51. Mularski RA, White-Chu F, Overbay D, Miller L, Asch SM, Ganzini L. Measuring pain as the 5th vital sign does not improve quality of pain management. J Gen Intern Med 2006;21:607–12.
52. Nasir D, Howard JE, Joshi GP, et al. A survey of acute pain service structure and function in United States hospitals. Pain Res Treat 2011:934932.
53. Office of the Assistant Secretary of Health at the USA Department of Health and Human Services. The national pain strategy. https://iprcc.nih.gov/docs/DraftHHSNationalPainStrategy.pdf.
54. Palmer RH. Considerations in defining quality of health care. In: Palmer RH, Donabedian A, Povar GJ, editors. Striving for quality in health care: an inquiry into policy and practice. Ann Arbor, Mich: Health Administration Press; 1991. p. 1–53.
55. Rabbitts JA, Aaron RV, Fisher E, Lang EA, Bridgwater C, Tai GG., Palermo TM. Long-term pain and recovery after major pediatric surgery: a qualitative study with teens, parents and peroperative care providers. J Pain 2017;18(7):778–86.
56. Rawal N. Organization of acute pain services – a low-cost model. Acta Anaesthesiol Scand Suppl 1997;111:188–90.
57. Rawal N. Acute pain services revisited – good from far, far from good? Reg Anesth Pain Med 2002;27(2):117–21.
58. Rawal N. Current issues in postoperative pain management. Eur J Anaesthesiol. 2016;33(3):160–71.
59. Ready LB, Oden R, Chadwick HS, Benedetti C, Rooke GA, Caplan R, Wild LM. Development of an anesthesiology-based postoperative pain management service. Anesthesiology 1988;68(1):100–6.
60. Rothaug J, Zaslansky R, Schwenkglenks M, Korman M, Alvin A, Backstrom R, Brill S, Bucholz IM, Engle C, Fletcher D, Foror L, Funk P, Gerbershagen HJ, Gordon DB, Konrad C, Kopf A, Leykin Y, Pogatzki-Zahn E, Puig M, Rawal N, Taylor RS, Ullrich K, Volk T, Yahiaoui-Doktor M, Meissner W. Patients' perceptions of post-operative pain management: validation of the International Pain Outcomes Questionnaire (IPO). J Pain 2013;14(11):1361–70.
61. Royal College of Anaesthetists Raising the Standard: a compendium of audit recipes for continuous quality improvement in anaesthesia, 3rd ed. 2012.
62. Schug SA, Palmer GM, Scott DA, Halliwell R, Trinca J, APM: SE Working Group of the Australian and New Zealand College of Anaesthetists and Faculty of Pain Medicine. Acute pain management: scientific evidence, 4th ed. Melbourne: ANZCA & FPM; 2015.

63. Spanjersberg WR, Reurings J, Keys F, van Laarhoven CJ. Fast track surgery versus conventional recovery strategies for colorectal surgery. Cochrane Database Syst Rev 2011;16(2):CD007635
64. Stamer UM, Mpasios N, Stüber F, Maier C. A survey of acute pain services in Germany and a discussion of international survey data. Reg Anesth Pain Med. 2002;27(2):125–31.
65. Tan M, Law LSC, Gan JF. Optimizing pain management to facilitate enhanced recover after surgery pathways. Can J Anesth 2015;62:203–18.
66. Taylor MJ, McNicholas C, Nicolay C, Darzi A, Bell D, Reed JE. Systematic review of the application of the plan-do-study-act method to improve quality in healthcare. BMJ Qual Saf 2014;23(4):290–8.
67. Titsworth WL, Abram J, Guin P, Herman MA, West J, Davis NW, Bushwitz J, Hurley RW, Seubert CN. A prospective time-series quality improvement trial of a standardized analgesia protocol to reduce postoperative pain among neurosurgery patients. J Neurosurg 2016;125(6):1523–32.
68. Van Boekel RLM, Vissers KCP, van der Sande R, Bronkhorst E, Lerou JGC, Steegers AH. Moving beyond pain scores: multidimensional pain assessment is essential for adequate pain management after surgery. PLoS One 2017;12(5):e0177345.doi:10.1371/journal.pone.0177345.
69. Vetter TR, Boudreaux AM, Jones KA, Hunter Jr JM, Pittet J-F. The perioperative surgical home: how anesthesiology can collaboratively achieve and leverage the Triple Aim in health care. Anesth Analg 2014;118(5):1131–6.
70. Vila Jr H, Smith RA, Augustyniak MJ, Nagi PA, Soto RG, Ross TW, Cantor AB, Strickland JM, Miguel RV. The efficacy and safety of pain management before and after implementation of hospital-wide pain management standards: is patient safety compromised by treatment based solely on numerical pain ratings? Anesth Analg 2005;101:474–80.
71. Wilmore DW, Kehlet H. Management of patients in fast track surgery. BMJ 2001;322(7284):473–6.
72. Zaslansky R, Rothaug J, Chapman CR, Bäckström R, Brill S, Fletcher D, Fodor L, Gordon DB, Komann M, Konrad C, Leykin Y, Pogatski-Zahn E, Puig MM, Rawal N, Ullrich K, Volk T, Meissner W. PAIN OUT: the making of an international acute pain registry. Eur J Pain 2015;19:490–502.
73. Zheng H, Li W, Harrold L, Ayers DC, Franklin PD. Web-based comparative patient-reported outcome feedback to support quality improvement and comparative effectiveness research in total joint replacement. EGEMS (Wash DC) 2014;2(1):1130.
74. Zoega S, Gunnarsdottir S, Wilson ME, Gordon DB. Quality pain management in adult hospitalized patients: a concept evaluation. Nurs Forum 2016;51(1):3–12.

INDEX

Note: Page numbers followed by "f" indicate figures and "t" indicate tables.

A

Acceptance and commitment therapy (ACT), 274
Acetaminophen (paracetamol), 293
Acid-sensing ion channels (ASICs), 19, 72
Acid sensitization, 48
Acupuncture, 160–161
Acute Pain Service (APS), 303
Acute postsurgical pain, 217, 219–220
Adductor longus tendon injections, 27
Adenosine triphosphate (ATP), 18
Adenylyl cyclases, 88
Adenylyl cyclase subtype 1 (AC1), 87
α2-Adrenoreceptor agonists, 213
Advanced cardiac life support (ACLS), 263
Afferent drive, periphery
   brain mechanisms, 76
   descending controls
      brain circuitry, spinal transmission, 75
      diffuse noxious inhibitory controls (DNIC), 75
      monoamine systems, 76
      noradrenergic controls, 75
   ionophore
      inflammation and nerve injury elicit plasticity, 71
      sodium channels, 72–73
      transducers, 72
   long-term consequences, neurochemical changes, 78
   neurochemical alterations, chronic pain
      dopamine (DA) neurotransmitter system, 76–77
      glutamate, 76
      opioids, 77
      positron emission tomography (PET), 76
      presynaptic dopaminergic signaling, 76
   rodent models, chronic pain
      anterior cingulate cortex (ACC), 78
      evoked hypersensitivity, 77
      limitations, 77
      mesolimbic dopamine (DA) system, 77
      neurotransmitter systems, 77
      ongoing pain, motivational aspects, 78
   spinal cord
      calcium channels, 74
      central excitatory transmission, 74–75
      central inhibitory transmission, 74
      neuropathic pain, 73
      peripheral sensitization, 73
Aging
   and nociception, 290
   and physiology, 289
α2-Agonists, 253
Agranulocytosis, 252

Altered perioperative pain processing
   central sensitization, 177
   clinical factors, 177
   conditioned pain modulation (CPM), 178
   descending inhibitory controls, 177
   and drug effects
      antinociceptive, 196
      ascending pronociceptive, 196
      conditioned pain modulation (CPM), 195–196, 196f, 198
      cyclooxygenase 2 (COX2) inhibitors and gabapentin, 199
      descending pronociceptive, 196
      diabetic painful neuropathy, 200
      dual pronociceptive, 196
      "fix the dysfunction" concept, 198, 200
      mean preoperative pressure pain detection thresholds, 197, 197f
      opioid-induced hyperalgesia, 200
      pain modulation, 199–201, 199f
      pain thresholds, 195
      placebo-controlled studies, 200
      postherpetic neuralgia, 200
      postoperative pain outcomes, 200
      postthoracotomy pain, acute, 198
      preemptive analgesia concept, 199
      pregabalin (PGB), 199
      pronociceptive pain-perceiving system, 195
      serotonin–norepinephrine reuptake inhibitor (SNRI), 198
      suprathreshold stimuli, 195
      temporal summation (TS), 195–196, 196f
      test-stimulus and conditioning-stimulus, 196
      total knee replacement (TKR), 198
   early postoperative period
      electric pain tolerance thresholds, 179, 179f
      ketorolac supplementation, positive effect, 179, 180f
      pre- and intraoperative analgesic supplementation, 179
      secondary mechanical hyperalgesia, 180, 181f
   late postoperative period
      central pain processing, 181
      cyclooxygenase 2 (COX2) inhibitors, 182
      postoperative time course *vs.* preoperative values, 180, 182f
   mapping techniques, 178
   Nijmegen–Aalborg Screening QST (NASQ), 178
   ongoing nociception effects, 177, 178f
   preoperative pain management, 183
   preoperative pain modulation, 183
   quantitative sensory testing (QST) methods, 177–178

American Pain Society Patient Outcome
    Questionnaire-revised (APS-POQ-R), 308
α-Amino-3-hydroxy-5-methyl-4-isoxazole propionate
    (AMPA), 84, 90–92
Analgesia system, 60
Animal bone tumor models, 23
Animal joint sensitization models, 19
Antidepressants, 236–237, 253
Anti-inflammatory cytokines, 169
Antiopioid peptides (AOPs), 211–212
Anxiety, 71
Appendicitis, acute, 48
APS (Acute Pain Service), 304
ASICs (acid-sensing ion channels), 19, 72
ATP (adenosine triphosphate), 18
Attribution, definition, 33
Attribution error, 33

B

Basal pain sensitivity, 61
Behavioral hypersensitivity, 62, 74
Behavioral management, chronic pain, 273
Bilateral sagittal split osteotomy (BSSO), 227
Blind source separation algorithms, 47
Bone fracture, musculoskeletal pain, 15
Bone metastases, 27
    musculoskeletal pain, 15
Bone pain
    cancer, 17, 20
    nonmalignant, 22
Brain metabolism, 51
Brainstem modulatory systems, 59

C

Ca-CaM, 88
Calcitonin gene–related peptide (CGRP), 17–18
Calcium channels, 74
Calmodulin-dependent protein kinase IIα (CAMKIIα), 211
CaMKIV, 88–89
cAMP response element–binding protein (CREB), 86
    CREB binding protein (CBP), 89
    phosphorylation, 89
cAMP signaling pathways, 88
Cancer bone pain, 17, 20
Capsaicin-induced sensitization, 21
Capsaicin injection, 23
Cardiovascular dysfunction, 259
Catechol-O-methyltransferase (COMT) gene, 172
Cation channel receptors, 49
CBT (cognitive behavioral therapy), 172, 274
^{11}C-carfentanil, 154, 160
Ccentral pain hyperexcitability, 112
^{11}C-diprenorphine, 154, 159
Central excitatory transmission, 74–75
Central inhibitory transmission, 74
Central modulating mechanisms, 227
Central nervous system (CNS) effects
    afferent nerve supply, gut, 41, 42f
    central sensitization, 44
    esophageal afferents, 44
    experimental pain, healthy volunteers. *See* Human experimental pain models
    extrinsic afferents, 41
    intrinsic afferents, 41
    nociceptive signaling, 224
    peripheral nociceptor sensitization, 43
    referred pain, 43
    silent nociceptors, 44
    somatic system, 43
    spinal afferents, 42–43
    spinal dorsal horn neurons, 44
    to surgery and clinical visceral pain
        clinical pain, acute, 48–49
        clinical pain, chronic, 49–51
        electrophysiology, 51
        inverse modeling, electrical sources, 52
        peri- and postoperative pain, 49
    vagal afferents, 42
    visceral diseases treatment, 52
    visceral pain disorders, 41
    visceral *vs.* somatic fibers, 43
    viscerovisceral hyperalgesia, 43
Central poststroke pain (CPSP), 155
Central sensitization (CS), 124
    altered perioperative pain processing, 177
    central nervous system (CNS) effects, 44
    chronic postsurgical pain (CPSP), 207
    deep tissue damage, nociceptive pathways, 9, 10f
    extent and duration, 239
    hyperalgesia, 177
    vs. long-term potentiation (LTP), 83–84
        synaptic plasticity, 84, 85f
    preclinical models, 233–234
    secondary hyperalgesia, 190
Cerebrovascular accidents (CVAs), 260
CFA (complete Freund adjuvant), 91, 190
C-fiber afferent activity, 124
CGRP (calcitonin gene–related peptide), 17–18
Chemosensitivity, 9
Children's pain
    assessment
        health care professionals, 282
        neuroplasticity, 283
        numeric rating scales (NRSs), 282
        pain measurement, 282
        patient-reported outcomes measurement
            information systems (PROMIS), 283
    minimally invasive approaches, 281
    nonpharmacologic and biobehavioral
        treatments, 284
    pain scores, 284
    pharmacologic treatment
        chronic/neuropathic pain management, 284
        health care professional approach, 285
        hyperalgesia, 285
        multimodal analgesia, 285
        pain events, acute, 286
        safety profiles of, 285
    treatment disparity, 281
Cholecystitis, acute, 48
Chronic obstructive pulmonary disease (COPD), 260
Chronic postsurgical pain (CPSP), 266
    central sensitization, 207
    elderly patients, 289

exogenous opioids
    long-lasting hyperalgesia, surgical lesion, 213–215
    pre-/postsurgical environmental stress, 215, 216f–218f, 217
nociceptive and nonnociceptive postsurgical events, 207
opioid-induced hyperalgesia (OIH)
    α2-adrenoreceptor agonists, 213
    analgesic effect, 211
    antiopioid peptides (AOPs), 211–212
    Ca^{2+}/calmodulin-dependent protein kinase IIα (CAMKIIα), 211
    glutamatergic synaptic efficiency, 211, 213f
    homeostatic equilibrium, 213
    inducible nitric oxide synthase (iNOS), 211
    N-methyl-D-aspartate receptor (NMDA-R) antagonist, 211
    μ-opioid receptor (MOR) stimulation, 211
    pain development, 210
    protein kinase C (PKC), 211
    rostral ventromedial medulla (RVM), 213
    surgical injury–induced hyperalgesia amplification, 211, 212f
    thermal hyperalgesia, 211
    transient receptor potential vanilloid 1 (TRPV1), 211
PAIN OUT, 207
pain vulnerability
    immune system, 217
    negative hedonic processes, 219
    N-methyl-D-aspartate receptor (NMDA-R), 219–220
    positive hedonic processes, 219
    reduction/prevention of, 219
    risk concept, 219
pre- and perioperative factors, 207
psychological risk factors, 271, 276–277
reverse translational research, 207–208
risk factors, 207–208
tissue injury, latent pain hypersensitivity
    N-methyl-D-aspartate receptor (NMDA-R), 208
    by surgical lesion, 208, 209f–210f
Clonidine, 235, 264
Cluster headache, 156–157
    deep brain stimulation, 159
    occipital nerve stimulation, 159, 160f
C mechanoheat nociceptors, 3
CNS effects. *See* Central nervous system (CNS) effects
Cognitive-behavioral interventions, 305
Cognitive behavioral therapy (CBT), 172, 274
Cognitive dysfunction, 260
Complete Freund adjuvant (CFA), 91, 190
Complex regional pain syndrome (CRPS), 155
Computer-controlled cuff algometry technique, 16
Computer-controlled sequential pressure stimulation, 23
Conditioned pain modulation (CPM), 59, 64–65, 105, 170
    duloxetine, 171
    nociceptive withdrawal reflex (NWR), 124
    pain sensitivity, 183
Conditioned place preference (CPP), 4
    peripheral nerve block, 5, 6f
Continuous peripheral nerve block catheters (CPNBCs), 265–266
Cool-sensitive fibers, 135
Corticosteroids, 237, 253–254

CPM (conditioned pain modulation), 59, 64–65, 105, 170
    duloxetine, 171
    nociceptive withdrawal reflex (NWR), 124
    pain sensitivity, 183
CPP (conditioned place preference), 4
    peripheral nerve block, 5, 6f
CPSP. *See* Chronic postsurgical pain (CPSP)
CREB (cAMP response element–binding protein), 86
    CREB binding protein (CBP), 89
    phosphorylation, 89
CRPS (complex regional pain syndrome), 155
CS. *See* Central sensitization (CS)
CVAs (cerebrovascular accidents), 260
Cuff algometry
    with arthritis, 22
    lateral epicondylalgia, 23
    pain sensitivity assessment, 16
    quantitative sensory testing (QST), 109, 110f
Cut injury, C mechanoheat nociceptors, heat sensitivity, 3
Cyclic AMP response elements (CRE), 89
Cyclooxygenase 2 (COX2) inhibitors, 199, 237

D

Deep brain stimulation, 159
Deep somatic postoperative pain, 15
Deep tissue damage, nociceptive pathways
    C mechanoheat nociceptors, 3
    human studies
        anti–nerve growth factor, guarding pain, 11
        central sensitization, 9, 10f
        chemosensitivity, 9
        forearm skin incision, 8
        heat hyperalgesia, 8
        hydrogen peroxide, 9
        incision-induced peripheral nociceptive mediators, 9
        ischemic-like signal, 9, 9f
        local anesthetic nerve blockade, 8–9
        mechanosensitive response, 9, 10f
        minimally invasive approach, 8
        nonsteroidal anti-inflammatory drugs, 11
        pain ratings, 8
        pain scores and opioid utilization, 8
        peripheral sensitization, 9, 10f
        plantar incision model, 9
        spontaneous activity, 9
    incisional postoperative pain. *See* Rat plantar hindpaw model
    incisional-type injuries, 3
    vs. mini-incision total hip arthroplasty, 8
    needle penetrations, 3
Degenerative animal joint models, 18
Delayed onset muscle soreness (DOMS), 19–20
Depression, 71
Descending control mechanisms
    ascending transmission pathways, 59
    brain circuitry, spinal transmission, 75
    diffuse noxious inhibitory controls (DNIC), 75
    inflammatory and neuropathic pain, 59
    monoamine systems, 76
    nociceptive primary afferents, 59
    noradrenergic controls, 75

Descending control mechanisms *(Continued)*
   rostral ventromedial medulla (RVM), 59, 60f
      analgesia system, 60
      ascending nociceptive information, 60
      behavioral hypersensitivity, 60
      "bottom-up" recruitment, normal and potentiated pain states, 61–64
      cognitive and emotional factors, 60
      conditioned pain modulation (CPM), 64–65
      endogenous analgesia, 60
      inflammatory and neuropathic pain, 60
      microinjection/single-cell recording approach, 61
      NEUTRAL-cells, 61
      nocifensor reflexes, 61
      OFF-cells and ON-cells, 61
      opioid analgesic drugs, 60
      pain-modulating network, 60
      physiology and function, 59
      supraspinal system, 60
      "top-down" engagement, 64
      withdrawal reflex, 61
Descending pain modulation mechanisms, 61, 111, 159
Dexamethasone, 253
Diffuse noxious inhibitory control (DNIC), 65, 75, 111, 224
Diffusion tensor imaging, 46, 50
Dipyrone (metamizole), 252
DOMS (delayed onset muscle soreness), 19–20
Dopamine (DA) neurotransmitter system, 76–77, 156
Duloxetine, 171, 198, 237
Dysmenorrhea, 33, 35–36, 35t, 38

E

Early long-term potentiation (E-LTP), 84
EEG. *See* Electroencephalography (EEG)
EFIC (European Pain Federation), 276
Egr 3, 89–91, 90f
Elderly patients
   acetaminophen (paracetamol), 293
   aging
      and nociception, 290
      and physiology, 289
   chronic postsurgical pain (CPSP), 289
   multimodal analgesia, 292
   nonopioid analgesics, 292–293
   nonsteroidal anti-inflammatory drugs (NSAIDs), 293
   opioid analgesics
      epidural opioids, 293
      fentanyl, 294
      hydromorphone, 294
      morphine, 294
      opioid-induced adverse effects, 295
      patient-controlled analgesia, 295–296
      patient-controlled analgesia (PCA), 293
      tramadol, 294–295
   opioid-naïve patients, 290
   pain assessment barriers, 291
   pain management, discharge plan, 297–298
   pharmacodynamic changes, 290
   pharmacokinetic changes, 290
   pharmacologic therapies, 292
   regional analgesic techniques
      epidural analgesia, 296
      intraoperative periarticular infiltration, 297
      nociceptive afferent pathways, 296
      peripheral nerve blocks (PNBs), 297
      wound infiltration, 297
   self-reported pain assessment tools, 291
   transcutaneous electrical nerve stimulation (TENS), 292
Electrical facet joint stimulation, 26
Electrical monopolar/bipolar cauterization, 34
Electric pain tolerance thresholds, 179, 179f
Electroencephalography (EEG), 45, 187
   acid sensitization, 48
   advantage, 46
   blind source separation algorithms, 47
   evoked potentials (EPs), 46, 47f, 48
   independent component analysis, 47
   inverse modeling algorithms, 46, 48
   low-resolution electromagnetic tomographic analysis (LORETA), 46, 47f
   multichannel recordings, 46
   neuronal pain networks, 46
   nociceptive withdrawal reflex, 48
   pain matrix, 48
   secondary pinprick hyperalgesia, 190–191, 192f
   signal decomposition procedures, 46–47
   somatic sensory system, 48
   visceral homunculus, 48
Electromyography (EMG), 121
Electrophysiologic techniques
   cool-sensitive fibers, 135
   disadvantages, 122
   electrical activity, 133
   electrical stimulation, 122
   event-related brain potentials (ERPs), 133, 138
   heat conduction and transduction, 144
   infrared laser stimulation (LS), 134, 134f
   intraepidermal electrical stimulation (IES), 135
   laser-evoked brain potentials (LEPs), 138
      Aδ and C nociceptors coactivation, 137–139
      C nociceptors, selective activation, 139–141
      intracranial recordings, 142–143
   laser-evoked magnetic fields
      Aδ and C nociceptors coactivation, 141–142
      C nociceptors, selective activation, 142
      electrocortical activity, 141
      MEG recordings, 141
   mechanical pinprick stimuli, 137
   neural activity, 133
   nociceptive afferent volley, 134
   nociceptive event-related potentials (EVPs), 135, 136f
   nonnociceptive mechanoreceptors, 135
   ongoing oscillatory activity, 144–145
   pain intensity, 144
   pain receptors, skin, 122
   postsynaptic potentials, 133
   quantification of, 122
   reflex receptive field (RRF)
      acquisition and recording of, 122, 123f
      bidimensional interpolation and extrapolation, 122
      detection of, 123
      quantitative features, 122
      reliability of, 123
   skin temperature profile, 134, 135f

spinal nociception. *See* Spinal nociception
steady-state evoked potentials (SS-EPs), 145–146, 146f
stimulus-evoked activity, 133
surface electromyography (EMG), 122
thermal activation threshold, 134
time-locked and transient brain responses, 134, 134f
Electrothermal stimulation, 27
EMG (electromyography), 121
Endogenous analgesia, 60
Endogenous opioidergic system, 159
Endogenous pain control system, 154–155
Endogenous pain inhibitory mechanisms, 50
Endometriosis
   dysmenorrhea, 35–36, 35t
   electrical monopolar/bipolar cauterization, 34
   nonacute pelvic pain, 34
   nonvisible pain process, 34
   pain sensitization, 33
      abdomen examination, 37, 37f
      allodynia/muscle hyperalgesia assessment, 37
      benefit of, 38
      definition, 36
      detection of, 38
      history of, 38
      hyperalgesic priming, 37
      hyperesthesia, 36
      pain pressure thresholds, 37–38
      postcholecystectomy syndrome, 37
      randomized controlled trial, 35
Enhanced recovery after surgery (ERAS) pathways, 261, 303–304
Epidural analgesia, 254, 296
   vs. peripheral nerve blocks, 266
Epidural opioids, 293
Epinephrine, 264
Escitalopram, 237
Esophageal afferents, 44
Esophagus sensitization, 45
European Pain Federation (EFIC), 276
Event-related brain potentials (ERPs), 133, 138
Evoked brain potentials, 51
Evoked potentials (EPs), 46, 47f, 48
Excitatory synaptic transmission, 84, 91
Exogenous opioids
   long-lasting hyperalgesia, surgical lesion, 213–215
   pre-/postsurgical environmental stress, 215, 216f–218f, 217
Experimental pain, healthy volunteers. *See* Human experimental pain models
Extracorporeal shock wave lithotripsy, 48
Extrinsic afferents, 41

F

Fast Accurate Cortical Extraction (FACE), 50, 50f
Fentanyl, 294
^{18}F-fluoroethyl-diprenorphine, 155
Fibromyalgia, 21–22, 24
   glutamate, 76
   opioids, 77
   positron emission tomography (PET), 156, 157f
Forearm skin incision, 8
Fracture pain, 17
Fragile X mental retardation protein (FMRP), 89

Freund adjuvant, 62
Functional magnetic resonance imaging (fMRI), 45–46, 76
Functional visceral pain disorders, 49

G

Gabapentin, 199, 236, 252
Gastrointestinal (GI) stimulations, 51
Generator potentials, depolarizing currents, 72
Gene-related proteins, 89
German Society for Anaesthesiology and Intensive Care, 309
GluR1-PDZ interaction, 88
GluR1 receptors, 91–92
Glutamate, 76, 84
   receptors, 94
Glutamatergic synapses, 84
Green fluorescent protein (GFP), 84
Groin herniotomy, 223–224
Guarding behavior, rat plantar hindpaw model, 4f
   conditioned place preference (CPP), 5, 6f
   contralateral unincised hindpaw, 4
   cutaneous injury elicits, 5
   in vivo neurophysiology, 5, 7, 7f
   ketoprofen, 4
   morphine, 4
   patient-controlled analgesia, 4
   sham incision, 5, 7f
   skin incision *vs.* skin plus deep tissue injury, 4
   spontaneous activity, 5, 7, 7f
Guarding pain, anti–nerve growth factor, 11
Gynecologic laparoscopy
   attribution, definition, 33
   attribution error, 33
   cognitive error, 33
   endometriosis, 34
      dysmenorrhea, 35–36, 35t
      electrical monopolar/bipolar cauterization, 34
      nonacute pelvic pain, 34
      nonvisible pain process, 34
      pain sensitization, 33, 36–38
      randomized controlled trial, 35
   "negative" rate of, 34

H

Heat hyperalgesia, 8
Heat-insensitive nociceptors, 188–189, 188f–189f
   heat stimulation, skin, 189, 189f
   high-frequency electrical stimulation (HFS), 188, 188f
   high-threshold mechanoreceptors (HTMs), 189
   TRPV1 receptor, 188
   type I mechano- and heat-sensitive A δ fibers (type I AMH), 189
Heat pain detection threshold (HPDT), 224
Heat sensitivity, C mechanoheat nociceptors, 3
Heat-sensitive nociceptive afferents, 134, 134f
Hemicrania continua, 156
Hemidiaphragmatic paresis (HDP), 263
Heterosynaptic long-term potentiation, 86
High-frequency electrical stimulation (HFS), 188, 188f
High-threshold mechanoreceptors (HTMs), 189
Homosynaptic long-term potentiation
   α-amino-3-hydroxy-5-methyl-4-isoxazole propionate (AMPA), 84
   formalin/sciatic nerve jury, 86

Homosynaptic long-term potentiation *(Continued)*
    glutamate, 84
    injury-related synaptic plasticity, 84
    N-methyl-D-aspartate (NMDA) receptors, 84, 86
    mitogen-activated protein (MAP) kinase, 84
HPDT (heat pain detection threshold), 224
5-HT and 5-HT(3) receptor antagonist, 19
5-HT-induced protein kinase C (PKC) activation, 86
HTMs (high-threshold mechanoreceptors), 189
Human experimental pain models
    analgesic effects, 44
    diffusion tensor imaging, 46
    electroencephalography (EEG), 45
        acid sensitization, 48
        advantage, 46
        blind source separation algorithms, 47
        evoked potentials (EPs), 46, 47f, 48
        independent component analysis, 47
        inverse modeling algorithms, 46, 48
        low-resolution electromagnetic tomographic analysis (LORETA), 46, 47f
        multichannel recordings, 46
        neuronal pain networks, 46
        nociceptive withdrawal reflex, 48
        pain matrix, 48
        signal decomposition procedures, 46–47
        somatic sensory system, 48
        visceral homunculus, 48
    functional magnetic resonance imaging (fMRI), 45–46
    magnetoencephalography, 48
    neuroimaging, 45
    nociceptive reflex, 45
    nonpainful visceral stimulus, 45
    psychological processes, 45
    reciprocal interactions, 45
    referred pain, 44
    visceral pain neuromatrix, 45
    viscerovisceral hyperalgesia, 44
Human sacroiliac join ligament, 23
Human surrogate model, 187
Hydromorphone, 294
5-Hydroxy-tryptamine (5-HT), 86
Hyperalgesia
    central sensitization, 177
    human surrogate model, 187
    mechanical, 191
    osteoarthritis (OA), 171
    primary, 187
    priming, 37
    quantitative sensory testing (QST), 108
    secondary, 187, 234
        central sensitization, 190
        heat-insensitive nociceptors, 188–189, 188f–189f
        pinprick-evoked brain potentials (PEPs), 190–191, 192f
        pinprick stimulator, characteristics, 190, 191f
Hyperesthesia, 36
Hypersensitivity
    behavioral, 62, 74
    latent, 64
    localized
        bone, 20
        connective tissue, 20–21
        joint, 19–20
        muscle, 18–19
    mechanical, 72
    spreading
        bone, 22–23
        connective tissue, 23
        joint, 22
        muscle, 21–22
Hypertonic saline, 15–16
Hypnosis, 273
Hypoalgesia, 225, 228
Hypothalamic dysfunction, 158

I

IASP (International Association for the Study of Pain), 167, 276
IES (intraepidermal electrical stimulation), 135
Ilioinguinal/iliohypogastric nerves, 227
Incision-induced pain, 187
Incision-induced peripheral nociceptive mediators, 9
Independent component analysis, 47
Inducible nitric oxide synthase (iNOS), 211
Inferior alveolar nerve (IAN), 227
Inflammatory and neuropathic pain, 60
Inflammatory animal joint models, 19
Inflammatory bowel disease, 51
Inflammatory pain, 71
Infraclavicular blocks, 263–264
Infrared laser stimulation (LS), 134, 134f
Inguinal herniotomy
    bilateral sagittal split osteotomy (BSSO), 227
    central modulating mechanisms, 227
    deep *vs.* superficial pain, 228–229
    degree of sensory hyperexcitability, 227
    heterogeneous pain processing, 226
    ilioinguinal/iliohypogastric nerves, 227
    inferior alveolar nerve (IAN), 227
    intercostobrachial nerve (ICBN), 228
    late sensory function
        pain-free patients, 225
        pain patients, 226
    mesh-based herniotomy, 228
    nociceptive heterogeneity, 226
    pain-related functional impairment, 227
    preoperative sensory function, 223–224
    sensory dysfunction, 227
        acute, 224–225
    in thoracotomy, 228
Injury-related synaptic plasticity, 84
Insult, acute, 62, 63f
Intense sensitization model, 44
Intercostobrachial nerve (ICBN), 228
International Association for the Study of Pain (IASP), 167, 276
International Pain Outcomes Questionnaire (IPO-Q), 308
Interscalene block, 263–264
Intra-articular stimulation, 16
Intraepidermal electrical stimulation (IES), 135
Intraoperative nerve injury, 223–229
Intrathecal analgesia, 254
Intravenous lidocaine, 238
Intrinsic afferents, 41

Inverse modeling
 algorithms, 46, 48
 electrical sources, 52
In vivo neurophysiology, rat plantar hindpaw model, 5, 7, 7f
Ionophore
 inflammation and nerve injury elicit plasticity, 71
 sodium channels, 72–73
 transducers, 72

J

Joint surgery. See Osteoarthritis (OA)

K

Ketamine, 74, 171, 236, 253
Ketoprofen, 4
Knee osteoarthritis (KOA), 167, 168

L

Laser-evoked brain potentials (LEPs), 138, 187
 Aδ and C nociceptors coactivation, 137–139
 C nociceptors, selective activation, 139–141
 intracranial recordings, 142–143
Laser-evoked magnetic fields
 Aδ and C nociceptors coactivation, 141–142
 C nociceptors, selective activation, 142
 electrocortical activity, 141
 MEG recordings, 141
Late long-term potentiation (L-LTP), 84
Latent hypersensitivity, 64
Latent pain sensitization, 215
Late sensory function
 pain—pain-free patients, 225
 pain—pain patients, 226
Lidocaine, 75
α2δ Ligands, 252
Liposomal bupivacaine, 265
Local anesthetic systemic toxicity (LAST), 262–263
Localized hypersensitivity
 bone, 20
 connective tissue, 22–23
 joint, 19–20
 muscle, 18–19
Long-lasting muscle hypersensitivity, 21
Long-term potentiation (LTP), 74
 vs. central sensitization (CS), 83–84
  synaptic plasticity, 84, 85f
 chronic pain reduction, 92–93
 microglia
  activation, 94, 95f, 97f
  activity-dependent synaptic plasticity, 94
  neuromodulators, 94
  in pain-related cortices, 94, 96f
 molecular mechanisms, cortical
  adenylyl cyclases, AC1, AC8, 88
  Ca-CaM, 88
  CaMKIV, 88–89
  Egr 1, 89–91, 90f
  fragile X mental retardation protein (FMRP), 89
  gene expression, 89
  GluR1-PDZ interaction, 88
  N-methyl-d-aspartate (NMDA) receptors, 87
  postsynaptic enhancement, 87
  presynaptic enhancement, 87
  "silent" synapses/synaptic trafficking, 87
  synaptic potentiation, 89
 neuropathic pain
  cortical glial cells, 94, 96
  spinal microglia, 93–94
 pain-related cortex
  anterior cingulate cortex (ACC), 86
  cAMP response element–binding protein (CREB), 86
  insular cortex (IC), 86
  L-type voltage-gated calcium channel (L-VGCC) dependent, 86–87
  N-methyl-d-aspartate (NMDA) receptor dependent, 86–87
  presynaptic LTP (pre-LTP), 86
  protein synthesis L-LTP, 87
 spinal cord dorsal horn
  heterosynaptic LTP, 86
  homosynaptic LTP, 84, 86
 synaptic responses measurement
  ACC plasticity, 91
  AMPA receptors, 91–92
  in vivo electrophysiology, 91
  NMDA GluN2B receptors, 92
  postsynaptic and presynaptic changes, 91
  presynaptic release, 92
 tissue injury, latent pain hypersensitivity, 208
Low-back pain, 27
 musculoskeletal pain, 15
Low-resolution electromagnetic tomographic analysis (LORETA), 46, 47f
LTP. See Long-term potentiation (LTP)
L-type voltage-gated calcium channel (L-VGCC) dependent, 86–87

M

Magnetoencephalography, 48
MAP (mitogen-activated protein) kinase, 84
Mapping joint pain sensitivity, 16
Mechanical hyperalgesia, 191
Mechanical hypersensitivity, 72
Mechanical nociceptive pathways, 187
Mechanical nociceptive threshold, 215, 216f–217f
Mechanism-based approaches, 103
Mechanistic pain phenotyping. See Quantitative sensory testing (QST)
Mechanosensitive receptors, 17
Melatonin homeostasis, 157
Mesh-based herniotomy, 228
Mesolimbic dopamine (DA) system, 77–78
Metamizole (dipyrone), 252
N-Methyl-d-aspartate (NMDA) receptor, 19–20, 74, 84, 86–89
 antagonist, 211
 GluN2B receptors, 92
 ketamine, 236
 multimodal analgesia, 253
 nitrous oxide, 237
 tissue injury, latent pain hypersensitivity, 208
Microglia
 activation, 94, 95f, 97f
 activity-dependent synaptic plasticity, 94
 neuromodulators, 94
 in pain-related cortices, 94, 96f

Microglia-specific antigens, 93
Microinjection/single-cell recording approach, 61
Migraine, 158
Mineralized bone, 17
Minimally invasive approach, 8, 49
Minocycline, 238
Mitogen-activated protein (MAP) kinase, 84
Monoamine systems, 76
MOR (μ-opioid receptor) stimulation, 211
Morphine, 4, 294
Multielectrode array (MED64), 87
Multimodal analgesia, 234
    α2-agonists, 253
    antidepressants, 253
    "antihyperalgesic" action, 250
    benefits of, 249
    clinical implications, 256
    components of, 250, 251f
    corticosteroids, 253–254
    elderly patients, 292
    α2δ ligands, 252
    neuraxial regional analgesia, 254
    N-methyl-D-aspartate (NMDA) receptor antagonists, 253
    nonopioid analgesics, 251–252
    opioid analgesics, 250
    opioid-free analgesia, 256
    opioid-induced ventilatory impairment (OIVI), 249
    patient-controlled analgesia (PCA), 249
    peripheral regional analgesia, 255
    peripheral sensitization, 250
    postoperative parecoxib/valdecoxib vs. placebo, 249, 250f
    postoperative period, 250
    procedure-specific evidence-based guidelines, 255
    spinal cord and brain nociceptive mechanisms, 250
    systemic local anesthetics, 253
Muscle nociceptors, 15
    sensitization of, 18
Musculoskeletal pain, 15
    bone, 17
    chronic, 18
    connective tissue, 18
    joint, 16–17, 17f
    muscle, 15–16
Myofascial and muscle injury/overuse, musculoskeletal pain, 15
Myofibrillar contractile mechanism, 21

N

Nerve growth factor (NGF), 17, 72
    injection, fascial tissue, 21
    long-lasting muscle hypersensitivity, 21
    microneuromas, nerve sprouting and formation, 20
Neuraxial regional analgesia, 254
Neurofilament 210
    sensory receptors, 17
Neurokinin-1 receptors, 51, 62
Neuromatrix, 50
Neuronal pain networks, 46
Neuropathic pain, 71
    cortical glial cells, 94, 96
    positron emission tomography (PET), 155
    spinal microglia, 93–94

Neuroplasticity, children's pain, 283
Neurotransmitter serotonin, 158
Nijmegen–Aalborg Screening QST (NASQ), 178
NMDA receptor. See N-Methyl-D-aspartate (NMDA) receptor
Nociceptive heterogeneity, 226
Nociceptive neuroplasticity, 104
Nociceptive primary afferent fibers, spontaneous activity, 5
Nociceptive reflex, 45
Nociceptive system modalities, 104
Nociceptive withdrawal reflex (NWR), 48
    disadvantages, 122
    electrical stimulation, 122
    pain receptors, skin, 122
    quantification of, 122
    reflex receptive field (RRF)
        acquisition and recording of, 122, 123f
        bidimensional interpolation and extrapolation, 122
        detection of, 123
        quantitative features, 122
        reliability of, 123
    spinal nociception. See Spinal nociception
    surface electromyography (EMG), 122
Nocifensor reflexes, 61
Nonopioid analgesics, 251–252
    elderly patients, 292–293
Nonpharmacologic modalities, 292
NR2B inhibitors, 92
Nonsteroidal anti-inflammatory drugs (NSAIDs), 11, 237
    elderly patients, 293
Numeric rating scales (NRSs), 282

O

OA. See Osteoarthritis (OA)
Occipital nerve stimulation, 159, 160f
Operculoinsular cortex, 154
Opioid analgesics, 250
    epidural opioids, 293
    fentanyl, 294
    hydromorphone, 294
    morphine, 294
    opioid-induced adverse effects, 295
    patient-controlled analgesia (PCA), 293, 295–296
    tramadol, 294–295
    usage, 260–261
Opioidergic receptor function, 155
Opioid-free analgesia, 256
Opioid-induced hyperalgesia (OIH), 62, 200, 234, 238
    α2-adrenoreceptor agonists, 213
    analgesic effect, 211
    antiopioid peptides (AOPs), 211–212
    Ca^{2+}/calmodulin-dependent protein kinase IIα (CAMKIIα), 211
    glutamatergic synaptic efficiency, 211, 213f
    homeostatic equilibrium, 213
    inducible nitric oxide synthase (iNOS), 211
    N-methyl-D-aspartate receptor (NMDA-R) antagonist, 211
    μ-opioid receptor (MOR) stimulation, 211
    pain development, 210
    protein kinase C (PKC), 211
    rostral ventromedial medulla (RVM), 213

surgical injury–induced hyperalgesia amplification, 211, 212f
thermal hyperalgesia, 211
transient receptor potential vanilloid 1 (TRPV1), 211
Opioid-induced ventilatory impairment (OIVI), 249
μ-Opioid receptor (MOR) stimulation, 211
Opioid-sparing anesthesia, 238–239
Organic visceral diseases, 50
Osteoarthritis (OA)
    articular cartilage and subchondral bone pathogenesis, 16
    calcium channels, spinal cord, 74
    clinical assessment, 168
    comorbidities, 169
    definition, 167
    genetics and joint pain, 171–172
    hip joint, 26
    hyperalgesia, 171
    inflammation, 169
    mapping joint pain sensitivity, 16
    musculoskeletal pain, 15
    nonsurgical methods, 167
    pain duration, 24
    pain intensity and scores, 20
    peripatellar hypersensitivity, 19
    psychological factors, 172
    quantitative sensory testing (QST), 108
        measurements, 170
        pain mechanisms, 170
        peripheral and central sensitization, 170
        preoperative screening, 169
    sensitization patterns, 20
    total joint arthroplasty (TJA)
        central nervous system, 171
        comorbidities, 169
        inflammation, 169
        knee osteoarthritis (KOA), 167
        pain-free recovery, 171
        patients phenotyping, 170
        pharmacologic and nonpharmacologic treatment guidelines, 167
        preoperative risk factors, 167, 168f
        social factors, 167
        total hip arthroplasty (THA), 167–168
        total knee arthroplasty (TKA), 167–168
    total knee replacement, 22
Osteoporosis, musculoskeletal pain, 15

P

Pain
    acute, 48–49
    children's pain. *See* Children's pain
    chronic, 63–64, 83
        after total joint arthroplasty (TJA). *See* Total joint arthroplasty (TJA)
        anterior cingulate cortex (ACC), 78
        brain metabolism, 51
        cation channel receptors, 49
        cognitive/evaluative functions, 50
        diffusion tensor imaging, 50
        dopamine (DA) neurotransmitter system, 76–77
        endogenous pain inhibitory mechanisms, 50
        evoked hypersensitivity, 77
        Fast Accurate Cortical Extraction (FACE), 50, 50f
        functional visceral pain disorders, 49
        glutamate, 76
        heat stimulation, 49
        inflammatory bowel disease, 51
        limitations, 77
        long-term potentiation (LTP), 92–93
        mesolimbic dopamine (DA) system, 77
        neurokinin-1 receptor, 51
        neuromatrix, 50
        neurotransmitter systems, 77
        ongoing pain, motivational aspects, 78
        opioids, 77
        organic visceral diseases, 50
        pain matrix, 50
        positron emission tomography (PET), 76
        presynaptic dopaminergic signaling, 76
        referred pain, 49
        visceral hypersensitivity, 50
        viscerasomatic convergence, 49
        visceromotor responses, 50
    chronification, 15
    health care quality. *See* Quality improvement (QI)
    inflammatory, 83
    management and prevention, 103
    neuropathic, treatments for, 83
    neuroplasticity, 105–106
    pathologic, 83
    physiologic, 83
    positron emission tomography (PET). *See* Positron emission tomography (PET)
    pre- and postsurgical psychological assessment and management. *See* Pre- and postsurgical psychological assessment and management
    sensitization, 33. *See also* Chronic postsurgical pain (CPSP)
        abdomen examination, 37, 37f
        acute, 59
        allodynia/muscle hyperalgesia assessment, 37
        assessment, 16
        benefit of, 38
        definition, 36
        detection of, 38
        history of, 36
        hyperalgesic priming, 37
        hyperesthesia, 36
        pain pressure thresholds, 37–38
        postcholecystectomy syndrome, 37
    signaling systems, 73
    vulnerability
        immune system, 217
        negative hedonic processes, 219
        N-methyl-D-aspartate receptor (NMDA-R) antagonist, 219–220
        positive hedonic processes, 219
        pre-/postsurgical environmental stress, exogenous opioids, 215, 216f–218f, 217
        reduction/prevention of, 219
        risk concept, 219
"Pain-inhibits-pain" paradigm, 111
Pain mapping technique, 111

Pain matrix, 44, 48, 50
   afferent drive, periphery, 76
   long-term consequences, neurochemical changes, 78
PAIN OUT, 309
Pain referral
   from bone, 27
   connective tissue, 27
   from joint, 26–27, 26f
   from muscle, 25–26
Pain-related cortex
   anterior cingulate cortex (ACC), 86
   cAMP response element–binding protein (CREB), 86
   insular cortex (IC), 86
   L-type voltage-gated calcium channel (L-VGCC) dependent, 86–87
   N-methyl-D-aspartate (NMDA) receptor dependent, 86–87
   presynaptic LTP (pre-LTP), 86
   protein synthesis L-LTP, 87
Paired-pulse facilitation (PPF), 92
Pancreatitis, chronic, 51–52
Paracetamol, 251
Paroxysmal hemicrania, 156
Patient-controlled analgesia (PCA), 214, 249, 293, 295–296
Patient-controlled epidural analgesia (PCEA), 296
Patient registries
   German Society for Anaesthesiology and Intensive Care, 309
   PAIN OUT, 309
   Plan-Do-Study-Act (PDSA) cycles, 309
   Quality Improvement in Postoperative Pain Management (QUIPS), 308–309
   Stanford Collaborative Health Outcomes Information Registry (CHOIR), 309
   US National Pain Strategy, 308
Patient-reported outcomes (PROs), 305
   factor analysis, 308
   goal of, 307
   perioperative pain registries, 308
Patient-reported outcomes measurement information systems (PROMIS), 283
Pediatric pain. *See* Children's pain
Pelvic pain
   acute, 34
   attribution, definition, 33
   attribution error, 33
   chronic, 33–34
      endometriosis, 34–35
   cognitive error, 33
   "negative" rate of, 34
Periaqueductal gray (PAG), 155
Perigenual ACC (pACC), 155
Perioperative pain, 49
Perioperative surgical home (PSH), 305
Periosteum, 17
Peripheral nerve blocks (PNBs), 78, 297
   vs. epidural analgesia, 266
Peripheral nerve injury (PNI), 263
Peripheral nociceptor sensitization, 43
Peripheral prostaglandins, 5
Peripheral regional analgesia, 255
Peripheral sensitization, 250

Persistent postoperative pain, 191
Persistent postsurgical pain (PPSP) prevention
   acute and subacute postoperative pain control, 240–241
   anesthesiologic aspects of, 241, 242t
   central sensitization, extent and duration, 239
   emotional distress, 233
   long-term pain, 233
   orthopedic procedure, 240
   perioperative drugs and techniques
      antidepressant drugs, 236–237
      corticosteroids, 237
      cyclooxygenase 2 (COX2) inhibitors, 237
      gabapentin, 236
      glial activation, 235
      inflammatory reaction, 234
      intraoperative opioid administration, 238
      intravenous lidocaine, 238
      ketamine, 236
      locoregional analgesia, 235–236
      minocycline, 238
      multimodal/balanced analgesia, 234
      neuronal-based phenomenon, 234
      nitrous oxide, 237
      nonsteroidal anti-inflammatory drugs, 237
      opioid-induced hyperalgesia (OIH), 234, 238
      opioid-sparing anesthesia, 238–239
      perioperative opioid use, 238
      pregabalin, 236
      sevoflurane inhaled anesthesia, 237
   perioperative risk factors, 239, 240t
   preclinical models, 233–234
   quantitative sensory testing (QST), 240
   risk-factor index, 239
   risk factors, 233
PET. *See* Positron emission tomography (PET)
Pinprick-evoked brain potentials (PEPs), 190–191, 192f
   persistent postoperative pain, 191
Plan-Do-Study-Act (PDSA) cycles, 309
Pneumothorax, 264
Polymodal muscle nociceptors, 15
Polysynaptic reflex, 121
Polysynaptic spinal pathway, 45
Positron emission tomography (PET), 76
   acupuncture, 160–161
   brain function, 153
   clinical pain conditions
      cluster headache, 156–157
      fibromyalgia, 156, 157f
      migraine, 158
      neuropathic pain, 155
   cortical glucose consumption, 153
   deep brain stimulation, 159
   endogenous pain control system, 154–155
   endurance training, 160
   in healthy brain, 154
   limitations, 153
   motor cortex stimulation, 159
   neuronal activity patterns, 153
   neurotransmitter systems in vivo, 153
   occipital nerve stimulation, 159, 160f
   pain-processing networks, 153
   radioactively labeled glucose, 153

Postanesthesia care unit (PACU), 261
Postcholecystectomy syndrome, 37, 49
Postherniotomy pain, 226
Postoperative cognitive dysfunction (POCD), 260
Postoperative nausea and vomiting (PONV), 251–252, 262
Postoperative pain, 49
    control
        acute and subacute, 240–241
        multimodal drug therapies, adults. *See* Multimodal analgesia
        for older persons. *See* Elderly patients
        regional anesthesia (RA), adults. *See* Regional anesthesia (RA)
    deep tissue damage, nociceptive pathways. *See* Deep tissue damage, nociceptive pathways
    human surrogate model, 187
    localized hypersensitivity. *See* Localized hypersensitivity
    musculoskeletal pain. *See* Musculoskeletal pain
    pain referral. *See* Pain referral
    spreading hypersensitivity. *See* Spreading hypersensitivity
    temporal summation. *See* Temporal summation
Postoperative patient-controlled analgesia (PCA)
    morphine, 105
Postsurgical pathophysiology, 71
Postsynaptic membrane GluA1 receptors, 92
PPSP prevention. *See* Persistent postsurgical pain (PPSP) prevention
Pre- and perioperative pain control, 103
Pre- and postsurgical psychological assessment and management
    barriers
        cost, 276
        patient adherence, 275–276
        postsurgical factors, 275
        provider-related barriers, 276
        resources, 275
        stigma, 276
    behavioral management, chronic pain, 273
    comprehensive behavioral treatment interventions, 274
    depression treatment, 274
    depressive symptoms/clinical depression, 271
    high-dose chronic opioid therapy, 272
    hypnosis, 273
    non-pharmacological and biobehavioral interventions, 273
    opioid management, 274
    pain-related outcomes, 271
    patient-specific functional activity goals, 275
    presurgical depression, 272
    psychological risk factors, 271
        chronic postsurgical pain (CPSP), 271, 276–277
    relaxation/mindfulness, 273
    screening and treatment planning, 272–273
    tapering, 274
    total joint arthroplasties, 271
Preemptive analgesia, 234
Pregabalin (PGB), 199, 236, 252
Preoperative peripheral sensory function, 224
Pressure algometry, 16
Pressure hyperalgesia, 224
Pressure-induced muscle pain, 23
Pressure pain thresholds, 170

Presynaptic LTP (pre-LTP), 86
Preventive analgesia, 234
Proinflammatory cytokines, 19–20, 169, 170f
PROs (patient-reported outcomes), 305
    factor analysis, 308
    goal of, 307
    perioperative pain registries, 308
Prostaglandin synthesis, 252
Protective analgesia, 234
Protein kinase C (PKC), 211
Pulmonary dysfunction, 260

Q

Quality improvement (QI)
    Acute Pain Service (APS), 304
    analgesic team concept, 304
    clinical practice guidelines, 304
    cognitive-behavioral interventions, 305
    continuous improvement, outcomes, 302–303
    elements, 301, 302f
    enhanced recovery after surgery (ERAS) pathways, 303–304
    health care quality, definition, 301
    pain trajectory, 307
    patient registries
        German Society for Anaesthesiology and Intensive Care, 309
        PAIN OUT, 309
        Plan-Do-Study-Act (PDSA) cycles, 309
        Quality Improvement in Postoperative Pain Management (QUIPS), 308–309
        Stanford Collaborative Health Outcomes Information Registry (CHOIR), 309
        US National Pain Strategy, 308
    patient-reported outcomes (PROs), 305
        factor analysis, 308
        goal of, 307
        perioperative pain registries, 308
    perioperative surgical home (PSH), 305
    in production process, 302–303
    in standardization, 302–303
    structural and process parameters, 302
    Structure-Process-Outcome model, 301
    technical quality, 301
    University of Washington Harborview Medical Center Perioperative Integrated Pain Care Pathway, 305, 306f
    workflow redesign, 305
Quality Improvement in Postoperative Pain Management (QUIPS), 308–309
Quality-of-life parameters, 235
Quantitative sensory testing (QST), 177–178, 214
    assessment methods, 104
    central pain hyperexcitability, 112
    deep *vs.* superficial pain, 228
    late sensory function and pain—pain patients, 226
    nerve identification and handling, 227–228
    nociceptive neuroplasticity, 104
    nociceptive system modalities, 104
    osteoarthritis (OA)
        measurements, 170
        pain mechanisms, 170

Quantitative sensory testing (QST) *(Continued)*
    peripheral and central sensitization, 170
    preoperative screening, 169
  pain neuroplasticity, 105–106
  peripheral and central spreading sensitization
    application, 106
    cuff algometry, 109, 110f
    deep somatic structures, 107
    descending modulation, neuronal excitability, 111–112
    dorsal horn neurons/nociceptive withdrawal reflex, 109
    heat stimulation, 109
    hyperalgesia, 108
    pain mapping technique, 107
    periosteal pain mechanisms, 107
    preoperative monitoring, 110
    pressure algometry, 107
    pressure stimulation, 107
    psychophysical assessment principles, 106, 106f
    receptive fields expansion, 108–109
    somatic pain, 108
    spatial integration, 110–111
    von Mises stress, finite element estimation, 107, 108f
    windup mechanism, 109
  peripheral nociceptors, 104–105
  persistent postsurgical pain (PPSP) prevention, 240
  postoperative patient-controlled analgesia (PCA)
    morphine, 105
  stimulus modalities, 104
  suprathreshold nociceptive processing, 104
  target structures, 104
  threshold determination, 104

R

RA. *See* Regional anesthesia (RA)
Randall–Selitto test, 215, 216f–217f
Raphe–spinal projection pathway, 86
Rat plantar hindpaw model
  behavioral effects, 3
  characteristics, 4
  guarding behavior, 4f
    conditioned place preference (CPP), 5, 6f
    contralateral unincised hindpaw, 4
    cutaneous injury elicits, 5
    ketoprofen, 4
    morphine, 4
    patient-controlled analgesia, 4
    sham incision, 5, 7f
    skin incision *vs.* skin plus deep tissue injury, 4
    spontaneous activity, 5, 7, 7f
    in vivo neurophysiology, 5, 7, 7f
Rectal hyperalgesia, 44
Referred hyperalgesia, 27
Referred pain, 43, 44, 49. *See also* Pain referral
  acid sensitization, 48
  clinical pain
    acute, 48
    chronic, 49
  peri- and postoperative pain, 49
  quantitative sensory testing (QST), 112
  somatic and visceral structure, 43
  and viscerovisceral hyperalgesia, 44

Reflex receptive field (RRF), 109, 121
  acquisition and recording of, 122, 123f
  bidimensional interpolation and extrapolation, 122
  detection of, 123
  quantitative features, 122
  reliability of, 123
Regional analgesic techniques
  epidural analgesia, 296
  intraoperative periarticular infiltration, 297
  nociceptive afferent pathways, 296
  peripheral nerve blocks (PNBs), 297
  wound infiltration, 297
Regional anesthesia (RA)
  additives usage, 264–265
  benefits of
    cardiovascular dysfunction, 259
    cognitive dysfunction, 260
    economic outcomes/time to discharge, 261
    enhanced recovery after surgery (ERAS), 261
    functional outcomes, 260
    immunologic outcomes, 260
    mortality, 259
    neurologic outcomes, 260
    opioid analgesic use, 260–261
    patient satisfaction, 261
    pulmonary dysfunction, 260
  chronic postsurgical pain (CPSP), 266
  contraindications, 262
  indications, 261–262
  infraclavicular blocks, 263–264
  interscalene block, 263–264
  local anesthetic systemic toxicity (LAST), 262–263
  peripheral nerve blocks *vs.* epidural analgesia, 266
  pneumothorax, 264
  risk factors, 264
  single injection *vs.* continuous peripheral nerve block catheters (CPNBCs), 265–266
  supraclavicular blocks, 263–264
Relaxation/mindfulness, 273
Rheumatoid arthritis (RA), 20, 155
  musculoskeletal pain, 15
  opioids, 77
  total joint arthroplasty (TJA), 169
Rostral ventromedial medulla (RVM), 59, 60f
  analgesia system, 60
  ascending nociceptive information, 60
  behavioral hypersensitivity, 60
  "bottom-up" recruitment, normal and potentiated pain states
    basal pain sensitivity, 61
    Freund adjuvant, 62
    hyperalgesic effect, 62
    NMDA and neurokinin-1 receptors, 62
    opioid, antinociception action, 62
    opioid-induced hyperalgesia, 62
    pain, chronic, 63–64
    pain/inflammation, acute, 62, 63f
  cognitive and emotional factors, 60
  conditioned pain modulation (CPM), 64–65
  endogenous analgesia, 60
  inflammatory and neuropathic pain, 60
  microinjection/single-cell recording approach, 61
  NEUTRAL-cells, 61

nocifensor reflexes, 61
OFF-cells and ON-cells, 61
opioid analgesic drugs, 60
opioid-induced hyperalgesia (OIH), 213
pain-modulating network, 60
physiology and function, 59
supraspinal system, 60
"top-down" engagement, 64
withdrawal reflex, 61
RRF. See Reflex receptive field (RRF)

S

Saline-induced pain, 26, 26f
Secondary pinprick hyperalgesia. See Hyperalgesia
Serotonin–norepinephrine reuptake inhibitor (SNRI), 198, 253
Sevoflurane inhaled anesthesia, 237
Short-lasting muscle hyperalgesia, 19
Silent nociceptors, 44
"Silent" (ineffective) synapses, 21
"Silent" synapses/synaptic trafficking, 87
Single nucleotide polymorphism (SNP), 172
Single-sweep analysis, 51
Skin dermatome, 21
Sodium channels, ionophore
    activity-dependent changes, 73
    cyclooxygenase (COX) inhibitors, 72
    glial cell–derived neurotrophic factor (GDNF), 73
    single nucleotide polymorphism (SNP), 73
    transcriptional regulation, 73
    voltage-gated sodium channels (VGSCs), 72
Somatic hyperalgesia, 112
Somatic sensory system, 43, 48
Somatosensory cortex, 154
Somatosensory sensitivity, 16
Spinal afferents, 42–43
Spinal cord
    calcium channels, 74
    central excitatory transmission, 74–75
    central inhibitory transmission, 74
    glutamatergic synapses, 84
    neuropathic pain, 73
    pain signaling systems., 73
    peripheral sensitization, 73
Spinal nociception
    hyperexcitability assessment
        central pain processing, 125
        chronic pain conditions, 128
        grand mean reflex receptive fields, 127, 127f
        synaptic sensitivity, 127
        temporal summation mechanisms, 126
    modulation of, 124–125, 126f
    reflex pathway, 124
    stimulus–response function, 124
    temporal summation, 124
Spinal sensory synapses, 86
Spreading hypersensitivity
    bone, 22–23
    connective tissue, 23
    joint, 22
    muscle, 21–22
Stanford Collaborative Health Outcomes Information Registry (CHOIR), 309

Steady-state evoked potentials (SS-EPs), 145–146, 146f
Stress-induced analgesia (SIA), 215
Stress-induced hyperalgesia, 64
Structure-Process-Outcome model, 301
Substance P (SP) immunoreactivities, 18
Sumatriptan, 158
Supraclavicular blocks, 263–264
Surgical pain models, 223
Synaptic plasticity, 84, 85f
Synaptic proteins, 89

T

Temporal summation (TS), 195–196, 196f
    bone pain, 24–25, 24f
    connective tissue pain, 25
    cuff algometry, 109, 110f
    definition, 23
    dorsal horn neurons/nociceptive withdrawal reflex, 109
    heat stimulation, 109
    joint pain, 24
    muscle pain, 23–24
    preoperative monitoring, 110
    spinal nociception modulation, 124
    windup mechanism, 109
Temporal summation of pain (TSP), 170
Tendinopathies, musculoskeletal pain, 15
TENS (transcutaneous electrical nerve stimulation), 292
Thoracoscopic splanchnic denervation, 52
Tibial fractures, 20
Tonic muscle hyperalgesia, 19
Total hip arthroplasty (THA), 167–168, 260
    inflammation, 169
    pain-free recovery, 171
Total joint arthroplasty (TJA), 271
    central nervous system, 171
    comorbidities, 169
    inflammation, 169
    knee osteoarthritis (KOA), 167
    pain-free recovery, 171
    patients phenotyping, 170
    pharmacologic and nonpharmacologic treatment guidelines, 167
    preoperative risk factors, 167, 168f
    social factors, 167
    total hip arthroplasty (THA), 167–168
    total knee arthroplasty (TKA), 167–168
Total knee arthroplasty (TKA), 167–168, 260
    inflammation, 169
    pain-free recovery, 171
Total knee replacement (TKR), 198
Tramadol, 294–295
Transcutaneous electrical nerve stimulation (TENS), 292
Transducers, 72
Transduction process, muscle pain, 16
Transient receptor potential ankyrin 1 (TRPA1) ion channel, 72
Transient receptor potential vanilloid 1 (TRPV1), 72, 188, 211
Trigeminal neuralgia, 155
TrkA receptors, 17
TS. See Temporal summation (TS)
Type I mechano- and heat-sensitive A δ fibers (type I AMH), 189

U

University of Washington Harborview Medical Center Perioperative Integrated Pain Care Pathway, 305, 306f
US National Pain Strategy, 308

V

Vagal afferents, 42
Venlafaxine, 237
Visceral homunculus, 48
Visceral hypersensitivity, 50
Visceral pain disorders, 41
Visceral pain neuromatrix, 45
Visceral pain processing, 52
Visceral pain syndromes, 25
Visceral tissues damage. *See* Central nervous system (CNS) effects
Viscerovisceral hyperalgesia, 43, 44
von Mises stress, finite element estimation, 107, 108f

W

Warmth detection threshold (WDT), 224
Whiplash pain, 21, 24
Whole-cell patch-clamp recording, 88
Windup mechanism, 109

Z

Zinc finger transcription factor, 89
Zygapophysial joint pain, 27